Manual of Pediatric Anesthesia

With an Index of Pediatric Syndromes

Manual of Pediatric Anesthesia, Sixth Edition

With an Index of Pediatric Syndromes

Jerrold Lerman, M.D., F.R.C.P.C., F.A.N.Z.C.A.
Clinical Professor of Anesthesiology
Women & Children's Hospital of Buffalo
SUNY at Buffalo
Clinical Professor of Anesthesiology
University of Rochester School of Medicine and Dentistry
Rochester, New York

Charles J. Coté, M.D.
Professor of Anaesthesia
Harvard Medical School
Director of Clinical Research
Division of Pediatric Anesthesia
Department of Anesthesia, Critical Care and Pain Management
MassGeneral Hospital for Children
Massachusetts General Hospital
Boston, Massachusetts

David J. Steward, M.B., F.R.C.P.C.
Honorary Professor of Anaesthesia
University of British Columbia
Vancouver, British Columbia, Canada
Formerly Director of Anesthesiology
Children's Hospital Los Angeles
Los Angeles, California

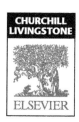

CHURCHILL
LIVINGSTONE

ELSEVIER

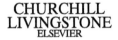

CHURCHILL
LIVINGSTONE
ELSEVIER

1600 John F. Kennedy Blvd.
Ste 1800
Philadelphia, PA 19103-2899

MANUAL OF PEDIATRIC ANESTHESIA   ISBN: 978-1-4377-0988-9

NOTICE

Knowledge and best practice in this field are constantly changing. As new research and experience broaden our knowledge, changes in practice, treatment and drug therapy may become necessary or appropriate. Readers are advised to check the most current information provided (i) on procedures featured or (ii) by the manufacturer of each product to be administered, to verify the recommended dose or formula, the method and duration of administration, and contraindications. It is the responsibility of the practitioner, relying on his or her own experience and knowledge of the patient, to make diagnoses, to determine dosages and the best treatment for each individual patient, and to take all appropriate safety precautions. To the fullest extent of the law, neither the Publisher nor the Authors assume any liability for any injury and/or damage to persons or property arising out of or related to any use of the material contained in this book.

The Publisher

Library of Congress Cataloging-in-Publication Data

Lerman, Jerrold.
   Manual of pediatric anesthesia : with an index of pediatric syndromes / Jerrold Lerman, Charles J. Coté, David J. Steward. —6th ed.
      p. ; cm.
   Rev. ed. of: Manual of pediatric anesthesia / David J. Steward, Jerrold Lerman. 5th. c2001.
   Includes bibliographical references and index.
   ISBN: 978-1-4377-0988-9
1. Pediatric anesthesia—Handbooks, manuals, etc. I. Coté, Charles J. II. Steward, David J. III. Steward, David J., Manual of pediatric anesthesia. IV. Title.
   [DNLM: 1. Anesthesia—methods—Handbooks. 2. Child. 3. Infant. WO 231 L616m 2010]
RD139. S84 2010
617.9'6083—dc22   2009022841

Executive Publisher: Natasha Andjelkovic
Editorial Assistant: Bradley McIlwain
Publishing Services Manager: Anitha Rajarathinam
Project Manager: Beula Christopher
Design Manager: Steven Stave

Cover photograph and design courtesy: Brian Smistek, Director of Medical Media,
                                Women and Children's Hospital of Buffalo, Buffalo, NY

Printed and bound by CPI Group (UK) Ltd, Croydon, CR0 4YY

Transferred to digital print 2013

Working together to grow
libraries in developing countries
www.elsevier.com | www.bookaid.org | www.sabre.org

ELSEVIER   BOOK AID   Sabre Foundation
           International

Preface

In the tradition of the previous five editions, this sixth edition of the *Manual of Pediatric Anesthesia* is designed as a concise but comprehensive pocketbook guide to pediatric anesthesia practice. It is a book to be kept in the pocket or on the desk for handy reference. It outlines management problems and presents a course of action for treating many of your pediatric patients and will also direct you to further reading. For the resident in training, it provides a source of current information about the special considerations of anesthesia for infants and children.

We are very pleased to add Dr. Charles J. Coté from Massachusetts General Hospital in Boston to the team of authors for this edition of the Manual. With Dr. Coté's extensive experience in pediatric anesthesia, sedation and clinical research, the three authors of this sixth edition have a combined total of almost a century of experience of providing intra-operative and postoperative care for children of all ages having all types of surgical procedures. More recently, along with our colleagues, we have extended our practices outside the operating rooms to care for children having a wide variety of procedures, or requiring pain relief throughout the hospital. We have incorporated our own experiences together with the information gleaned from many published studies in order to compile this manual. The information presented has been reviewed by all the authors and a consensus achieved. In many instances, we recommend a course of action for a given clinical situation. When we do this, it is based on what has worked well for us. However, we recognize that others may have other ideas and other constraints on their practice.

It is now thirty years since the first edition of this book appeared. Many changes in our practice have occurred during this time. Some developments were in response to the expanding scope of pediatric surgery in this period. It is satisfying that many were a result of the simultaneous proliferation of clinical investigations relating to anesthesia care for infants and children. Unlike thirty years ago, we are now in the fortunate position of being able to practice evidence-based pediatric anesthesia most of the time.

Children remain the most rewarding patients to manage. There is great satisfaction in the successful management of the tiny infant, the reticent child, or the many other children that you will meet in your practice. We hope that our handbook will help you to achieve this satisfaction.

JERROLD LERMAN
CHARLES J. COTÉ
DAVID J. STEWARD

Abbreviations and Acronyms

$A\text{-}aDO_2$	alveolar-arterial oxygen tension gradient
$A\text{-}aDN_2$	alveolar-arterial nitrogen difference
ACE	angiotensin-converting enzyme
ACT	activated clotting time
ASD	atrial septal defect
AV	arteriovenous (**AVM** arteriovenous malformation)
BP	blood pressure
BSA	body surface area
CBF	cerebral blood flow
CF	cystic fibrosis
CHD	congenital heart disease
CHF	congestive heart failure
CK	creatine kinase
CL	lung compliance
$CMRO_2$	cerebral metabolic rate for oxygen
CNS	central nervous system
CO	carbon monoxide
CoHb	carboxyhemoglobin
CPAP	continuous positive airway pressure
CPB	cardiopulmonary bypass
CPK	creatine phosphokinase
CPP	cerebral perfusion pressure
CSF	cerebrospinal fluid
CT	computed tomography
CV	closing volume
CVP	central venous pressure
DDAVP	1-deamino-8-D -arginine vasopressin
DIC	disseminated intravascular coagulation
DN	dibucaine number
2,3-DPG	2,3-diphosphoglycerate
EACA	epsilon-aminocaproic acid
EBV	estimated blood volume
ECF	extracellular fluid

ECG	electrocardiogram
ECHO	echocardiography
ECMO	extracorporeal membrane oxygenation
ED$_{95}$	effective dose in 95% of patients
EDTA	ethylenediaminetetraacetic acid
EEG	electroencephalography
EMG	electromyography
ETT	endotracheal tube
EUA	examination under anesthesia
FFP	fresh frozen plasma
FIO$_2$	fraction of inspired oxygen
FN	fluoride number
FRC	functional residual capacity
GFR	glomerular filtration rate
Hb	hemoglobin
HbA	adult hemoglobin
HbC	hemoglobin C
3-HBDH	3-hydroxybutyrate dehydrogenase
HbF	fetal hemoglobin
HbS	sickle cell hemoglobin
Hct	hematocrit
HME	heat and moisture exchanger
HpD	hematoporphyrin derivative
ICF	intracellular fluid
ICP	intracranial pressure
ICU	intensive care unit
ID	internal diameter
IJV	internal jugular vein
IOP	intraocular pressure
IPPB	intermittent positive-pressure breathing
IPPV	intermittent positive-pressure ventilation
IVAC	intravenous accurate control [device]
IVH	intraventricular hemorrhage
LDH	lactate dehydrogenase
LMA	laryngeal mask airway
L/S	lecithin-sphingomyelin [ratio]
LV	left ventricle
MAC	minimum alveolar concentration
MEP	motor evoked potential
MetHb	methemoglobin
MH	malignant hyperthermia or hyperpyrexia

MHS	malignant hyperthermia-susceptible
MRI	magnetic resonance imaging
NEC	necrotizing enterocolitis
NGT	nasogastric tube
NO	nitric oxide
N_2O	nitrous oxide
NSAID	nonsteroidal antiinflammatory drug
OSA	obstructive sleep apnea
OR	operating room
P_{50}	PO_2 with 50% hemoglobin saturation
PA	pulmonary artery
PaO_2	arterial oxygen pressure
PACU	postanesthesia care unit
PAR	postanesthesia room
PC	partition coefficient (λ)
PCA	patient-controlled analgesia
pCO_2	partial pressure of carbon dioxide (**$PaCO_2$** arterial carbon dioxide; **$PetCO_2$** end-tidal carbon dioxide)
PDA	patent ductus arteriosus
PEEP	positive end-expiratory pressure
PGE_1	prostaglandin E_1
PIP	peak inspiratory pressure
PNF	protamine neutralization factor
pO_2	partial pressure of oxygen
PONV	postoperative nausea and vomiting
PPM	parts per million
PT	prothrombin time
PTT	partial thromboplastin time
PVC	polyvinyl chloride
PVOD	pulmonary vascular obstructive disease
PVR	pulmonary vascular resistance
$\dot{Q}$	perfusion
Qp:Qs	ratio of pulmonary to systemic blood flow
RA	right atrium
RAST	radioallergosorbent testing
RBC	red blood cell
RDS	respiratory distress syndrome
REM	rapid eye movement
RES	reticuloendothelial system
ROP	retinopathy of prematurity
RSI	rapid sequence induction

RV	right ventricle
SaO_2	arterial oxygen saturation
SBE	subacute bacterial endocarditis
SCIWORA	spinal cord injury without radiologic abnormality
SGOT	serum glutamic oxaloacetic transaminase
SIADH	syndrome of inappropriate antidiuretic hormone secretion
SNP	sodium nitroprusside
SpO_2	saturation pulse oximetry
SSEP	somatosensory evoked potentials
SVR	systemic vascular resistance
TCI	target controlled infusion
TEE	transesophageal echocardiography
TEF	tracheoesophageal fistula
TGA	transposition of the great arteries
TLC	total lung capacity
V_A	alveolar ventilation
V_D	dead space volume
$\dot{V}$	ventilation
$\dot{V}O_2$	rate of metabolism (or consumption) for oxygen
$(\dot{V}/\dot{Q})$	ventilation-perfusion [matching]
V_t	tidal volume
VAE	venous air embolism
VATER association	vertebral defects, anal atresia, tracheoesophageal fistula, esophageal atresia, radial and renal dysplasia
VACTERL association	the VATER association with added cardiac and limb defects
VATS	video-assisted thorascopic surgery
VIP	vasoactive intestinal polypeptide
VSD	ventricular septal defect
WBC	white blood cell

Contents

Foundations of
Pediatric Anesthesia

Psychological Aspects

PSYCHOLOGICAL ASPECTS OF ANESTHESIA FOR CHILDREN

Hospitalization and/or medical procedures can have profound emotional consequences for infants and children. Some children demonstrate behavior disturbances that persist long after the event. The extent of the upset is determined by several factors, the most important of which is the child's age.

Infants younger than six months of age are not upset by separation from parents and readily accept a nurse as a substitute mother. From a psychological viewpoint, this is probably a good age for major surgery, although prolonged separation may impair parent-child bonding.

Older infants and young children (six months to five years) are much more upset by a hospital stay, especially with separation from family and home; ambulatory surgery is much less upsetting. Separation of a preschool age child from their parents at the time of surgery, even ambulatory surgery, is a stress that requires consideration. Explanations of procedures and the need for them are difficult at this age, and not surprisingly, these children show the most severe behavior regression after hospitalization.

School-age children are usually less upset by separation and more concerned with the surgical procedure and its possible mutilating effect. They often have the wildest misconceptions of what their operation involves. In contrast, adolescents fear the process of narcosis, the loss of control, waking up during the surgery and the possibility of not being able to face the process calmly. It is for these reasons that providing as much information as possible is essential along with assuring them that they will not awaken during anesthesia and feel the pain of surgery, and that they will awaken at the end.

The type and extent of the surgery is an important factor. Major surgery, craniofacial surgery, and amputation of a limb are especially distressing, and appropriate psychiatric support is encouraged. Surgery of the genitalia in particular may have important psychological implications in children over 18 months of age.

Factors other than age also influence the child's emotional response. For example, a prolonged hospitalization is much more disturbing than a brief admission, although the former has been mitigated in part by having parents "live-in" with their children during hospital stays. Ambulatory surgery usually has a negligible emotional effect on most children whereas repeated hospitalizations and surgeries may cause significant psychological disturbance; a previous bad experience may be long remembered.

Children vary in their responses to impending hospitalization or medical intervention. Some seek information and participate keenly in preparation programs; they have an active coping style. These children are likely to benefit from psychological preparation and can be expected to cooperate. Others maintain an air of disinterest; they have an avoidant coping style (the "silent child"). Children in the latter group may not benefit and indeed may be further sensitized by efforts at psychological preparation. They may benefit more from an effective anxiolytic premedication (see later discussion).

Psychological Preparation

Preoperative psychological preparation is very important and has been clearly demonstrated to be beneficial to many children. Usually this is accomplished by the parents, although the extent of preparation possible is determined by the child's age. The basic objective is to explain to the child in simple, understandable, and reassuring terms what will happen at the hospital. Older children and adolescents should be prepared well in advance, as soon as hospitalization is arranged. Younger children should not be prepared too far in advance—it is unnecessary and will be a continuing source of worry for them. Rather, they should be prepared a day or so beforehand.

Hospital tours, puppet shows, and/or audiovisual presentations should be available, as all have been shown to be beneficial. Videotapes are most useful and may be loaned to parents. In some cities, prehospital preparation programs for children have been televised via community television stations on a weekly basis. In this way, a whole population of children can be prepared for the possibility of hospitalization, rather than just those scheduled for surgery.

Meeting with the Parents

"Being unable to choose parents for your patients, you must make do with those who come with the child … ; it would be abnormal if they showed no anxiety"

Mellish, 1969

Parents are playing an increasingly active role in the perioperative care of their children; many expect to be present at induction of anesthesia and in the recovery room. However, some parents are more anxious than others, and this is readily perceived and may further upset the child. Good preparation of the parents reduces parental anxiety and indirectly helps the child.

There are many factors that influence the extent of parental anxiety when a child requires surgery. Even parents of children with only minor problems may initially be very anxious. Complete explanations and good communication with the medical and nursing teams usually do much to reduce their anxiety level. In particular, it is important to describe to parents how their child could respond during induction of anesthesia (eyes rolling up, movements of the arms and legs and turning of the head) and to reassure them that these are normal and expected responses.

Obtaining Consent

The anesthesiologist is placed in a difficult situation when obtaining informed consent for general anesthesia; providing information on all the potential risks before a minor surgical procedure might well be expected to increase the level of anxiety of the parents. However, parents appear to benefit from an appropriate discussion of the risks of anesthesia in that this fulfills their own needs of responsibility and understanding. The parents should be permitted to dictate the extent of the information they wish to be given. Most parents of children having minor procedures accept that there are risks, including death, and prefer to have the opportunity for discussion of these risks. Such discussions should, of course, be outside the earshot of the young child.

In general, the anesthesiologist should rely on some well-established general principles in dealing with anxious parents. An approach that has been found most helpful in decreasing parental anxiety is one built on genuine warmth and friendliness, empathy, and understanding. Parents like to be listened to; discussions should allow ample time for questions and for the parents to express their concerns and ideas about the child and the proposed anesthesia process. Parents particularly wish to know about premedication, how their child will be anesthetized, monitored, and provided with postoperative pain relief. A videotaped explanation may be helpful, but should be augmented by a personal interview. An overall discussion of risks, in particular those specific to their child, helps to place risk in perspective. Assurance that their child's anesthesia will be specifically designed with their child's safety and the surgeon's needs in mind also helps to relieve anxiety. Every parent will be pleased if you communicate the message, "We will take very good care and will be with your child all the time!"

Parental Presence at Induction

The question of the parents' accompanying the child during induction of anesthesia requires special consideration. Many parents express a strong wish to be present, and many facilities routinely allow them to stay with their child. Studies are inconclusive as to the extent to which a parent's presence can positively influence the emotional outcome for the child, but it may help the parent achieve satisfaction. Certainly many parents of handicapped children can often be of great assistance to the anesthesiologist. Many parents are calm and supportive of their child and appear to benefit from participating in the induction process.

The overanxious parent requires special consideration. Excessive anxiety is often of multifactorial origin and may not be entirely related to the child's present surgical condition. These parents may not gain much reduction in their anxiety levels from additional information about the forthcoming procedure. An anxious parent who insists on remaining with the child may do more harm than good and may increase the child's anxiety level. Such anxious parents should be counseled and excluded if possible. Adequate preoperative sedation of the child may help them to agree to this course. Certainly there is no benefit for parental presence for a neonate or infant who is not fearful of strangers due to their young developmental level or for the child in need of a rapid sequence induction. It must be clear that parental presence during induction for older children is a privilege given at your discretion in what you deem to be for the best interests of the child and the child's safety.

The Anesthesiologist and the Child

Anesthesia, and particularly the induction period, is recognized to have the potential to cause psychological trauma. Studies indicate that anesthesiologists vary in their ability to relate to children and minimize this upset. An *empathic approach* to the child before and during medical procedures is preferred (e.g., *"This may be a little uncomfortable and I know you are scared, but we are going to do all we can to help and it will soon be over. We don't mind if you cry."*). The alternative *directive approach* (*"Hold still and be big and brave."*) is generally condemned.

Premedication with an oral anxiolytic is beneficial in decreasing anxiety during separation, increasing cooperation during induction, and decreasing posthospitalization behavior disturbance.

Caution should be exercised in caring for the silent child who has an avoidant coping style, especially the child who must undergo repeat procedures because such a child may not respond as well to routine preparation methods. Some may respond more favorably if they are allowed to continue with their avoidant coping pattern but are given a well-chosen preoperative medication.

Preparing Infants and Children for an Operation

1. Try to meet the young child with the parents so that the child can see them accept you.
2. Direct most of your attention at all times to the child, even if he or she is developmentally delayed. Try to maintain eye contact; it helps to sit alongside the child, on the floor if necessary.
3. Talk to the child in simple terms that the child can understand.
4. Pay special attention to the silent child and recognize that he or she may be very upset. Consider the use of a suitable sedative premedication if not otherwise contraindicated.
5. Truthfully explain all the procedures to be undertaken in clear and simple terms, but avoid unnecessary alarming details. Some children may ask about the operation: try to help them understand what is to be done, using drawings if necessary. In many cases children grossly overestimate the extent of the procedure and must be reassured, for instance, about the small size of the incision.
6. Do not use the phrase "put you to sleep"—this may worry some children if they recall a family pet that never came back! It may also cause them to worry that they might wake up from their "sleep" when the operation starts or while it is still in progress.
7. Do not present the child with unpleasant and difficult choices. For example, avoid questions such as, "Do you want the needle or the mask?" Tell the child what you intend to do and then try to meet any special requests (e.g., "I do not want a needle, I want to go to sleep with the mask" or "I'd like to hold the mask myself").
8. Avoid uncovering the child more than is necessary to complete the physical examination; many children get upset at being disrobed.
9. Television and especially hand-held computer games are wonderful distractions for the older child waiting in the preoperative area.

10. Allow the young child to bring a favorite toy or other security object to the operating room (OR). Label the toy with the child's name; if it is a doll, suggest that perhaps the doll should also get a cast or a dressing applied during the operation. If the child is able, let him or her walk to the OR rather than be carried or wheeled: children are quite independent and feel more at ease walking.

11. If possible, allow those parents who are judged to be calm and supportive to accompany their child during the induction. If this is not possible, both the child and the parents may be helped by premedicating the child (e.g., oral midazolam, see page 88). The parents are much happier seeing their child leave them if he or she is very well sedated. It is sometimes useful to start an intravenous infusion away from the OR with the parents present, especially for handicapped or developmentally delayed children. The intravenous route can then be used for induction as soon as the child is taken to the OR. Always use local analgesia to insert the intravenous cannula; topical anesthetic cream is ideal if it can be applied well in advance (see page 634).

12. An empathic approach should be used to prepare the child. Small children who are crying during venipuncture can often be calmed by telling them, "We will put on a Band-Aid in a minute."

13. Reassure older children and adolescents and provide them with careful explanations. They may be quite scared and have many questions. It is important to reassure them of the safety of the procedure and to emphasize that they will not wake up during the operation but will definitely wake up when it is over. Older children may also benefit from premedication (see page 87).

14. Use premedicant drugs whenever indicated; most young children will benefit.

15. Select the most appropriate induction technique for each child and proceed without delay. Cooperative children may be given a choice of one of three flavors to apply to the facemask to flavor the "magic laughing gas." Do not allow a child to wait on the OR table longer than is absolutely necessary for the application of basic monitors. A pulse oximeter may be the only monitor that can be maintained during induction of anesthesia in a combative child.

16. Talk to the child throughout the induction period to explain or distract him or her from the procedures that are required. Ensure that all extraneous noises and conversations are excluded during this time. Only one person should be talking to the child. Quiet soothing music may help.

17. Tell the child what to expect during the recovery, where recovery will take place, and what discomfort they may experience. Carefully explain such items as eye patches, nasogastric tubes, and catheters as necessary and that they will be inserted while the child is anesthetized. A urinary catheter may look like a giant worm to an unprepared child! Assure the child that any pain will be treated.

18. Discuss in advance with the family and child the plan for optimal postoperative pain relief.

Postoperative Care

The parents should be allowed to be with their child as soon as it is practical—before the child awakens, if possible. Every effort should be made to provide good, but safe, analgesia. Regional nerve blocks, opioid infusions, patient-controlled analgesia, epidural opioids, and all ancillary techniques used for adults should be considered, discussed with the parents, and provided for infants and children when appropriate.

In the intensive care unit (ICU), the child's problems are similar to those for adults: pain, lack of sleep, and later, boredom. In addition, children have their own special concerns, such as separation from the family. Special attention should be directed to pain relief, regular visitation by the parents, and provision of toys, games, and other distractions (e.g., television) as the child's condition improves. Parents of children in the ICU benefit by being kept very well informed of their child's condition and progress, and they must also be continuously updated on the treatment plans for their child.

Suggested Reading

Caldas JCS, Pais-Ribeiro JL, Caneiro SR: General anaesthesia, surgery and hospitalization in children, and their effects upon cognitive, academic, emotional and sociobehavioural development, Paediatr Anaesth 14:910–915, 2004.

Kain ZN, Caldwell-Andrews AA: Preoperative psychological preparation of the child for surgery: an update, Anesthesiol Clin North America 23:597–614, 2005.

Wisselo TL, Stuart C, Muris P: Providing parents with information before anaesthesia: what do they really want to know? Paediatr Anaesth 14:299–307, 2004.

For Parents: When your child needs anesthesia. Brochure of the American Society of Anesthesiologists. www.asahq.org/patientEducation/WhenYourChild NeedsAnesthesia.pdf.

2 Anatomy and Physiology

CENTRAL NERVOUS SYSTEM

The central nervous system in the neonate differs from that in the older child: the myelination of nerve fibers is incomplete, and the cerebral cortex is less developed; its cellular elements continue to increase during the first years of life. Reflexes not seen in older children may be elicited. In the preterm, brain stem evoked potentials are prolonged, and the normalization of these coincides with maturation of respiratory control mechanisms.

Sensitivity to Pain

Until quite recently, little was understood of the ability of infants and small children to appreciate pain. As a result there was an unfortunate tendency to ignore the need for analgesia during painful procedures; even during and after surgical operations. It is now well established that neonates, including those born prematurely, may have increased sensitivity to pain and will react to it with tachycardia, hypertension, increased intracranial pressure, and a neuroendocrine response that exceeds that reported in adults. Infants demonstrate measurable behavioral responses to pain (e.g., crying, grimacing, restlessness); these responses have been used as a basis for pain scoring systems. Evidence suggests that infants who are subjected to painful procedures (e.g., circumcision) without adequate analgesia may experience an increased sensitivity to pain as older children. This has been attributed to the persistence of alterations in the infant's central processing of painful stimuli. Control of intraoperative and postoperative pain, by modifying stress responses, may possibly even improve survival in infants with critical illness. It is for these reasons that we provide optimal analgesia or anesthesia for all infants and children during and after *any* painful procedure with the same care as we do for adults. As children grow from infancy into early childhood, their pain threshold remains reduced compared with that of older children or adults.

Suggested Reading

Ghai B, Makkar JK, Wig J: Postoperative pain assessment in preverbal children and children with cognitive impairment, Pediatr Anesth 18:462–477, 2008.
Walker SM: Pain in children: recent advances and ongoing challenges, Br J Anaesth 101:101–110, 2008.

CRANIUM AND INTRACRANIAL PRESSURE

The skull is less rigid in infants than in adults. As a result, an increase in the volume of its contents—blood, CSF, and brain tissue—can be accommodated to some extent by expansion of the fontanelles and separation of the suture lines. Palpation of the fontanelles can be used to assess intracranial pressure in infants.

CEREBRAL BLOOD FLOW AND INTRAVENTRICULAR HEMORRHAGE

Autoregulation of cerebral blood flow is impaired in sick neonates and blood flow is pressure dependent. Hypotension may lead to cerebral ischemia, and pressure fluctuations are transmitted to the capillary circulation. In the preterm infant, the cerebral vessels are very fragile, especially in the region of the germinal matrix overlying the caudate nucleus. Rupture of these vessels leads to intracerebral hemorrhage, which often extends into the ventricular system as an IVH.

Small preterm infants are very prone to IVH, which usually occurs during the first few days after birth and is a leading cause of morbidity and mortality. Potential predisposing factors to IVH include hypoxia, hypercarbia, hypernatremia, fluctuations in arterial or venous pressure, low hematocrit, overtransfusion, and rapid administration of hypertonic fluids (e.g., sodium bicarbonate).

The anesthesiologist should avoid precipitating these factors in the small preterm infant: airway manipulations, including awake endotracheal intubation and suctioning have been shown to increase blood pressure and anterior fontanelle pressure to similar extents. "Awake" intubation should be avoided whenever possible (even though a definite relationship between "awake" tracheal intubation and IVH has never been established). If the airway is known or appears to be difficult to secure or maintain by facemask, then an "awake" or preferably sedated tracheal intubation is a reasonable choice. If an awake tracheal intubation is planned, topical analgesia to the mouth and palate (using weight appropriate doses of local anesthetic [see page 145]) may attenuate the infant's physiologic responses.

To further prevent blood pressure fluctuations during surgery or painful procedures, adequate anesthesia and analgesia should be provided. Rapid injections of undiluted hypertonic solutions, such as dextrose or sodium bicarbonate, should be avoided. Care should be taken to replace blood losses accurately. Severe anemia and/or coagulopathy should be corrected promptly. Periventricular white matter injury is a major cause of persistent brain injury in small preterm infants, and may follow IVH or may be a direct consequence of prematurity, hypoxia, ischemia, and inflammation. Indomethacin therapy may reduce the incidence of severe IVH.

Suggested Reading

Shalak L, Perlman JM: Hemorrhagic-ischemic cerebral injury in the preterm infant: current concepts, Clin Perinatol 29:745–763, 2002.

Back SA, Rivkees SA: Emerging concepts in periventricular white matter injury, Semin Perinatol 28:405–714, 2004.

CEREBROSPINAL FLUID AND HYDROCEPHALUS

The CSF, which occupies the cerebral ventricles and the subarachnoid spaces surrounding the brain and spinal cord, is formed by choroid plexuses in the temporal horns of the lateral ventricles, the posterior portion of the third ventricle, and the roof of the fourth ventricle. Meningeal and ependymal vessels and blood vessels of the brain and spinal cord also contribute small volumes of CSF.

The choroid plexuses are cauliflower-like structures consisting of blood vessels covered by thin epithelium through which CSF continuously exudes. The rate of secretion is about 750 ml/day in the adult (i.e., about five times the intracavity volume). Except for the active secretion of a few substances by the choroid plexus, CSF is similar to interstitial fluid.

CSF flow is initiated by pulsation in the choroid plexus. From the lateral ventricles, CSF passes into the third ventricle via the foramen of Monro and along the aqueduct of Sylvius into the fourth ventricle, each ventricle contributing more fluid by secretion from its choroid plexus. CSF then flows through the two lateral foramina of Luschka and the midline foramen of Magendie into the cisterna magna and throughout the subarachnoid spaces. CSF is reabsorbed into the blood by hydrostatic filtration through the arachnoid villi, which project from the subarachnoid space into the venous sinuses. Hydrocephalus is an abnormal accumulation of CSF within the cranium that may be either obstructive or nonobstructive.

Obstructive hydrocephalus is caused by a blockage in the flow of CSF. It may be communicating (e.g., when the CSF pathway into the subarachnoid space is open, as after chronic arachnoiditis) or noncommunicating (e.g., when the fluid's pathway proximal to the subarachnoid space is obstructed, as in aqueduct stenosis or Arnold-Chiari malformation).

Nonobstructive hydrocephalus is caused by a reduction in the volume of brain substance, with secondary dilation of the ventricles; by overproduction of CSF (e.g., in choroid plexus papilloma); or by diminished reabsorption of CSF due to scarring.

EYES

Retinopathy of Prematurity

Retinopathy of prematurity (ROP), which is caused by retinal vessel proliferation and retinal detachment, is a leading cause of blindness. Improved survival of very-low-birth-weight infants increased the incidence of this condition. ROP is most common in neonates weighing less than 1500 g. Increased oxygen tension in the retinal arteries was thought to be the principal cause of ROP, although more recent research points to an effect on the processes of angiogenesis and vasculogenesis as the leading cause. These processes are stimulated by hypoxia. Exposure of the retina of the preterm to tissue oxygen levels in excess of the usual fetal levels interrupts normal vasculogenesis and may lead to subsequent hypoxic-ischemic tissue damage. At this stage additional oxygen may not cause further damage.

The cause of ROP is multifactorial; risk factors include hypoxia, hypercarbia, or hypocarbia; blood transfusion; exposure to light; recurrent apnea; sepsis; and other systemic illness. Occasionally ROP occurs in infants who have never been given supplemental oxygen and even in infants with cyanotic congenital heart disease. A major multi-institutional study of tight control of oxygen administration failed to reduce the incidence of ROP. Nevertheless, the inspired oxygen concentration should be carefully controlled in all preterm infants to avoid unnecessary hyperoxia. The safe level of Pao_2 is now considered to be 50 to 70 mm Hg. Large fluctuations in inspired oxygen concentrations should be avoided. Monitoring oxygen saturation at a preductal site (right hand or earlobe), maintaining the SaO_2 at 90% to 95%, and avoiding major fluctuations in oxygenation are recommended. On occasion, it may still be necessary to err on the side of safety and administer high inspired oxygen concentrations. Major surgical procedures do not appear to predispose infants to ROP.

Suggested Reading

Hutcheson KA: Retinopathy of prematurity, Curr Opin Ophthalmol 14:286–290, 2003.

Rubaltelli DM, Hirose T: Retinopathy of prematurity update, Int Ophthalmol Clin 48:225–235, 2008.

THE RESPIRATORY SYSTEM

The respiratory system is of special interest to the anesthesiologist since this is the route of administration of inhaled anesthetic agents, and its functions may be significantly compromised during and after anesthesia. Changes in the respiratory system occur continuously from infancy to about age 12 years as the child grows to maturity.

Anatomy

There are major anatomic differences in the airway between the neonate, the small infant, and the adult that are important for the safe conduct of anesthesia:

1. The head is relatively large and the neck is short, which may contribute to difficulty in laryngoscopy.

2. The tongue is relatively large and readily blocks the pharynx during and after anesthesia: therefore, an oropharyngeal airway or a jaw thrust is often needed. The large tongue may also hamper attempts to visualize the glottis at laryngoscopy.

3. The nasal passages are narrow and may be blocked by secretions or edema, which may cause serious problems. Neonates were previously described as "obligate nose-breathers," but whether this is always true has been questioned. It is certain that some neonates may not immediately convert to mouth breathing if the nasal passages are obstructed. Upper airway obstruction is more likely to occur when the neck is flexed. The anesthesiologist should extend the infant's neck after extubation until the infant completely recovers from anesthesia. Insertion of a nasogastric tube (NGT) increases total airway resistance; if the nares are of unequal size, the NGT should be inserted into the smaller nostril where it will have the least adverse effect.

4. The larynx is situated more cephalad (C4) and anteriorly, and its long axis is directed inferiorly and anteriorly. The high cervical level of the larynx in the infant means that elevation of the head to the "sniffing position" during laryngoscopy will not assist in visualization of the glottis as it does in the adult. In the infant, if the head is elevated, the larynx also moves anteriorly (See page 94).

5. The airway is narrowest at the level of the cricoid cartilage just below the vocal cords. This cartilage is the only solid circumferential component of the airway. The lining of the airway here is pseudostratified, ciliated epithelium that is loosely bound to the underlying tissue. Trauma to these tissues causes edema, and even a small amount of circumferential edema significantly compromises the already small cross-sectional area of the infant's airway. The net effect is an increase in the resistance to airflow (which is turbulent [i.e., Reynold's number >2500]) resulting in stridor, where: $R \propto 1/r^5$, (R is the resistance and r is the radius of the airway). Insertion of an ETT similarly encroaches on this space, as the internal diameter of the ETT becomes the area for gas flow; hence, airway resistance increases. This is more significant in smaller children (<3 yr). This is the reason that thinner uncuffed tubes used to be advocated in pediatric cases. Today, the wall thickness of cuffed and uncuffed tubes is the same.

6. The epiglottis is relatively long and stiff. It is U-shaped and projects posteriorly at an angle of approximately 45° above the glottis. Often,

it must be lifted by the tip of a laryngoscope blade before the glottis can be seen. For this reason, a straight-blade laryngoscope is recommended for use in infants and children.

7. The trachea is short (approximately 5 cm in the neonate), so precise placement and firm fixation of the ETT are essential. The tracheal cartilages are soft and can easily be compressed by the fingers of an anesthesiologist holding a mask or collapsed (dynamic compression) by the infant's vigorous attempts to breathe against an obstructed airway.

8. The right main bronchus is larger than the left and is less acutely angled at its origin. For this reason, if the ETT is advanced too far, it almost invariably enters the right main bronchus. This most often occurs while taping the tube in place or with changes in position for surgery after tracheal intubation. It is therefore essential to reassess the equality of bilateral breath sounds after repositioning for surgery (see Chapters 4 and 8).

9. Because the ribs are almost horizontal, ventilation is mainly diaphragmatic. The abdominal viscera are bulky and can hinder diaphragmatic excursion, especially if the gastrointestinal tract is distended.

Table 2-1 lists the approximate airway dimensions in infants and children.

Suggested Reading

Pohunek P: Development, structure and function of the upper airways, Paed Resp Rev 5:2–8, 2004.

Physiology

Breathing movements begin in utero and are characteristically rapid, irregular, and episodic during late pregnancy. Normally, they are present 30% of the time in the third trimester, vary with the sleep state of the fetus and are subject to diurnal variation. Fetal breathing movements may play a role in lung development and provide exercise for the muscles of respiration. Monitoring of these movements may provide information on fetal health: hypoxemia leads to a decrease in fetal breathing, and severe hypoxemia leads to gasping movements. The fetal lungs are filled with fluid, which is moved by this respiratory muscle activity. After 26 to 28 weeks of gestation, production of surface-active substances (surfactants) is established in the type II pneumocytes. Surfactant is secreted into the lung and can be detected in amniotic fluid samples, providing a diagnostic index of lung maturity and hence neonatal prognosis.

TABLE 2-1 Approximate Airway Dimensions in Infants and Children

Age (yr)	Tracheal Length (cm)	Trachea (AP)	Diameter (mm) Right Bronchus	Left Bronchus
>0.5	5.9	5.0	4.5	3.5
0.5–1	7.2	5.5	4.8	3.7
1–2	7.5	6.3	5.1	3.9
2–4	8.0	7.5	6.4	4.9
4–6	8.6	8.0	6.7	5.3
6–8	9.5	9.2	7.9	6.1
8–10	10	9.75	8.4	6.5
10–12	11.5	10.5	9.2	6.8
12–14	13.5	11.5	9.8	7.5
14–16	14.5	13.2	11.5	8.8

Passage of the fetus through the birth canal compresses the thorax, forcing much of the fluid from the lungs through the nose and mouth. On delivery, this compression is relieved and some air is sucked into the lungs. Peripheral (cold, touch, temperature, etc.) and biochemical (respiratory and metabolic acidosis) stimuli have been thought to initiate the onset of regular, continuous breathing. Other factors may be important, such as an increase in the Pao_2 or removal of central biochemical inhibitors. The first few spontaneous breaths are characterized by increased transpulmonary pressures (more than 50 cm H_2O). They establish the FRC of the neonate's lungs. Remaining lung fluid is removed over the first few days of life by the pulmonary lymphatics and blood vessels. Infants who are delivered by cesarean section are not subjected to the same thoracic squeeze and may have more residual fluid in the lungs. This may cause them to have transient respiratory distress (transient tachypnea of the neonate).

The stability of the alveolar matrix in the neonate depends on the presence of adequate amounts of surfactant, which may be deficient in the preterm infant. Lack of surfactant leads to collapse of alveoli, maldistribution of ventilation, impaired gas exchange, decreased lung compliance, and increased work of breathing (i.e., RDS). Not surprisingly, pneumothorax occurs more commonly during the neonatal period than at any other age.

Control of Respiration in the Neonate

Control of respiration, which involves biochemical and reflex mechanisms, is well developed in the healthy full-term neonate but exhibits several differences from adults. Respiration in the infant in relation to body mass is greater for any given arterial carbon dioxide tension ($PaCO_2$), reflecting a greater metabolic rate. The ventilatory response to hypercapnia is less in the neonate than in older infants, and less still in the preterm neonate. Any increase in the work of breathing is not well sustained. The slope of the carbon dioxide response curve is decreased in infants displaying episodes of apnea and hypoxemia decreases the response of the neonate to hypercapnia.

The neonate is sensitive to changes in arterial oxygen tension (PaO_2). Administration of 100% oxygen decreases ventilation, indicating the existence of tonic chemoreceptor activity. The ventilatory response of the neonate to hypoxia is modified by many factors, including gestational and postnatal age, body temperature, and sleep state. Preterm and full-term infants younger than 1 week of age who are awake and normothermic usually demonstrate a biphasic response to hypoxemia—a brief period of hyperpnea followed by ventilatory depression. Hypothermic infants and very small preterm infants respond to hypoxemia with ventilatory depression without the initial hyperpnea. This depression of ventilation has been attributed to the central effects of hypoxia on the cortex and medulla. The peripheral chemoreceptors, although active in neonates, are unable to maintain a significant influence on this hypoxic response. Infants show a less sustained response to hypoxia during REM sleep. In neonates, hypoxia also depresses the ventilatory response to carbon dioxide. Hypoxia may induce periodic breathing in infants, and this may be abolished by oxygen administration. Full-term infants older than 2 to 3 weeks of age demonstrate hyperpnea in response to hypoxia, probably as a result of maturing of the chemoreceptor function.

Reflexes that arise from the lung and chest wall are probably more important in maintaining ventilation in the neonate, possibly compensating for inadequacies in other control mechanisms. They primarily determine the rate *(f)* and V_t but are also important for maintaining lung volume (i.e., terminating expiration). The Hering-Breuer inflation reflex, which is active in the neonate, is even more powerful in the preterm infant. This reflex disappears during REM sleep and progressively fades during the early weeks of life. The paradoxical "Head" reflex, a large inspiration triggered by a small lung inflation, is active in the neonate. It may play a role in maintaining lung volumes in the neonate, and may be present during anesthesia.

Periodic breathing (rapid ventilation alternating with periods of apnea lasting 5 to 10 seconds) occurs in many preterm and some full-term infants. It is associated with increased peripheral chemoreceptor activity. In the preterm infant, the $PaCO_2$ is greater than normal during these episodes of periodic breathing, but the heart rate does not change significantly. In the full-term infant, hypocapnia may occur during periodic breathing, which seems to have no serious physiologic consequences and usually ceases by 44 to 46 weeks of postconceptual age. Periodic breathing generally only occurs about 3% of the time in full-term infants; a greater fraction of periodic breathing in a full-term infant is a warning sign of possible abnormal control of ventilation. Some preterm infants demonstrate far more serious and indeed life-threatening episodes of apnea. These commonly exceed 20 seconds and may be accompanied by bradycardia (possibly due to a chemoreceptor mediated reflex) and hemoglobin oxygen desaturation. Brief apnea spells (<20 seconds) may also be accompanied by significant bradycardia (<80 beats/min). The pathogenesis of apnea in preterm infants is not fully understood. Apnea may reflect an immature central respiratory control system because it tends to resolve as the brain matures. However, a variety of pathophysiologic mechanisms are involved. Apneic episodes may result from a failure of central control mechanisms (central apnea); in such instances, there is no ventilatory effort. It may also result from airway obstruction (obstructive apnea), in which case ventilatory effort may be observed but there is no gas exchange. Obstruction usually occurs in the infant's nasopharynx, pharynx, or hypopharynx. Mixed apnea (a combination of central and obstructive) may also occur and one type may progress to another (i.e., obstructive apnea may progress to central apnea). Apnea may also result from failure of the ventilatory muscles. Many apneic episodes occur during REM sleep, when it is possible that fatigue of the ventilatory muscles is an important factor. Although neonatal apnea may be idiopathic, it may also be symptomatic of an underlying disease process, such as sepsis, intracranial bleeding, anemia, hypoglycemia, hypothermia, sensitivity to sedating medications, or patent ductus arteriosus.

Preterm infants must be carefully monitored to detect apneic episodes. Treatment is by tactile stimulation or, if this fails, by bag-mask resuscitation. The incidence of apneic episodes is decreased by therapy with aminophylline or caffeine (central stimulation) or by institution of continuous positive airway pressure (increased reflex activity of lung and chest wall reflexes and "splinting" of the airway). Preterm and former preterm infants up to 60 weeks postconceptual age, particularly those with anemia, are at risk for postoperative apnea even if apnea-free at the time of anesthesia.

These infants will benefit from appropriate postoperative monitoring in an ICU or similar close observation unit with apnea monitoring.

Suggested Reading

Givan DC: Physiology of breathing and related pathological processes in infants, Semin Pediatr Neurol 10:271–280, 2003.

Baird TM: Clinical correlates, natural history and outcome of neonatal apnea, Semin Neonatol 9:205–211, 2004.

Muscles of Respiration

The muscles of respiration in the neonate are subject to fatigue, a tendency that is determined by the types of muscle fiber present. In the diaphragm, 10% of the muscle fibers are type I (slow-twitch, highly oxidative, fatigue-resistant) in preterm infants, which increases to 25% in full-term infants, and reaches a maximum of 55% (the adult level) after 8 months postpartum. In the intercostals, 20%, 46%, and 65% of the fibers are type I for the same age groups, with the maximum reached by 2 months postpartum. Thus the preterm infant is prone to ventilatory muscle fatigue, a predisposition that progressively disappears with maturity. Ventilation is also affected by changes that occur during changing sleep states. The preterm infant spends 50% to 60% of this time in REM sleep, during which time, intercostal muscle activity is inhibited and paradoxical movement of the soft chest wall occurs. The reduced intercostal muscle activity is offset in part by an increase in diaphragmatic activity. Much of this activity is wasted when the ribs move paradoxically and may lead to diaphragmatic fatigue.

Suggested Reading

Gaultier C: Respiratory muscle function in infants, Eur Respir J 8:150–153, 1995.

Respiratory Mechanics

The specific CL increases slowly after birth as fluid is removed from the lung. The chest wall compliance of the infant (especially the preterm infant) is great, so that total compliance approximates CL. This highly compliant chest wall provides a relatively weak force to maintain the FRC and to oppose the action of the diaphragm. The FRC of the small infant is maintained by a rapid respiratory rate, the point of termination of expiration, controlled expiration ("laryngeal braking"), and the tonic activity of the ventilatory muscles. This being so, it is not surprising that large decreases in FRC occur with apnea and during anesthesia when inhalation agents depress intercostal muscle function.

These large decreases in FRC are accompanied by airway closure and impaired oxygenation. Intercostal muscle inhibition during REM sleep or with inhaled anesthetic agents compounds the weakness of the chest wall and results in paradoxical movement. This paradoxical chest wall movement is markedly augmented by any airway obstruction. It may be inferred that infants generally require controlled ventilation during anesthesia and benefit from rapid respiratory rates or use of positive end-expiratory pressure to maintain the lung volume, avoid airway closure, and pharyngeal collapse during mask ventilation. As the child grows through infancy and childhood, the rib cage stiffens so that it becomes better able to oppose the action of the diaphragm and less reliant on intercostal muscle tone.

The transpulmonary pressures needed to optimally inflate the lungs are remarkably similar in healthy infants, children, and adults. During artificial ventilation, peak inspiratory pressures of 15 to 20 cm H_2O are normal.

The nasal air passages contribute up to 50% of the total airway resistance in infants and slightly less in African American infants. Insertion of an NGT increases this resistance by as much as 50%. The nasal passages are usually of unequal size; if an NGT is inserted, it should be placed through the smaller nostril, so as to have a lesser effect on total nasal airway resistance. The resistance of the neonate's peripheral airways is small but increases with age.

Lung Volumes

In the full-term infant, TLC is approximately 160 ml; the FRC is about half this volume. The V_t is approximately 16 ml (6 to 7 ml/kg), and V_D is about 5 ml (30% of the V_t). Relative to body size, all of these volumes are similar to adult values. Note, however, that any dead space in anesthesia or ventilator circuits is much more significant in relation to the small volumes of the infant (e.g., a 5 ml apparatus dead space would increase the total effective V_D by 100%).

In contrast to the static lung volumes, V_A is proportionally much greater in the neonate ($\sim$100 to 150 ml/kg/min) than in the adult ($\sim$60 ml/kg/min). This high V_A in the infant results in a V_A:FRC ratio of 5:1, compared with 1.5:1 in the adult. Consequently, the FRC is a much less effective "buffer" in the infant, so that changes in the concentration of inspired gases (including anesthetic gases) are more rapidly reflected in alveolar and arterial values.

The CV is relatively greater in infants and young children than in young adults; it may exceed the FRC to encroach on the V_t during normal respirations. Airway closure during normal respirations may explain the reduced normal values for PaO_2 in infants and neonates (Table 2-2). A decrease in FRC, which usually occurs during general anesthesia and persists into the postoperative period, further increases the significance of the large CV and increases the A-aDO_2. The younger the infant or child, the greater the decrease in FRC. The intraoperative decrease in FRC may be partially reversed by continuous positive airway pressure.

The total surface area of the air-tissue interface of the alveoli is small in the infant ($2.8\ m^2$). When this area is related to the high metabolic rate for oxygen, it is apparent that the ratio between surface area and rate of oxygen consumption is smaller in the infant than the adult. As a result, the infant has a reduced reserve capability for gas exchange. This developmental fact assumes greater significance in the presence of congenital pulmonary hypoplasia or lung damage (e.g., from meconium aspiration). In such cases, the remaining healthy lung tissue may be inadequate to sustain life.

Work of Breathing

The muscles of respiration generate the force necessary to overcome the resistance to airflow and the elastic recoil of the lungs and chest wall. These two factors dictate an optimal rate of ventilation and a V_t that delivers a given V_A while expending minimal muscular energy for each child. Because the time constant of the infant's lung is relatively small, efficient alveolar ventilation can be achieved at high respiratory rates. In the neonate, a respiratory rate of 37 breaths/min has been calculated to be most efficient, a rate that is close to the rate in healthy neonates. Full-term infants are similar to adults in that they require 1% of their metabolic energy to maintain ventilation; the oxygen cost of breathing is 0.5 ml / 0.5 L

TABLE 2-2   Arterial Oxygen Tension in Healthy Infants and Children

Age	Normal Arterial Oxygen (mmHg) in Room Air
0–1 wk	70
1–10 mo	85
4–8 yr	90
12–16 yr	96

of ventilation. The preterm infant has a greater oxygen cost of breathing (0.9 ml/0.5 L), which is greatly increased if the lungs are diseased, as in RDS or bronchopulmonary dysplasia.

Ventilation-Perfusion Relationships in the Neonatal Lung

Ventilation (V) and perfusion (Q) are imperfectly matched in the neonatal lung. This may be in part a result of gas trapping in the lungs. $\dot{V}/\dot{Q}$ mismatch is evident in the alveolar-arterial nitrogen difference (A-aDN$_2$), which is 25 mm Hg immediately after birth and declines to about 10 mm Hg within the first week. The normal PaO$_2$ in an infant breathing room air is about 50 mm Hg just after birth and increases to 70 mm Hg by 24 hours of age. The large A-aDO$_2$ in infants is mainly caused by persisting anatomic shunts (see page 26) and the relatively large CV.

Lung Surfactant

Surfactants in the alveolar lining layer stabilize the alveoli, preventing their collapse on expiration. Reducing the surface tension at the air-liquid interface in the alveoli also reduces the force required for their re-expansion. The principal surfactant in the lung is lecithin, which is produced by type II pneumocytes. The quantity of lecithin in the fetal lung increases progressively, beginning at 22 weeks of gestation and increasing sharply at 35 to 36 weeks as the lung matures. The lecithin production of the lung can be assessed by determining the lecithin/sphingomyelin (L/S) ratio in amniotic fluid and this is used as a measure of lung maturity and predictor of RDS. The L/S ratio is usually less than 1 until 32 weeks gestation, reaching 2 by 35 weeks, and 4 to 6 by full term.

Preterm infants with inadequate pulmonary lecithin production suffer from RDS. The biochemical pathways for surfactant production may also be depressed by hypoxia, hyperoxia, acidosis, or hypothermia; therefore, early correction of these abnormalities in the sick neonate is vitally important. Inhaled anesthetic agents seem to have little effect on surfactant production. Maturation of biochemical processes in the lungs of the fetus in utero may be accelerated by the administration of corticosteroids to the mother. The use of exogenous surfactant therapy to treat RDS is now well established.

Suggested Reading

Been JV, Zimmermann LJ. What's new in surfactant? A clinical view on recent developments in neonatology and paediatrics, Euro J Pediatr 166:889–899, 2007.

Lung Growth and Development

The lungs continue to develop during the first 2 decades of life. The number of alveoli increases rapidly over the first 6 years, almost reaching adult levels, but growth continues into adolescence. In young children, the small size of the peripheral airways may predispose to obstructive lung diseases such as bronchiolitis.

Pulmonary Function Testing in Children

Children older than 6 years of age may cooperate sufficiently to enable standard tests of pulmonary function to be performed, and these may be an important part of the preoperative assessment. However, they should be interpreted within the context of their cooperation. Maximum expiratory and inspiratory flow-volume curves may be useful in determining the site and nature of airway obstruction; for example, they can differentiate between intrathoracic and extrathoracic obstruction. Such studies may be most useful in the preoperative assessment of children with a mediastinal mass. Spirometric studies may provide useful information as to the degree of reversible airway obstruction present in those with a disease such as asthma and may assist in preoperative planning. They also may indicate the extent of restrictive disease such as accompanies scoliosis, thereby predicting the likelihood of postoperative pulmonary insufficiency.

Suggested Reading

Beydon N, Davis SD, Lombardi E, et al: An official American Thoracic Society/ European Respiratory Society Statement: pulmonary function testing in preschool children, Am J Respir Crit Care med 175:1304–1345, 2007.

Larson GL, Kang JA, Guilbert T, et al: Assessing respiratory function in young children: developmental considerations, J Allergy Clin Immunol 115:657–666, 2005.

Respiratory System Changes with Anesthesia

The following is a summary of some of the major changes that occur in the respiratory system during and after anesthesia.

1. Spontaneous ventilation is decreased by the potent inhalational anesthetics. This is thought to occur because of the combined effects of anesthetic drugs on the central chemical control of respiration and on the muscles of respiration. Intercostal muscle activity is inhibited by inhalational anesthetics; consequently, diaphragmatic breathing

predominates and the chest wall may move paradoxically, even if the airway is only partially obstructed. Surgical stimulation tends to increase ventilation back toward normal levels. The effect of intravenous agents on ventilation in children is variable and not fully documented.

2. The FRC is reduced during general inhalation anesthesia with or without neuromuscular block. This reduction is greatest in the youngest children and is caused by elevation of the diaphragm and loss of chest wall stability. As the FRC decreases, airway closure may occur during tidal ventilation, resulting in impaired oxygenation. It is for this reason that 5 cm PEEP is commonly advocated during anesthesia in infants and toddlers.

3. The ratio of physiologic dead space to tidal volume (V_D:V_t) remains constant in children breathing spontaneously but may increase in those whose ventilation is controlled. During controlled ventilation, major alterations in gas distribution within the lungs occur as a result of changes in the action of the diaphragm. This effect tends to markedly unbalance the $\dot{V}/\dot{Q}$ matching within the lungs. Apparatus dead space may assume considerable significance given the small physiologic V_D and rapid rate of ventilation.

4. Compliance is little changed and airway resistance is generally reduced by the bronchodilator action of inhalational anesthetics. Insertion of an ETT increases total flow resistance (see page 15), especially in children less than 3 years of age.

5. The efficiency of gas exchange may be impaired by the effects of anesthetic drugs on the physiologic process that normally controls the regional distribution of inspired gases and blood flow throughout the lung (hypoxic pulmonary vasoconstriction).

6. Laryngospasm occurs more frequently in children compared with adults, especially those with an active or recent upper respiratory infection (URI), particularly during induction of anesthesia and after extubation (see page 92). Laryngeal closure results from apposition of the vocal cords and supraglottic structures. The reason for the increased incidence of laryngospasm in children is unknown.

CARDIOVASCULAR SYSTEM

The Fetal Circulation

The fetal cardiovascular system perfuses the low-resistance placental circulation, directing 36% to 42% of the combined ventricular output to this organ; only 5% to 10% goes to the lungs. The high pulmonary vascular resistance limits flow to the fetal lungs resulting in blood bypassing the lungs via the foramen ovale and the ductus arteriosus. Most of the blood returning from the placenta bypasses the liver via the ductus venosus. The pattern of flow from the inferior vena cava into the right atrium (RA) ensures that about one third of the oxygenated placental blood (partial pressure of oxygen [pO_2], 28 to 30 mm Hg) is directed through the foramen ovale into the left atrium. This blood, which combines with the limited venous return from the lungs, is pumped by the left ventricle into the ascending aorta and thence to the coronary, cerebral, and forelimb circulations. Blood returning via the superior vena cava (pO_2, 12 to 14 mm Hg) passes through the RA into the right ventricle, from which most of the output flows through the ductus arteriosus into the descending aorta. Thus blood supplied to the heart and upper body has a greater oxygen content (saturation, 65%; pO_2, 26 to 28 mm Hg) than that supplied to the abdominal organs, lower limbs, and placenta (saturation, 55% to 60%; pO_2, 20 to 22 mm Hg). In utero, the right ventricle pumps about 66% of the combined ventricular output, and the left ventricle pumps the remaining 34%.

Circulatory Changes at Birth

At birth, pulmonary ventilation is normally established quickly, and blood flow to the lungs is greatly increased while placental flow ceases. When the lungs expand and fill with gas, pulmonary vascular resistance (PVR) decreases markedly as a result of mechanical effects on the vessels and relaxation of pulmonary vasomotor tone when the pO_2 increases and the partial pressure of CO_2 decreases in alveolar gas. PVR decreases by 80% from prenatal levels within a few minutes after normal initiation of respirations. As PVR decreases, blood flow to the lungs and then via the pulmonary veins into the left atrium increases, increasing left atrial pressure above that in the RA and closing the atrial septum over the foramen ovale.

Simultaneously, as flow to the placenta ceases because of clamping or umbilical artery constriction, a large, low-resistance vascular bed is excluded from the systemic circulation. This activity results in a large increase in systemic vascular resistance (SVR) and a decrease in inferior vena cava blood flow and RA pressure. The increase in SVR and the simultaneous decrease in PVR increase the aortic pressure above that in the pulmonary artery. Blood flow through the ductus arteriosus reverses (i.e., becomes left to right), and the ductus fills with oxygenated blood. This increased local pO_2 (to levels greater than 50 to 60 mm Hg) causes the muscular wall of the ductus arteriosus to constrict secondary to a prostaglandin-mediated response. Shunts may persist through the ductus for some hours after birth, producing audible murmurs. Normally, however, flow through the ductus is insignificant by 15 hours. Permanent closure of the ductus is usually complete within 5 to 7 days but may not be complete until 3 weeks.

The ductus venosus, which communicates between the umbilical veins, the portal vein, and the inferior vena cava, also remains patent for several days after birth. This channel provides a shunt past the hepatic circulation and therefore may delay the clearance of drugs metabolized in the liver (e.g., opioid analgesics).

The Transitional Circulation

During the early neonatal period, reversion to the fetal circulatory pattern is possible under some circumstances. If hypoxia occurs, PVR increases, the foramen ovale opens and the ductus arteriosus may also reopen; a significant proportion of blood then again bypasses the (now high-resistance) pulmonary circulation, causing a rapid decline in arterial oxygenation. Impaired tissue oxygenation then results in acidosis, which causes a further increase in PVR, establishing a vicious circle of hypoxemia $\Rightarrow$ acidosis $\Rightarrow$ impaired pulmonary blood flow $\Rightarrow$ hypoxemia. Reversion to a fetal pattern of circulation may complicate any condition that causes hypoxemia or acidemia (e.g., RDS, or congenital diaphragmatic hernia).

The Neonatal Cardiovascular System

In healthy neonates, the wall thickness of the right ventricle exceeds that of the left. This preponderance is evident in the ECG, which shows an axis of up to +180° during the first week of life. After birth the left ventricle enlarges disproportionately. By 3 to 6 months, the adult ratio of ventricular size is established (axis approximately +90°). During the immediate neonatal period, the heart rate is between 100 and 170 beats/min and the rhythm is regular. As the child grows, the heart rate gradually decreases (Table 2-3). Sinus arrhythmia is common in children. All other irregular rhythms must be considered abnormal.

Systolic blood pressure is approximately 60 mm Hg in the full-term neonate, and the diastolic pressure is 35 mm Hg. These pressures vary considerably and may be 10 to 15 mm Hg more if clamping of the umbilical cord is delayed or the cord is "stripped," causing an increase in circulating blood volume. In either case they decrease to normal values within 4 hours. Preterm infants have reduced arterial pressures, as low as 45/25 mm Hg in a 750-g infant (Table 2-4).

TABLE 2-3   Normal Heart Rate

Age	Heart Rate (beats/min)	
	Average	Range
Neonate	120	100–170
1–11 mo	120	80–160
2 yr	110	80–130
4 yr	100	80–120
6 yr	100	75–115
8 yr	90	70–110
10 yr	90	70–110
14 yr		
Boys	80	60–100
Girls	85	65–105
16 yr		
Boys	75	55–95
Girls	80	60–100

TABLE 2-4   Normal Blood Pressure*

Age	Blood Pressure (mmHg)		
	Systolic	Diastolic	Mean
Neonate			
Preterm (750 g)	44	24	33
Preterm (1000 g)	49	26	34.5
Full term	60	35	45
3–10 d	70–75	57	
6 mo	95		
4 yr	98		
6 yr	110	60	
8 yr	112	60	
12 yr	115	65	
16 yr	120	65	

* Reported normal blood pressure values for infants and children must be considered in light of their methods of determination. These values should serve as a guide only (see Monitoring During Anesthesia, page 116).

The myocardium of the neonate contains less contractile tissue and more supporting tissue than the adult heart. Consequently, the neonate's ventricles are less compliant when relaxed and generate less tension during contraction. Because the reduced compliance of the relaxed ventricle tends to limit the size of the stroke volume, the cardiac output of the neonate is rate dependent. Bradycardia is invariably accompanied by reduced cardiac output. The less compliant ventricle of the neonate is also dependent on an adequate filling pressure, so that hypovolemia is followed by a decrease in cardiac output. Thus cardiac output is both rate dependent and volume dependent. Reduced compliance and contractility of the ventricles also predisposes the infant heart to failure with increased volume load. In the infant, failure of one ventricle rapidly compromises the function of the other, and biventricular failure results.

The reduced contractility of the neonatal heart is also thought to be secondary to the immaturity of the myofibrils and to the less developed sarcoplasmic reticulum. It is postulated that the cyclic calcium flux within the neonatal myocardium is more dependent on exchange across the cell membrane (sarcolemma) and less a function of the sarcoplasmic reticulum, thus a greater dependency upon ionized calcium. As the infant grows, the myocardial sarcoplasmic reticulum expands and progressively assumes a dominant role in intracellular calcium regulation, which is typical of the adult heart. The greater role of the sarcolemma in calcium regulation within the myocyte may explain the greater sensitivity of the neonate to myocardial depression because of inhalational anesthetics (calcium channel blocking activity). It may also explain the severe cardiac depressant effects of calcium channel-blocking drugs or the rapid administration of citrated blood products such as fresh frozen plasma or platelets in the neonate.

The autonomic innervation of the heart is incomplete in the neonate and there is a relative lack of sympathetic elements. This may further compromise the ability of the less contractile neonatal myocardium to respond to stress. The differences in the neonate's myocardium are all particularly marked in the preterm infant.

In the neonate, shunts hamper the precise measurement of cardiac output, which averages two to three times that of the adult on a milliliter per kilogram body weight basis and is appropriate for the metabolic rate. The total systemic vascular resistance is reduced, reflecting the great proportion of vessel-rich tissue in the neonate (18%—twice that in the adult) and resulting in a reduced systemic arterial pressure despite the large cardiac output.

The Pulmonary Circulation

The changes in the pulmonary circulation that occur at birth continue with a slower progressive decrease in PVR over the first 3 months of life.

This is associated with a parallel regression in the thickness of the medial muscle layer of the pulmonary arterioles. During the neonatal period, PVR is still high and the muscular pulmonary vessels are highly reactive. Hypoxia, acidosis, and stress (e.g., from endotracheal suctioning) may all increase PVR. If the increase in the PVR is sustained by such stimuli, right-sided intracardiac pressures may exceed those on the left and right-to-left shunting may ensue via the ductus arteriosus or foramen ovale. Right ventricular failure, rapidly progressing to biventricular failure, may occur.

In some circumstances, the normal regression of the muscular layer of the pulmonary vessels and the associated decrease in PVR may not occur. Continued hypoxemia, caused for example by continued high altitude or cyanotic heart disease (e.g., tetralogy of Fallot) or excessive pulmonary blood flow as a result of left-to-right shunts (ventricular septal defect, patent ductus arteriosus, etc.) may lead to persistence of a high PVR into childhood and beyond. Initially, this high PVR is reversible (e.g., with pulmonary vasodilators) and correction of the underlying defect. Later, this high PVR results in structural changes in the pulmonary vascular bed that are irreversible, causing pulmonary vascular obstructive disease.

Nitric oxide has been identified as an endothelium-derived relaxing factor that is normally produced continually in the lung to regulate pulmonary vascular tone. This has led to the use of nitric oxide inhalation to treat increased pulmonary vascular resistance.

Blood Volume

The blood volume varies considerably during the immediate postnatal period (the primary variable being the amount of blood drained from the placenta before the cord is clamped) and during the first year of life. Delay in clamping or stripping the cord at delivery may increase the blood volume by more than 20%, resulting in transient respiratory distress. Conversely, fetal hypoxia during labor may vasoconstrict the cord, shift blood to the placental circulation, and cause hypovolemia in the already asphyxiated neonate.

The Response to Hypovolemia

The response to hypovolemia and restoration of the blood volume are of great importance to the anesthesiologist because surgery in the neonate may be accompanied by significant blood loss. Withdrawal of blood during exchange transfusion causes a progressive parallel decrease in systolic blood pressure and cardiac output. Reinfusion of an equal volume of blood restores these parameters to their original values. The changes in arterial blood pressure are proportional to the degree of hypovolemia. The capacity of the neonate to adapt the intravascular volume to the available blood volume is very limited, perhaps due to less efficient control of capacitance vessels. The baroreflexes of the infant, especially the preterm infant, are inactive during anesthesia, further compromising the response to hypovolemia.

In summary, the infant's systolic arterial blood pressure is closely related to the circulating blood volume. Blood pressure is an excellent guide to the adequacy of blood replacement during anesthesia, a fact that is amply confirmed by extensive clinical experience. The hypovolemic infant is unable to maintain an adequate cardiac output; hence, accurate early volume replacement is essential.

Table 2-5 shows approximate normal values for blood volume in infants and children. Values may be greater however, particularly in preterm infants.

The Response to Hypoxia

Because of the high $\dot{V}O_2$, hypoxemia can develop rapidly in the neonate. The first observed response is usually bradycardia in contrast to the tachycardia observed in the adult. The anesthesiologist should treat any episode of unexplained bradycardia by immediately ventilating the child with 100% oxygen. During hypoxemia, pulmonary vasoconstriction occurs and the pulmonary artery pressure increases more than in adults. The foramen ovale and the ductus arteriosus may reopen resulting in a large right-to-left shunt, further decreasing SaO_2. Changes in cardiac output and SVR in infants also differ from those in older children and adults. During hypoxemia, the principal response in adults is systemic vasodilation, which together with an increased cardiac output, helps to maintain oxygen transport to the tissues. The fetus and some neonates respond to hypoxemia with systemic vasoconstriction. During fetal life this directs more blood to the placenta, but after birth this response may reduce cardiac output, further limiting oxygen transport and forcing the heart

TABLE 2-5 Normal Blood Volume of Children

Age	Blood Volume (ml/kg)
Neonate	80–85
6 wk to 2 yr	75
2 yr to puberty	72

to work harder. In the infant, the early and pronounced bradycardia in response to hypoxia may be caused by myocardial hypoxia and acidosis.

Neonates exposed to hypoxemia experience pulmonary and systemic vasoconstriction, bradycardia, and decreased cardiac output. Rapid intervention is necessary to prevent this state from proceeding to cardiac arrest.

Oxygen Transport

Blood volume in the neonatal period is approximately 80 ml/kg in the term infant and about 20% greater in the preterm infant (Table 2-5). The hematocrit (Hct) may be as great as 60%, and the hemoglobin (Hb) 18 to 19 g/dl. The values for blood volume, hematocrit, and Hb vary from infant to infant, depending on the time of clamping of the umbilical cord. These values change little during the first week of life, after which the Hb level starts to decrease. This change occurs more rapidly in the preterm infant.

Most (70% to 90%) of the Hb present at birth in a full-term infant is HbF. The affinity of HbF for oxygen is greater than that of HbA, primarily because of a lack of effect of 2,3-DPG on the HbF-O_2 interaction. HbF combines with more oxygen but releases it less readily in the tissues than does HbA. The P_{50} for HbF is approximately 20 mm Hg, in contrast to 26 to 27 mm Hg for HbA. Adequate oxygen transport to the tissues of the neonate therefore demands a greater Hb concentration. Less than 12 g/dl constitutes anemia, and greater levels are very desirable in hypoxic states. However, there are many risks associated with transfusion. Current thought is that correction of anemia by blood transfusion may be indicated to maintain the Hct greater than 40% in cases of severe cardiopulmonary disease, 30% in moderate cardiopulmonary disease or major surgery, and 25% in symptomatic anemia (apnea, tachycardia, lethargy, poor growth).

Transfusion with HbA-containing erythrocytes may improve oxygen transport to the tissues in the sick preterm infant. However, this treatment has also been reported to increase the risk of ROP. During the first weeks of life, the hematocrit and Hb levels decline steadily, in part because of a progressive increase in blood volume but also a result of suppression of erythropoiesis caused by improved tissue oxygenation (see Table 4-10). This physiologic anemia of infancy reaches a nadir at 2 to 3 months of age, with Hb levels of 9 to 11 g/dl. At this time the HbF content of the blood has been largely replaced by HbA. Thus oxygen delivery at the tissues is improved. Provided that nutrition is adequate, the Hb level now increases gradually over several weeks to 12 to 13 g/dl, which is maintained during early childhood.

The preterm infant demonstrates an earlier and greater decrease in Hb concentration, reaching 7 to 8 g/dl in infants weighing less than 1500 g at birth. This is the result of a short erythrocyte life span, rapid growth, and decreased erythropoietin production. The early "physiologic" anemia of the preterm infant is often followed by a continuing "late" anemia, which is secondary to nutritional deficiencies. In the infant in the neonatal intensive care unit, this anemia is accentuated by repeated blood sampling. Iron therapy is not effective in correcting this anemia and may cause other problems (e.g., hemolysis, infection). Anemia of the preterm infant may lead to tachycardia, tachypnea, poor feeding and growth, diminished activity, and apnea. In severe states, congestive heart failure may occur.

Suggested Reading

Hutton EK, Hassan ES: Late vs early clamping of the umbilical cord in full-term neonates: systematic review and meta-analysis of controlled trials, JAMA 297(11):1241–1252, 2007.

METABOLISM: FLUID AND ELECTROLYTE BALANCE

Glucose Homeostasis

The term neonate has stores of glycogen that are located mainly in the liver and myocardium. These are used during the first few hours of life until gluconeogenesis becomes established. Small-for-gestational-age and preterm infants may have inadequate glycogen stores and may fail to establish adequate gluconeogenesis. Hence, they are very dependent upon IV infusions to prevent hypoglycemia.

Hypoglycemia is common in the stressed neonate (Table 2-6). Blood glucose levels should be measured frequently in sick neonates, and if they decrease to less than 40 mg/dl or 2.2 mmol/L, they should be corrected by a slow continuous infusion of 10% dextrose (5 to 8 mg/kg/min). Symptoms of hypoglycemia (jitteriness, convulsions, apnea) should be treated immediately by slow injection of 10% dextrose (1 to 2 ml/kg). Neurologic damage occurs in up to 50% of infants with symptomatic hypoglycemia. Infants of diabetic mothers and those with Beckwith-Wiedemann syndrome must be treated with particular care because a bolus dose of intravenous glucose may precipitate hyperinsulinemia and serious rebound hypoglycemia. In these infants, a slow infusion of glucose as outlined above is recommended. Older infants and young children rarely become hypoglycemic even during an excessively long preoperative fasting period. Current pediatric practice minimizes preoperative fasting (see page 77).

TABLE 2-6   Factors Associated With Hypoglycemia in Neonates

Prematurity
Perinatal stress
Sepsis
Small for gestational age
Polycythemia
Hypoxia
Excess insulin
Infant of diabetic mother
Beckwith-Wiedemann syndrome

Hyperglycemia is a common iatrogenic problem of small infants receiving intravenous therapy, probably as a result of inadequate insulin release and continued hepatic glucose production. The effects of hyperglycemia can be serious. Osmotically induced cerebral fluid shifts may lead to cerebral hemorrhage, and glycosuria may cause diuresis resulting in water and electrolyte depletion. Hyperglycemia (glucose values >200 mg/ dl) may also increase the extent of neurologic damage during a cerebral hypoxic-ischemic event. It is essential that glucose therapy be carefully controlled to avoid hyperglycemia. We recommend the use of a continuous infusion pump for maintenance glucose containing fluids with other intraoperative losses replaced with balanced salt solutions "piggy backed" to the maintenance fluids.

Suggested Reading

De Lonlay P, Giurgea I, Touati G, et al: Neonatal hypoglycemia: aetiologies, Semin Neonatol 9:49–58, 2004.
Leelanukrom R, Cunliffe M: Intraoperative fluid and glucose management in children, Paediatr Anaesth 10:353–359, 2000.

Calcium Homeostasis

Calcium is actively transported across the placenta to meet the needs of the fetus. This transport accelerates near term and may cause a decline in maternal calcium levels. After birth, the infant must depend on its own calcium reserves. However, parathyroid function is not fully established, and vitamin D stores may be inadequate. As a result, hypocalcemia must be anticipated—especially in the preterm infant—after birth trauma, neonatal asphyxia, any severe neonatal illness, or blood transfusion (especially fresh frozen plasma or platelets). Correction of metabolic acidosis in the neonate by administration of sodium bicarbonate may precipitate a significant decrease in ionized calcium levels.

Symptoms of hypocalcemia include twitching, increased muscle tone, and seizures (hypocalcemia is not always easily distinguished from hypoglycemia). The Chvostek sign may be present, but confirmation depends on laboratory test results (total serum calcium, less than 7 mg/dl or 1.75 mmol/L; ionized calcium, less than 4 mg/dl or 1.0 mmol/L) or on the response to therapy. The infant prone to hypocalcemia is treated with continuous calcium chloride infusion at a rate of 5 mg/kg/hr. Symptomatic hypocalcemia requires a slow infusion of either 10% calcium chloride (10 to 30 mg/kg) or 10% calcium gluconate (30 to 90 mg/kg), with continuous ECG monitoring. Note that calcium-containing solutions may cause severe skin damage, leading to sloughing if they leak into adjacent tissues. They should preferably be given through a central line.

Suggested Reading

Hsu SC, Levine MA: Perinatal calcium metabolism: physiology and pathophysiology, Semin Neonatol 9:23–36, 2004.

Kossoff EH, Silvia MT, Maret A, et al: Neonatal hypocalcemic seizures: Case report and review of the literature, J Child Neurol 17:236–239, 2002.

Magnesium Homeostasis

Magnesium and calcium metabolism are closely related: an imbalance in one may affect the other. Magnesium levels affect parathyroid hormone secretion, and the renal excretion of calcium and that of magnesium are interrelated. Chronic hypomagnesemia is commonly accompanied by hypocalcemia secondary to the effect on parathyroid function.

Hypomagnesemia is more common in preterm infants, small-for-gestational-age infants, infants of diabetic mothers, and infants with intestinal disease. It may also complicate massive blood transfusion. Hypomagnesemia results in abnormal muscle activity, tremors, seizures, and cardiac arrhythmias, and may alter sensitivity to muscle relaxant drugs.

Hypermagnesemia may complicate renal failure, or, in the neonate, it may be a consequence of the administration of magnesium sulfate to the mother. It may result in depression of the central nervous and respiratory systems, hyporeflexia, and hypotension.

Bilirubin Homeostasis

In the full-term neonate, unconjugated hyperbilirubinemia during the first week of life (physiologic jaundice) occurs secondary to an increased bilirubin load, limited hepatic cell uptake of bilirubin, and deficient hepatic conjugation to the water-soluble glucuronide. Serum bilirubin levels seldom exceed 7 mg/dl or 103 μmol/L. In preterm infants, greater levels (10 to 15 mg/dl or 170 to 255 μmol/L) are commonly reached. These persist for a longer period, owing to a greater bilirubin load and delayed maturation of the hepatic conjugation pathway. The preterm infant may sustain neurologic damage (kernicterus) at reduced serum bilirubin levels (6 to 9 mg/dl) than does the full-term infant (20 mg/dl). This predisposition is a result of the preterm infant's less effective blood-brain barrier and may be exacerbated by hypoxia, acidosis, infection, hypothermia, or a low level of serum albumin and hence decreased binding sites. The preterm infant must be carefully monitored for increased serum bilirubin levels, and specific treatment should be administered as required. Treatment includes phototherapy and possibly exchange transfusion. Some drugs (e.g., diazepam, sulfonamides, furosemide) displace protein-bound bilirubin (i.e., "acidic" binding sites for albumin) and therefore increase the danger of neurologic damage. There are no reports of anesthetic drugs (except benzodiazepines) producing adverse changes in bilirubin levels, but hypoxia, acidosis, hypothermia, and hypoalbuminemia may all increase the danger.

Suggested Reading

Stevenson DK, Wong RJ, Desandre GH, et al: A primer on neonatal jaundice, Adv Ped 51:253–288, 2004.

COMPOSITION AND REGULATION OF BODY FLUIDS

Body Water

The amount of total body water in neonates and infants is relatively greater than in adults. Its distribution also differs, the proportion of ECF being greater in neonates and young children. In the preterm infant, the ECF exceeds the ICF, whereas in the older child and adult the ECF is only half the volume of the ICF (Table 2-7). Normal levels of serum electrolytes in the neonate are listed in Table 2-8.

TABLE 2-7   Extracellular and Intracellular Fluid Compartments

Fluid	Preterm Neonate	Full-term Neonate	Infant (7–8 Mo)	Adult
ECF	50	35–40	30	20
ICF	30	35–40	35	45

TABLE 2-8   Normal Blood Chemistry

Parameter	Preterm Neonate	Full-term Neonate	2 Yr to Adult
Serum chloride (mEq/L)	100–117	90–114	98–106
Serum potassium (mEq/L)	4.6–6.7	4.3–7.6	3.5–5.6
Serum sodium (mEq/L)	133–146	136–148	142
Blood glucose (mg/dl)	40–60	40–80	70–110
Total protein (g/dl)	3.9–4.7	4.6–7.7	5.5–7.8
Pa_{CO_2} (mmHg)	30–35	33–35	35–40

Neonatal Renal Function and Water Balance

In the neonate, renal function is limited by immaturity of tubular function and an increased renal vascular resistance, which results in reduced renal blood flow and GFR. GFR rapidly increases after birth as renal blood flow increases. The preterm infant has an even lower GFR, which increases less rapidly over the first weeks of life than it does in the full-term infant. The GFR of the neonate increases with fluid loading, but only to a limited capacity. Consequently, the infant cannot readily handle an excessive water load and may be unable to excrete excess electrolytes or other substances dependent on glomerular filtration. The GFR is further decreased by hypoxia, hypothermia, congestive cardiac failure, or mechanical ventilation; adult values are usually achieved by approximately 1 year of age.

The limited tubular function impairs the infant's ability to modify the glomerular filtrate for conservation or excretion. For this reason, sodium losses may be large, especially in the preterm infant, and must be balanced by intake. These losses are further increased if the GFR is increased by a high fluid intake; hence, the tendency of the neonate to hyponatremia. Glucose reabsorption is limited in the preterm infant, and glycosuria may occur. In the child with marked hyperglycemia, the resultant osmotic diuresis may lead to severe dehydration. The ability of the tubule to excrete acid is reduced in the preterm infant, thus impairing renal compensation during acidosis. The capacity to excrete H^{++} increases with gestational age. The renal threshold for bicarbonate excretion is less in infants than adults, and this leads to reduced serum bicarbonate levels. The limitations of renal function summarized above necessitate careful fluid and electrolyte replacement therapy planned to match losses. Renal vascular resistance decreases and renal function matures rapidly over the first few weeks after birth in the full-term infant. Preterm infants show less rapid changes in renal function.

Fluid loss and hence the required replacement is related to insensible fluid losses, urine output, and metabolic rate. Insensible fluid losses are relatively great during infancy, major factors being the increased alveolar ventilation and the thin skin of low-birth-weight infants. Fluid losses are markedly increased by the use of radiant heat and/or phototherapy. Because of the infant's proportionally greater water turnover and the limited ability to concentrate urine and conserve water, dehydration develops rapidly when intake is restricted or losses occur.

Maintenance Requirements

Although maintenance requirements are directly related to the metabolic rate and caloric expenditure and are more accurately expressed in milliliters per square meter of surface area, it is most convenient to relate them to body weight. Fluid requirements for full-term neonates are reduced (40 to 60 ml/kg per 24 hours) during the first few days of life as excess fluid present at birth is being excreted. By 1 week of age, the requirements are increased. Table 2-9 shows the volumes of fluid required during the period of great metabolic activity in infants weighing 4 to 20 kg.

Intraoperative fluid management in the neonate must include replacement of fluid deficits, third space losses, blood loss, and maintenance fluid therapy. Fluid deficits and losses are generally replaced with a balanced salt solution such as lactated Ringer's solution whereas maintenance therapy is replaced with an infusion of 5% glucose and one half to one fourth normal saline, containing 20 mEq of K^+ per liter. If high-concentration glucose solutions (D-10 or D-20) are infusing preoperatively, these solutions should be continued either at the same or at a somewhat reduced rate throughout surgery. In critically-ill neonates, balanced salt solutions should be replaced with colloid solutions or plasma early, as hypoproteinemia is common.

TABLE 2-9 Daily Maintenance Requirements for Fluid, Electrolytes, and Carbohydrates in Relation to Weight

Weight	H_2O (ml/kg)	Na^+ (mEq/kg)	K^+ (mEq/kg)	Carbohydrate (g/kg)
Neonate*				
1000 g	≤200	3.0	2.0–2.5	≤10
1000–1499 g	≤180	2.5	2.0–2.5	
1500–2500 g	≤160	2.0	1.5–2.0	≤8
2500 g	≤150	1.5–2.0	2.0	≤5
4–10 kg	100–120	2.0–2.5	2.0–2.5	5–6
10–20 kg	80–100	1.6–2.0	1.6–2.0	4–5
20–40 kg	60–80	1.2–1.6	1.2–1.6	3–4
Adult	30–40	50 mEq total	50 mEq total	100–150 g total

* Adjust according to postnatal age, exposure to phototherapy, reduced insensible losses with assisted ventilation, etc.
(From The Hospital for Sick Children: Residents' Handbook of Pediatrics, 6th ed. Toronto, Canada, 1979, with permission.)

Suggested Reading

Hartnoll G: Basic principles and practical steps in the management of fluid balance in the newborn, Semin Neonatol 8:307–313, 2003.

PHYSIOLOGY OF TEMPERATURE HOMEOSTASIS

Because of their large surface area relative to body weight and their lack of heat-insulating subcutaneous fat, infants lose heat rapidly via four routes in order of importance: radiation (39%) > convection (34%) > evaporation (24%) > conduction (3%). Evaporative heat is lost into the respiratory tract and through the skin, the latter being related to increased skin permeability and is thus a particularly important factor in preterm infants. When heat loss occurs, heat production within the body must increase to maintain a normal core temperature. In adults and older children, this heat production is principally a function of involuntary muscular activity (shivering) accompanied by increased oxygen consumption, both of which can be prevented by the administration of a neuromuscular blocking drug. Infants rely primarily on nonshivering thermogenesis to generate heat. This mechanism, which also results in increased oxygen consumption, occurs mainly in the brown adipose tissue, which makes up 2% to 6% of the full-term infant's body weight (less in the preterm infant) and is located around the scapulae, in the mediastinum, and surrounding the kidneys and adrenal glands. The cells of this "brown fat" have many mitochondria and fat vacuoles, and the tissue has a rich blood and autonomic nerve supply. Increased metabolic activity in brown fat is initiated by norepinephrine released at the sympathetic nerve endings. Hydrolysis of triglyceride to fatty acids and glycerol occurs with associated increased $\dot{V}O_2$ and heat production. Brown fat deposits decline during the first weeks of extrauterine life.

Exposure to a cool environment together with a decrease in central temperature normally triggers thermoregulatory vasoconstriction in unanesthetized infants and children. This vasoconstriction tends to limit further heat loss from the body surface. It is now recognized that the mechanisms for controlling body temperature are well developed in the full-term neonate. However, a decrease in core temperature results when compensatory increases in heat production cannot match heat losses. On exposure to a cool environment, increased metabolic activity is initiated in the brown fat so as to maintain the core temperature. This is accompanied by a progressive increase in oxygen consumption as the temperature gradient between the skin and the environment increases. Oxygen consumption is minimal when this gradient is less than

TABLE 2-10 Neutral Thermal Environment Temperatures (°C)

Age	Weight			
	1200 g	1200-1500 g	1500-2500 g	>2500 g
0-6 hr	34-35.4	33.9-34.4	32.8-33.8	32.0-33.8
6-12 hr	34-35.4	33.5-34.4	32.2-33.8	31.4-33.8
12-24 hr	34-35.4	33.3-34.3	31.8-33.8	31.0-33.7
24-36 hr	34-35	33.1-34.2	31.6-33.6	30.7-33.5
36-48 hr	34-35	33.0-34.1	31.4-33.5	30.5-33.3
48-72 hr	34-35	33.0-34.0	31.2-33.4	30.1-33.2
72-96 hr	34-35	33.0-34.0	31.1-33.2	29.8-32.8
4-12 day	—	33-34*	31-33.2	29.5-31.4
2-3 wk	—	32.2-34*	30.5-33.0	—
3-4 wk	—	31.6-33.6*	30.0-32.7	—

*1500 g

2° C (i.e., neutral thermal environment). Exposure to a cool environment also leads to increased glucose use and acid metabolite formation.

The physiologic responses to cooling lead to increased oxygen and glucose use and result in acidosis, all of which may compromise the sick infant. The infant with chronic hypoxemia (e.g., cyanotic congenital heart disease) is unable to compensate if exposed to a cool ambient temperature and cools rapidly. To eliminate the need for compensatory responses, sick neonates should be maintained in a neutral thermal environment (i.e., in an ambient temperature that minimizes oxygen consumption [Table 2-10]).

During anesthesia the normal thermoregulatory response of the infant to cold stress is lost and oxygen consumption is unchanged in response to a cool environment. In addition, normal thermoregulatory skin vaso-constriction is inhibited. There is also a redistribution of body heat away from the central core to the periphery. Therefore anesthetized infants and children have increased heat loss and a decrease in body temperature. Measures to minimize heat loss and avoid cold stress (warmed operating room, warmed preparation and irrigation solutions, convective forced air warmers) are important during anesthesia and are outlined on page 124.

Suggested Reading

Luginbuehl I, Bissonnette B: Thermal regulation. Chap 25. In Cote CJ, Lerman J, Todres ID (eds.): A practice of Anesthesia for Infants and Children, 4th ed., Elsevier, Philadelphia, 2009, pp 557–567.

Clinical Pharmacology 3

ROUTES OF ADMINISTRATION

Intravenous. The intravenous route is the most certain route to deliver drugs to the bloodstream under all conditions and is the principal route for all anesthetic drugs given parenterally. Be very careful to check all drugs (i.e., *read the label*) and doses before administration. In the case of less commonly used drugs (e.g., antibiotics), ensure that the manufacturer's directions as to route of administration, speed of injection, and dilution are carefully followed. Rapid injection of some drugs (e.g., vancomycin) may cause severe physiologic effects (e.g., cardiac arrest, "red man syndrome"). Administration of drugs using tuberculin syringes or when diluted is very important in neonates and infants. It is essential to eject all air bubbles from the syringe before administration. Be very careful that all intravenous tubing is flushed after all drugs are administered to ensure that no drugs remain in the tubing or the dead space of the injection port. Serious incidents have occurred when neuromuscular blocking drugs or anesthetics/opioids have been flushed into the child after a procedure has ended.

N.B. Drugs should not be injected into infusions of *hyperalimentation* fluids because infection or thrombosis of the line may result. However, some children will have had a central line inserted for the specific purpose of providing for repeated anesthesia/sedation procedures. In this case, access the line using appropriate connectors and with careful aseptic technique. In other cases, it may be appropriate to "Hep-Lok" a peripheral IV for use in subsequent procedures.

Intramuscular. Drugs administered intramuscularly are rapidly absorbed, especially in small children and preferably should be given in the lateral aspect of the thigh. *(Absorption is more rapid from the arm [deltoid] muscle than from the leg muscle; however, it carries a risk of nerve damage).* Intramuscular injections are much less reliable in children in shock or who are hypovolemic, and there is a danger that repeated doses may have a cumulative effect when muscle tissue perfusion improves. Intramuscular injections are painful and generally avoided in conscious children.

Intralingual. Injections into the tongue have been recommended for use in an emergency (e.g., succinylcholine) when parenteral access is limited. Systemic absorption is rapid via this route. *However, we have never found a need for this technique and do not recommend it* (see page 69).

Intratracheal. Drugs sprayed into the trachea through a tracheal tube are quite rapidly absorbed, and this may be a useful in an emergency if an intravenous route is not available (e.g., to administer atropine or epinephrine during cardiopulmonary resuscitation). However, this route is no longer recommended as a first choice for resuscitation; if it is used, larger drug doses are required. It is important to either dilute the drug to a larger volume or flush the drug into the tracheobronchial tree with 3 to 5 ml of saline to ensure delivery to a mucosal surface. Beware that local anesthetics sprayed into the trachea are rapidly absorbed; always check to ensure that the total dose given is safe.

Rectal. Use of suppositories (acetaminophen) or rectal administration of drugs (e.g., pentobarbital, methohexital) is usually well accepted by children under 3 years of age. Absorption is less certain than with other routes, in part because of the partial first-pass effect of the liver when absorption occurs through the inferior/middle hemorrhoidal veins and the variable volume and pH of the rectal milieu. Unanesthetized children older than 3 years of age may be upset if medications are administered via this route.

Oral. Preoperative medication and postoperative analgesics may be given to selected children by this route. The oral route cannot be used if vomiting or other gastrointestinal dysfunction exists. Many drugs are very rapidly and predictably absorbed across the oral mucous membrane (e.g., fentanyl, midazolam) if administered as a lozenge or placed under the tongue. The oral transmucosal route is a potentially very useful route for drug therapy in children.

Intranasal. Some drugs are well absorbed across the nasal mucous membrane and are rapidly effective by this route (e.g., sufentanil, midazolam). However, many children are upset at having nose drops instilled, and this route has not gained wide acceptance. There is also a concern that some drugs or their preservative (e.g., midazolam) might be neurotoxic if they penetrate the cribriform plate into the brain.

Intraosseous. This route is recommended for use during resuscitation in all age groups when an intravenous route is not available. Drugs are rapidly absorbed by this route and may be given in the usual doses. This route is now advocated for pediatric resuscitation if initial attempts at venous access fail (see Chapter 4, page 128).

DISTRIBUTION OF ADMINISTERED DRUGS

In infants and young children, the relative sizes of the body fluid compartments differ from those in the adult. The extracellular fluid compartment is large; hence, drugs that are distributed throughout this space (e.g., succinylcholine) are required in larger doses.

Protein binding is less in neonates because of reduced total serum protein concentrations and reduced concentrations of specific proteins (e.g., α_1-acid glycoprotein). More of the administered drug is free in the plasma to exert a clinical effect. For this reason, reduced doses of such drugs as barbiturates and local anesthetics are indicated.

The composition of the body also has an influence on drug distribution; neonates have little fat or muscle tissue. Drugs normally distributed throughout these tissues will have greater plasma concentrations and prolonged duration of action.

METABOLISM AND ELIMINATION OF DRUGS

The half-lives of drugs that are metabolized in the liver in the neonate and small infant are generally greater than in the adult (e.g., opioid analgesics). Hepatic blood flow and hepatocellular enzymatic activity are the primary determinants of the rate of metabolism of a drug by the liver. Hepatic blood flow may be reduced in the small infant because of increased intraabdominal pressure and congestive cardiac failure. In the first few postnatal days, blood may shunt past the liver via a patent ductus venosus. The conjugation pathways for drug metabolism are immature in preterm infants and are not fully active until several months of age. Hence, the elimination half-life of drugs such as morphine in this age group is increased. In addition, alternative pathways for drug metabolism may result in the accumulation of metabolites, some of which may be pharmacologically active (e.g., morphine-3- and 6-glucuronide).

Older infants and young children demonstrate a rapid elimination of some drugs, reflecting the greater hepatic blood flow and enhanced metabolic activity in the child's liver.

Drugs excreted via the kidney (e.g., most antibiotics) depend on the glomerular filtration rate or tubular secretion capacity, both of which are reduced during the first few weeks of postnatal life, thus necessitating greater intervals between drug dosing.

Suggested Reading

Anand KJS, Anderson BJ, Holford NHG, et al: Morphine pharmacokinetics and pharmacodynamics in preterm and term neonates: secondary results from the NEOPAIN trial, Br J Anaesth 101:680–689, 2008.

DRUGS USED IN ANESTHESIA

Inhalation Agents

The concentration of inhaled anesthetics in the alveoli increase more rapidly with decreasing age: infants > children > adults. This is the result of the increased alveolar ventilation to functional residual capacity ratio, the greater proportion of vessel-rich tissues that rapidly equilibrate with blood concentrations, and the reduced blood-gas and tissue-gas partition coefficients (λ) of the inhaled anesthetics (except sevoflurane) in infants. Therefore, induction of anesthesia is more rapid in infants and small children. The rapid increase in alveolar, blood, and tissue concentrations of inhaled anesthetics may account in part for the precipitous decreases in blood pressure that occur when greater concentrations of these anesthetics are given to infants, particularly during controlled ventilation.

Excretion of inhaled anesthetic agents, and therefore recovery, is also more rapid in infants and small children than in adults, provided that ventilation is not depressed. The alveolar concentration of N_2O decreases to 10% within 2 minutes after discontinuation of 70% N_2O, a level not reached until 10 minutes in adults.

The minimum alveolar concentration (MAC) of inhaled anesthetics is greater in infants than in older children and adults (Table 3-1); the reasons for this are unknown. MAC values have been determined for a number of anesthesia interventions including tracheal intubation and extubation, and for LMA insertion and removal (Table 3-2).

All inhaled anesthetics depress ventilation to a similar degree as evidenced by CO_2 response curves. A dose related decrease in V_t and minute ventilation is accompanied by an increase in $PaCO_2$. Intercostal muscle activity is inhibited, particularly during halothane anesthesia. This contributes to the depressed ventilation, and may lead to paradoxical chest wall movement, especially if any degree of airway obstruction occurs.

Inhaled anesthetics are myocardial depressants due to their calcium channel blocking activity; this is most marked with halothane, less with isoflurane, and least with sevoflurane or desflurane. Halothane frequently, and sevoflurane rarely, causes bradycardia, which may be corrected by atropine administration. Inhaled anesthetics may prolong the Q-Tc interval (halothane > sevoflurane > isoflurane) in some children, especially young infants. Although this may be insignificant, in many children it may predispose those with long Q-T syndrome to serious arrhythmias. Recent evidence points to the dispersion of repolarization (defined as the difference between the maximum and minimum Q-T interval) as predisposing to ventricular arrhythmias.

TABLE 3-1   Minimum Alveolar Concentration MAC (%) of Inhalational Agents

Age	Halothane	Isoflurane	Sevoflurane	Desflurane
Preterm neonate	0.55	1.3–1.4	Not available	Not available
Full-term neonate	0.87	1.6	3.3	9.1
Infant	1.2	1.8	3.2	9.4
Child	0.95	1.6	2.5	8.5

TABLE 3-2   MAC for Anesthesia Interventions in Children

	MAC (%)
Tracheal intubation	Halothane: 1.3 Enflurane: 2.93 Sevoflurane: 2.7
Tracheal extubation	Isoflurane: 1.4 Sevoflurane: 1.70, 2.3 Desflurane: 7.7
LMA insertion	Halothane: 1.5 Sevoflurane: 2.0
LMA extubation	Sevoflurane: 1.84
Tracheal intubation/ skin incision ratio*	Halothane, enflurane, sevoflurane: 1.33
Awake	Sevoflurane: 0.3

* Calculated using the above MAC data.
From Coté CJ, Lerman J, Ward RM et al. Chapter 6. In: A practice of Anesthesia for Infants and Children. Coté CJ, Lerman J, Todres D (eds), 4th ed, 2009, p. 108.

Inhaled anesthetics inhibit hypoxic pulmonary vasoconstriction and thereby disrupt the mechanism that normally redistributes perfusion away from underventilated alveoli. This increased shunt may cause a clinically significant decrease in arterial oxygen saturation, especially in infants with lung disease (e.g., bronchopulmonary dysplasia).

All of the inhaled anesthetics reduce the requirements for nondepolarizing neuromuscular blocking drugs (NMBDs) to produce a standard degree of block. This relaxant enhancing effect may be useful in reducing the total dose of NMBDs administered and facilitating antagonism of the neuromuscular blockade.

All inhaled anesthetics are capable of triggering MH and should be avoided in a child with an MH history. Controversy exists regarding the risk of rhabdomyolysis in children anesthetized with inhalational anesthetics.

Nitrous Oxide (N₂O)

N_2O is commonly used in pediatric anesthesia to speed and facilitate induction and to provide analgesia/amnesia during maintenance. It may also be administered to sedate and to provide analgesia before intravenous induction of anesthesia. N_2O is odorless and insoluble (blood/gas partition coefficient ($\lambda_{b/g}$) is 0.47) with a MAC of 104% in adults. In large concentrations, it enhances the rate of uptake of the inhaled anesthetics into the alveoli, accelerating induction of anesthesia (second-gas effect). The analgesic effects of N_2O may complement the anesthetic regimen during maintenance. The effects of N_2O on ventilation appear to equal those of equipotent concentrations of halothane. N_2O mildly depresses cardiac output and systemic blood pressure in infants, but it has little effect on pulmonary artery pressure or pulmonary vascular resistance, even in those with pulmonary vascular disease. In infants and small children, the cardiovascular effects of N_2O combined with either halothane or isoflurane to 1.5 MAC are similar to those of equipotent (1.5 MAC) concentrations of either halothane or isoflurane in oxygen. N_2O rapidly diffuses into any gas-containing space within the body; this contraindicates its use in those with lung cysts, pneumothorax, lobar emphysema, necrotizing enterocolitis, bowel obstruction, and any other gas filled cavity. N_2O (70%) doubles the size of a pneumothorax in 12 minutes and that of gas containing bowel in 120 minutes. The tenfold difference in doubling time is the result of the shrinking blood supply to the bowel, as the lumen of the bowel expands, and unchanged blood flow to the chest wall/pleura with expansion of the pneumothorax. N_2O also diffuses into the middle ear and may displace the graft during tympanoplasty. In some children with a normal ear and an intact eardrum, postoperative absorption of N_2O from the middle ear results in atelectasis of the drum and a later complaint of earache. N_2O does not appear to increase postoperative vomiting in children. However, when treating children for procedures that are associated with a high incidence of PONV, it may be prudent to avoid nitrous oxide.

Sevoflurane

In the past decade, sevoflurane has become the agent of choice for inhalational induction in children. A fluorinated methyl isopropyl ether, it has a low solubility in blood ($\lambda_{b/g}$ is 0.68), a not-unpleasant odor, and is the least irritating to the airway of the inhaled anesthetics. Thus it is the ideal agent for inhalational induction. Induction of anesthesia can most rapidly be achieved by administering the maximum deliverable initial concentration (8%); it is not necessary to introduce sevoflurane in slow stepwise increases in inspired concentration except as a means of reducing its pungency for the child. Slowly increasing the inspired concentration of sevoflurane only prolongs the excitement period. To minimize the response to 8% sevoflurane during induction, the mask should be flavored and 70% N_2O in oxygen administered first until the child stops responding. For older, cooperative children, the so called "single breath induction" (i.e., a vital capacity breath) using an anesthesia circuit primed with 8% sevoflurane in 66% nitrous oxide and fitted with a large reservoir bag will induce anesthesia rapidly and smoothly. The effect of age on the MAC of sevoflurane differs from that of the other anesthetics: it is 2.4% in children 6 months to 10 years and 3.2% in neonates up to 6 months of age. The large MAC limits the magnitude of the overpressure technique that is possible with an 8% vaporizer. The addition of 60% N_2O to sevoflurane in children only decreases the MAC by 23%. Attempts at intravenous cannulation should not be made until the child is adequately anesthetized and unresponsive. Satisfactory conditions for endotracheal intubation without neuromuscular blocking agents can be achieved quite rapidly as anesthesia is deepened especially if a single dose of propofol is administered before intubation or ventilation is controlled for a brief period.

During sevoflurane anesthesia there is a dose related decrease in tidal volume, respiratory frequency, and minute ventilation, which is reversed by surgical stimulation. In practice, the addition of nitrous oxide to sevoflurane decreases the MAC of the latter and thus minimizes respiratory depression in the spontaneously ventilating child.

Sevoflurane causes less myocardial depression than halothane, isoflurane, or desflurane and arrhythmias are uncommon, even when epinephrine-containing solutions are injected. An increase in heart rate and a slight decrease in blood pressure usually occur after induction of anesthesia. Occasionally bradycardia occurs during induction of anesthesia in infants and particularly in children with trisomy 21, but this may be prevented by pretreatment with an anticholinergic. Compared with halothane, sevoflurane causes less hypotension in children with congenital heart disease and less desaturation in those with cyanotic CHD.

Epileptiform EEG activity and myoclonic jerking movements have been reported exceedingly rarely during sevoflurane anesthesia in children. The combination of high concentrations of sevoflurane and hyperventilation appear to increase the epileptiform activity, although frank seizures are exceedingly rare. Epileptiform EEG activity during sevoflurane may cause paradoxical readings on "depth of anesthesia" monitors (e.g., the BIS monitor). Caution should be exercised when interpreting BIS values during sevoflurane anesthesia at higher concentrations.

Emergence from sevoflurane anesthesia is smooth and rapid, although emergence agitation may occur in some children, especially preschool-age children (see page 216). This transient phenomenon is characterized by restless and inconsolable behavior, inability to establish eye contact, lack of purposeful movement, and lack of interaction with their surroundings. To reduce the incidence of agitation, care must be taken to ensure adequate analgesia during emergence by means of a regional block or systemic analgesics. Antinociceptive strategies combined with midazolam premedication, propofol, or an alpha$_2$ agonist (e.g., dexmedetomidine) all reduce the risk of emergence agitation. There is some evidence that recovery of fine coordination over the first few hours after sevoflurane is more complete than it is after isoflurane or halothane.

Sevoflurane is metabolized (5%) in vivo by CYP450 2E1 releasing inorganic fluoride; maximum plasma concentrations occur within 2 hours of terminating the anesthetic. Although large plasma inorganic fluoride concentrations after methoxyflurane were associated with nephrotoxicity, this does not occur after sevoflurane. Nephrotoxicity depends on the affinity of renal CYP450 2E1 for the ether anesthetic, which locally releases inorganic fluoride that may impair renal tubular function. In the case of CYP450 2E1, the affinity for sevoflurane is one fifth that of methoxyflurane, hence nephrotoxicity does not occur with the former despite similar plasma concentrations of inorganic fluoride to those after methoxyflurane. Sevoflurane is also degraded in vitro in the presence of some carbon dioxide absorbents (baralyme > soda lime>>Amsorb Plus). The extent of degradation in vitro increases at low fresh gas flows and in desiccated absorbent. Degradation of sevoflurane in vitro yields five compounds, the most common being Compound A, a potentially nephrotoxic vinyl compound. Compound A production varies directly with the weight of the child. Absorbents that are free of KOH and NaOH such as Amsorb Plus do not degrade sevoflurane. In some countries, a minimum fresh gas flow and concentration-time exposure have been recommended for sevoflurane although there is limited evidence that very low fresh gas flows present any risk to humans. The combination of desiccated baralyme and sevoflurane resulted in an absorber fire (the result of hydrogen production from degradation of sevoflurane in the presence of desiccated baralyme at temperatures >200 °C) that led to the withdrawal of baralyme from the market. To date, neither sevoflurane nor its degradation products have been shown to be toxic in humans.

Isoflurane

Isoflurane is a polyhalogenated methyl ethyl ether. It is a stable compound that is metabolized less than 0.2% in vivo, although it is degraded to carbon monoxide in the presence of some desiccated CO_2 absorbents. It is eliminated almost completely unchanged via the lungs; therefore recovery should be very complete.

The $\lambda_{b/g}$ of 1.43 dictates that wash-in to the alveoli is slower than that of sevoflurane. In addition, isoflurane is not suited as an induction agent because its pungent odor irritates airway reflexes (coughing, laryngospasm, and breath holding). Nonetheless, isoflurane can be successfully introduced after an intravenous induction, provided the concentration is increased slowly. Alternatively, for more prolonged surgery, anesthesia may be maintained with isoflurane after induction has been successfully completed with sevoflurane. Recovery after isoflurane anesthesia is slower than after sevoflurane although emergence agitation appears to be less of a problem. The incidence of laryngospasm during extubation and emergence is similar to that with halothane (see later discussion). Isoflurane depresses the respiratory system to a similar extent as sevoflurane.

During isoflurane anesthesia, blood pressure decreases although heart rate does not change substantively. The decrease in blood pressure is due in part to myocardial depression, but also to peripheral vasodilation. Infusion of intravenous fluids tends to restore the blood pressure. The vasodilating effect of isoflurane may be useful to control blood pressure, such as during induced hypotension. Isoflurane depresses the baroreflex in the neonate. This impairs the ability to compensate for changes in arterial blood pressure and for hypovolemia. Isoflurane does not sensitize the myocardium to the effects of catecholamines or theophylline.

Isoflurane potentiates nondepolarizing neuromuscular blocking drugs to a greater extent than sevoflurane or halothane, thus allowing reduced doses of relaxant drugs to be used. The neuromuscular effects of isoflurane are reversible when isoflurane is withdrawn, thereby facilitating reversal of neuromuscular blockade.

Halothane

Halothane was considered to be an ideal anesthetic for children, although its popularity in pediatric anesthesia has waned since the introduction of sevoflurane into clinical practice. Indeed, many recent North American trainees have never used halothane in children, unless they have administered anesthesia overseas. Nonetheless, halothane is inexpensive and is still used in some parts of the world where more expensive anesthetics are less available. Pediatric anesthesiologists familiar with halothane consider that it may have some advantages over sevoflurane when a more prolonged emergence is needed to facilitate endoscopy with spontaneous ventilation (e.g., for laryngoscopy, bronchoscopy), or when managing a difficult airway. Its use will therefore be discussed.

With a $\lambda_{b/g}$ of 2.3 the wash-in of halothane is slow compared with sevoflurane. However, with a 5% maximum inspired concentration and a MAC in children of approximately 1%, greater MAC-multiples of halothane can be delivered than of sevoflurane. The MAC in children who are cognitively challenged may be 25% less than in children who are not challenged. Halothane provides a smooth inhalation induction with minimal irritation of the airways.

During halothane anesthesia, a dose-dependent depression of spontaneous ventilation occurs; there is usually an increase in respiratory rate, but tidal volume and minute ventilation decrease considerably. This increases the end-tidal carbon dioxide concentration but prevents anesthetic overdose as long as respirations are not assisted or controlled (see later discussion). Alveolar ventilation returns toward normal during surgical stimulation but is variable throughout anesthesia. Halothane inhibits intercostal muscle activity. Diaphragmatic ventilation predominates, and paradoxical movement of the chest wall may occur. Even very low blood levels of halothane severely depress the ventilatory response to hypoxia in young adult volunteers. It is likely that this effect also occurs in children of all ages. Laryngospasm may occur during light planes of halothane anesthesia, especially during extubation of the trachea. This effect can be avoided by extubating the trachea while the child is either still deeply anesthetized or completely awake. Lidocaine (1 to 2 mg/kg IV) given slowly before extubation may reduce coughing but will not prevent laryngospasm. Halothane is a potent bronchodilator and is very useful in children with asthma.

Halothane depresses myocardial contractility, especially in small infants. It also produces bradycardia and thus causes a decrease in cardiac output. Atropine prevents the bradycardia and tends to maintain cardiac output, but does not reverse the reduced myocardial contractility. Neonates are especially sensitive to the myocardial depressant effects of halothane. Severe hypotension may ensue if large concentrations of halothane are administered to infants and children, particularly when ventilation is controlled. This is a result of myocardial depression and, with the subsequent decreased cardiac output, the concentration of halothane rapidly increases in the child's myocardium, leading to electromechanical dissociation/cardiac arrest.

The infant's blood pressure is very sensitive to changes in cardiac output. Vasoconstriction is less effective than in the adult. Halothane also depresses reflex baroresponses. Inspired halothane concentrations are usually limited to 0.5% to 1% during controlled ventilation, and the blood pressure should be carefully monitored. In children with cardiac failure, the myocardial depressant effects of halothane are prominent, and severe hypotension may occur.

Arrhythmias also occur during halothane anesthesia. Ventricular premature beats are common, especially during spontaneous ventilation in the presence of hypercarbia. If they occur, ventilation should be assisted or controlled; if they persist, another inhalational anesthetic (e.g., isoflurane) should be substituted for halothane. Junctional rhythm and wandering pacemaker also occur during halothane anesthesia. This is usually of little consequence but might compromise the child with congenital heart disease. Halothane sensitizes the myocardium to exogenous catecholamines, and arrhythmias may occur when these compounds are injected (e.g., to infiltrate the skin). Studies indicate that children tolerate greater doses of injected epinephrine than adults. Epinephrine in doses up to a maximum of 10 µg/kg mixed with local anesthetic or saline and injected into the tissues of healthy children appears to be safe. Serious arrhythmias may occur if halothane is administered to children who have been receiving theophylline medication chronically; other agents should be used.

Halothane, like most other inhalational anesthetics, increases cerebral blood flow and therefore may increase ICP. At small concentrations, this effect is minimal, and if hyperventilation is employed, the increase is insignificant even in those with intracranial space-occupying lesions.

Shivering and muscle rigidity are common during emergence from halothane anesthesia. These effects may be of concern after orthopedic surgery and in children in whom the additional oxygen demands of shivering might be detrimental. In such cases, an alternative anesthetic technique may be more appropriate.

Halothane is metabolized 15% to 20% in adults in vivo, but the extent of metabolism is less in infants and small children. Occasional cases of hepatic failure have been reported in adults, but many fewer have been reported in children, despite its wide and often repeated use in the latter age group. These rare cases of halothane hepatitis in children have been confirmed by the presence of halothane-related antibodies. Most episodes of halothane hepatitis in children run a less fulminant course than in adults. The reason for the reduced susceptibility of prepubertal children to halothane hepatitis is not known. Contraindications to halothane include a history of unexplained postoperative jaundice.

Desflurane

Desflurane is a fluorinated ether with a boiling point of 23 °C and the smallest $\lambda_{b/g}$, 0.42. In addition, it is the least soluble anesthetic in all tissues. It is a very stable compound, with less than 0.02% metabolized in vivo, although it is degraded to carbon monoxide in the presence of some desiccated absorbents. Desflurane is a less potent anesthetic agent with a MAC of 7% to 9.5% in children. MAC increases with decreasing age, peaking in infants 6 to 12 months of age. The effects of desflurane on the cardiovascular system at 1 MAC anesthesia are similar to those of other ether inhalational anesthetics, although bradycardia is rare. In adults, when desflurane is the sole anesthetic agent, sudden increases in the inspired concentration can lead to profound central sympathetic discharge, resulting in sudden increases in blood pressure and heart rate.

Desflurane is very pungent and causes airway irritation; breath holding and laryngospasm are very common and for these reasons desflurane is not recommended for inhalational inductions in children. It can, however, be safely used for maintenance after induction with other agents in children whose airways are intubated. There are limited data on airway responses to desflurane in children managed with either a mask or an LMA. Emergence is very rapid as a result of its limited solubility. To prevent the sudden onset of acute pain, analgesics should be administered before emergence. Emergence agitation has also been reported after desflurane, particularly if pain is present. The very rapid recovery may be useful in some children (e.g., small infants at risk for postoperative apnea, although this does not eliminate this risk).

Desflurane increases intracranial pressure more than isoflurane and sevoflurane, although this effect may be attenuated by hyperventilation before introducing the desflurane.

Desflurane is less convenient to use than other agents because its low boiling point demands a specially designed, electrically heated vaporizer. A greater concentration is required to maintain anesthesia (because of its greater MAC), necessitating small fresh gas flows to limit the cost.

Enflurane

This inhaled agent has several disadvantages compared with other agents and, as a result, is not commonly administered to children.

Summary

1. The MAC values of inhalational anesthetics increase with decreasing age from adults to infancy at which age these peak and decrease as age further decreases in neonates and preterm infants.
2. The smaller the child, the more rapid the uptake of inhalational anesthetics.
3. Large concentrations of inhalational anesthetics can cause serious hypotension in infants and young children, particularly when ventilation is controlled. *Beware: overdose of inhaled agents is a leading cause of serious complications.*

4. Sevoflurane is currently the most commonly used induction agent in infants and children.
5. All inhalational anesthetics may be used for maintenance, although recovery is more rapid with those of reduced solubility: desflurane < isoflurane ~ sevoflurane < halothane.
6. Halothane remains a useful alternative to sevoflurane and is less expensive. It may be useful during endoscopy and in the management of the difficult airway.
7. Halothane-induced hepatic failure is rare in children younger than 14 years of age.

Suggested Reading

Coté CJ, Lerman J, Ward RM, et al: Pharmacokinetics and pharmacology of drugs used in children. In: Coté CJ, Lerman J, and Todres ID, (eds.). A Practice of Anesthesia for Infants and Children, Chapter 6. 4th ed., Elsevier, Philadelphia, 2009, pp 89–146.

Intravenous Agents

If the child arrives in the operating room (OR) with peripheral intravenous access, this route can be used to induce anesthesia. In general, injections should not be made into central or peripheral lines that are infusing intralipid or other hyperalimentation fluids to minimize the risk of sepsis. If there is no intravenous access, then a skillful, painless intravenous induction may cause fewer psychological sequelae than an inhalation induction. Needles and syringes should be kept out of the child's sight at all times, and the word *needle* specifically should be avoided. Music, pictures, television, or bubble blowing are helpful distractions during venipuncture. A disposable 27-gauge "butterfly" needle is easy to conceal during insertion and to leave in place for brief procedures (e.g., myringotomy and tubes). Use of appropriately applied topical local anesthetic (see Appendix 3, page 634) facilitates painless venipuncture or intravenous cannula insertion. Alternatively, N_2O (inspired concentration, 50% to 70%) may be given by mask to sedate the child and provide analgesia for venous cannulation. "Poorly visible veins" may be improved by warming the site or applying nitroglycerine cream.

Propofol

Propofol (2,6-diisopropylphenol) is a short-acting hypnotic that is associated with a very rapid onset and offset of anesthesia and pleasant recovery. Although recovery after a single dose of propofol is more rapid than after thiopental, propofol has less advantage over thiopental if the duration of the anesthetic exceeds 1 hour. Propofol has rapidly replaced thiopental as the induction agent of choice. Propofol is hydrophobic and therefore must be suspended in an emulsion of soybean oil. Asepsis is especially important to avoid rapid bacterial contamination when handling this anesthetic, although all contain an antibacterial agent (EDTA, sodium metabisulfite, or benzyl alcohol). Benzyl alcohol may trigger bronchospasm in asthmatic children. Anaphylactoid reactions have been reported after the use of the metabisulfite formulations. Unused propofol should be discarded after the vial has been opened or the syringe loaded for 6 hours. The dose of propofol to induce anesthesia ranges from 1 to 5 mg/kg; larger doses may be required for younger infants and unpremedicated children (Table 3-3). The respiratory and cardiovascular effects of a sleep dose (2.5 to 3.5 mg/kg) are similar to those of thiopentone; a short period of apnea may occur, and there is a slight decrease in blood pressure. Insertion of an LMA is usually possible after a dose of 3.5 mg/kg. If a dose is given to facilitate tracheal intubation during a sevoflurane induction without a muscle relaxant, up to 3 mg/kg appears to facilitate laryngoscopy without a prolonged apnea.

Airway reflexes and oropharyngeal muscle tone are depressed by propofol; this is useful for cases involving airway instrumentation (e.g., laryngeal mask insertion, intubation without muscle relaxant, difficult airway) and generally results in a good airway during emergence. The hypertensive response to instrumenting the airway is less after an induction sequence with propofol plus relaxant than after thiopental plus relaxant. In the presence of a difficult airway, small incremental doses of propofol may be used after an inhalational induction to facilitate tracheal intubation. Extraneous limb movements may occur during induction of anesthesia with propofol, especially if smaller doses are administered.

Pain is common at the site of IV injection of propofol, although it is less severe if propofol is injected into a free-flowing infusion or into a large antecubital vein. Pain is thought to be due to trace concentrations

TABLE 3-3   Effect of Age on the Effective Dose (ED_{50}) of Common IV Induction Agents

Age	Thiopental	Propofol
Neonate	3–4	—
Infant	6–7	3–5
Child	4–5	1–2.5

Doses are mg/kg.
N.B. These are the ED_{50} values; larger doses are required to reliably induce anesthesia.

of propofol in the aqueous egg lecithin outer layer of the emulsion droplets. Either administration of 70% N_2O by mask or application of a "mini Bier block" with 0.5 mg/kg lidocaine for 30 seconds before IV administration of propofol eliminates the pain of injection. Newer preparations of propofol with increased concentrations of medium chain triglycerides also have reduced or no pain during IV induction. Microemulsions of propofol (droplet diameter <50 nm) in aqueous solutions are under investigation; these formulations may not cause pain on injection.

Propofol may be infused continuously for maintenance of anesthesia in children to provide total intravenous anesthesia. This approach may offer the advantage of rapid recovery with minimal sequelae and may also facilitate anesthesia in special locations where space is limited.

The infusion rates for children vary depending on concurrent medications, but they tend to be greater than those in adults. In the case of preterm and full-term neonates, propofol clearance is dramatically reduced; there is a risk of accumulation after repeated doses or an infusion in this age group. When infusions are used to maintain anesthesia, the administration rate should be adjusted to match the predicted elimination of the drug (to maintain a constant blood level) and to prevent light anesthesia. The infusion may be adjusted manually or controlled by a computer, TCI. In either case, the rate should be dictated by the pharmacokinetic parameters for the child's age group. Although these parameters vary considerably more in children than in adults, clinically useful dosage schedules for children have been developed (Table 3-4). For brief or minor surgeries, intermittent intravenous boluses of propofol proved to be both effective and efficient. Experience with propofol in pediatric hospitals suggests that it has widespread applications outside the operating room—in MRI and other radiological studies, radiotherapy, and invasive procedures that include medical procedures, burn dressing changes, and endoscopies.

TABLE 3-4   Infusion Regimen for Propofol in Children

No other opioid or anesthetic agents used
Loading sleep dose: 2.5–5 mg/kg
Initial infusion rate (first 20 min): 200–300 µg/kg/min or 12–18 mg/kg/hr
Subsequent infusion rate (next 20 min): 200 µg/kg/min or 12 mg/kg/hr
Final infusion rate: 150 µg/kg/min or 9 mg/kg/hr
These rates must be adjusted or supplemental doses administered if signs of light anesthesia appear.
If an opioid is used, these infusion rates may be reduced by 25%.

Propofol has a potent antiemetic effect and has been used in children with persistent postoperative vomiting after anesthesia or when the risk of vomiting is substantial.

Propofol has been quite widely used in the neonate (e.g., before intubation in the NICU), however, there have been rare reports of severe hypotension in neonates given propofol and one unpublished report of a subsequent cardiac arrest. Propofol should be used with caution in the neonate.

Propofol is no longer recommended for prolonged sedation in the pediatric intensive care unit. Propofol infusion syndrome (PRIS), which consists of acute refractory bradycardia progressing to asystole, associated with severe metabolic acidosis and other metabolic derangements, has been reported in children after prolonged propofol infusions (>5mg/kg/hr for 48 hours), although PRIS has been diagnosed after exposures of several hours and during anesthesia. Watch for unexpected arrhythmias and metabolic acidosis as signs that PRIS may be developing; the infusion rate should be decreased or discontinued. The mechanism underlying PRIS is unclear but may be due to impaired active transport of long chain triglycerides into myocardial mitochondria and to an interruption of the respiratory chain at complex II by propofol.

Suggested Reading

Kam PC, Cardone D, Propofol infusion syndrome, Anaesthesia 63:690–671, 2007.

Allegaert K, deHoon J, Versesselt R, et al: Maturational pharmacokinetics of single intravenous bolus of propofol, Pediatr Anesth 17:1028–1234, 2007.

Thiopental

Thiopental has been supplanted by propofol as the primary intravenous induction agent in infants and children in many centers. Induction dose depends on age (see Table 3-2). Onset of anesthesia is rapid and smooth, without pain but usually accompanied by a very brief period of apnea. Cardiovascular changes are minimal in the healthy child. Neonates are especially sensitive to barbiturates because of reduced protein binding. Contraindications to thiopental are similar to those in adults. Intravenous induction with thiopental should be avoided in children with a difficult airway. Barbiturates should not be used for children with porphyria and should be administered with caution in children who may be hypovolemic and in those with limited cardiac reserve. Thiopental reduces intraocular and cerebrospinal fluid pressure and hence may be especially useful for induction of anesthesia in children having ocular or neurosurgical procedures. Thiopental may cause arterial spasm if injected into an artery; injections should not be made into the antecubital fossa of infants or children. Extravasation into tissues should be avoided but does not usually cause any serious problem in children. Thiopental precipitates if it is mixed/followed by an acidic drug (i.e., muscle relaxant rocuronium), as the former requires an alkaline pH (>11) to remain soluble in water. Since the precipitate can completely block a small gauge IV catheter, the IV tubing should be flushed between administration of thiopental and the acidic drug.

Methohexital

Methohexital is rarely used for induction of anesthesia, although some authors have reported that recovery after methohexital is faster than after thiopental. Methohexital often causes muscle twitching or hiccups— effects that can be minimized by avoiding large doses. Intravenous injection of 1% methohexital commonly causes pain along the injected vein; this can be minimized by adding a small amount of plain lidocaine (e.g., 1 mg lidocaine /ml solution).

Methohexital is most effective for sedation/induction of anesthesia in apprehensive children younger than 3 years of age by the rectal route, although it is rarely used today. Children may remain in their mother's arms until they fall asleep. Doses of 20 to 30 mg/kg of a 10% solution or 15 mg/kg of a 1% solution induce sedation/anesthesia in 6 to 8 minutes. Methohexital should be administered from a syringe, using a well-lubricated No. 10 catheter, which should be inserted into the rectum only 3 to 4 cm. A diaper should be placed under the child, because soiling sometimes occurs. Rarely, ventilatory obstruction or depression may occur; therefore children must be observed closely by an anesthesiologist with equipment to establish an airway should loss of consciousness occur. Once the child is anesthetized, induction may be continued with an inhalational anesthetic; gently assisted ventilation may be needed at this stage.

Etomidate

Etomidate is not widely used in children. The single induction dose recommended is 0.3 mg/kg IV. It causes pain on injection and extraneous movements, myoclonus, and laryngospasm. Pretreatment with lidocaine may attenuate these effects. This drug should not be given by continuous infusion or repeatedly. Its main advantage is cardiovascular stability in hypovolemia patients or those with cardiovascular disease (e.g., cardiomyopathy). Etomidate has been used to sedate children for CT scans and emergency room procedures. However, suppression of adrenocortical function may persist for 24 hours even after a single dose. This suppression may have clinical implications for critically ill children.

Midazolam

Midazolam is a water-soluble benzodiazepine that has been used for pre-medication (0.5 to 0.75 mg/kg PO), for sedation during endoscopic procedures (in a dose of 0.2 to 0.3 mg/kg IV), and as an amnesic supplement to general anesthesia. Ventilation and cardiovascular homeostasis are generally maintained. Midazolam produces satisfactory sedation in children in pediatric intensive care units; the loading dose is 0.2 mg/kg followed by an infusion at 0.4 to 2 μg/kg/min. It is not an effective agent for induction of anesthesia because of the large doses required and the variability in response. Midazolam has been most widely used as an oral premedication in children, although other routes including the nasal and rectal routes have been used (see Table 4-5, page 87). It should be noted that severe hypotension might occur in neonates when it is combined with fentanyl.

Ketamine Hydrochloride

Ketamine, a phencyclidine derivative, has been used for sedation and general anesthesia since 1964. It has been used extensively in pediatric anesthesia for a wide variety of situations, although its appeal has been diminished with the introduction of propofol.

Ketamine 1 to 2 mg/kg IV induces general anesthesia within 1 minute. For sedation, 3 to 10 mg/kg IM has a 2 to 5 minute onset and about a 30 to 60 duration of action. Oral ketamine (5 to 6 mg/kg) may be useful as a premedication or combined with midazolam (Table 4-5, page 87). These doses should be supplemented with atropine (0.02 mg/kg) or glycopyrrolate (0.01 mg/kg) to prevent excessive secretions. Low-dose ketamine has also been used for perioperative analgesia, particularly after tonsillectomy in children with OSA (see page 284). The effects of ketamine on the central nervous system are unlike those of any other anesthetic in common use. It produces profound analgesia, unconsciousness, cataleptic state, and amnesia. Ketamine increases cerebral blood flow, ICP, and cerebral metabolic rate. The airway is usually well maintained, but secretions are increased (give atropine!) and airway obstruction or laryngospasm may occur. A mild degree of respiratory depression with brief periods of apnea may occur after induction. Because the protective laryngeal reflexes are depressed, gastric contents may be regurgitated and aspirated. Ketamine increases both the heart rate and the mean arterial pressure, although its direct effect on the isolated heart is a depressant one. In healthy subjects, cardiac output is increased and peripheral vascular resistance is little changed. These indirect cardiovascular responses are mediated by adrenergic pathways.

Ketamine has limited gastrointestinal effects, although hypersalivation, nausea, and vomiting may occur. There have been no reports of hepatic or renal damage after its administration. Ketamine is associated with emergence phenomena, including hallucinations and nightmares. These emergence phenomena may be reduced by pretreatment with benzodiazepines and allowing the child to recover in a quiet area. The effects of ketamine on ICP and cerebral blood flow have led most to abandon this drug during neuroradiologic or similar procedures although it remains in use for cardiac catheterization. Ketamine has no effect on visceral pain and therefore is unsatisfactory for abdominal surgery, unless regional analgesia is also provided.

Ketamine has been widely used for children with burns for dressing changes and for minor skin grafting procedures. For prolonged procedures, the advantage of an early return to normal nutrition is outweighed by the slow emergence (particularly if given in a prolonged infusion and in combination with a benzodiazepine). It is also useful for minor superficial procedures in infants. Ketamine may also be valuable for anesthesia in children with right-to-left intracardiac shunt, epidermolysis bullosa, or Stevens-Johnson syndrome; for induction of anesthesia in children in severe shock; for general anesthesia when facilities are limited as in some underdeveloped countries; and in large-scale disasters.

Alpha-2 Agonist Drugs

This class of drugs acts at presynaptic alpha-2 receptors in sympathetic nerves and postsynaptic sites in the central nervous system to inhibit the release of norepinephrine and other neurotransmitters; thus affecting the level of consciousness and perception of pain.

Clonidine

Clonidine is used most commonly in pediatric anesthesia as an adjunct to neuraxial blockade with local anesthetics. It is also used as an oral premedication to reduce postsevoflurane delirium, to reduce shivering, and to augment induced hypotensive regimens (see Table 4-5, page 87).

When combined with local anesthetics via the epidural route, clonidine 2 µg/kg has been reported to extend the duration of caudal epidural analgesia by approximately 3 hours without side effects. However, there are reports of apnea in preterm infants after the use of epidural clonidine.

For oral premedication, 4 µg/kg clonidine produces sedation similar to that of midazolam, but requires 60 to 90 minutes to reach its full effect. Oral atropine should be added to prevent bradycardia. Mild hypotension may also follow its use. Clonidine reduces the cardiovascular responses to tracheal intubation and decreases the MAC for inhaled anesthetics. Analgesic and sedative effects may persist into the postoperative period, decrease delirium, and reduce analgesic requirements. Residual sedation from clonidine may be a safety concern for outpatient surgery.

Dexmedetomidine

Dexmedetomidine is eight times more specific for the α_2-receptor than clonidine with similar physiologic effects. It has been used in the ICU, in the operating room, and in remote sites offering the advantage of sedation without respiratory depression. It is administered commonly as a continuous IV infusion after a loading dose. The elimination half-life in children is approximately 2 hours. Various regimens have been proposed for effecting sedation with this drug. For MRI, 1 µg/kg loading dose over 10 minutes combined with 0.1 mg/kg midazolam and followed by an infusion at 0.7 µg/kg/hr is effective. Recovery after this regimen in children is slightly delayed when compared with propofol. Its role in the care of children continues to evolve. It has also been used for sedation to secure a difficult airway and to promote hypotension for large blood loss surgery and for cardiovascular stability during CV surgery.

As an oral premedication, it has a faster onset than clonidine. Recently, intranasal dexmedetomidine has been used for premedication, although the permeable cribriform plate may facilitate its transfer into the central nervous system (see Table 4-5).

Opioid Medications

Morphine, meperidine, and fentanyl have been administered extensively as part of balanced anesthesia in children. Alfentanil, sufentanil, and remifentanil have also been used; the latter drug may be particularly useful in a TIVA protocol. Administration by infusion after loading doses is optimal, although intermittent bolus doses are often preferred intraoperatively. In addition to providing analgesia, fentanyl and sufentanil, when given in adequate doses, may block neuroendocrine and pulmonary vascular responses to intraoperative stress. Meperidine use in children is now limited to single dose administration to treat shivering in PACU; chronic administration is contraindicated due to accumulation of normeperidine, which may cause seizures, particularly in children with compromised renal function.

Morphine

Morphine provides excellent analgesia and sedation and remains a most satisfactory agent for postoperative systemic analgesia. A standard initial dose of morphine in children during surgery is 0.05 to 0.1 mg/kg IV with additional doses as indicated. Neonates have been considered more sensitive to the ventilatory depressant effects of morphine than to those of meperidine (pethidine). Various factors have been postulated to account for this apparent sensitivity, including differences in permeability of the blood-brain barrier. Probably the most important factor is the relatively slower, less predictable clearance of morphine in the neonate, which tends to accumulate in the blood during continuous infusions. The decrease in the blood concentration after discontinuation of a morphine infusion may also be delayed in small infants. Indeed, sometimes a transient increase may be observed, possibly as a result of enterohepatic recirculation. Provided that careful monitoring and suitably low infusion rates are used, morphine can be safely administered by continuous infusion even in the neonate. The infant should be monitored for 24 hours after discontinuation of a morphine infusion.

Codeine

Codeine is a naturally occurring opium alkaloid constituting approximately 0.5% of raw opium. The drug as supplied is essentially methylated morphine. It is widely accepted that the analgesic properties of codeine are a result of the systemic O-demethylation of codeine with the release of morphine (5% to 15% of the administered dose of codeine) that occurs via the CYP2D6 pathway. The metabolic pathways for demethylation are less active in the neonate and young child than in the adult. This may explain the relative tolerance to codeine in children. However, there are populations that show variations in the activity of these metabolic pathways and very rarely children may have little analgesic effect (slow or no conversion to morphine) or opioid toxicity (rapid or accelerated conversion to morphine) from a standard dose. Several genetic polymorphisms of CYP2D6, which is the enzyme responsible for converting codeine to morphine, have been identified that explain these variable responses. According to the polymorphisms, up to 10% of the Caucasians and 30% of Hong Kong Chinese have a 2D6 variant that results in poor conversion of codeine to morphine and therefore limited analgesia from a standard dose of codeine. Conversely, 29% of Ethiopians and 1% of Swedes and Germans have a variant that results in ultrarapid metabolism of codeine that may cause excessive doses of and possible toxicity from morphine. In our clinical experience in North America, these variable responses are uncommon. On rare occasion, a child may be very sensitive to codeine—presumably as a result of a hyperactive metabolic pathway.

Codeine may be administered by the oral, rectal, or IM route. It should not be administered IV; severe hypotension may result, possibly as a result of histamine release.

Suggested Reading

William DG, Hatch DJ, Howard RF: Codeine phosphate in paediatric medicine, Br J Anaesth 86(3):413–421, 2001.

Fentanyl

Fentanyl is a potent but short-acting synthetic opioid. Its metabolism in infants is age dependent: neonates, and especially preterm infants, metabolize fentanyl more slowly than older infants. Increased intraabdominal pressure (e.g., repaired omphalocele, intestinal obstruction) further slows the clearance of fentanyl by reducing hepatic blood flow. As a sole analgesic agent during anesthesia, 12 to 15 µg/kg is required to prevent cardiovascular responses to surgery in neonates and infants. Supplemental fentanyl may not be required for 60 to 90 minutes. If extubation is planned after surgery, an infusion of 2 to 4 µg/kg/hr may be used to supplement N_2O during balanced anesthesia. Larger doses should not be given to small infants unless they are ventilated or closely monitored postoperatively. The context-sensitive half-life of fentanyl after continuous infusion increases rapidly with the increased duration of the infusion. Rebound of fentanyl blood levels may occur and may cause depression of ventilation; therefore, if large doses have been given, the child must be carefully monitored. Infants older than 3 months of age may be less sensitive to fentanyl-induced ventilatory depression and have been demonstrated to metabolize the drug more rapidly. Bradycardia may occur after use of fentanyl unless it is preceded by a vagal blocking drug (e.g., atropine, pancuronium). Chest wall (muscle) rigidity may occur but occurs infrequently in infants and children.

Infants who receive large doses of fentanyl over a prolonged period may develop tolerance and a significant number may also show signs of dependence. This effect is common in infants who have been treated with a fentanyl infusion for a period of days. Such infants subsequently require escalating doses to prevent responses to stimulation. It may then be appropriate to substitute another anesthetic or analgesic drug. A methadone program may be required to wean the child off opioid dependency. Neonatal abstinence syndrome may occur when fentanyl is withdrawn after continued use for as little as 7 days; it is characterized by crying, hyperactivity, fever, tremors, abdominal distention, poor feeding and sleeping, and—in the extreme case—vomiting and convulsions. These sequelae can be avoided by careful tapering the opioid dose slowly, but may require intervention with methadone.

Remifentanil

Remifentanil, an ultrashort-acting synthetic opioid, represents a new class of opioids that must be administered as a continuous intravenous infusion. It is available as a lyophilized powder and requires reconstitution. The intravenous loading dose is 0.5 to 2.0 µg/kg, and the maintenance dose is 0.05 to 2.0 µg/kg/min. The maintenance dose may be reduced by half if a potent inhaled agent is administered. The kinetics of remifentanil are unique: its elimination half-life, which is 3 to 10 minutes, is independent of both the dose and the duration of administration of the infusion. Its context-sensitive half-life is constant, approximately 4 minutes. Its action is terminated by hydrolysis of an ester bond by ubiquitous tissue esterase enzymes, and is therefore independent of hepatic and renal dysfunction. As an analgesic, the potency of remifentanil is twentyfold to thirtyfold greater than that of alfentanil. The side effects of remifentanil are similar to those of other opioids and include bradycardia, apnea, chest wall rigidity, and vomiting. The rapid offset of the analgesic effect of remifentanil once an infusion is discontinued demands that an alternative analgesic be administered before emergence to prevent severe acute pain. A vagolytic agent may be indicated when remifentanil is given to infants and children. This is the only opioid with a shorter elimination half-life in neonates and infants less than 4 months of age than adults; this may offer a great advantage in instances where an intense but brief opioid effect is desired. This drug should only be administered by an infusion pump, and in neonates and infants is best diluted to 5 µg/ml compared with the usual adult dilution of 50 µg/ml. Remifentanil is a very useful component of a total intravenous anesthetic (TIVA) protocol (see page 141).

Sufentanil

Sufentanil is 10 times more potent than fentanyl and has a smaller elimination half-life. The clearance rate is slower in infants younger than 1 month of age. Sufentanil has been administered in large doses during cardiac surgery in infants, producing cardiovascular stability with minimal depression of ventricular function. Sufentanil in large doses may favorably influence the metabolic and neuroendocrine response to major cardiovascular surgery in infants.

Alfentanil

Alfentanil has a more rapid onset and a shorter duration of action than fentanyl and a greater incidence of vomiting than other opioids. It is less lipid soluble than fentanyl and is highly protein bound. Most of the drug is metabolized in the liver; less than 1% is excreted via the kidney unchanged. Clearance is slower and more variable in young infants, especially preterm infants. Otherwise, in older infants and children, the pharmacokinetics are similar to those in adults. The drug has minimal cardiovascular effects. Alfentanil, 35 µg/kg as a bolus followed by intermittent doses of 10 µg/kg every 10 to 15 minutes, has been suggested as suitable for children. A continuous infusion may be used but in this case remifentanil (see previous discussion) may be the preferred drug. Recovery after alfentanil is reported to be very rapid and complete. However, this is a very potent drug and all children should be closely observed for signs of residual or recurring respiratory depression.

Neuroleptics

Droperidol

Droperidol is a powerful tranquilizer that potentiates sedatives and hypnotics. It has a potent antiemetic effect when administered in small doses. Droperidol was the subject of a "black box" warning by the U.S. Food and Drug Administration after reports of Q-T interval prolongation and torsades de pointes surfaced in adult patients given inappropriately large doses of the drug.

Many anesthesiologists believe that this remains a very useful drug when given in appropriate doses. Droperidol and fentanyl have been given together to produce tranquility and analgesia during procedures performed using local analgesia (neuroleptanalgesia) or to supplement N_2O (neuroleptanesthesia). Neuroleptanalgesia is most useful when the child's cooperation is required during major surgery. The child should be monitored very closely afterward because droperidol potentiates all other depressant drugs and its effects may continue for some hours.

Opioid Antagonists

Provided opioids are carefully administered, it is rare that they need to be antagonized after general anesthesia. Remember that if you completely antagonize the opioid, your patient may experience severe pain.

Naloxone Hydrochloride

Naloxone hydrochloride (Narcan), an *N*-allyl derivative of oxymorphone HCl, antagonizes opioids, but unlike previous agents it has no opioid effects. In addition (unlike *N*-allyl-normorphine or levallorphan), it also antagonizes the opioid effects of pentazocine. Because naloxone selectively reverses opioid effects, it may be useful to identify the class of drugs responsible for an unwitnessed drug overdose. Respiratory depression may be reversed with as little as 0.5 to 1.0 µg/kg, although larger doses (up to 100 µg/kg) may be required. We prefer to give repeated small doses to reverse the respiratory depression without affecting the analgesia. The naloxone dosage should always be titrated slowly until the desired effect is achieved unless apnea has occurred in which case a full dose is indicated. The same cumulative dose that reversed the respiratory depression should also be administered intramuscularly to prevent recrudescence. Naloxone is contraindicated in children who may be opioid dependent.

Benzodiazepine Antagonists

Flumazenil

This reversal agent for the benzodiazepines has a rapid onset of action reaching its full effect within 5 to 10 minutes. A dose of 2 to 20 µg/kg IV may be repeated as required to reverse the sedative/respiratory effects of the benzodiazepine and then repeated IM to prevent recrudescence. Children who receive flumazenil should be observed for a minimum of two hours.

Neuromuscular Blocking Drugs

Neuromuscular blocking drugs are widely used in pediatric anesthesia both to facilitate tracheal intubation and to provide muscle relaxation during controlled ventilation and surgery. These drugs require special attention because their pharmacodynamic effects in infants often differ compared with adults. The neuromuscular junction in infancy has less reserve than that of the adult. Fade occurs at high rates of stimulation. This has led to the suggestion that infants show a myasthenic response and would be sensitive to nondepolarizing relaxants. In fact, to produce a similar degree of block, infants and adults require similar doses of relaxants on a milligram-per-kilogram basis. This may be attributed to the combined effects of a larger volume of distribution plus a greater degree of block for a specific plasma concentration in the infant. It is important to note that although the average doses of nondepolarizing relaxants in infants are similar to those in adults, the variability in dose requirements is much greater. This may be related to the larger number of extrajunctional receptors in the skeletal muscles of infants. It is prudent to monitor the degree of neuromuscular block carefully as a guide to dosage.

Depolarizing Muscle Relaxant

Succinylcholine

Succinylcholine is the only depolarizing relaxant in clinical use. Its onset and offset of action are still more rapid than those of any other relaxant. Succinylcholine is metabolized by pseudocholinesterase of which there are five major (and several minor) alleles: typical (E^u), atypical (E^a), fluoride resistant (E^f), silent gene (E^s), and C_5 variant (or Cynthiana). E^a, E^f, and E^s have reduced pseudocholinesterase activity, with the homozygote genotypes expressing less activity than the heterozygote. The C_5 variant is an ultrarapid metabolizer.

Succinylcholine may be administered by any one of three routes: intravenously, intramuscularly, or intralingually. Intravenous succinylcholine (2 mg/kg) has an onset of action of 20 to 30 seconds and reaches its maximum effect within 40 seconds. Intramuscular administration of succinylcholine (4 to 5 mg/kg) has a slower onset of action compared with the intravenous route. Intralingual or submental succinylcholine has been used for emergencies when other routes are not accessible; we do not recommend this route as puncture of the vascular supply could cause a lingual hematoma. Infants require a relatively higher dose of succinylcholine than adults (2 versus 1 mg/kg, respectively) due to the distribution of the drug throughout the relatively large extracellular fluid compartment. Reduced plasma cholinesterase activity in infants younger than 6 months of age does not significantly affect the drug's clinical duration of action.

Bradycardia occurs commonly after a single dose of intravenous succinylcholine in infants and children. This can be prevented by prior administration of intravenous atropine (0.02 mg/kg) or glycopyrrolate (0.01 mg/kg). Intramuscular succinylcholine (4 to 5 mg/kg) changes the heart rate and rhythm minimally, even in anesthetized children who have not received atropine.

Although myoglobinemia and myoglobinuria occur more commonly after succinylcholine in children than in adults, especially if halothane precedes succinylcholine, the incidence of strong fasciculations and muscle pain is less. Nonetheless, children who are ambulatory should be pretreated with a nondepolarizing relaxant (10% of an intubating dose) to prevent postoperative muscle pain. Serious rhabdomyolysis, severe myoglobinuria, and hyperkalemic cardiac arrest may occur in children with myopathies (including Duchenne muscular dystrophy).

Masseter spasm has been reported in 1% of children who received intravenous succinylcholine after a halothane induction. In such children, the halothane-caffeine contracture test was positive for MH in 50% yielding an apparent incidence of MH of 1:200 (in contrast to the epidemiological evidence for MH in children of 1:15,000 to 1:25,000). There is no satisfactory explanation for this apparent discrepancy. In contrast, masseter spasm is extremely rare after an intravenous induction of anesthesia with thiopental (with atropine) followed by succinylcholine (1:3000). If masseter spasm occurs in this situation, it must be considered a significant warning sign of possible MH. The sequence of thiopental (or propofol), atropine and succinylcholine do not commonly result in masseter spasm and remains the most effective means of securing the airway rapidly. In very rare instances, the masseter spasm is of such severity that a laryngoscope blade cannot be inserted into the mouth and even if it is, the jaw cannot be pried from the maxilla. This condition, also known as the "jaws of steel," is strongly associated with MH and the child should be monitored and investigated accordingly (see Chapter 6, page 197).

Succinylcholine does not decrease the gastric-esophageal barrier pressure. In part, because some muscles of the crura of the diaphragm are not skeletal in origin. Intraocular pressure increases transiently after succinylcholine administration (5 to 10 mm Hg) because of greater tension in the smooth muscles lining the globe of the eye and possible dilation of the choroidal blood vessels. Although succinylcholine has been reported to transiently increase intraocular pressure, studies have indicated that high doses of thiopental attenuate this response. If intraocular pressure is to be measured (i.e., in glaucoma), or if forced duction testing is planned (i.e., in strabismus surgery), it may be best to avoid succinylcholine. If succinylcholine is considered for a child with an open globe injury, the ophthalmologist should be consulted first. Pinpoint punctures of the globe are less likely to lead to extrusion of intraocular contents after succinylcholine than are large (>4 mm) lacerations. Alternatively, high-dose rocuronium (1.2 mg/kg) provides similar intubating conditions in children 45 seconds after administration.

Serum potassium levels increase after succinylcholine administration in children with burns beyond the first 24 hours, crush injury, major neurologic diseases (upper and lower motor neuron lesions), chronically bedridden, and renal failure. These increases in K^+ may result in ventricular tachycardia. Intravenous calcium and other measures to treat hyperkalemia and restore cardiac rhythm and output must be initiated immediately.

Nondepolarizing Neuromuscular Blocking Agents—Intermediate Duration

Vecuronium

Vecuronium (lyophilized powder), a steroidal relaxant, is an intermediate-acting nondepolarizing neuromuscular blocking agent. Its duration of action in children is 35 to 45 minutes but in neonates, its duration is much greater, 70 minutes or more. The ED_{95} for vecuronium is: infants, 47 μg/kg; children 2 to 10 years old, 81 μg/kg; and adolescents, 55 μg/kg. It is a highly specific drug, devoid of cardiovascular effects and histamine release. The duration of action of vecuronium increases in the presence of some forms of liver disease or impaired renal function. Because vecuronium has no vagal blocking effect, bradycardia may occur if vagotonic drugs (e.g., fentanyl, halothane) are coadministered; atropine may be required. Vecuronium may also be administered as an infusion. Infants require a considerably smaller infusion rate, 60 μg/kg/hr, than older children, 150 μg/kg/hr.

Rocuronium

Rocuronium, a steroid-based relaxant, differs from vecuronium in its potency (one sixth as potent as vecuronium) and in its availability as a solution that is stable at room temperature. The onset of block is more rapid than after vecuronium and is dose dependent; larger doses speed its onset of action. The intubating dose is 0.6 mg/kg, with a dose of 1.2 mg/kg recommended for a rapid-sequence induction. With greater doses, a prolonged duration of effect must be anticipated. It is devoid of cardiovascular and histamine effects. Recovery after 1.2 mg/kg requires about 75 minutes, although this dose may be antagonized earlier. Elimination is unchanged in renal failure but may be prolonged by up to 100% in hepatic failure. Low dose rocuronium (0.3 mg/kg) provides satisfactory intubating conditions after 3 minutes and can usually be antagonized within 15 to 20 minutes. It should be noted that coadministration of thiopentone and rocuronium precipitates thiopentone blocking the IV. Rocuronium may also be administered as a continuous infusion (10 μg/kg/min and adjusted up or down by 2 to 3 μg/kg/min according to the train-of-four response). Rocuronium may cause pain on injection if the child is not adequately anesthetized.

Atracurium

Atracurium, a benzylisoquinolonium, is a nondepolarizing neuromuscular blocking agent with an intermediate duration of action (~30 minutes). It is a mixture of 10 stereoisomers that vary in potency and side effects. It is used infrequently now, having been replaced by *cis*-atracurium (see later discussion). Atracurium degrades spontaneously at physiologic pH to inactive compounds (Hofmann elimination) and hence has a predictable rate of elimination that is unaffected by the presence of severe hepatic or renal disease. Its brief duration of action and constant rate of metabolism made this drug ideal for administration by continuous infusion. In children, an initial bolus of 0.3 mg/kg followed by an infusion of 6 mg/kg/hr (and the adjusted up or down by 1 to 2 µg/kg/min according to the train-of-four response) provides satisfactory relaxation. Slightly larger doses are required if opioids are substituted for inhaled agents. Atracurium usually has little effect on the cardiovascular system. It does release histamine, especially if large doses are given rapidly, and should not be given to children with asthma. Bronchospasm has been described after use in adults and children. A rash is common, but significant hypotension is uncommon. Rarely, precipitous and severe hypotension has occurred after atracurium, especially when it has been given in a large dose (more than 0.4 mg/kg) and preceded by thiopental. Anaphylaxis was reported in an infant after induction with thiopental and paralysis with atracurium.

Cis-atracurium

Cis-atracurium is 1 of the 10 stereoisomers of atracurium besylate. It was isolated and purified because it conferred the most stable hemodynamics and least histamine release of the isomers; it has now largely supplanted atracurium in clinical practice. It has a relatively slow onset of action. The dose for tracheal intubation is 0.15 to 0.2 mg/kg, which yields a duration of action of approximately 35 minutes. Cis-atracurium may also be administered by infusion at a dose of 1.5 µg/kg/min. Termination of its action is similar to atracurium, via Hofmann elimination and ester hydrolysis. The duration of action of cis-atracurium is unaffected by renal or hepatic failure; therefore it is a drug of choice in such situations and in neonates with immature renal and hepatic function.

Prolonged Duration Relaxants

Pancuronium

Pancuronium is the only nondepolarizing relaxant with a prolonged duration of action. An initial dose of 0.1 mg/kg permits intubation in about 2 minutes. Supplementary doses should be given carefully, using a nerve stimulator for guidance; each dose should be only 10% to 20% of the initial paralyzing dose. Pancuronium has a vagolytic effect and causes an increase in heart rate and blood pressure, particularly when given as a rapid intravenous bolus. These effects are more pronounced in younger patients. In preterm infants, pancuronium causes a sustained tachycardia and hypertension and increased plasma epinephrine level. In practice, if pancuronium is combined with fentanyl, their effects on heart rate offset one another resulting in a relatively stable hemodynamic situation. Pancuronium causes little histamine release, and is the preferred relaxant for prolonged surgery in children with asthma.

Pancuronium is excreted principally via the kidney and should not be given to children whose renal function is impaired, as prolonged neuromuscular block may occur.

Antagonism of Neuromuscular Blockade

Nondepolarizing neuromuscular blocking agents should always be antagonized unless the child has completely recovered normal neuromuscular function as documented with a blockade monitor. Antagonism may not be fully effective in children who are hypothermic (less than 35 °C); therefore controlled ventilation is often continued until they are rewarmed. Rarely, antibiotics potentiate the neuromuscular blocking drugs in infants or children to the extent that they cannot be antagonized. This possibility must be considered, especially in those receiving aminoglycoside derivatives (e.g., neomycin, gentamicin, tobramycin).

The adequacy of antagonism of relaxants may be difficult to judge, especially in infants. The train-of-four should demonstrate four equal contractions. Muscle tone can be examined and is often best judged in neonates and infants by flexion of the elbows and hips. The ability to generate a negative inspiratory pressure of 25 cm H_2O has also been suggested as a useful index. When any doubt whatsoever exists about the adequacy of the antagonism, controlled ventilation should continue and recovery of neuromuscular function should be reevaluated periodically. Antagonism of neuromuscular blockade is recommended for all neonates and infants below 2 years of age.

Commonly used regimens to antagonize the nondepolarizing muscle relaxants in infants and children are as follows:

1. Neostigmine (0.05 mg/kg) mixed with atropine (0.02 to 0.025 mg/kg) is most effective and results in few and insignificant cardiac arrhythmias even in those with congenital heart disease. Glycopyrrolate does not have any advantage over atropine during antagonism and may not prevent neostigmine-induced bradycardia.
2. Edrophonium (1 mg/kg) after atropine (20 µg/kg) may be used. Edrophonium has a more rapid onset of action than neostigmine, and its vagotonic action appears early. These findings have led to the practice of administering atropine before the edrophonium.
3. Sugammadex is a cyclodextrin that has been developed to irreversibly trap rocuronium and eliminate it. It has been approved to reverse rocuronium in adults in Europe but not in the United States. Sugammadex can reverse large doses of rocuronium within 3 minutes in adults, although data in children are currently lacking.

Nonsteroidal Antiinflammatory Drugs

Acetaminophen

Acetaminophen is an analgesic and antipyretic drug without antiinflammatory actions, but is commonly grouped with the NSAIDs. It is metabolized well by infants and children of all ages. It is useful as an analgesic for mild pain and is also useful as an opioid-sparing adjunct for more severe pain. It is usually given in doses of 10 to 15 mg/kg PO q 4 to 6 hours. If given rectally, a loading dose of 35 to 45 mg/kg is recommended followed by 20 mg/kg PR q6h. The time to peak effect after oral administration is 10 to 20 minutes and after rectal administration is 60 to 180 minutes. The total daily dose should not exceed 100 mg/kg. *Beware: hepatic failure may occur with overdose and is a particular risk in the seriously ill debilitated child.*

Proparacetamol is a water-soluble parenteral prodrug formulation of acetaminophen that is available in Europe and many other countries outside of North America. Rapid hydrolysis by nonspecific esterases yields paracetamol within 10 to 30 minutes of IV administration. The pharmacokinetics are independent of age (beyond neonates) and the drug should be administered on a weight basis. In neonates, clearance is markedly diminished but increases with age. A dose of 30 mg/kg IV (15 mg/kg acetaminophen equivalent) provides adequate relief for mild to moderate pain in children. In adults and volunteers, proparacetamol has been shown to have a morphine-sparing action and no ceiling effect (in contrast to oral paracetamol).

Suggested Reading

Allegaert K, Van der Marel CD, Debeer A, et al: Pharmacokinetics of single dose intravenous propacetamol in neonates: effect of gestational age, Arch Dis Child Fetal Neonatal Ed 89:F25–F28, 2004.

Ibuprofen

Ibuprofen (4 to 10 mg/kg PO q6h max. 40 mg/kg/day) reduces postoperative morphine requirements and improves pain relief in children. Ibuprofen may be a useful alternative to acetaminophen with codeine after tonsillectomy in small children.

Suggested Reading

Charles CS, Matt BH, Hamilton MM, et al: A comparison of ibuprofen versus acetaminophen with codeine in the young tonsillectomy patient, Otolaryngol Head Neck Surg 117:76–82, 1997.

Diclofenac

Diclofenac is a nonsteroidal antiinflammatory agent that is available in oral (25 to 75 mg tablets) and rectal formulations (50 or 100 mg suppositories). Outside of North America, rectal formulations as small as 12.5 mg per suppository are available for use in children. Absorption and bioavailability after rectal administration is greater than after oral administration. Pediatric dosing for oral and rectal diclofenac is 1 mg/kg every 8 hours. It provides similar analgesia to proparacetamol. Rectal diclofenac is widely used in Europe for children after minor superficial surgery. Its effect on platelet activity is intermediate between placebo and ketorolac.

Ketorolac

Ketorolac is a nonsteroidal analgesic racemic mixture that is available for parenteral use either intramuscularly or intravenously. It is considered a moderately potent analgesic that is devoid of respiratory depression, vomiting, sedation, and urinary retention effects. In clinical trials ketorolac has been shown to be effective and opioid-sparing. The usual dose for children more than 6 months and less than 50 kg is 0.5 mg/kg IV up to 15 mg/dose, repeated every 6 hours up to a maximum 24-hour dose of 60 mg. The dose for children greater than 50 kg is 0.5 mg/kg IV up to 30 mg/dose or 120 mg/24 hours. The elimination half-life of ketorolac in children is similar to that in adults: approximately 4 hours.

Ketorolac should be used only for brief periods (i.e., several days at a time) because of the risk of nephrotoxicity. Ketorolac should be administered with caution to children with impaired renal or hepatic function. Like most nonsteroidal antiinflammatory drugs (NSAIDs), ketorolac reversibly inhibits platelet function and may cause increased bleeding, especially if it is administered before or early in the surgical procedure. Postoperatively, ketorolac does not appear to increase bleeding, although most clinicians avoid it for surgeries where bleeding may be a problem (adenotonsillectomy, cleft palate, and so forth). There are limited data in animal studies that suggest ketorolac may impair bone healing; prompting some orthopedic surgeons to avoid this agent.

4 Techniques and Procedures

ROUTINE PREPARATION FOR SURGERY

Preoperative Assessment

A careful assessment of the child must be made at the time of the pre-operative visit. Although many children are healthy, some have diseases with significant implications for the anesthesiologist. A thorough history is obtained from the child's chart and the parents. Review the systems and search for special problems that may complicate anesthesia (Table 4-1). When a significant history is obtained, it is important to establish the current status of the disease; this may require consultation with the pediatrician, the surgeon or radiologist, and other physicians. Although most children take no medications, some may be taking medications that have implications for management during the perioperative period. Document all medications, neutraceuticals, and drug allergies. Common medications for children and their significance to anesthetic management are detailed in Table 4-2; (**N.B.** Some herbal preparations may have anesthetic implications [Table 4-3]). Throughout the preoperative interview, strive to gain the confidence of the child and the parents; always invite questions from both the parents and the child so as to help establish rapport and confidence.

Preoperative Feeding Orders

Infants and children should not be subjected to prolonged preoperative fasting. Excessive fluid restriction rapidly leads to dehydration and hypovolemia because of their high metabolic rate; hypotension in infants during induction of anesthesia has been shown to be directly related to the duration of fasting. In addition, excessive fasting may precipitate hypoglycemia and/or metabolic acidosis, particularly in young infants. Studies have shown that healthy children may safely be given unlimited clear fluids up to 2 hours before induction of general anesthesia. The volume and acidity of the gastric contents are not increased when this regimen is used. Indeed, clear fluids 2 hours before anesthesia may reduce gastric contents at induction, possibly by stimulating gastric emptying. Furthermore, this practice reduces hunger and thirst and makes for a happier child! Fasting guidelines are presented in the Table 4-4.

Children who are scheduled for afternoon surgery may have a light breakfast (dry toast and black tea) early in the morning. These rules must, of course, be modified in special cases (e.g., for diabetics). Children who require emergency surgery, those with gastrointestinal disease, and any others at increased risk for vomiting during induction should receive

TABLE 4-1 Review of the Medical History—Possible Implications for Anesthesia

Systems	History	Concerns for the Anesthesiologist
Central nervous system	Seizures	Adequacy of seizure medication, recent control of convulsions. Phenytoin increases nondepolarizing relaxant and fentanyl requirements, produces gingival hyperplasia and bleeding, and may cause hepatic dysfunction. Ketamine, enflurane, and methohexital are relatively contraindicated.
	Hydrocephalus	Possible raised intracranial pressure. Repeated anesthesias. Possible need for prophylactic antibiotics to prevent shunt infection.
	Head injury	Possible raised intracranial pressure. Current status. Possible danger of hyperkalemia with succinylcholine.
	Cerebral tumor	Possible raised intracranial pressure, vomiting, change in electrolyte status. Chemotherapeutic agents and possible drug interactions.
	Cerebral palsy	Nutritional status, presence of chronic infections. Possible history of chronic aspiration and difficulties with positioning. Intelligence may be normal—careful psychological preparation needed.
	Down syndrome	Optimal cooperation at induction may be a problem. (Possibly get help from parent.) Airway (large tongue, subglottic stenosis). Heart disease. Evidence of joint hypermobility and indications of atlantoaxial instability.
	Neuromuscular disease	Difficulty positioning. Repeated surgery—careful psychological preparation needed.
	Meningomyelocele	Associated hydrocephalus. History suggesting latex allergy. Renal infections. Impaired renal function.
Cardiovascular system	Heart murmur	Innocent murmur vs. significant lesion. Need for prophylactic antibiotics. Risk of paradoxic embolism. Hemoconcentration—avoid fluid restriction; risk of hyperviscosity. Coagulopathy secondary to hyperviscosity; check coagulogram. Reduced response to hypoxemia—caution with premedication.

	Cyanosis	Evidence of congestive cardiac failure. History of digoxin and/or diuretic therapy. Digoxin level. Electrolyte levels.
	Dyspnea, tachypnea	Previous heart surgery
	Sweating	Need for prophylactic antibiotics. Cardiac conduction defects. Pacemaker. History of arrhythmias.
	Hypertension	Renal disease, coarctation of the aorta, endocrine disease.
Respiratory system	Prematurity	Risk of perioperative apnea.
	Respiratory distress syndrome	Present postconceptual age, gestational age at birth. Anemia. History of apnea, residual chronic respiratory disease, impaired gas exchange. History of prolonged ventilation, residual subglottic stenosis.
	Recent upper respiratory tract infection	Evidence of acute infection. Pyrexia. Lower respiratory tract infection. Reactive airways prone to secondary infection. Increased risk of laryngospasm, bronchospasm and oxygen desaturation.
	Bronchiolitis	Reactive airways, evidence of bronchospasm.
	Croup	Possible subglottic stenosis. Avoid intubation, use LMA.
	Asthma	Reactive airways. Current status. Theophylline therapy (blood level). β-Agonist drug therapy, history of corticosteroid therapy (prescription supplements). Develop a plan to ensure optimal status preoperatively.
	Cystic fibrosis	Present pulmonary function. Any acute infection? Can condition be improved? Can regional analgesia be used? Present drug therapy. Nutritional status. Emotional status.
Gastrointestinal system	Gastroesophageal reflux	Evidence of aspiration pneumonia. Reactive airways and bronchospasm. Recent food intake, risk of regurgitation, and need for antacid and H_2-blockers. Evidence predicting difficult intubation.
	Vomiting	Nutritional and hydration status. Electrolyte values. Urine output. Immediate full stomach danger.
	Diarrhea	Nutritional, fluid, and electrolyte status. Risk of hypoglycemia and hypovolemia.

Continued

TABLE 4–1 Review of the Medical History—Possible Implications for Anesthesia—Cont'd

Systems	History	Concerns for the Anesthesiologist
	Liver disease	Drug metabolism. Increased requirements for nondepolarizing relaxants
Genitourinary system	Renal failure	Anemia and coagulopathy, electrolyte abnormality, volume status. Acid-base status. Hypertension, pericardial effusion and incipient congestive cardiac failure. Date of last dialysis. History of infection? Impaired immunity? Psychological status.
	Bladder surgery	Is history suggestive of latex allergy?
	Bladder Extrophy	Is history suggestive of latex allergy?
Endocrine system	Diabetes mellitus	Current status and therapy. Plans for perioperative management. Need for planning with surgeon and endocrinologist.
	Thyroid disease	Current status and medication? Euthyroid? Enlarged thyroid effect on the airway.
	Pituitary disease	Intracranial pressure? Adrenal insufficiency? Thyroid function? Diabetes insipidus?
	Adrenal disease	Need for corticosteroid therapy? Volume and electrolyte status.
Hematopoietic system	Anemia	What is cause? Possible medical therapy. Urgency of surgery. Will anemia affect the course of anesthesia? Is transfusion indicated?
	Bruising or bleeding	Is coagulopathy present? Are further tests required? Preoperative therapy? Order products.
	Sickle cell disease	Trait or disease? Are other abnormal hemoglobins present (Hb electrophoresis results)? Is preoperative preparation required?
Muscular system	Muscular dystrophy	Risk of hyperkalemia with succinylcholine. Avoid nondepolarizing relaxants if possible. Ventilatory reserve? Cardiac function? Will postoperative ICU admission be necessary?
Immune system and allergy	Latex allergy	Allergy to bananas, eggplant, passion fruit, and other fruits/vegetables Possibility of concurrent latex allergy (see page 205 for further details)

TABLE 4-2 Concurrent Medication—Possible Implications for Anesthesia

Drug	Implications for Anesthesia
Analgesic, antiinflammatory Acetylsalicylic acid (ASA, aspirin)	Prolonged bleeding time due to platelet inactivation; check bleeding time if ASA given within 10 days.
Nonsteroidal antiinflammatory drugs (NSAIDs; e.g., ibuprofen, ketorolac)	Affect platelet aggregation and prolong bleeding time. Effect of antihypertensive agents may be decreased. Ketorolac decreases diuretic effect of furosemide
Antibiotics	Many of the "mycins" may potentiate neuromuscular blockade. Monitor neuromuscular block, check reversal carefully.
Aminoglycosides	May potentiate succinylcholine and nondepolarizing relaxant drugs. Renal toxicity.
Clindamycin	Cardiac depression when given rapidly. May potentiate nondepolarizing relaxant drugs.
Erythromycin	May prolong the effect of alfentanil and midazolam. Decreases theophylline clearance rates. Potentiates anticoagulant effect of warfarin.
Gentamicin	May prolong the effect of succinylcholine. Potentiates nondepolarizing relaxant drugs.
Vancomycin	Potentiates nondepolarizing relaxant drugs. Rapid administration (<1 hr) may cause "red man syndrome" with severe cardiovascular collapse.
Anticancer agents	All may cause blood dyscrasia, coagulopathy, anorexia, nausea, stomatitis, and reduced resistance to infection.
Doxorubicin (Adriamycin)	Cardiotoxic, may cause arrhythmias.
Daunorubicin (Cerubidine)	Severe cardiac depression with halothane, especially likely when cumulative dose exceeds 250 mg/m^2 (or 150 mg/m^2 plus radiation).

Continued

TABLE 4-2   Concurrent Medication—Possible Implications for Anesthesia—Cont'd

Drug	Implications for Anesthesia
Bleomycin	Pulmonary fibrosis—may be exacerbated by excess oxygen. Limit carefully.
Busulfan	Inhibits plasma cholinesterases. May prolong the effect of succinylcholine.
Cyclophosphamide	Inhibit plasma cholinesterases; prolonged effect of succinylcholine or mivacurium.
Anticonvulsants Phenytoin	May cause blood dyscrasia, hypotension, bradycardia, arrhythmia.
Mephenytoin	May increase requirements for nondepolarizing relaxants and may cause peripheral neuropathy.
Valproic acid	May cause hypotonia. Hepatotoxic.
Antihypertensive drugs	Severe hypotension may occur with potent anesthetics, especially if dehydrated.
Captopril	Hyperkalemia with potassium-sparing diuretics (spironolactone). Indomethacin reduces antihypertensive effect.
Clonidine	Must not be abruptly withdrawn—severe hypertension may result. Interaction with β-blockers—bradycardia, hypotension.
Hydralazine (Apresoline)	May cause systemic lupus erythematosus (SLE)-type syndrome. Decreases tachycardia with atropine.
Labetalol	Cimetidine may potentiate labetalol action.
Prazosin (Minipress)	May potentiate effects of ketamine. Diuretics potentiate antihypertensive effect
Antiviral agent Acyclovir	Nephrotoxic, bone marrow depression.
β-Agonist agents (e.g., albuterol, Alupent)	May cause tachycardia, hypertension, arrhythmia. Albuterol has increased effect with tricyclic antidepressants or monoamine oxidase inhibitors. Blocked by β-blocking drugs.

Continued

TABLE 4-2   Concurrent Medication—Possible Implications for Anesthesia—Cont'd

Drug	Implications for Anesthesia
β-Blocking drugs	May cause bronchospasm, block effects of albuterol. Potentiate cardiac depression caused by halothane. May cause bradycardia with anticholinesterase drugs (e.g., neostigmine) and hypoglycemia.
Calcium channel blockers	Potentiate nondepolarizing relaxant drugs. Severe bradycardia or heart block with β-blocking drugs.
Verapamil, nifedipine	May interact with β-blockers to cause severe cardiac depression.
Corticosteroid preparations	Chronic therapy may lead to depression of the hypothalamic pituitary axis; severe collapse may occur perioperatively. Supplemental steroid therapy should be ordered preoperatively.
Digoxin	May potentiate bupivacaine toxicity. Hypokalemia, if induced (e.g., by hyperventilation), predisposes to arrhythmias.
Diuretics	All may result in electrolyte disturbances.
Acetazolamide (Diamox)	Produces hyperchloremic metabolic acidosis.
Furosemide	Hypokalemia, if present, may prolong action and delay reversal of relaxant drugs.
Ophthalmic topical drugs Echothiophate (anticholinesterase)	Inhibits plasma cholinesterases. Prolonged apnea with succinylcholine.
Phenylephrine	May cause tachycardia and hypertension.
Timolol (β-blocker)	May exacerbate asthma.
Theophylline	Severe arrhythmias may occur with halothane; check blood level

TABLE 4-3 Some Herbal Preparations and Their Anesthesia Implications

Herbal Preparation	Reason for Use	Anesthesia Implication
Echinacea	URI prophylaxis	Increased sedation with midazolam. Decreased metabolism of phenobarbital, phenytoin, rifampin. Increases liver damage with hepatotoxic agents. Immunosuppression with long-term use.
St John's wort	Anxiety, depression, sleep problems, etc.	Cardiovascular collapse, delayed awakening due to effect on GABA neurotransmitter. Severe interactions with antidepressants. Induces CYP3A4 system leading to increased dose requirements of many drugs (including midazolam).
Gingko	Improves memory and concentration	Increased surgical bleeding due to antiplatelet effects. Concurrent use of NSAIDs not recommended. Decreases effect of anticonvulsants.
Garlic	Cardiac health	Increased surgical bleeding. Augments ASA, warfarin, and heparin.
Ginseng	General health	Hypoglycemic effects in diabetics. Antiplatelet effects and bleeding. Hypertension, headaches, and vomiting.
Aloe	Skin problems	Allergic skin reactions. GI constipation bleeding, renal damage with oral use.

TABLE 4-4 Preoperative Fasting Intervals

	Fasting Interval	Comments
Clear fluids	2 hr	Water, ginger-ale, apple juice; any particle-free fluids
Breast milk	4 hr	
Formula/cow's milk	6 hr	Also dry toast, black tea
Solids	8 hr	

N.B: Chewing gum should be expectorated; if swallowed the anesthetic should be delayed 8 hours.

intravenous fluids and a rapid sequence induction. When evaluating injured children, the interval between last food or fluid and the injury is the best predictor of the likely stomach contents. Children for whom any period of fluid deprivation might pose a risk (e.g., those with cyanotic heart disease) should have an intravenous infusion established at the commencement of any prolonged period of restricted oral intake.

Prophylaxis Against Hemorrhage for Infants

Ensure that the neonate undergoing surgery has been given vitamin K_1 to prevent Vitamin K deficiency bleeding (VKDB). Aqueous vitamin K_1 (1 mg IM or IV) corrects the deficiency within a few hours and therefore should be given as early as possible. Late onset VKDB may occur in breast-fed infants who were never given vitamin K; check the history.

Basic Laboratory Tests

Preoperative laboratory tests are considered unnecessary for most children; however, in some regions, these tests are legislated requirements. Preoperative urinalysis has not been found useful in detecting significant diseases or in routine screening of children. However, because a history is unreliable, urine (or blood) for pregnancy testing has become mandatory in many centers for all females who have reached menses. Hemoglobin (Hb) determination is likewise of little value in otherwise healthy children. Mild degrees of anemia have not been shown to increase the risk of anesthesia and do not alter the anesthesia technique selected. Most authorities now recommend that these tests may be omitted in healthy children undergoing minor surgery. All small infants, especially those who were born preterm, should have a preoperative Hb determination to exclude anemia, which is more common in such infants and may increase the risk of complications. Older children with systemic diseases, those with a history of anemia, and those who may lose significant amounts of blood intraoperatively should also have a preoperative Hb determination. A sickle cell test is now performed routinely in neonates immediately after birth in many regions. Older infants and children whose sickle status is unknown should be tested with a Sickledex and if that is positive, a hemoglobin electrophoresis should be performed.

Premedication

Drugs may be given preoperatively to block unwanted autonomic reflex (vagal) responses, produce preoperative sedation and tranquility, facilitate separation from parents if necessary, and smooth the induction of anesthesia.

Topical Local Anesthetics

For topical local anesthetics, see Appendix 3, page 634.

Vagal Blocking Drugs

Vagal blocking drugs (atropine, hyoscine, glycopyrrolate) are no longer routinely given to children preoperatively; however, they may be useful to decrease secretions for specific procedures such as bronchoscopy, to smooth induction in the child with a suspected difficult airway or to reduce secretions in neurologically impaired children.

Brisk vagal responses may occur during anesthesia in infants and children. Atropine should immediately be available for injection (preferably IV) should it become necessary. Serious bradycardia may occur in young children and may lead to significant hypotension or more dangerous arrhythmias. This can result from instrumentation of the airway, manipulation of the eye, traction of the peritoneum, or administration of cholinergic drugs (i.e., halothane, succinylcholine). If bradycardia occurs, it must be treated promptly; ventilate with 100% oxygen, withdraw the precipitating stimulus, and give intravenous atropine.

Atropine is the preferred anticholinergic in children. It is more effective in blocking the cardiac vagus nerve and causes less drying of secretions than hyoscine or glycopyrrolate. Respiratory tract secretions, in fact, are not a serious problem with current inhalational anesthetics.

Children require larger doses of atropine than adults to achieve the same effect on the heart rate. If indicated, atropine (0.02 mg/kg; maximum, 0.6 mg) may be given IV at induction. This is the preferred route of administration since it ensures effective drug action and spares the child a painful intramuscular injection and a preoperative dry mouth. If successful venipuncture is in doubt, the same dose of atropine may be given orally 90 minutes or IM 30 minutes preoperatively to ensure a peak effect at the time of induction. Atropine may also be given per rectum if a rectal barbiturate is used for induction of anesthesia. In an emergency, the usual dose of atropine diluted in 2 ml of saline is rapidly effective by the intratracheal route.

Infants with established bradycardia have a longer onset time for the chronotropic effect of intravenous atropine because of their reduced cardiac output. Therefore, if bradycardia is attributed to a vagal response, atropine should be given as early as possible. *A very common cause for intraoperative bradycardia in infants or children is hypoxia, so the first treatment for any unexpected bradycardia is ventilation with 100% oxygen.*

Contraindications to the use of atropine are few in the pediatric age group; infants and children tolerate tachycardia much better than bradycardia. Children with heart disease who might tolerate tachycardia poorly (e.g., aortic stenosis or cardiomyopathy) require special attention; if bradycardia develops; small incremental doses of atropine should be given until the desired heart rate is reached. Studies have failed to confirm a reputed increased sensitivity of children with Down syndrome to atropine and as such they should be given the usual doses if indicated.

True allergy to atropine is extremely rare (if it exists), but it is common for parents to state that their child is "allergic" to atropine. This claim has usually been prompted by the appearance of a rash after a previous atropine administration. This erythematous rash commonly involves the upper part of the body and is thought to be caused by histamine release.

Sedatives and Tranquilizers

There is a voluminous literature and many widely divergent opinions concerning the use of sedative premedications for children (Table 4-5). Sedatives, opioids, or hypnotics may not ensure calm cooperation at the

TABLE 4-5   Premedications and Route of Delivery

	Midazolam (mg/kg)	Ketamine (mg/kg)	Clonidine (µg/kg)	Dexmedetomidine (µg/kg)
Intravenous	0.05–0.15	1–2		
Intramuscular	0.1–0.2	2–10		
Oral	0.25–0.75	3–6	4	2.6
Nasal	0.1–0.2	2–4	4	1
Rectal	0.75–1.0	6–10		
See Chapter 3 for further discussion of medications.				

time of induction, but they may be associated with postoperative respiratory depression, slowed emergence, delirium, and vomiting.

The oral route has become most popular for administering premedication to healthy children. Midazolam is the most widely prescribed sedative premedication for children. Given orally, it is effective in calming the child, easing separation from parents, and smoothing induction of anesthesia. Recently, oral clonidine was reported to produce good preoperative tranquility, reduce anesthetic drug requirements and smooth emergence; however, it requires a 90 minute onset time and if larger doses are used, may cause postoperative sedation.

Midazolam. Midazolam is a water-soluble benzodiazepine with a shorter duration of action than diazepam. It may be given orally, nasally, rectally, or intravenously. For healthy infants and children up to 6 years of age, the oral route is preferred; a dose of 0.5 to 0.75 mg/kg produces sedation and tranquility in greater than 95% of children within 10 to 15 minutes, after which time its effects start to wane. Older children (>6 years) require smaller mg/kg doses (0.3 to 0.4 mg/kg, maximum dose of 20 mg) than children less than 6 years of age. In infants, midazolam may be applied sublingually with a medicine dropper; this technique ensures rapid oral transmucosal absorption. However, children with OSA may be at risk; 3% of children with OSA who received oral midazolam desaturated. Children with confirmed OSA should be premedicated with great caution and observed closely.

Oral midazolam produces sedation and tranquility with an approximate 50% incidence of antegrade amnesia, does not significantly affect the volume or acidity of gastric fluid, but does improve cooperation on separation from parents and during induction. Recovery is not delayed after surgeries lasting 1 hour, but after a brief procedure, early recovery may be delayed. Some children given midazolam are more restless during emergence after a brief procedure possibly because of paradoxical excitation.

There is some evidence that effective midazolam premedication reduces the incidence of emergence agitation after sevoflurane administration and also adverse behavioral outcomes after hospitalization; however, it is also suggested that some children have an increased incidence of bad dreams.

Intranasal midazolam (0.2 mg/kg) is effective particularly in the uncooperative child who will not swallow an oral premedication, although giving it by this route is unpleasant and usually makes the child cry. As a result, it is not recommended. Rectal midazolam (0.3 to 1 mg/kg) may be useful for small infants who cannot take the drug orally, but the onset of sedation is less predictable. Children with established intravenous access may be given midazolam 0.05 to 0.1 mg/kg IV immediately before arrival in the operating room for a rapid calming effect. It should be noted that the peak brain effect after IV administration is slower than that of diazepam occurring at approximately 5 minutes vs. approximately 1.5 minutes for diazepam.

Lorazepam. Lorazepam is very useful for adolescents greater than 12 years of age. In an oral dose of 1 to 2 mg, it produces good anxiolysis with a significant degree of amnesia. There is insufficient data to recommend its use in children less than 12 years of age.

Ketamine. Ketamine may be given orally in doses of up to 6 mg/kg but must be accompanied by oral atropine if excessive secretions are to be avoided. The combination of oral midazolam (0.3 to 0.5 mg/kg) and oral ketamine (3 to 5 mg/kg) produces very effective sedation for the more disturbed child. If this combination is used, the child should be closely observed as the drugs become effective. The combination should not be used when heavy sedation might be dangerous (e.g., in the child with a difficult airway). Immediate postoperative emergence agitation has been reported in a 12-year-old given 6 mg/kg oral ketamine after surgery that lasted less than 1 hour.

Clonidine. Clonidine 4 µg/kg may be used as a premedication, but given orally requires a 90 minute onset time, much greater than oral midazolam (10 to 15 minutes). It reduces anesthesia requirements and smoothes emergence, prevents agitation after sevoflurane and enhances analgesia. In addition, clonidine diminishes cardiovascular responses to endotracheal intubation and facilitates planned induced hypotension. Clonidine may result in unwanted postoperative sedation and this may be a disadvantage in the outpatient.

Dexmedetomidine. Intranasal dexmedetomidine (1.0 µg/kg) has been reported to be effective as a premedicant in children when given 60 minutes before separation from parents. Neither pain nor discomfort was reported. Neurotoxicity studies of dexmedetomidine have not been forthcoming; because it is unclear whether dexmedetomidine may cause nerve damage, this unapproved route of administration should be viewed with caution.

Opioids

Opioids are rarely used as premedications in children unless pain is present. Opioids have traditionally been given intramuscularly, which children find unpleasant. Dizziness, nausea, and vomiting are common after their use. Fentanyl in the form of an Oralet (lozenge) is available as a premedication in some countries. This formulation takes advantage of the rapid effect that may be obtained by oral transmucosal absorption of the drug. The fentanyl Oralet produces good sedation together with analgesia that complements the anesthesia regimen and may extend into the postoperative period. Provided the total dose administered is 15 µg/kg, significant respiratory depression is unlikely, but the child should be continuously monitored with pulse oximetry. As with all opioids, fentanyl may increase the incidence of nausea and/or vomiting.

Special Considerations

1. Neurosurgical patients who may have increased ICP should not receive any sedative premedication.
2. Children with a suspected difficult airway or OSA should be sedated with caution because it could lead to respiratory depression or airway obstruction.
3. Atropine should not be given intramuscularly to children with a fever because it may exacerbate the fever by abolishing sweating. If needed, it may be given intravenously at the time of induction.
4. Some children undergoing correction of strabismus are assessed by the ophthalmologist immediately before the operation and should not be premedicated with atropine. They may receive atropine (0.02 mg/kg intravenously) at induction to block the oculocardiac reflex.

MANAGEMENT OF THE AIRWAY

Mask Anesthesia

1. During mask anesthesia, always have age and size appropriate equipment for endotracheal intubation immediately at hand:
   a. A selection of suitably sized tracheal tubes with connectors in place (Table 4-6)
   b. Two properly functioning laryngoscope handles with several suitable blades
   c. Labeled syringes containing atropine, succinylcholine, and induction agent (propofol, thiopental, ketamine, etomidate)
2. Select a mask that fits the contours of the child's face and minimizes the dead space if possible. The Rendell Baker mask is ideal for infants

TABLE 4-6   Approximate Diameter of Pediatric
Endotracheal Tubes* and Insertion Depth

Age of Child (yr)	Internal Diameter (ID) (mm)[†]	Approximate depth of insertion (cm) to mid-trachea* from: Teeth	Nares
Premature	2.5 (for infants <1500 g) to 3.0 (for infants >1500 g)	6-9	8-11
Neonate	3.5	9-10	12
1	4.0	11	13
2	4.5	12	14
4	5.0	14	16
6	5.5	15	17
8	6.0	16	18
10	6.5	17	19
12	7.0	18	20
14	7.5	19	21
16	8.0	20	22

* See also page 97.
[†] Formula: (age of child (≥2 yr) in years ÷ 4) + 4.0 = size of tube ID in millimeters. The tube diameters listed are given only as a guide. Always prepare a selection of tubes, and use the one with the best fit (see text).

and small children; however, the anesthesiologist may find it easier to achieve a good seal with a cushion-type mask.

3. The relatively large tongue in infants and adenoid or tonsillar hypertrophy in older children may cause airway obstruction. If obstruction occurs, insert an oropharyngeal or nasopharyngeal airway of suitable size. Alternatively, sublux the temporomandibular joint by applying digital pressure to the apex of the ascending rami (behind the pinna) directing the force towards the frontal hairline. This maneuver translocates the mandible anteriorly and rotates the joint, thereby lifting the tongue and intraoral tissues off the posterior pharyngeal wall and opens the airway and the mouth.

4. Infants have soft laryngeal cartilages and tracheal rings. Therefore the anesthesiologist should avoid applying pressure over the airway in the neck during mask anesthesia. Monitor breath sounds, $EtCO_2$, and the movement of the reservoir bag continuously.

Laryngospasm

Laryngospasm occurs most commonly during induction of anesthesia, but also during emergence and occasionally during maintenance of anesthesia if the child is stimulated while lightly anesthetized. It occurs more commonly in infants (compared with older children), in preterm infants, children with recent URIs, children with reactive airways disease, after airway surgery and in those exposed to second-hand smoke. The clinical hallmarks of laryngospasm include high-pitched sounds with inspiratory stridor that may progress to silence as the glottic aperture closes. Suprasternal and supraclavicular retractions occur with paradoxical chest wall motion, increased diaphragmatic excursions and if the spasm persists, hemoglobin desaturation and bradycardia/asystole. As soon as laryngospasm is suspected, the precipitating event (such as secretions, blood, or other foreign material) should be cleared. Initial treatment should include the application of a facemask to deliver 100% oxygen with positive end-expiratory pressure (maximum pressure of 10 to 15 cm H_2O) (Figure 4-1). If laryngospasm continues, the mandible should be displaced by transiently applying pressure to the superior end of the ascending ramus of the mandible (i.e., the condyles) using a single digit behind each pinna (see previous discussion). Although subluxing the mandible, the thumbs should seal the facemask to the face. Oral airways must be used with great caution in these circumstances as short oral airways may push the tongue into the glottic opening and long airways may push the epiglottis into the opening, in both instances obstructing rather than helping the airway. An additional benefit from pressing on the ascending ramus of the mandible is that the stimulation incurred increases respiratory effort. However, if these measures fail and the oxygen saturation and heart rate continue to decrease, early treatment should include IV atropine (0.02 mg/kg) followed by IV propofol (1 to 2 mg/kg) and/or succinylcholine (1 to 2 mg/kg IV or 4 to 5 mg/kg IM) and intubation. If the child is in extremis (i.e., bradycardia and hypoxic) from laryngospasm, then intubate the trachea immediately, and ventilate the lungs with 100% oxygen.

Postobstructive Pulmonary Edema

Postobstructive pulmonary edema is a complication that may occur after relief of acute (laryngospasm) or chronic upper airway obstruction (tonsillectomy). The mechanism of this pulmonary edema appears to be the generation of extreme negative intrathoracic pressure against a closed glottis and its sudden release causing a dramatic increase

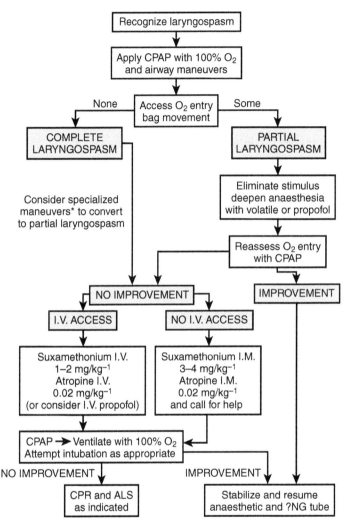

Figure 4-1.   Laryngospasm algorithm. *(From Hampson-Evans D, Morgan P, Farrar M: Pediatric laryngospasm. Pediatr Anesth 18:303-307, 2008.)*

in pulmonary blood flow resulting in low pressure, noncardiogenic pulmonary edema. This complication should be suspected when pink frothy sputum appears in the tracheal tube and oxygen desaturation continues unabated. Treatment is to continue positive pressure ventilation and IV lasix as needed.

Postintubation Croup

Postintubation croup or subglottic edema is associated with traumatic intubation, tight-fitting endotracheal tubes, coughing on the tube, a change in the child's position, prolonged intubation, surgery of the head and neck, and a history of croup. Treatment includes the inhalation of cool mist, steroids, and racemic epinephrine. Inhalation of racemic epinephrine (0.5 ml in 3 ml normal saline over 10 minutes) is usually effective although its effects are temporary and its use may be followed by rebound edema. Prolonged observation or overnight admission may be required.

Laryngoscopy

1. Ensure that the head is correctly positioned and supported.
   a. For infants and children younger than 6 years of age, the head should be on the level of the table and supported in a low head ring. At this age, the larynx is positioned high in the neck and there is no advantage to anterior displacement of the cervical spine because the relatively large head accomplishes this naturally. Extension of the neck at the atlanto-occipital joint aligns the oral, pharyngeal, and tracheal axis for optimal visualization. External pressure (so called optimal external laryngeal manipulation [OELM]) applied to the thyroid cartilage region of the anterior aspect of the neck (applied most effectively by the anesthesiologist using their second hand, in a posterior and cephalad direction) may further improve the view of the glottic aperture.
   b. For older children and adolescents, place a folded sheet or blanket under the head as a pillow to cause anterior displacement of the cervical spine and improve the alignment of the airway and the view of the glottis as in adults.
   c. Beware of conditions that may be associated with an unstable cervical spine (e.g., Down syndrome, Marfan syndrome). In such cases, note the range of spontaneous motion of the neck when the child is awake and inquire about the presence of neurologic symptoms preoperatively (wide based gait, urinary or fecal/urinary incontinence). There is no evidence that cervical spine films are

helpful in ruling out unstable cervical vertebra; however, we advise extreme care be taken to limit neck movement during intubation or surgical positioning.

2. Examine the teeth carefully; many young children have loose deciduous teeth. The teeth must be kept in view throughout laryngoscopy: retract the lip with your thumb and exert no pressure on the teeth during laryngoscopy. If loose teeth are present, it should be noted pre-operatively and the parents should be informed that it may be safer to remove them once the child is anesthetized. If teeth are removed, they should be retained and given to the parents after the anesthetic. A plastic tooth guard may be applied to the maxillary teeth and is particularly useful for older children and adolescents when a Macintosh (curved) blade is used.

3. In infants and children, the anesthesiologist's view of the glottis may be obscured by the epiglottis unless it is raised with the tip of the straight blade. (This is why we advocate the use of a straight blade in this age group.) In small infants, it is sometimes a problem to lift the epiglottis without it slipping off the laryngoscope blade. If this happens, advance the blade into the hypopharynx (with the entire tongue to the left of the blade) and slowly withdraw it until the glottis slips off the blade and the base of the epiglottis is firmly held. Alternatively, a straight blade may be used as would a curved blade and slowly advanced along the surface of the tongue. As the tip of the blade enters the vallecula, lift the base of the tongue to avoid trauma to other laryngeal structures.

4. Insufflation of oxygen into the pharynx during laryngoscopy (especially in infants or those with a difficult airway) improves oxygenation during attempts at intubation. Specially designed blades with an oxygen port are available (Oxyscope, Anesthesia Medical Specialties, Santa Fe Springs, Calif.), or an oxygen catheter may be taped to the side of any blade so as to deliver approximately 2 L/min of oxygen.

Tracheal Intubation

1. The optimal size of the tube is the largest one that passes easily through the glottis and subglottic regions without incurring resistance. The presence of a leak around an uncuffed tube at 20 cm H_2O positive pressure depends on a number of factors (including head position and muscle relaxation). A leak should be tested and achieved between 20 and 30 cm H_2O peak inflation pressure. If the leak is too large, the next half size larger tube may be inserted. If there is no leak at 30 cm H_2O, then a smaller diameter tube should be considered. In deciding that the tube size is appropriate, many clinicians depend more on the

absence of any resistance when the tube passes through the cricoid region than on the presence of an audible leak. There is increasing use of cuffed tracheal tubes in children in the operating room (OR) and PICU but these tubes should also have a leak when the cuff is deflated (see later discussion).

2. Clear, thin-walled polyvinyl chloride (PVC) tubes (Z79-approved) are preferred.

3. Cuffed tubes may be preferred for major surgery in children whose lungs may be difficult to ventilate and who may be at increased risk for regurgitation of gastric contents. Even in infants and young children, the use of an appropriately sized cuffed tracheal tube does not increase postoperative morbidity. The use of a cuffed tube reduces the need to change tubes, reduces OR pollution, and may reduce the risk of aspiration. It also obviates the need to have a close fit in the subglottic region to ensure effective ventilation. For this reason it may be preferable, in children with a known tendency to subglottic stenosis (e.g., Down syndrome), to use a tube of smaller diameter together with a cuff to seal the airway. Small-sized cuffed tubes are now available with a wall thickness similar to that of uncuffed tubes. In infants and small children when a cuffed tube is used, the cuff may not require inflation to achieve an adequate seal for ventilation. However, positioning the cuff below the cords places the tip of the tube much closer to the carina in small infants and may increase the risk of an endobronchial intubation. The new MicroCuff tubes have addressed these shortcomings by designing a high compliance, better shaped cuff that is more distally attached to the tube.

4. Endotracheal connectors must have a lumen at least equal to the internal diameter (ID) of the tube and must be firmly inserted. Tracheal tube connectors (particularly in small diameter tubes) should be removed, moistened with an alcohol swab, and reinserted into the tube up to the shoulder.

5. The correct positioning of the tracheal tube should be immediately confirmed by observation of the chest excursion, the presence of humidity within the lumen of the tube, the capnograph trace, and chest auscultation. Ventilation should be auscultated in both axillae. The length of the trachea of the infant and young child is short, only 5 cm in the neonate. The tip must be accurately placed at midtracheal level to minimize the risk of an endobronchial intubation or accidental extubation. Note carefully the length of tube that is passed through the cords, and check the tube length marking at the teeth. An easy method of determining the correct depth of insertion of the tracheal

tube when it is even with the teeth or alveolar ridge is 10 cm in a neonate, 11 for a 1-year-old and 12 for a 2-year-old (**N.B.** The second digit is the child's age in years.); beyond 2 years, halve the child's age and add 12 cm (see Table 4-6). Tubes must be firmly taped in place, preferably near the middle of the mouth, where they are less likely to kink. When cuffed tubes are used, the cuff should be positioned just past the vocal cords; check for bilateral ventilation and secure the tube carefully. As previously mentioned, the margin of safety before the tip passes into the bronchus is shorter with cuffed tubes.

6. Avoid pressure by anesthetic hoses and other equipment on the child's face or head by the use of suitable padding. Facial nerve palsy has been reported after anesthesia because of pressure of anesthesia equipment.

7. The anesthesia circuit and tube must be carefully positioned and supported to prevent any traction on the tube that might cause it to kink or become dislodged. *Endotracheal tubes used in children kink very easily, and this is a potential cause of disastrous accidents.*

8. Remember that extension of the neck withdraws the tip of the tube proximally in the trachea and flexion advances the tube; 1 to 3 cm of movement may occur between full flexion and full extension in infants. Position the tube carefully and consider the effects of changing the head position. Always reassess bilateral ventilation after repositioning the child.

9. Be aware that some neonates and infants have a congenitally short trachea, which increases the danger of endobronchial intubation (e.g., DiGeorge syndrome).

Nasotracheal Intubation

If the nasal route is chosen, the child should be prepared as outlined earlier. When performing nasotracheal intubation it is not unusual to cause some bleeding from the nose. As a result, several strategies have been developed to reduce this risk. Although warming the tip of the tube softens it, this has not been shown to be effective in reducing nose bleeding. Two effective strategies are application of a vasoconstrictor (e.g., oxymetazoline) to the nares and/or telescoping the tip of the tube into the flange end of a smooth red rubber catheter. With the latter, the catheter tip should be lubricated and passed along the floor of the (preferably left) nostril followed by the tube. (The left nostril aligns the tip of the tube [bevel on the left] directly with the glottic opening and aligns the bevel of the tube on the turbinate side.) The catheter is then advanced into the oropharynx where it is visualized in the hypopharynx and pulled off the endotracheal tube with McGill forceps. The tube is then directed using McGill forceps into the trachea.

A Note on Awake Intubation in the Neonate. It was common practice to intubate the neonate awake; however, it is now usual to induce anesthesia first. Intubation is more likely to be successful and less desaturation to occur if the neonate is first anesthetized. Awake intubation might be considered in neonates who are hemodynamically unstable, have micrognathia or a difficult airway, or who are extremely premature. To perform an awake intubation, pretreat the neonate with oxygen and atropine, have a styletted tube available, and have an assistant position the neonate's arms fully abducted against the head to stabilize the neonate's head. With the laryngoscope in one hand and the tube in the second, remove the facemask and intubate the trachea rapidly. Awake intubation increases blood pressure and intracranial pressure to a similar extent as crying and coughing. There has been a concern raised regarding an increased risk of IVH in preterm infants whose tracheas were intubated awake; however, this risk has never been confirmed. If awake intubation is deemed to be necessary, a local anesthetic solution (diluted, with upper limits predetermined) may be applied to the oropharynx and palate to reduce the infant's distress and struggling. Small doses of fentanyl (0.5-1 µg/kg) and midazolam (0.05-0.1 mg/kg) may also facilitate the process. The use of a laryngeal mask airway (LMA) to establish the airway before anesthesia may also be considered (see later discussion).

Rapid Sequence Induction (RSI)

RSI is an intravenous induction technique used to rapidly and safely secure the airway with a tracheal tube when there is a risk of vomiting or regurgitation and aspiration. Careful preparation for a RSI is essential and requires the following:

1. Equipment; anesthesia machine, age appropriate laryngoscopes and tracheal tubes, functioning suction.
2. Predetermined drugs in weight-appropriate doses.
3. Skilled anesthesiologist and skilled assistant.

The equipment must include all standard monitors and the necessary airway instruments and supplies. The airway equipment should include two functioning laryngoscope blades and handles, two sets of suction tubing, cuffed tracheal tubes of age appropriate size (plus a half-size larger and smaller diameters) and a stylet. Predetermined drugs include 100% oxygen to be given before the sequence begins, an intravenous induction agent (propofol 3 to 4 mg/kg, ketamine 1 to 2 mg/kg, or etomidate

0.2 to 0.3 mg/kg) in predetermined doses according to weight and physical status (**N.B.** Severity of dehydration and sepsis, etc.), atropine (0.02 mg/kg), and a muscle relaxant (succinylcholine 2 mg/kg or rocuronium 1.2 mg/kg). The child's head is optimally positioned during preoxygenation and as anesthesia is induced, cricoid pressure (see below) is applied by the assistant. (Before commencing, ensure that your assistant is instructed in the effective application of cricoid pressure.) Once paralyzed, the trachea is intubated without delay and the cuff inflated. In the modified RSI technique, the lungs may be ventilated manually with 100% oxygen while maintaining cricoid pressure (see later discussion).

Cricoid Pressure

Cricoid pressure (Sellick maneuver) should be applied to the cricoid ring with thumb and long finger as anesthesia is induced and should be maintained until tracheal position is confirmed. Cricoid pressure has been popularized as an adjunct to the RSI to prevent passive regurgitation of gastric contents during induction of anesthesia. The use of this technique is widely advocated. However, evidence has not been forthcoming to support the effectiveness of cricoid pressure to either occlude the lumen of the esophagus or prevent passive regurgitation of gastric contents. MRI evidence indicates that the lumen of the esophagus is lateral to the cricoid ring in 50% of patients and is laterally displaced with cricoid pressure in 90%. Moreover, studies of the force required to occlude the lumen in adults report that inadequate force is applied in the majority of patients. Surveys indicated that cricoid pressure is used in only half of those children in whom it is indicated. In adults, 30 to 40 Newton (3 to 4 kg of force) must be applied to the esophagus; there are no comparable data in children. Cricoid pressure is known to relax lower esophageal sphincter tone. If mask ventilation is ever necessary in a child with a full stomach, it is probably prudent to continue to apply cricoid pressure to prevent gastric inflation and maintain small peak inflation pressures. Contraindications to cricoid pressure should be recognized (Table 4-7). Excessive cricoid pressure may increase the difficulty of laryngeal visualization; OELM combined with cricoid pressure may be needed.

The Laryngeal Mask Airway

The LMA is an oropharyngeal tube provided with an anatomically conforming elliptical inflated rim designed to encircle the laryngeal inlet. If correctly inserted, the mask tip lies against the upper esophageal sphincter, the sides against the pyriform fossa, and the upper border against

TABLE 4-7   Contraindications to Cricoid Pressure

Contraindication	Potential Complication
Active vomiting	Rupture of the esophagus
Airway issues	Fractured cricoid cartilage ⇒ may be worsened Sharp foreign body in the airway may perforate airway
Esophageal issues	Regurgitation from a Zenker diverticulum Sharp foreign body may perforate esophagus, larynx, aorta, or spinal canal
Vertebral/neurologic issues	Unstable C-spine may cause disruption of spinal cord Sharp foreign body may perforate spinal cord
Education	Lack of knowledge, expertise, and/or ability to apply cricoid pressure

Adapted from Thiagarajah S, Lear E, Keh M: Anesthetic implications of Zenker's diverticulum. Anesth Analg 70;109-11, 1990.

the base of the tongue. It was primarily designed as a substitute for mask anesthesia in spontaneously ventilating adults, but more recently its use has been extended to some children whose lungs were ventilated. In children, controlled ventilation without distention of the stomach may be possible if peak airway pressures are maintained at approximately 15 cm H_2O. The LMA does not protect the airway should vomiting or regurgitation occur. LMAs are sized according to the child's weight (Table 4-8).

Insertion of the LMA is performed after induction of adequate anesthesia by inhalation or by an intravenous injection of propofol (3 to 4 mg/kg for children). The cuff should be checked before it is inserted. After the cuff has been completely deflated and the mask well lubricated, it is inserted blindly along the curve of the palate into the pharynx, with the aperture positioned anteriorly, until resistance is felt. If the LMA becomes "hung up" on the posterior pharyngeal wall, a finger should be inserted into the mouth to lift the tip of the LMA and continue insertion. The LMA is then advanced using gentle pressure. When the cuff is inflated, the LMA should rise slightly out of the mouth. The adequacy of ventilation and fit are checked. Generally, a leak will become obvious at approximately 15 cm H_2O peak inflation pressure. An alternative method of insertion in children has also been suggested: with the cuff partly inflated, the LMA is inserted with the mask facing posteriorly and then rotated 180° as it enters the pharynx. In either case, a black guideline on the proximal visible tube should lie against the central incisors when the LMA is in place

TABLE 4-8 Size Selection and Recommended Cuff Volumes for the Laryngeal Mask Airway

Mask Size	Child's Weight	Maximum Cuff Volume (ml)	Largest ETT (ID, mm) Inside Classic LMA	Largest ETT (ID, mm) Inside Unique LMA*	Largest Endotracheal Tube (ID, mm) Proseal LMA*	Largest FOB Inside ETT (mm)
1	<6.5 kg	4	3.5	3.5	N/A	2.7
1.5	5–10 kg	7	4.0	4.0	4.0, some manufacturers	3.5
2	10–20 kg	10	4.5	4.5	3.5	4
2.5	20–30 kg	14	5.0	5	4.0	5
3	30–50 kg	20	6.0, cuffed	5.0, cuffed	4.5	5
4	50–70 kg	30	6.0, cuffed	5.5, cuffed	5.0	
5	70–100 kg	40	7.0, cuffed	6.0, cuffed	5.0, cuffed	
					6.0, cuffed	

* Note that these sizes differ from the manufacturers recommendations, but have been found by us to be the better alternatives to ensure easy passage of the endotracheal tube through the LMA. In some cases the tubes listed are smaller, in some cases a cuffed alternative is given as an option rather than an uncuffed tube.

* Olympus Surgical Inc., Orangeburg, NY.

Fiberoptic bronchoscopes:

Olympus LF-P: (Outside diameter 2.2 mm) will pass through ETT 3-mm ID or larger. Will pass through 26 fr double lumen tube. (No suction channel)

Olympus LF-2: will pass through 5-mm ID ETTs or larger. (1.5 mm suction channel)

and correctly oriented. Coughing and laryngospasm may occur if insertion is attempted at too light a level of anesthesia; such complications may be more common in infants and small children than in adults.

Studies have shown that, when the LMA is in position, the tip of the tube lies in the hypopharynx but the relationship of the cuff to the epiglottis and laryngeal aperture may vary somewhat despite an apparently good airway.

Some difficulty with insertion may be encountered in up to 25% of children; this is more likely in the smaller child having a size 1 or size 1.5 LMA inserted. In a very small percentage of children, it may be impossible to place the LMA correctly.

When correctly positioned, the LMA provides a good airway with less resistance than an endotracheal tube. It avoids instrumentation through the glottis and frees the anesthesiologist from holding a facemask. It is particularly useful during imaging procedures, radiotherapy, and for other short procedures where mask anesthesia with spontaneous ventilation might be used. Somewhat surprisingly, some have found the LMA to be useful during adenotonsillectomy, and it has been suggested that less aspiration of blood occurs with the LMA than with an uncuffed endotracheal tube. (We, and most ENT surgeons prefer to intubate the trachea). A special application of the LMA is to use it as a guide to assist management of the child with a difficult airway, where it may be used as a prelude to fiberoptic endoscopy and intubation. The LMA can be inserted in awake infants (e.g., with Pierre Robin syndrome) after inhalation of nebulized lidocaine, and used to provide an airway to induce and deepen anesthesia before fiberoptic intubation. The LMA is useful when difficulty with ventilation occurs in a child during attempts at intubation. The LMA may also be advantageous in infants with tracheal stenosis, in whom passage of an endotracheal tube would severely reduce an already compromised airway diameter. It must be remembered that the LMA does not guarantee the airway as does an endotracheal tube, and it does not protect against aspiration. The ProSeal LMA provides a better seal (average leak at ~25 cm H_2O peak inflation pressure) and a means for venting the stomach; this device may be optimal for management of the difficult airway in a situation where the child has a full stomach.

At the end of the procedure, the LMA may be left in place until protective reflexes have returned, or it may be removed while the child is still deeply anesthetized. Removal while the child is anesthetized results in fewer airway complications and less desaturation, but a facemask should be applied until the child is able to maintain a safe airway. The incidence of postoperative sore throat is similar whether an LMA or an endotracheal tube is used. Other supraglottic devices are available and each practitioner should decide which is best in their hands.

"Difficult Tracheal Intubation"

Preoperative Assessment

It is most important that the anesthesiologist carefully assess the airway before administering anesthesia to determine the likelihood of obstruction during anesthesia and to judge the likely ease of endotracheal intubation.

Beware of any child who does not look quite normal or who has any syndrome or association of defects. Always anticipate the possibility of an abnormal airway. When there is any doubt, assume the airway will be difficult and be prepared. Review the history and examine the child carefully. Always review any previous anesthesia records—but do not be lulled into a false sense of security by a previous uneventful anesthetic. First, not all anesthetic difficulties are detailed in the record or child's chart. But even if they were, the ease of intubation may change as the child grows. In some cases, intubation may become easier, as in the child with a cleft palate and Pierre Robin sequence. In others, it becomes more difficult, as in the child with Treacher Collins, Goldenhar, or Klippel-Feil syndrome.

The examination of the child may provide clues as to the likely ease of intubation:

1. Assess the extent of mouth opening.
2. Check the extent of neck flexion and extension.
3. Check the shape and size of the mandible and maxilla (profile view).
4. Examine the mouth, tongue, and palate.
5. External ear deformities are often associated with mandibular hypoplasia.
6. Assess the distance between the ramus of the mandible and the thyroid cartilage.

Limited mouth opening, restricted neck extension, a large tongue, or a short ramus of the mandible predicts difficulty with laryngoscopy and tracheal intubation in children. Inability to fully visualize the fauces and uvula suggests difficult intubation, although the Mallampati scoring system does not predict a difficult laryngoscopy in children. Successful laryngoscopy depends on the ability to displace the soft tissues of the oropharynx into the mandibular space. Any deformity that limits this space (short or shallow mandible) or increases oropharyngeal tissue (large tongue) can be expected to compromise efforts to see the glottis.

Management Strategies

It is most important to be prepared for every option when facing a difficult airway in a child. Confirm that all the equipment you may require is
readily available. It is essential to keep all the "difficult pediatric airway"
supplies on a special cart that is located centrally and can be wheeled
into any room where it is required. It is always advantageous to have
expert assistance on hand. If there are other members of the department with special skills, do not hesitate to enlist their aid, even if their
initial role is simply to stand by, provide moral support, and be ready to
intervene.

Preoperative administration of an anticholinergic drug may be advantageous to decrease secretions in the mouth and pharynx and minimize
the possibility of laryngeal spasm. No heavy sedation should be admin-
tered; small doses of anxiolytics might be administered when necessary,
using suitable caution and appropriate monitoring. Children who cannot
be fasted and require emergency surgery may be prepared with the use of
histamine$_2$-blocking drugs and intravenous metoclopramide.

A recommended sequence to follow is outlined in the Pediatric
Difficult Airway Algorithm (Figure 4-2).

The choice of anesthetized versus awake intubation is quite simple:
children, unlike adults, almost always require general anesthesia. Children
are very easily upset and will not cooperate during attempts at an awake
intubation (even after local anesthesia is applied to the airway). Small
infants may be severely stressed by attempts at awake intubation and are
more easily and rapidly intubated when they are anesthetized. An exception is advised for certain small infants (i.e., those with Pierre Robin syndrome), in whom intubation may be very difficult and who may be more
safely managed by topical anesthesia of the mouth and insertion of a well-
lubricated LMA while the infant is awake. The LMA can then be used as
a route to induce anesthesia and, if necessary, as a conduit for fiberoptic
intubation (see Table 4-8).

Standard Management

The classic traditional approach to the management of the difficult pediatric airway is by inhalational induction, deep inhalational anesthesia,
continued spontaneous ventilation, and direct laryngoscopy. This method
is advantageous in that it does not require complex equipment and does
immediately determine the status of the airway and the degree of difficulty
of direct laryngoscopy. These details, along with the type of laryngoscope
blade used and other data, can then be clearly recorded in the anesthesia
record. *Although this procedure is still recommended as a standard basic*

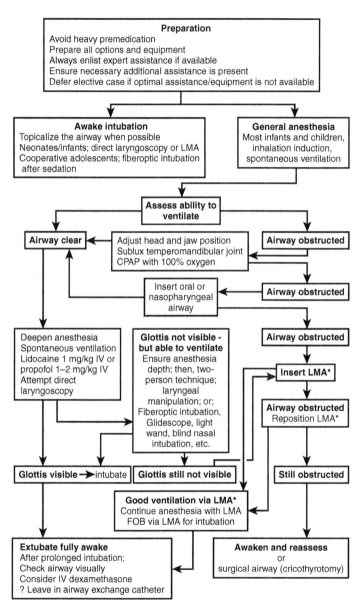

Figure 4-2. Difficult airway algorithm.

*management plan, some children may be more effectively managed by early insertion of the LMA or other techniques (*see Alternative Methods*).*

Induction of anesthesia should be performed by inhalation; intravenous relaxant drugs are generally contraindicated. Sevoflurane is preferred for a smooth, rapid induction. If halothane is available, its greater solubility facilitates a more prolonged laryngoscopy than is possible with sevoflurane. As anesthesia is induced, the muscles of the tongue and pharynx relax. At this time, obstruction may occur, and immediate measures may be required to re-establish a clear airway.

1. Adjust the position of the head with increased jaw thrust to lift the tongue off the posterior pharyngeal wall and open the upper airway. A two-handed method is preferred, with one digit behind the most cephalad tip of the ascending ramus on each side of the mandible. The finger is wedged in the triangle formed at the base of the skull between the ascending ramus of the mandible anteriorly and the mastoid process posteriorly, immediately behind the tragus. Pull the mandible towards the frontal hairline. This maneuver subluxes the mandible anteriorly and rotates the temporomandibular joint, thereby opening the mouth. At the same time, two thumbs hold the mask on the face. With this maneuver, an oropharyngeal airway is often unnecessary.

2. If necessary, insert an oropharyngeal airway (see previous discussion); but be aware that if the child is too lightly anesthetized this may result in coughing and laryngospasm. Make sure that the airway is appropriately sized for the child; measure it against the outside of the face (the tip should extend just to the angle of the mandible).

When an airway is established, anesthesia is deepened with 8% sevoflurane in oxygen. Before the first attempts at laryngoscopy and intubation, 1.5 mg/kg of intravenous lidocaine and/or 1 to 3 mg/kg propofol are administered slowly to reduce the likelihood of breath holding or coughing during instrumentation. During laryngoscopy, oxygen may be insufflated into the pharynx via a catheter or by the use of a special laryngoscope blade. If an adequate view of the glottis is obtained, intubation can be performed; if not, other manipulations are required:

a. With the laryngoscope in place, apply posterior and cephalad pressure on the cricoid region of the neck to bring the larynx into view (OELM). In children with severe retrognathia, consider pushing the larynx to the right to visualize the glottis.

b. In some cases, a "two-person approach" to intubation is preferable. One person who holds the laryngoscope with one hand also applies pressure (as described previous discussion) to align the axes of the larynx and oropharynx. Once the glottis is visualized, the laryngoscopist tilts his head to the left to enable the second person to pass the tube through the cords.

c. A retromolar or paraglossal approach may be indicated. Insert a straight blade at the extreme right side of the mouth behind the bicuspid or last molar tooth while rotating the head to the left and retracting the corner of the mouth with a small surgical retractor. The epiglottis is visualized and the tracheal tube advanced off a stylet.

d. An alternative approach after induction of anesthesia and after confirming the ability to ventilate the child with bag and mask is to administer succinylcholine. Laryngoscopy can then be attempted during apnea with complete muscular relaxation. This may facilitate laryngoscopy and tracheal intubation, but at the same time, it limits the time available for each intubation attempt. Infants and small children desaturate more rapidly during apnea than do older children or adults. (**N.B.** Administration of a relaxant drug might result in a "can't intubate/can't ventilate" situation with an apneic child.)

If laryngoscopy proves impossible by direct vision, the mask should be reapplied, deep anesthesia continued, and other options considered (see Figure 4-2). It is wise not to persist with prolonged attempts at direct laryngoscopy because these may become traumatic and result in bleeding, thus compromising the chances of success with other methods or by other individuals.

Alternative Techniques

Laryngeal Mask Airway. The introduction of the LMA has made possible many new approaches to management of the difficult airway, provided the mouth and pharynx are of adequate size. If intubation under direct vision is impossible, the LMA may be inserted without delay. Insertion of an LMA at any stage is usually successful in establishing a patent upper airway, but laryngeal spasm may occur if the child is inadequately anesthetized. Once in place, the LMA can be used as a route for ventilation and oxygenation, to continue anesthesia, and as a conduit for flexible bronchoscopes, endotracheal tubes, airway catheters, light wands, or other equipment needed to complete intubation (see Table 4-8).

Flexible Bronchoscope. In some children it is impossible to insert an LMA (i.e., very small or scarred mouth) and it may be necessary to perform flexible bronchoscopy via the mouth or nose. The use of fiberoptic laryngobronchoscopes in children has been facilitated by the development of small-diameter scopes that accommodate small endotracheal tubes. The smallest scopes do not have a suction channel (see Table 4-8). A suction channel on the scope is a very desirable feature because secretions frequently obscure the view and this channel may also be used to administer oxygen in children who are breathing spontaneously; external suction may then be required to clear secretions.

If the nasal route is chosen, anesthesia should be cautiously induced with sevoflurane and spontaneous ventilation as previously described. The flexible bronchoscope should be prepared in advance by sliding an appropriate size tracheal tube (without the connector) over the scope. When the child is adequately anesthetized, the flexible bronchoscope is passed through the left nostril, to the glottis and into the trachea. The tube should then be passed over the scope and into the trachea. If the tube does not pass the cords, the tube should be rotated 90° so that the tip of the tube is midline. Practicing flexible fiberoptic bronchoscopy in children with normal airways is essential if the anesthesiologist is to become adept at a similar intubation technique with a difficult airway. When a very small endoscope is not available, alternative methods for children have been suggested including visualizing the glottis with a larger scope to pass an airway exchange catheter into the trachea under direct vision, over which the endotracheal tube can subsequently be threaded.

Bullard Laryngoscope. The Bullard laryngoscope and other similar devices are designed to indirectly view the glottis and thereby make it possible to direct the tracheal tube. All of these devices require practice, especially in the manipulation of the tube once the glottis is visualized. Initial experience should be gained with children who have a normal airway. The success rate for the experienced operator is reported to be high.

The Glidescope. (Verathon Inc., Bothell, WA, 98011) This device incorporates a small video camera to observe the glottis on a monitor screen. The "Glidescope small GVL" is recommended for children 1.5 to 20 kg.

Light Wand Intubation. The use of a malleable lighted stylet, passed blindly into the trachea, makes it possible, with practice, to rapidly secure the airway. The stylet should be curved to suit the predicted shape of the child's airway, and a suitable endotracheal tube is mounted on it. Always check that the lamp is screwed firmly in place. As the light passes into the trachea, the anterior neck can be seen to transilluminate. This is more easily seen with the room lights dimmed. The endotracheal tube can then be advanced over the stylet into the trachea. The method requires practice but may be successful in many children with a difficult airway. It is limited by the size of tube that can be passed over the stylet

(5.0 to 5.5 mm with the Flexi-Lum*); the Trachlight[†] has two sizes: child accommodating tubes 4 to 6 mm ID and infant accommodating tubes 2.5 to 4 mm). This technique can be used with general anesthesia, appropriate sedation, and regional or topical analgesia. The use of a light wand via the LMA has also been described. The Optical Stylet[‡] provides a further advance since this device will accommodate a 2.5 mm ID tracheal tube with a video camera and monitor to facilitate visualization of the laryngeal inlet. The Shikani optical stylet best accommodates a 3.0 tracheal tube.

Blind Nasotracheal Intubation. This is a technique that requires much practice. It is an art that few acquire in an era when advances in technology offer so many alternative methods. Blind nasotracheal intubation may still be necessary if all else fails, or when equipment fails, and the child's glottis cannot be visualized (see **N.B.** after item 7 next). The following are some hints:

1. It is essential to understand the anatomy of the nose. The septum is always angled; if the nares is open anteriorly, it is narrowed posteriorly and vice versa. The turbinates, which arise from the lateral wall, may be damaged (resulting in bleeding) or dislodged as the tube passes through the nose. To minimize damage to the turbinates and nasopharyngeal mucosa during passage through the nostril, consider instillation of vasoconstrictors (i.e., oxymetazoline) into the nares and/or the tube should be telescoped into a red rubber catheter (as described previously). The success rate for blind nasotracheal intubation increases if the left nostril is used because the leading tip of standard tracheal tubes is on the right and this tip will advance along the midline into the glottis. (Special tubes are made with the bevel on the right for use in the right nostril.)

2. Prepare and lubricate suitable tubes (ID 0.5 mm smaller than for oral intubation).

3. Use an inhalation induction (i.e., O_2, + sevoflurane or halothane); if available, 5% CO_2 may be added to increase the tidal volume before intubation attempts. *Do not use intravenous induction agents or muscle relaxants.*

4. When the child is deeply anesthetized, position the head slightly extended, as in the sniffing position.

5. Insert the tracheal tube through the nostril and advance it as described previously. There are five possible outcomes:
   a. Larynx-desired location.

---

* Concept Corp., Clearwater, Fla.
[†] Laerdal Inc., Long Beach, Calif.
[‡] Storz, Inc., Endoscopy-America Inc, Culver City, Calif.

    b. Right of larynx—withdraw the tracheal tube slightly; turn it to the left and turn the child's head to the right.

    c. Left of larynx—withdraw the tracheal tube slightly; turn it to the right and turn the child's head to the left.

    d. Esophagus—withdraw the tracheal tube slightly and extend the head maximally before advancing the tube again.

    e. Anterior to epiglottis—withdraw the tracheal tube slightly and flex the head.

6. If unsuccessful, repeat, using the other nostril.

7. Other useful maneuvers include:

    a. Connecting the capnogram for the largest signal or listening at the end of the tracheal tube for maximal gas exchange to reach the larynx.

    b. Passage of a second tube through the other nostril to block the esophagus.

    c. External pressure to the neck which may direct the glottis toward the tip of the tube.

    d. An angled stylet passed through the tube to direct the tip toward the glottic aperture. Usually this requires a 90° bend right at the tip of the tracheal tube.

    e. Use of a smaller-size tube for initial intubation; the tube can then be changed up in size by passing an airway exchange catheter and leaving it in place to guide the larger tube.

8. At the glottic aperture, the tip becomes lodged at the anterior commissure of the cords and fails to advance. To advance the tube, three possible maneuvers may be used:

    a. Rotate the tube 90° clockwise (so the bevel points superior)

    b. With McGill forceps, grab the tube 2 to 4 cm proximal to the end, withdraw the tube several centimeters and then bend it downwards as the tube is advanced, or

    c. Flex the child's neck (by raising the child's head and resting it onto your chest) while you perform laryngoscopy and maneuver the tube with McGill forceps (most difficult maneuver)

N.B. The technique of blind intubation requires considerable skill, which can be acquired only by extensive practice. It is a method that cannot be learned in a lecture but must be mastered by repeated practice. If the anesthesiologist is not sufficiently experienced and has no skilled assistant at hand, some other technique may be preferable or further attempts at intubation are abandoned and the child awakened from anesthesia.

As a means to simpler blind intubation, an endotracheal tube or an airway exchange catheter passed blindly through an LMA frequently passes into the trachea. Monitor end-tidal CO_2 via the catheter or tube to confirm its position.

Retrograde Intubation. This technique depends on threading a wire proximally through the vocal cords into the pharynx via a needle passed percutaneously into the trachea. This is a very dangerous technique with a reduced success rate particularly in infants and small children because of their compliant tracheas and the very small tracheal dimensions that together increase the risk of tracheal and extratracheal tissue injury. If cannulated successfully, the wire is then retrieved in the mouth and used to guide a tube into the trachea. A modification of this technique passes the retrieved wire retrograde up the suction port of a bronchoscope. The scope is then guided into the trachea by the wire and can be used to position the tube.

Failed Intubation. If intubation options are failing, consider the following:

1. Should we awaken the child and reschedule?
2. Can this case be done safely with mask anesthesia?
3. Can this case be done safely with an LMA for airway support?
4. Do we need a surgical airway?

Extubation of the Trachea

1. Children are prone to laryngeal spasm during extubation, especially if extubated during a light plane of anesthesia. Therefore,
   a. Before extubation, ensure that all airway equipment to ventilate with oxygen and to reintubate if necessary are available.
   b. Extubate when the child is fully awake (or, if indicated, deeply anesthetized).
   c. Some children should not cough or strain with the endotracheal tube in situ during emergence (e.g., those having neurosurgery or intraocular surgery). This may be achieved with a planned "deep" extubation, preceded by careful suctioning of the stomach and pharynx. Lidocaine, 1 to 2 mg/kg IV administered slowly before extubation, also decreases the risk of coughing and breath holding. After the tracheal tube is removed, a facemask should be applied, the airway maintained, and oxygen administered until the child is awake. Studies suggest that oxygen saturation (Sao_2) levels

are better maintained if extubation is performed while the child is still anesthetized and oxygen is then given by mask until the child is fully awake.

d. When judging whether the child is "awake" enough for awake extubation, wait until the eyes and mouth open spontaneously, all limbs are moving, and the child resumes regular spontaneous ventilation after coughing.

e. Do not disturb the child unnecessarily during the awaking stage, so as to minimize coughing and bucking on the tube before the child is fully awake. A "No touch" technique while waiting to extubate awake is very successful in many children.

f. All monitors should be left in place until successful extubation is complete.

2. Severe laryngospasm upon extubation may be followed by pulmonary edema as the laryngospasm is relieved. If this occurs, it should be treated by continued positive pressure ventilation, a diuretic (e.g., Lasix) and morphine.

3. The following children should be fully awake before extubation:

a. All those in whom tracheal intubation was difficult.

b. All those having emergency surgery; these children may vomit gastric contents during emergence from anesthesia.

c. All infants.

4. Children who have had a mouth gag with tongue blade inserted by the surgeon (e.g., for cleft palate repair) are at risk for postoperative swelling of the tongue; always inspect the mouth before extubation.

Extubation of the Difficult Pediatric Airway

Extubation should be performed as a well-planned exercise, with the necessary equipment and personnel to reintubate the child readily available. In selected children a trial extubation, leaving an airway exchange catheter in situ, may be indicated.

All children with difficult airways should be extubated or have the LMA removed only after they have fully regained consciousness and when all danger of swelling in the region of the airway has passed. Corticosteroids (dexamethasone) have been used before extubation to decrease the likelihood of stridor, and all children should be given humidified oxygen after the tracheal tube is removed.

The golden rule: If there is any doubt about the airway, leave the trachea intubated.

Pediatric Anesthetic Circuits

The ideal anesthetic circuit for children should be lightweight; with low resistance and dead space; with low compliance; adaptable to spontaneous, assisted, or controlled ventilation; and readily humidified and scavenged. These conditions are most nearly met by the T-piece systems; however, modified circle systems are now extensively used for children.

The T-Piece and its Variants

The T-piece, originally described by Ayre in 1937, was modified by Jackson Rees to provide for artificial ventilation. The T-piece relies on continuous flow from the fresh gas limb to flush expired gases from the expiratory limb, thus its performance depends on the rate of fresh gas flow and the minute ventilation of the child. Setting the fresh gas flow to target a specific $Paco_2$ has proven to be unreliable and superseded by capnography.

Small fresh gas flows that permit some rebreathing are well tolerated by children provided a capnograph is used to maintain the $EtCO_2$ tension within acceptable limits. Indeed, it has become environmentally, economically, and physiologically rational to decrease the fresh gas flow and permit rebreathing with these circuits. If capnography is not available, then minimum fresh gas formulas should be used to reduce the risk of rebreathing exhaled gases; for mask anesthesia greater than 8 L/min and for ETT greater than 6 L/min.

Because the T-piece has no valves, it cannot malfunction and has a very low resistance. However, kinking or obstruction of the expiratory limb can lead to high pressure within the circuit and might cause barotrauma. Because it is also lightweight and convenient and has minimal dead space, it is considered by many to be the ideal circuit for transporting infants and young children, especially during spontaneous ventilation to and from the ICU. The Bain coaxial system is a modification of the T-piece. It has essentially the same characteristics and requires the same fresh gas flows.

Circle Absorber Semi-Closed System

The adult circle absorber semi-closed system can be modified for use in children by incorporating a smaller-diameter breathing circuit. The circle system is more economical and provides limited humidification of inspired gases, but the greater circuit resistance and the possibility of valve malfunction lead some to prefer the T-piece system for infants and small children, especially during spontaneous ventilation. From a practical point of view today, this does not appear to be a substantive concern in clinical pediatric anesthesia. The circle system facilitates $EtCO_2$ monitoring because there is less mixing of expired and inspired gases than occurs in the open T-piece system. The integrity of the circle system and the presence and correct functioning of the valves must be carefully checked before each use.

Humidification of Anesthetic Gases

Humidification of inspired gases during anesthesia in the past was recommended to prevent damage to the respiratory tract by dry gases and to minimize heat loss via the respiratory tract and thereby assist in maintaining normothermia. Dry gases inhibit ciliary activity and lead to the accumulation of inspissated secretions, which may, in the extreme, progress to obstruct the endotracheal tube. Degenerative changes in cells exfoliated from the trachea after exposure to dry gas have been described, but an increased incidence of postoperative morbidity from pulmonary complications remains unproved. However, the use of circle systems, particularly with low flows has reduced the need for a humidifier. Gases should be humidified during very prolonged surgery and in the intensive care unit to reduce the risk of tube blockage from inspissated secretions.

Humidified anesthetic gases significantly reduce heat loss during surgery, particularly in neonates and infants. However, heated humidifiers are not as easily incorporated into circle circuits and accumulated water may plug capnogram tubing. Humidifiers are less frequently used in pediatric anesthesia since other effective means for maintaining body temperature are now available. An alternative means of humidification for older children is the use of a heat and moisture exchanger (HME) inserted at the connection of the endotracheal tube to the circuit. The HME conserves approximately 50% of the water normally lost via the respiratory tract and thus prevents a corresponding heat loss. The HME is most efficient with smaller tidal volumes and greater respiratory frequency, so it is quite useful in pediatric cases. These normally are very low resistance, but if blocked by secretions will significantly increase airway resistance; always monitor ventilation carefully when an HME is used.

Controlled Ventilation During Anesthesia

During anesthesia, ventilation may be controlled using manual or mechanical ventilation.

Manual Ventilation

This is used at times, especially during induction and when there is doubt about the adequacy of ventilation. It has been claimed that manual ventilation enables the anesthesiologist to monitor compliance continuously and to compensate rapidly for changes. Although this may be true for the experienced pediatric anesthesiologist, there is some question about the ability of individual anesthesiologists to detect even complete airway obstruction just by the feel of the bag. However, if there is any doubt about the adequacy of ventilation or in the event of sudden deterioration in the child's vital signs, it is wise to switch to manual ventilation. Then the adequacy of ventilation should be further confirmed by auscultation of the lungs, observation of chest movement, and the $EtCO_2$ monitor.

Rapid ventilation with small tidal volumes provides optimal results in the neonate because this pattern of ventilation tends to maintain the functional residual capacity and prevent airway closure. $EtCO_2$ levels should be monitored continuously because it is very easy to overventilate small infants. Hyperventilation (and consequent respiratory alkalosis) should be avoided.

Mechanical Ventilation

Mechanical ventilators have the advantage of maintaining a relatively constant level of ventilation while freeing the anesthesiologist to perform other functions. Remember that in small children the compression volume of the anesthesia circuit may exceed the tidal volume that is delivered to the lungs. Therefore the volume readings on the ventilator may be meaningless. The adequacy of ventilation must be judged by auscultation of the chest and observation of chest movement, along with $EtCO_2$ or arterial carbon dioxide levels.

Controlled ventilation with the circle system permits the use of extremely small fresh gas flows while monitoring the adequacy of ventilation by capnography. Several strategies for mechanical ventilation have been introduced into clinical anesthesia.

1. Volume cycled ventilation. In this mode, the ventilator delivers the prescribed tidal volume (unless it reaches the pressure relief limit—usually 40 mm Hg). Therefore during surgeries in which the compliance of the chest/abdomen changes, the delivered tidal volume remains relatively constant. (Tidal volume may decrease slightly because of the large volume of gas compressed in the anesthesia circuit as compliance decreases).

2. Pressure cycled ventilation. In this mode, the ventilator delivers a volume until the preset pressure is reached (usually 20 to 40 mm Hg). In this mode, if the pressure is reached before a desired tidal volume is

delivered, the ventilator switches into expiration. During surgeries in which the compliance of the chest/abdomen changes, the delivered tidal volume varies from breath to breath as compliance changes. Hence, without an accurate capnogram, tidal volume delivered cannot be estimated. We find this mode only acceptable during minor peripheral surgery.

3. Pressure assisted ventilation—new ventilators incorporate the potential for various modes of ventilation. The place of these in pediatric anesthesia is undetermined at the present time.

Monitoring During Anesthesia

Routine Monitoring Methods

Monitoring during anesthesia must always include the following:

1. Pulse oximeter: apply before induction and leave in place during transport and during the recovery room stay. The light source and sensor must be positioned to transilluminate a part of the body (earlobe, finger, toe, palm of hand, or sole of foot, depending on the size of the child). Placement on the earlobe or buccal angle rather than the finger or foot may result in a slightly faster initial response time during acute desaturation. Placement at a preductal site (head or right hand) is desirable in infants with any potential for patency of the ductus arteriosus. A second postductal oximeter probe is useful to detect shunting. The sensor(s) should be protected to prevent outside light or pressure from interfering with the reading. Pulse oximetry has proved most effective in providing an early warning of developing hypoxemia. Failure of the pulse oximeter to detect and record a pulsatile flow may provide useful warning information about the child's circulatory status. However, if the pulse oximeter fails, check the child first (color of mucus membranes or nailbeds, heart rate, breath sounds, blood pressure); then, if necessary, troubleshoot the equipment.

   Pulse oximetry is relatively accurate throughout a wide variation in hematocrit. In children with cyanotic congenital heart disease the oximeter tends to overestimate saturation at lower readings (below Spo_2 70%). Similarly, the faster the rate of desaturation, the more the oximeter underestimates the true hemoglobin saturation.

   Fetal hemoglobin (HbF), hemoglobin SS, and hyperbilirubinemia do not affect the pulse oximeter measurement.

   Nail polish or disease of the nails may affect the performance of the monitor (blue or green nail polish); the accuracy is unaffected by pigmented skin. Methemoglobin (MetHb) and carboxyhemoglobin (CoHb) affect the accuracy of readings: the former has a nonlinear effect, either underestimating or overestimating saturation and the latter overestimates saturation.

An arterial saturation of 80% to 95% reflects a Pao_2 of 40 to 80 mm Hg—a safe range for the preterm infant. But because of the slope of the Hb/O_2 association curve, pulse oximetry is less precise in the assessment of hyperoxia than it is in hypoxia. If considered necessary, an arterial sample can be obtained to confirm which level of saturation is appropriate in terms of Pao_2 for each child. This level of saturation can then be maintained by varying the fraction of inspired oxygen (Fio_2).

The complications of pulse oximetry are few, but severe burns have occurred when an incorrect sensor from a different manufacturer has been substituted. Burns may also occur when pulse oximetry is incorrectly used in the magnetic resonance imaging suite (see Chapter 18).

2. Stethoscope, precordial or esophageal: there must be provision to monitor heart and breath sounds throughout anesthesia. Recently, there has been a trend away from the use of a stethoscope; however, should there be an equipment failure, this is an essential aid. If the monitors stop working, check the child first.

3. Blood pressure (BP) cuff of suitable width: the cuff should occupy two thirds of the upper arm. If the cuff is too narrow, the BP readings are falsely high; if it is too wide, they are falsely low. A width of 4 cm is recommended for full-term neonates. A noninvasive blood pressure device (i.e., Dinamap) may be used, but ensure that it is set to provide readings at a maximum of 5 minute intervals.

4. Electrocardiogram: It is standard to monitor the EKG; however, the EKG is of limited value in pediatric cases. Any arrhythmias that occur are usually benign and bradycardia on the EKG is a very late sign that the child is in trouble.

5. Thermistor probe (axillary, esophageal, or rectal) (see Management of Body Temperature).

6. End-tidal carbon dioxide: This device noninvasively reflects the adequacy of ventilation and pulmonary perfusion. It also provides the most reliable indicator of successful endotracheal intubation and should be used whenever intubation is performed. Two types of monitors are available: measuring carbon dioxide "in-line" at the connector or by sidestream sampling from the circuit. The latter method is more commonly used. However, it is not as easy to apply in infants

and small children owing to the small size of the ventilatory volumes. When a partial rebreathing circuit is used (i.e., a T-piece plus ventilator), end-tidal sampling must be obtained from within the lumen of the endotracheal tube for all small children (i.e., those weighing less than 12 kg) if useful numbers are to be obtained. When a circle circuit is used, proximal sampling at the endotracheal connector gives valid results even for small infants. The presence of a leak around the endotracheal tube may also affect end-tidal sampling, especially when positive end-expiratory pressure is applied; with a very large leak, the $EtCO_2$ waveform may disappear completely.

$EtCO_2$ measurements correlate poorly with the $Paco_2$ in children who have congenital heart disease with a right-to-left shunt or mixing lesion; the lower the saturation, the greater the $Paco_2$-$EtCO_2$ gradient. In those with left-to-right shunting, the accuracy of $EtCO_2$ readings is unaffected.

A decrease in the $EtCO_2$ provides a very early indication of a reduction in pulmonary blood flow. This may be useful in the early diagnosis of cyanotic spells in the child with tetralogy of Fallot. A decrease may also be diagnostic of pulmonary embolism, air embolism, or a low cardiac output state.

7. Peripheral nerve stimulator: should be used whenever nondepolarizing muscle relaxants are administered.

8. Arterial catheter: should be inserted for direct measurement of BP and to provide for intermittent blood gas analysis when required. The radial or femoral artery is usually cannulated (see later discussion); rarely, the axillary artery may be used. We recommend checking for collateral flow from the ulnar artery when cannulating the radial artery. Do not use the brachial artery, which has poor collateral vessels. (See Precautions with Arterial Lines.) Cannulation of the superficial temporal artery has been described but this introduces the possibility of retrograde intracranial embolization. Children with Down syndrome may have a single (median) artery in the wrist, in which case cannulation should be avoided. (Always check the wrist vessels before attempting cannulation.)

9. Urine output: record this at regular intervals for all children undergoing major surgery and all who have hypovolemic shock or whose renal function may be impaired.

10. Central venous pressure (CVP): record from a catheter inserted centrally via the internal or external jugular vein (see later discussion). The external jugular is a less reliable route for CVP monitoring but is often useful for fluid replacement and drug infusions. The CVP

should always be monitored in children in whom major blood loss and/or impaired cardiac performance is anticipated.

Cannulation Techniques

Radial Artery Cannulation

The left radial artery is often preferred for arterial puncture (in right-handed children).

1. Locate the artery by palpation; if this is difficult, use the Doppler flow meter or ultrasound, or in small infants, transilluminate the wrist with a bright cold light.
2. Use careful aseptic technique and prepare the skin with povidone-iodine (Betadine).
3. Make a small skin incision over the artery with an 18-gauge needle. This prevents damage to the tip of the cannula during skin puncture.
4. Perform arterial puncture; as soon as blood issues into the hub of the needle, turn the needle so that the bevel faces down.

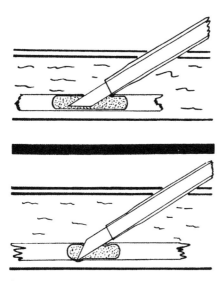

Figure 4-3. Advantage of turning the needle bevel down when inserting an intravenous cannula into a small vein or artery. *(From Filston HC, Johnson DG: Percutaneous venous cannulation in neonates and infants: a method for catheter insertion without cutdown. Pediatrics 48:896-901, 1971, with permission of the American Academy of Pediatrics.)*

5. Advance the cannula gently into the artery (Figure 4-3).
6. If it will not advance, withdraw until blood flows freely and carefully insert a fine guidewire,* then advance the cannula over the wire.
7. If you fail to enter the artery at all, remove the needle and palpate the artery again, critically evaluating its alignment with the skin puncture. Then try again.
8. Apply antibiotic spray or ointment to the skin puncture site and cover with a sterile dressing (e.g., Tegaderm, 3M Health Care Inc.).
9. Secure cannula carefully with adhesive tape. All connections should be Luer-Lok or similar to prevent accidental bleeding.
10. Place a red label indicating that this is an arterial line at the site of insertion and all connections to prevent confusion with a venous line.

Femoral Artery Cannulation

In some children the radial artery cannot be cannulated or is inappropriate (e.g., after surgery of the aortic arch). In such cases the femoral artery may be used.

1. Place a low pad under the child to elevate the pelvis.
2. Palpate the femoral artery *below* the inguinal ligament.
3. Use careful aseptic technique and prepare the skin with povidone-iodine (Betadine).
4. Using the Seldinger technique, puncture the artery *below* the inguinal ligament using an appropriate sized thin-walled needle. Punctures superior to the inguinal ligament introduce the risk of a retroperitoneal bleed.
5. Avoid needling the head of the femur; aseptic necrosis may result in infants and young children.
6. When the artery is entered, insert a guide wire and use it to introduce an appropriate size catheter. Secure the catheter carefully in place and cover it with antibiotic ointment and a clear plastic dressing.

If the artery is difficult to palpate, the use of a Doppler flow meter, a Doppler tipped-needle,[†] or ultrasound may facilitate arterial puncture.

Precautions With Arterial Lines. Regarding any arterial cannulation:

1. Insert the cannula with meticulous asepsis.

2. Secure all connections, using Luer-Lok fittings, to exclude the danger of accidental disconnection and hemorrhage. Plug sampling taps

---

* 0.018 (0.46 mm) dia. × 25 cm spring guide wire, AW -04018, Arrow International Inc., Reading, Pa.
† Smart Needle, Peripheral Systems Group, Mountainview, Calif.

when not in use. Tape stopcocks in the "line-open" position if they will be hidden under the drapes and inaccessible. Clearly indicate all access ports with red tape or label as "arterial line" so as to avoid accidental drug administration through the arterial line.

3. For radial lines, immobilize the forearm and wrist on a padded splint to prevent accidental decannulation.

4. Use a continuous flush device, but beware of accidental fluid overload. Use 1 N or 0.5 N saline with heparin (1000 IU/500 ml). Do not use dextrose because of increased risk of infection of the line.

5. Beware of embolization.
   a. Do not reinfuse blood removed during sampling into the arterial line. Return the blood to an IV line.
   b. Do not use high pressure to attempt to clear a blocked cannula.
   c. Infuse only small volumes of flush fluid after sampling. In small infants, volumes of only 0.5 to 1.0 ml injected into the radial artery may flow retrograde into the cerebral vessels.

6. Remove the arterial line as soon as it has served its purpose. Complications (especially arterial thrombosis and sepsis) increase with the duration of cannulation of the vessel.

Internal Jugular Vein Cannulation

The use of an ultrasound probe (Site Rite*) improves the success rate and decreases the incidence of complications.

1. Position the child—head to left, 20° Trendelenburg, with a rolled towel under the shoulders to reduce concavity of the neck.

2. If available, use the Site Rite*or other ultrasound probe to locate and mark the position of the internal jugular vein (IJV) at the level of the cricoid cartilage. It is helpful to also note the relation of the IJV to the carotid artery at this level.

3. Prepare skin and drape, and gown and glove. (Gowning and gloving to perform CVP catheter insertion has been demonstrated to decrease infection rates.)

4. Using the Seldinger technique, insert the thin-walled needle through the skin at 45° over the marked course of the IJV until the vein is punctured: a flow of venous blood is usually obtained as the needle is being slowly withdrawn.

5. Hold the needle very still, pass the guide wire; there should be no resistance to passage. The occurrence of premature ventricular beats indicates passage of the guide wire into the right ventricle; withdraw the

---

* Dymax Corp., Pittsburg, Pa.

wire several centimeters. Remove the needle, make a skin nick with a scalpel blade, and complete the cannulation after advancing and removing the dilator.

If ultrasound is not available, cannulation may be performed using anatomic landmarks; after positioning the child as described in 1 previously:

1. Palpate the carotid pulse medial to the sternocleidomastoid and pick this muscle up to identify its bulk at the level of the thyroid cartilage prominence (the midpoint between the mastoid process and the sternal notch).
2. At the level of the bifurcation of the sternomastoid into the sternal and clavicular heads, aim the finder needle under the medial border of the clavicular head aiming for the ipsilateral nipple. Gradually fan medially until the vein is found. Thread the guidewire down the needle and withdraw the needle. Using a scalpel to create free access through the subcutaneous tissue, insert a dilator over the wire. After withdrawing the dilator, insert the catheter over the wire until it is properly positioned and then remove the wire. Aspirate each lumen of the catheter and flush with heparizined saline. Throughout this procedure, steer clear of the carotid pulsation.
3. Suture the catheter in situ, cover with antibiotic ointment and a sterile dressing.

N.B. In cyanotic children, it is advisable to attach the needle or cannula to a transducer and confirm that the pressure is venous before using the dilator.

To position the tip of the catheter at the junction of the superior vena cava and right atrium, the length should be equal to the distance from skin penetration to a point 2 cm below the upper border of the manubrium.

The tip of the guide wire, accurately placed to just protrude from the catheter, may be used as an internal ECG electrode to position the catheter. Connect the L (leg) lead to the wire with a sterile alligator clip and look at lead II; a biphasic P wave is seen if the catheter is correctly placed.

Always check the position of the tip of the catheter on the radiograph if the catheter is to be left in place postoperatively. Catheters that extend into the right atrium may perforate the heart.

If IJV puncture cannot be performed and the external jugular vein is visible, it may provide a useful alternative route for CVP monitoring.

External Jugular Vein Cannulation

1. Position the child with a 20° head-down tilt and a small roll of towels under the shoulders.

2. Locate the external jugular vein, and prepare and drape the area.
3. Puncture the vein using a 22-gauge intravenous catheter.
4. Feed a J-wire through the catheter and advance it centrally, rotating as necessary. A J-wire with a 3 mm radius of curvature at the J* is most likely to pass easily into the subclavian and towards the heart. The wire must be manipulated gently to avoid the possibility of puncturing the vein. It may be advantageous to abduct the child's arm to direct the wire towards the heart.
5. When the wire has advanced, a dilator may be inserted gently, taking care not to pass it more than 1 to 2 cm into the external jugular vein, otherwise it might tear the vein at the junction with the subclavian.
6. Advance the soft central venous catheter over the guide wire until it is sited at the junction of the superior vena cava and right atrium. This distance can be judged by measuring the distance from skin puncture to manubriosternal junction.
7. The position of long-indwelling CVP lines should always be checked by radiography. Complications (including perforation) may occur if the line is advanced too far.

Other Important Forms of Monitoring

Blood Glucose. Infants, especially preterm or small-for-gestational-age infants are prone to hypoglycemia; their blood glucose levels should be checked frequently. This may be accomplished using an inexpensive hand-held glucometer. The results obtained are accurate enough to detect important abnormalities. Hypoglycemia (less than 40 mg/dl) should be corrected using a glucose infusion (6 mg/kg/min). Avoid excessive glucose administration; however, because it may result in hyperglycemia and glycosuria leading to dehydration and electrolyte losses. Hyperglycemia may increase the extent of cerebral damage should a hypoxic/ischemic episode occur.

Fluid Administration. The intravenous administration of fluids must be very carefully monitored to avoid overload. Syringe pumps or controlled intravenous infusion pumps are recommended for all children, and especially for preterm infants and neonates. Total all fluids given, including those given with drugs. The use of a low-volume remote injection site[†] or an injection cap at the infusion line site minimizes the need for large volumes of flushing fluid. Tuberculin syringes should be used to measure

---

* #C-Doc_18-50-0-2, Cook Medical, Bloomington, Ind.
† Mini-Vol micro bore extension sets, SIMS medical, Keene, N.H.

small doses accurately, avoiding the need to dilute drugs to give accurate doses. When medications are administered in small volumes, flush the IV line to be sure the medication reaches the bloodstream in a timely manner.

Anesthesia Chart. The anesthesia chart is an important monitor and, if well kept, permits the anesthesiologist to detect important trends in the child's progress.

Management Of Body Temperature

Monitoring

Continuous monitoring of body temperature with a thermistor probe is essential for all children undergoing general anesthesia. In larger children having minor surgery, the temperature is usually recorded from the axilla. This reflects the core temperature provided that the tip of the probe is close to the axillary artery and the child's arm is adducted. Adhesive skin temperature sensors (e.g., on the forehead) do not provide an accurate estimate of core temperature. In infants and children undergoing major surgery, core temperature is best monitored in the distal esophagus or rectum. Esophageal temperatures should be recorded at the lower third of the esophagus to avoid falsely low readings caused by gases flowing into the trachea. When using an esophageal stethoscope with a thermistor, adjust the position until the heart sounds are loudest; the thermistor is then optimally placed behind the left atrium.

Tympanic membrane probes have been used to monitor core temperature. The tympanic membrane temperature closely follows lower esophageal temperature, but care must be taken not to damage the ear. We prefer to take the safe, easy, and reliable course and monitor the esophageal temperature during major surgery.

Conservation of Body Heat in Neonates

The objective of body heat conservation is to prevent cold stress and to avoid hypothermia. A reduced body temperature affects recovery from anesthetic and relaxant drugs, impairs coagulation, may depress ventilation, may result in arrhythmias, and increases postoperative oxygen consumption.

The sources of body heat loss are: radiation (39%) > convection (34%) > evaporation (24%) > conduction (3%). Hence preheating the OR and wrapping the child reduces radiation heat loss; the use of a forced air warmer in a closed space decreases convection heat loss. The other sources of heat loss are relatively minor contributions to thermoneutrality.

Preoperatively. Adjust the OR ambient temperature to 24°C (75°F) or greater. Prepare a Bair Hugger* or similar forced air heater and mattress. Keep the child in the heated transport incubator until you are ready to induce anesthesia.

Intraoperatively. Position an infrared heating lamp at the correct distance over the child during induction and preparation for surgery. Keep a cap on the infant's head whenever possible. Use warmed intravenous solutions when large volumes will be infused. A heated humidifier (at 36°C) may be useful if an Ayre's T-piece breathing circuit is used. Warmed (40°C) skin preparation solution should be used, and any excess should be dried from the skin to prevent cooling by evaporation. The use of a forced hot air blanket is preferred during surgery. The use of plastic drapes creates a "warm tent" around the infant.

Postoperatively. Use the infrared heater during extubation and other procedures at the end of anesthesia. Place the infant in a warmed incubator and return the infant promptly to the postanesthesia care unit or the NICU.

Hyperthermia During Surgery

Hyperthermia sometimes develops during surgery if all of the described heat-conserving procedures are followed. If this occurs, the forced air heater should be discontinued. Other causes for hyperthermia during surgery include pyrexial reactions (e.g., from manipulation of an infected organ or a blood transfusion reaction) should be sought; very rarely, it is caused by malignant hyperthermia (MH) (see page 197), cocaine overdose and thyroid storm.

Intravenous Therapy

1. For all children weighing less than 20 kg, insert a buretrol or similar graduated reservoir between the intravenous bag and the administration set; this prevents accidental fluid overload and permits an accurate check of infused volumes.
2. Always use an infusion pump. This allows accurate control of the rate of infusion and easy monitoring of volumes administered. It also provides a warning if the infusion becomes obstructed.
3. Percutaneous insertion of a plastic cannula into a vein is considered optimal. If this is to be done with the child awake, apply a topical local anesthetic cream to the site (in advance, see page 634). Use a 22-gauge cannula or larger if blood transfusion may be required. Observe strict

---

* Augustine Medical Inc., Eden Prairie, Minn.

asepsis when performing cannulation; use Betadine skin preparation solution, and cover the puncture site with a sterile dressing. Label the intravenous line with the size of the cannula and the date and time of insertion.

4. For major abdominal surgery, intravenous access should be secured in the upper limbs.

5. Before surgery commences, ensure that the intravenous line is working well. Do not embark on any procedure with a doubtful intravenous line.

6. Do not be lulled into security if the child has a multilumen CVP since resistance to flow is so great that infusion of blood is impossible. It is unwise to rapidly infuse blood into CVP lines; the temperature or K^+ content of stored blood may cause serious arrhythmias.

Venipuncture for Induction of Anesthesia

The ability to perform a venipuncture painlessly and to cannulate small veins successfully is essential for the pediatric anesthesiologist. Some tips that may help follow.

For venipuncture:

1. Apply a topical local anesthetic cream in advance whenever possible (e.g., see page 634). Alternatively, nitrous oxide may be administered (50% to 75% inspired concentration) to sedate the child during venous cannulation. Make sure that you have a skilled assistant who can distract the child while gently restraining him.

2. Do not use tourniquets in awake children; have your assistant grasp the arm to gently impede venous return and gently squeeze the hand or foot to shift blood into the veins. Do not attempt venipuncture unless the vein is obviously well filled; filling can be facilitated by having the assistant hold the child's hand below body level and apply gentle manual constriction to the limb.

3. Avoid injecting medications into veins in the antecubital fossa or anatomical snuffbox, even if an intravenous catheter is sited in this location. Accidental intraarterial injection is more common here than at any other site and the consequences, which include arterial spasm, may be catastrophic. The risk is greater in young children because of the close proximity of arteries and veins, the small diameter cannulas that may preclude detection of an intraarterial puncture (even if a pump is infusing fluids) and the possibility that the child might move during the injection.

4. A vein on the dorsum of the hand is usually most suitable.

5. Use the smallest size needle and syringe possible, and keep the equipment from the child's view at all times.
6. Hold the needle and syringe firmly, and avoid accidentally touching the skin with the needle until ready to puncture the vein.
7. When ready, puncture the skin and vein firmly with one rapid movement, and then hold the butterfly needle firmly in place until the injection is completed.

Venous Cannulation

This may be performed after induction of anesthesia; otherwise, apply a topical local anesthetic cream in advance of the procedure (see Appendix 3).

1. Select a suitable vein. The best sites usually are the dorsum of the hand, the medial aspect of the ankle (saphenous vein), the lateral aspect of the foot, a scalp vein (in infants), or the lateral aspect of the wrist (in older children). Consider which sites are appropriate (i.e., children with abdominal trauma or a tumor must have intravenous access in an upper extremity. Those children who will be using crutches should not have an intravenous line in the back of the hand).
2. Use careful aseptic technique and prepare the skin with alcohol or Betadine solution.
3. Make sure the vein selected is well filled, and make a small incision over it with an 18-gauge needle.
4. Note the direction of the bevel on the cannula needle. After the initial venous puncture is made, turn the bevel face down before attempting to advance the cannula into the vein. This ensures that the point of the needle is unlikely to be in the distal wall of a small vein and that the cannula will advance unimpeded into the vein (see Figure 4-2). Alternately, when a flashback is observed (suggesting the needle tip is within the lumen), advance the entire unit gently (without excessive pressure) 2 to 3 mm into the lumen of the vein, so that the catheter actually enters the lumen. At that point, check that blood is still flowing back and advance the catheter into the vein.
5. When the cannula is in place, cover it with a sterile dressing. Tape the cannula firmly in place, and immobilize the limb on a splint.
6. When inserting a cannula into a very small vein it may help to pass a fine guidewire into the vein before attempting to advance the catheter:
   a. A 22-gauge Angiocath is inserted toward the vein at a shallow angle.
   b. As soon as there is a "flashback" of blood into the hub of the needle, the cannula is held absolutely still and the needle is very gently removed. Blood is usually seen flowing back into the cannula.

    c. A 0.018-inch (0.46-mm)* diameter spring wire guide is then gently advanced through the cannula into the vein. In most instances this guidewire is easily inserted, even into very small veins, and can be seen tracking inside the vein for some distance up the limb. The cannula is now advanced over the guidewire with full confidence that it will end up lying freely within the lumen of the vein and will provide a very reliable intravenous route.

Intraosseous Infusions

When venipuncture is impossible and urgent fluid or drug therapy is indicated, the intraosseous route should be employed. Any drug or solution that can be given intravenously can also be given by this route. Continuous infusions can be given. In "shock" or "arrest" states, absorption from the intraosseous site may be more rapid than from a peripheral intravenous line.

    The usual insertion sites are the distal femur (midline 1 cm above the patella) and the proximal tibia (medial on the tibial plateau 1 cm below the tuberosity); accidental injections into the epiphysis do not usually cause any harm. A bone marrow needle, a strong large-bore spinal needle, or a specifically designed intraosseous needle† is firmly advanced through the bone until a "give" is noted and the needle stands rigidly. At this point bone marrow can be aspirated and fluid can be injected with very little resistance and with no swelling or extravasations. After initial fluid resuscitation by this route, it is often possible to start an intravenous infusion into a peripheral vein.

Preoperative Fluid Replacement

Most children will have been taking oral fluids up until 2 hours before surgery and will be well hydrated. However, some infants may have serious fluid depletion secondary to their disease, which must be corrected before surgery. Preoperative dehydration in infants can be classified by the size of the deficit as mild, moderate, or severe:

Mild: 50 ml/kg (5% body weight loss) (poor skin turgor, dry mouth)
Moderate: 100 ml/kg (10% body weight loss)(sunken fontanelle, tachycardia, oliguria)
Severe: 150 ml/kg (15% body weight loss)(sunken eyeballs, hypotension, anuria)

---

* Arrow RA-04018, Arrow International Inc., Reading Pa.
† EZIO, Vidacare, San Antonio Tx or BIG, Bone Injection Gun, Waismed Ltd, New York, USA.

Replacement of water and electrolytes should proceed in three phases:

PHASE 1. *Treatment of overt or impending shock* (severe dehydration and hypovolemia): Start with balanced salt solution (lactated Ringer's solution or normal saline—20 ml/kg) while ordering packed cells (10 ml/kg) if anemia is present, plasma or 5% albumin (20 ml/kg) if anemia is not present.

PHASE 2. *Replacement of extracellular water and sodium:* Half the estimated fluid deficit should be replaced over the initial 6 to 8 hours as 0.3 N saline. If the deficit is severe, give an initial infusion of 1 N saline (20 ml/kg). The degree of success of this therapy can be gauged from the clinical signs (heart rate, arterial and venous pressures, and urine output). The following formula is useful in correcting sodium deficiency:

$$Na^+ \text{ deficit (mEq)} = [\text{normal } Na^+ \text{ (mEq)-measured } Na^+ \text{ (mEq)}] \times 0.6 \times \text{weight (kg)},$$

where 0.6 = diffusion constant.
Metabolic acidosis should be treated simultaneously, using the formula:

$$\text{Dose required (mEq of } HCO_3) = \text{base deficit} \times 0.3 \text{ (0.4 for infants)} \times \text{weight (kg)}$$

Give half the calculated requirement, then reassess the acid-base status.

PHASE 3. *Replacement of potassium:* Potassium (K^+) replacement should begin when a good urinary output has been established, according to the following:

1. Replace a maximum of 3 mEq/kg of potassium per 24 hours.
2. The rate of administration should not exceed 0.5 mEq/kg/hr.
3. Complete correction of severe K^+ deficiency may take 4 to 5 days.

These rates only serve as estimates and must be adjusted for changes in metabolic activity, clinical conditions, and extrarenal losses (i.e., gastric suction).

N.B. A neonate's insensible water loss decreases by 30% to 35% when nursed in a high-humidity atmosphere or ventilated with humidified gases. Insensible water loss is increased by crying, sweating, hyperventilation, and the use of a radiant heater or "bili" lights. Pyrexia increases water loss by 12% per 1 °C.

Intraoperative Fluid Management

Calculation of the volume and type of fluid for infusion must take into account:
1. Dehydration present *before* preoperative fasting.

2. Fluid deficit incurred *during* preoperative fasting. (To determine the fluid deficit, use the 4:2:1 rule for hourly requirements [see later discussion] and take the product of that requirement and the number of hours of fasting. Replace half that deficit in the first hour and one fourth the deficit in the subsequent 2 hours)
3. Maintenance fluid requirement during surgery.
4. Estimated extracellular third space fluid loss resulting from surgical trauma.
5. Replacement of blood loss.
6. Alterations in body temperature.

For brief surgical procedures (<10 minutes) in otherwise healthy children, intravenous fluids usually are not needed intraoperatively if the preoperative deficit was small, the fasting period was brief, blood loss or tissue trauma was minimal, and oral intake is likely to be reestablished early (e.g., myringotomy and tubes). An intravenous line should, however, be set up and ready for use should an emergency develop.

For surgical procedures of greater duration, and/or when reestablishment of oral intake may be delayed:

1. An intravenous infusion is established.
2. Fluid is administered intraoperatively and postoperatively until oral intake is reestablished.
3. Lactated Ringer's solution is usually given for simple procedures. For very preterm infants, cachectic children and those who were fasted for a prolonged period, a 1% dextrose solution in lactated Ringer's solution is usually sufficient to maintain normoglycemia. In contrast, 5% dextrose in lactated Ringer's solution may cause hyperglycemia during prolonged infusions.
4. For extensive surgery, especially in infants, it is advantageous to separate the administration of dextrose from other fluid therapy. An infusion of 5% or 10% dextrose can be established at a rate of 4 to 6 mg/kg/min (usually with an infusion pump). Blood glucose levels should be checked periodically. Other isotonic fluids given to replace losses should be free of dextrose. For older children, lactated Ringer's solution is sufficient for prolonged infusions.

The hourly rate of infusion is based on daily maintenance requirements (4:2:1 rule for a hypotonic glucose solution, see later discussion). Adjust the hourly rate if (1) factors affecting insensible fluid loss are present (e.g., increased body temperature) or (2) there are extrarenal losses (e.g., gastrointestinal).

Sufficient fluids should be given to compensate for preoperative fasting. The total volume to be administered during surgery is calculated by multiplying the number of hours (fasting + surgery) by the hourly maintenance requirement.

The 4:2:1 rule for maintenance fluids based on body weight:

4 ml/kg for the first 10 kg, 2 ml/kg for the second 10 kg, and then 1 ml/kg for >20 kg.

Additional Fluids

For surgical procedures causing significant tissue trauma and/or blood loss, give additional fluids to replace extracellular fluid lost in blood or sequestered into damaged tissue. This deficiency should be replaced with a multiple-electrolyte solution (e.g., lactated Ringer's solution) in which the electrolyte concentrations are similar to those in extracellular fluid (Table 4-9). Superficial or extremity surgery (in terms of minimal third space loss) requires only 5 ml/kg/hr fluid replacement, moderate procedures (e.g., spine surgery) requires 10 ml/kg/hr and major procedures (e.g., laparotomy) requires = 15 ml/kg/hr. Thoracotomy is associated with much less translocation of fluid, so smaller fluid volumes are required. When replacing blood loss with balanced salt solutions (such as lactated Ringer's solution), the volume of salt solution required is 3 ml for every milliliter of blood lost. As a general rule, we recommend sending coagulation indices when 75 ml/kg balanced salt solution has been infused. By 100 ml/kg balanced salt solution, consideration should be given to switching to colloid solutions (or blood products). Adequacy of fluid replacement is best judged by continuous monitoring of the cardiovascular indices and urine output. If urine output is less than 0.5 to 1 ml/kg/hr, the fluid infusion rate should be increased.

N.B. Postoperative hyponatremia is a real danger in children. It is usually associated with the intraoperative and postoperative use of hypotonic fluids and occasionally with inappropriate secretion of antidiuretic hormone. Children are much more susceptible than adults to brain damage from hyponatremia. Do not use hypotonic solutions during or after surgery for fluid resuscitation. If, however, balanced salt solutions are used, the postoperative infusion rate is one half that prescribed previously to avoid an excessive sodium load:

The 2:1:0.5 rule for postoperative maintenance fluids based on body weight (balanced salt solutions): 2 ml/kg/hr for the first 10 kg, 1 ml/kg/hr for the second 10 kg, and 0.5 ml/kg/hr for > 20 kg. Monitor serum electrolytes during and after major surgery.

TABLE 4-9 Composition of Electrolyte Solutions

| Solution | Concentration (mEq/L) | | | | | Concentration HCO₃⁻ (mEq/L) | | |
	Na⁺	K⁺	Mg⁺⁺	Ca⁺⁺	Cl⁻	Acetate	Gluconate	Lactate
Normal saline (0.9%)	154	—	—	—	154	—	—	—
0.3 N saline in D₅W	51	—	—	—	51	—	—	—
0.2 N saline in D₅W	34	—	—	—	34	—	—	—
Normosol-M	40	13	3	—	40	16	—	—
Normosol-R	140	5	3	—	98	27	23	—
Lactated Ringer's solution	130	4	—	3	109	—	—	28

Magnesium sulfate (2 ml amp., 50% w/v (where w/v is weight/unit volume)): 4.0 mEq Mg⁺⁺/ml
Sodium bicarbonate (50 ml amp., 7.5% w/v): 0.9 mEq HCO₃⁻/ml
Calcium gluconate (10 ml amp., 10% w/v): 0.447 mEq Ca⁺⁺/ml
Calcium chloride (10 ml amp., 10% w/v): 1.36 mEq Ca⁺⁺/ml
D₅W, 5% dextrose in water.

Suggested Reading

Holliday MA, Friedman AL, Segar WE, et al: Acute hospital-induced hyponatremia in children: a physiologic approach, J Pediatr 145:584–587, 2004.

Barcelona SL, Thompson AA, Coté CJ: Intraoperative pediatric blood transfusion therapy: a review of common issues. Part I: hematologic and physiologic differences from adults; metabolic and infectious risks, Pediatr Anesth 15:716–726, 2005.

Barcelona SL, Thompson AA, Coté CJ: Intraoperative pediatric blood transfusion therapy: a review of common issues. Part II: transfusion therapy, special considerations, and reduction of allogenic blood transfusions, Pediatr Anesth 15:814–830, 2005.

Blood Replacement

Preoperative Assessment

Although minor surgical procedures are commonly performed in children who are mildly anemic with no problems, a normal Hb level (Table 4-10) is desirable in every case of *major* elective surgery. If the child is anemic preoperatively, elective surgery sometimes may be delayed until the anemia has been investigated and treated. In other cases, surgery is more urgent; anesthesia for these children must be administered with a technique that is compatible with their anemia (see Chapter 6). When surgery cannot be delayed despite a very low Hb (e.g., 5 to 7 g/dl), packed cells should be infused preoperatively. Approximately 4 ml/kg of packed cells and 6 ml/kg of whole blood increase the Hb concentration 1 g.

TABLE 4-10 Normal Hemoglobin Levels

Age	Normal Hb Values* (g/dl)
1st day of life	20 (18–22)
2nd wk	17
3 mo	10–11
2 yr	11
3–5 yr	12.5–13.0
5–10 yr	13.0–13.5
10+ yr	14.5

* The Hb concentration declines gradually to about 10-11 g/dl during the first few months of life as fetal Hb is replaced. It then gradually increases and is maximal at about 14 years.

The hemoglobin content of stored whole blood is 12 g/dl; that of packed cells is 24 g/dl; and that of buffy-coat-poor washed cells is 28 g/dl.

When significant blood losses (10% of the estimated blood volume [EBV] or greater) are expected, the child's blood group should be determined and an appropriate number of units cross-matched. Insert a CVP line preoperatively in children who are hypovolemic and/or may require extensive blood replacement during surgery.

Perioperative Management

At commencement of the operation, record the EBV, the preoperative Hb level, and an estimate of the maximal allowable blood loss on the anesthesia record.

Assessment of Blood Loss

Accurate estimates of blood loss must be maintained throughout the surgery.

1. Monitor cardiovascular system indices; in infants, the systolic BP is the most reliable indicator of blood volume.
2. Measure blood loss from the surgical site:
   a. All sponges must be weighed before they dry out. This method is simple and accurate (assume 1 g = 1 ml blood and subtract the known dry weight).
   b. Measure blood from suction (in graduated flasks).
   c. Estimate blood on drapes.
3. Chart the running total continually.
4. Be aware of the possibility that blood losses may accumulate in body cavities (e.g., peritoneum, pleura) or on the surgical drapes and on the floor.

Blood Transfusion

The decision whether to transfuse blood must be based on the preoperative Hb level, the measured surgical blood loss, and the child's cardiovascular response. As a rough guide, in otherwise healthy children, blood replacement may be necessary after loss of 15% of the EBV. The need for blood transfusion can be determined more accurately from serial hematocrit (Hct) measurements. Normally, the Hct should be maintained at or greater than 30% to 40% in infants and in those children with significant cardiac or respiratory disease, and at approximately 25% in other healthy children.

Check each unit of blood against the child's identity bracelet and mix it well by repeated inversion of the bag. Blood should be warmed to 37° C before administration; it should not be heated to more than

38° C, otherwise red cells may be damaged. Packed red blood cells are commonly diluted in saline before administration. Massive blood transfusions in smaller children may require the packed cells to be diluted in fresh-frozen plasma to prevent a dilutional coagulopathy. Calcium is rarely necessary during massive transfusion in children but should be given if persistent hypotension follows apparently adequate volume replacement in infants. This is of particular concern after transfusing fresh frozen plasma (FFP) because it has the greatest concentration of citrate per unit volume of any blood product. If the FFP transfusion is =1 ml/kg/min, then ionized hypocalcemia is likely and exogenous calcium should be administered during the transfusion (5 mg/kg calcium chloride or 15 mg/kg calcium gluconate, repeat as needed). In severely shocked children who require rapid massive transfusion, be prepared to also give sodium bicarbonate if indicated by serial acid-base determinations. Avoid direct transfusion of cold blood products into the right atrium in infants, otherwise life-threatening arrhythmias may ensue.

Massive Blood Transfusion

If it becomes apparent that massive blood transfusion will be required (i.e., more than one blood volume), institute monitoring of coagulation indices. Platelet counts, prothrombin time, and partial thromboplastin time together with tests for fibrinolysis (determination of fibrin split products) should be repeated at least after every 50% blood volume replacement. It is helpful to have a preoperative platelet count if massive transfusion is a possibility. A low initial count may necessitate early platelet transfusion. Platelet counts of less than 50,000/mm³ increase clinical bleeding and should be corrected. In practice, if platelets are monitored during a continuing massive replacement, platelets should be ordered as the count decreases below 100,000/mm³. Infusion of 5 to 10 ml/kg of platelet concentrate increases the platelet count by 50,000 to 10,000/mm³. Platelets must be stored at room temperature, not refrigerated, and they should be rocked periodically. Other deficiencies that become apparent should be dealt with by appropriate therapy (e.g., fresh frozen plasma—10 to 15 ml/kg increases factor levels by 15% to 20%).

Cryoprecipitate may be required if bleeding persists despite all other measures in small infants (1 to 2 units/kg increase fibrinogen by 60 to 100 mg/dl). Remember that FFP, cryoprecipitate, and platelet solutions contain more citrate per unit volume than does whole blood. Therefore calcium infusions may be required if hypotension occurs as these products are given rapidly.

Alternatives to Blood Transfusion

The risk of infection through transfusion has prompted the search for alternatives, many of which may be applicable in children:

1. *Autologous transfusion of blood donated preoperatively:* Suitable size donations may be collected at 4- to 5-day intervals, preoperatively. If blood donation is combined with measures to increase erythropoiesis (oral iron 6 to 8 weeks in advance, erythropoietin 3 to 4 weeks in advance), significant volumes may be collected. These techniques are most applicable to older children and teenagers.

2. *Blood conservation:* Blood losses are minimized through the use of proper positioning, infiltration of vasoconstrictors, induced moderate hypotension, and meticulous surgical technique.

3. *Acute normovolemic hemodilution:* Blood is withdrawn after anesthesia but before surgery commences, and replaced with three times the volume of warmed lactated Ringer's solution. It has been suggested that hemodilution to a Hct of 25% is acceptable in otherwise healthy children. Blood is then reinfused as the surgery proceeds, saving the first collected unit of blood to be transfused last. The volume to be collected can be calculated from the following formulae:

$$EBV = weight(kg) \times 70 \text{ ml/kg (or Table 2-5)}$$

$$Volume = EBV \times [(\text{initial Hct-target Hct})/\text{average Hct}]$$

4. *Intraoperative autotransfusion of shed blood using a "cell saver":* This technique has limited application, but it may be useful in orthopedic surgery. Shed red cells may be collected by suction, washed, and reinfused. However, coagulation factors are discarded in the washing process, and extensive reinfusion of washed cells may lead to dilution of these factors and coagulopathy.

Special Considerations in Providing Anesthesia for the Preterm Infant

1. *Infection:* The immune system is immature, and the preterm infant is particularly prone to infection. Use careful aseptic technique for all invasive procedures.

2. *Intraventricular hemorrhage:* The preterm infant is prone to intraventricular hemorrhage. Avoid causing fluctuations in blood pressure, ensure adequate anesthesia, avoid overtransfusion, infuse hypertonic solutions slowly (e.g., dextrose, sodium bicarbonate), and treat anemia and coagulopathy.

3. *Apneic spells:* These are common in preterm infants, who must be monitored closely at all times and especially during and after anesthesia. Risk factors for perioperative apnea include:

   a. Preterm infants of less than 45 weeks postconceptual age are more likely to experience significant episodes of apnea than term infants; those less than 34 weeks gestational age at birth are at greater risk.
   b. Anemia (Hct <30%).
   c. A history of apnea episodes and use of an apnea monitor indicate greater risk.
   d. The presence of chronic lung disease increases the risk of apnea.
   e. The presence of any comorbidity.
   f. Parental cigarette smoking.

In very small infants, the risk of apnea may extend for as long as 72 hours into the postoperative period. The following are general recommendations:

   a. It is common practice to admit and monitor all preterm infants of less than 60 weeks postconceptual age after any general or regional anesthesia (see page 139).
   b. Older infants should also be admitted and observed if there is any evidence of ventilatory disturbance in the perioperative period.

N.B. Apnea may be less common after surgery performed under spinal analgesia, but it may still occur, so the child must still be admitted and monitored. Caffeine therapy (10 mg/kg IV administered slowly after induction) may prevent or reduce the incidence of apnea, but monitoring is still advised.

4. *Temperature control:* The preterm infant is extremely vulnerable to heat loss—even more so than the full-term neonate. The surface area is even larger relative to body mass, there are no insulating subcutaneous tissues and the brown fat stores are deficient. Be especially alert to prevent heat loss at all times because these infants cannot generate much heat.

5. *Oxygenation:* This must be very carefully controlled if hyperoxia is to be avoided and the risk of retinopathy of prematurity minimized. Inspired concentrations must be kept to the minimum that will allow safe conduct of general anesthesia. Monitor with a pulse oximeter and attempt to keep the saturation between 90% and 95%.

   a. Ascertain the Fio_2 required preoperatively that ensures satisfactory oxygenation. During nonthoracic surgery with controlled ventilation, continue with this Fio_2 and check saturation.

   b. Whenever N_2O is contraindicated, use an air-O_2 mixture to achieve the desired FIO_2 and saturation.
   c. During intrathoracic surgery it is often essential to increase the FIO_2; monitor saturation and limit the O_2 concentration as far as possible while avoiding the possibility of inducing hypoxemia.
6. ***Hypoglycemia and hyperglycemia:*** Preterm infants are prone to hypoglycemia. Blood sugar levels should be checked frequently, and hypoglycemia (less than 40 mg/dl) should be corrected by infusions of glucose. The preterm infant is also subject to hyperglycemia, which is usually iatrogenic but may also be caused by poor insulin response and continued glycolysis. Hyperglycemia leads to glycosuria, osmotic diuresis, and dehydration and should be avoided by frequent blood sugar determinations and controlled intravenous glucose administration.
7. ***Fluid administration:*** Avoid overload by very careful metering the infusion of intravenous fluids. Determine the total intravenous fluids given, including those given with drugs. Use small (1 ml) syringes to accurately measure small volumes of drugs. Syringe pumps and controlled infusion lines are essential.
8. ***Benzyl alcohol:*** This is used as a preservative in multidose vials of some medications and has been linked with kernicterus, intraventricular hemorrhage, and mortality in preterm infants. Preparations containing this substance should be avoided.
9. ***Coagulation:*** Ensure that vitamin K has been administered. The preterm infant is also subject to coagulopathy associated with shock and sepsis. Thrombocytopenia is common. Perform coagulation studies on all seriously ill preterm infants. Platelet concentrates, FFP, or exchange transfusion may be required.

ANESTHESIA FOR OUTPATIENT SURGERY

Advantages

1. The child's psychological upset is minimized.
2. There is less risk of hospital-acquired infection.
3. Cost of care is reduced; hospital beds are available for others.

Selection of Cases

1. The child must be healthy or have any chronic disease under good control.
2. The child's parents must be reliable and willing to follow instructions concerning preoperative and postoperative care.

3. The operation should be associated with minor physiologic upset, requiring no complex postoperative care or pain management.
4. Infants who were born preterm and are still less than 60 weeks post-conceptual age should be admitted and monitored for 12 hours for apnea.*

Suggested Reading

Coté CJ, Zaslavsky A, Downes JJ, et al: Postoperative apnea in former preterm infants after inguinal herniorrhaphy: a combined analysis, Anesthesiology 82:809–822, 1995.
Walther-Larsen S, Rasmussen LS: The former preterm infant and risk of postoperative apnoea: recommendations for management, Acta Anaesth Scand 50:888–893, 2006.

Preoperative Preparation

Preoperative preparation is the same as for inpatient surgery. The parents should be given written instructions concerning preoperative fasting and methods to prepare their child for a visit to the hospital. They should also be given a health questionnaire to complete and bring with them to facilitate obtaining a medical history for the child (Figure 4-4).

On the day of the operation, the child is brought to the outpatient department surgical unit. Routine Hb determination is not required for healthy children but should be obtained when the child appears anemic or chronic disease is present. A sickle cell preparation is obtained if indicated (i.e., in a child who has not been previously tested or whose status is unknown). The parent's or legal guardian's consent for operation must be properly obtained.

The anesthesiologist makes a preoperative assessment by taking the history, examining the child, and noting laboratory data. This may be done on the day of surgery or a few days before at the anesthesia assessment clinic.

Anesthetic Techniques and Tricks

Premedication is not routinely given to outpatients in order that the recovery phase is not prolonged. Many properly prepared children attending for outpatient surgery with their parents are not very upset,

---

* This remains the recommended practice in the United States. A recent meta-analysis suggested that completely healthy preterm infants who are more than 46 weeks PCA be monitored postoperatively for 6 hours apnea-free before discharge. However, until prospective studies confirm the safety of this strategy, we recommend 12 hours of monitoring.

Questionnaire for Outpatients

Please complete this form and bring it with you. This will assist in the preoperative evaluation of your child.

Has your child ever been hospitalized before?	yes/no
Why/when?_____	
Was your child premature?	yes/no
Has your child ever had an anesthetic before?	yes/no
Any problems?_____	
Has any family member had problems with anesthesia?	yes/no
Details:_____	
Is there any family history of muscle, nerve or bleeding disorders?	yes/no
Details:_____	
Does your child take any medicines or herbal remedies?	yes/no
Please list: _____	
Has your child ever been treated with prednisone or similar medicines?	yes/no
Does your child have allergies?	yes/no

If yes, please circle or list the relevant items:

      i. Latex or toy balloons, band-aids, bananas, eggplant, other fruit.

      ii. Antibiotics or other medicines.

          Type of allergic reaction: _____

      iii. Other foods or household items: _____

Is your child exposed to cigarette smoke at home?	yes/no
Has your child had a head cold recently?	yes/no
Has your child ever had asthma?	yes/no
Ever admitted to hospital with asthma?	yes/no
Does your child have loose teeth, dental plate, or dental appliance?	yes/no
Does your child bruise or bleed easily?	yes/no
Does your child have muscular dystrophy or other muscle disease?	yes/no
Any other medical issues we should know about your child's health?	yes/no
Details:_____	

For Adolescents

Do you smoke or take any drugs?	yes/no
Details:_____	
Do you have any ear-rings or other body piercings?	yes/no
Details:_____	
Has menstruation commenced?	yes/no
Date of last menstrual period _____	

      Child's name: _____

      Parent's name: _____

      Date: _____

Figure 4-4. Questionnaire for outpatients.

and premedication may not be necessary. In the event that the child is apprehensive, premedication may be administered, as described earlier (see page 86).

Use simple general anesthesia techniques that are likely to result in rapid recovery. Do not give unnecessary drugs that might increase postoperative morbidity (a single dose of any opioid increases the incidence of postoperative nausea and vomiting). Inhaled agents have been widely used for pediatric outpatients, sevoflurane being the agent of choice for short procedures. Simple inhalation anesthesia for brief procedures in children is followed by relatively rapid and complete recovery. TIVA using propofol, remifentanil, and a short-acting muscle relaxant is an alternative technique.

It is preferable, whenever possible, to supplement a light general anesthetic with the appropriate regional analgesia technique. If the block is established before surgery, it provides analgesia during and after surgery while reducing anesthetic requirements and the need for opioids. Regional block before surgery may also reduce the total pain experienced after surgery (preemptive analgesia) and reduce the incidence of postoperative nausea and vomiting.

The introduction of propofol has provided the alternative of using an infusion technique that is also followed by a rapid recovery and minimal morbidity. Propofol infusion may be used to supplement regional analgesia, or it may be combined with a short-acting opioid (e.g., alfentanil, remifentanil) and an intermediate-acting relaxant drug (e.g., rocuronium or cis-atracurium), depending on the surgical procedure. A suitable regimen for total intravenous anesthesia for children undergoing relatively short procedures would be the following:

Propofol: 2.5 to 3.5 mg/kg for induction, then infusion of
250 μg/kg/min for 10 minutes; 200 μg/kg/min for next 10 minutes and 150 μg/kg/min for remainder of operation
In addition, remifentanil-loading dose; 0.5 to 2 μg/kg infusion @ 0.1 to 2 μg/kg/minute
Rectal acetaminophen (35 to 45 mg/kg) and ketorolac (0.5 mg/kg IV, up to 15 mg for children <50 kg and up to 30 mg for those >50 kg) for mild to moderate pain (given after conferring with the surgeon and after hemostasis is achieved);

Tracheal intubation should be used whenever indicated; postintubation complications can be prevented by gentle laryngoscopy and by using a tracheal tube that passes easily through the glottis and subglottic space. A small leak should be present when the circuit is pressurized to 20 to 30 cm H_2O. In many cases the LMA is a suitable alternative for the healthy outpatient. For dental surgery, a nasotracheal tube is used (see previous discussion). At the end of the procedure, always perform a laryngoscopy, suction the pharynx well, and ensure that all throat packs and other items have been removed.

For strabismus surgery, a propofol infusion with oxygen/air is associated with less nausea and vomiting than when inhalational agents are used. Current antiemetic management for strabismus surgery when using inhaled agents includes ondansetron (0.05 mg/kg, maximum 4 mg) and dexamethasone (0.1 mg/kg, maximum 8 mg) IV.

Some procedures in older children may be performed under regional analgesia; when possible, this is ideal for the outpatient. For example, for superficial surgery on the limbs, an intravenous block may provide excellent results.

Postoperative Care for the Outpatient

Many children require no analgesics immediately after surgery, especially if a regional block has been performed (e.g., for hernia; see page 153 & 395), but beware of the "analgesic window," which may occur later at home as the block wears off. Analgesics should be ordered in anticipation of pain and should be administered by the clock rather than waiting for pain to occur. Plan for adequate continuing analgesia, and thoroughly instruct the parents on how to dose their child; provide written instructions. Acetaminophen and/or acetaminophen with codeine can be given in the usual dose depending on the surgery. More potent analgesics are seldom indicated for outpatients. It is important, however, to be aware that up to 10% of some ethnic groups poorly convert codeine to morphine and thus receive no analgesia from the codeine (see previous discussion).

Many children take and retain oral fluids well before discharge, but it is unwise to "push" oral fluids before the child is ready to drink; doing so increases the incidence of postoperative vomiting. A useful method of fluid administration is to offer Popsicles ad lib, especially to children who have undergone tonsillectomy or adenoidectomy (see Chapter 10).

Every child should be discharged from the postanesthesia care unit (PACU) by the anesthesiologist or his/her designee; in most cases standard discharge criteria may be used. Infants may be taken home when they have fully recovered. Children should be tested for street fitness and should be able to walk out; if dizzy or nauseated, they must stay longer. If the anesthesiologist determines that a child is unfit for discharge, overnight admission is recommended.

Children must be accompanied home by an adult, who preferably should not also be the driver of the vehicle. Warn the parents that their child must not ride a bicycle or engage in dangerous activities for 24 hours. A brochure containing basic information and a follow-up service should be provided. Parents should be carefully instructed regarding the treatment of postoperative pain. As more complex procedures are being performed in the day surgery unit, the need for effective postoperative analgesia is increasing. Parents should be instructed of the need to administer analgesic drugs before pain becomes severe. They can be instructed in the use of visual analog scores or other means to assess their child's pain, and provided with suitable charts to record this. Parents must be encouraged to seek advice from the hospital if problems develop during the postoperative period. A follow-up phone call should be made to the parents on the evening of surgery.

Complications After Pediatric Outpatient Surgery

Complications are rare after pediatric outpatient surgery, with fewer than 1% of children requiring overnight admission after a planned outpatient procedure. The most common reasons for admission are protracted vomiting or a complication of surgery. Nausea and vomiting are a predictable consequence of some types of surgery (i.e., correction of strabismus, tonsillectomy). In such cases the choice of anesthesia techniques (i.e., propofol) or the preemptive administration of effective antiemetic drugs are recommended.

Complications that may occur at home include vomiting, cough, sleepiness, sore throat, and hoarseness. If the parents are well prepared, these can usually be treated effectively in the home.

5 Regional Analgesia Techniques

LOCAL ANESTHETIC DRUGS

Local analgesic drugs are now very widely used in children, particularly in the management of postoperative pain (Table 5-1).

TABLE 5-1   Maximum Doses of Local Anesthetics*

Local Anesthetic	Dose (mg/kg)
Bupivacaine[†] Plain or with epinephrine	2.5
Ropivacaine[†] and levobupivacaine[†]	3.0
Lidocaine[†] Without epinephrine	4.5
With epinephrine	7
Mepivacaine[†] or prilocaine[†] Without epinephrine	5
With epinephrine	7
Tetracaine	1.5
Procaine	10
2-chloroprocaine[‡]	20

* Maximum dose may depend on site of injection.
[†] Doses for continuous infusions of amides should be reduced by 30% in infants <6 mos.
[‡] For children >3 yr.

Clinical Pharmacology

Local analgesic drugs are amino esters (procaine, chloroprocaine, tetracaine) or amino amides (lidocaine, bupivacaine, ropivacaine) that interrupt nerve conduction by blocking sodium channels.

The pharmacokinetics in infants differ from those in older children and adults:

1. Absorption of the drugs is rapid, the cardiac output and regional tissue blood flows are greater, and the epidural space contains less fat tissue to buffer uptake. Drugs sprayed into the airway are very rapidly absorbed.
2. The volume of distribution of the drug is larger. Plasma levels of bupivacaine after administration of a 2.5 mg/kg dose into the epidural space in infants are therefore significantly less than in young children and adults. This greater volume of distribution also prolongs the elimination half-life.
3. The extent of protein binding in the neonate is less than in children because serum albumin and α_1-acid glycoprotein levels are reduced. Bilirubin, which binds to the acidic sites on albumin, does not interfere with bupivacaine binding as the latter binds to the basic binding sites.
4. The rate of metabolism of local analgesic drugs is reduced in very young infants:

a. Plasma cholinesterase activity is reduced, which may prolong the metabolism of the ester type of drugs. For example, the plasma half-life of ester anesthetics is extended in the neonate. This is probably clinically insignificant.

b. The hepatic pathways (cytochrome P450) for conjugation of the amide local analgesics are immature. The neonate has a reduced capacity to metabolize bupivacaine; clearance at 1 month of age is only one third of adult rates, although, by 9 months, clearance reaches adults rates. This may lead to clinical problems in neonates during prolonged infusions of bupivacaine (i.e., limit infusions to 48 hours at 0.2 mg/kg/hr). Older infants and children metabolize drugs much more rapidly because of their relatively large liver size.

5. The metabolism of prilocaine may result in methemoglobinemia. This may be more important in infants with reduced levels of the enzyme methemoglobin reductase, and may be significant if large areas of skin are covered with EMLA cream.

Local Anesthetic Drugs

Lidocaine

Lidocaine is commonly used for local infiltration. Total dose should not exceed 4.5 mg/kg of the plain solution or 7 mg/kg if epinephrine is added. Epinephrine prolongs the block and decreases the peak serum concentration by about 40%.

Bupivacaine

Bupivacaine is a racemic mixture; the levo form is the clinically active form and the dextro form is the more toxic form. It has been widely used for peripheral and epidural blocks. It has the disadvantage that overdosing or accidental intravascular injection may lead to severe myocardial depression that may be prolonged and difficult to reverse (see Intralipid). Bupivacaine metabolism is reduced in small infants requiring close attention to dose (see Clinical Pharmacology). The addition of epinephrine to bupivacaine is less effective in prolonging the block and decreasing peak serum concentration than it is for lidocaine. However, epinephrine does extend the duration of action of bupivacaine to a greater extent in infants and young children than in older children.

Levobupivacaine

Levobupivacaine is the levo enantiomer of bupivacaine. It is less cardiotoxic, approximately 20% more potent than bupivacaine and may be more suitable for prolonged infusions.

Ropivacaine

Ropivacaine is also a levo enantiomer, but of the racemate termed ropivacaine. It too is less cardiotoxic than bupivacaine and produces an equal sensory block with a more rapid onset, less motor block, but similar duration of effect. It has gained popularity as an agent for caudal analgesia. Compared with bupivacaine, ropivacaine is less rapidly absorbed from the caudal epidural space, and peak plasma levels are less after an ilioinguinal nerve block. *Ropivacaine should not be used for penile or digital nerve blocks as vasoconstriction and ischemia have been reported.* Epinephrine does not prolong the duration of an epidural or other blocks with ropivacaine.

Toxicity

Maximum dosages of local anesthetics have been recommended to prevent overdoses (see Table 5-1).

Compared with adults, neonates may exhibit signs of central nervous system toxicity (jitteriness and seizures) at lower blood levels of a drug. Local analgesic blocks in children are commonly performed during general anesthesia. This practice tends to mask any signs of neurologic toxicity, but depending upon the anesthesia agent used might increase cardiac toxicity. If seizures occur, 100% oxygen should be administered, the airway secured, and medication to stop the seizure administered immediately: intravenous benzodiazepine (i.e., midazolam 0.05 to 0.2 mg/kg), thiopental (2 to 3 mg/kg), or propofol (1 to 2 mg/kg) in repeated doses as required. Because potent inhalational anesthetics (e.g., halothane) may augment the cardiac effects of the local anesthetic drugs, caution is advised.

N.B. Acute intravascular (intravenous or intraosseous) injection of bupivacaine (and less likely ropivacaine or levobupivacaine) may cause ventricular tachycardia and difficulty restoring normal sinus rhythm, both resulting in a low cardiac output state. To date, no pharmacologic intervention has reversed these cardiac effects of local anesthetics. However, anecdotal reports in adults and studies in animals suggest a role for intravenous Intralipid (20%) at 1 ml/kg loading dose followed by either 1 ml/kg every 3 to 5 minutes (total of 3 ml/kg) or an infusion of 0.25 to 0.5 ml/kg/min after an acute intravascular overdose of bupivacaine (and other local anesthetics) with acute myocardial dysfunction. The mechanism is believed to be elution of the local anesthetic from the myocardium by the lipid. To date, only one case reported successful recovery in a child given a toxic dose of bupivacaine. (**N.B.** Propofol should *not* be substituted for Intralipid if the latter is not available to resuscitate a local anesthetic toxicity.)

Intravenous lidocaine in normal doses may produce toxic effects in children with right-to-left cardiac shunting because the normal first-pass absorption within the pulmonary circulation is bypassed. The dose should be reduced by at least 50% in such cases.

Adjuvant Drugs

Epinephrine

Epinephrine is added to local anesthetic drugs to extend their duration of action, and to limit absorption of the drug into the intravascular space. It also acts as a marker for intravascular injection; peaked T waves and ST segment elevation are more reliable signs of intravascular injection than tachycardia, although this also may depend on the inhalational anesthetic administered. Certainly, tachycardia may be more difficult to assess and therefore is less sensitive a warning sign in children. Epinephrine may interact with halothane and precipitate arrhythmias, but doses up to 10 μg/kg by infiltration are considered safe in children.

Clonidine

Clonidine (1 to 2 μg/ml) may be added to local anesthetics for use in the caudal/epidural space. This will prolong the effect of the block approximately 3 hours (based on a systematic review), but has inconsistent effects on the rate of elimination of the local analgesic from the epidural space.

Apnea has been reported after epidural clonidine administration in preterm infants, although three toddlers who received a 100 fold overdose of clonidine experienced only prolonged postoperative sedation and no respiratory distress/apnea. Clonidine may also contribute to postoperative sedation (usually at doses >2 μg/kg) and this may be undesirable in outpatients.

Suggested Reading

Arsermino M, Basu R, Vanderbeek C, et al: Nonopioid additives to local anaesthetics for caudal blockade in children, Paediatr Anaesth 13:561–573, 2003.

Mazoit JX, Dalens BJ: Pharmacokinetics of local anaesthetics in infants and children, Clin Pharm 43:17–32, 2004.

Berde C: Local anesthetics in infants and children: an update, Paediatr Anaesth 14:387–393, 2004.

Mayer C, Cambray R: One hundred times the intended dose of caudal clonidine in three pediatric patients, Paediatr Anaesth 18:888–890, 2008.

REGIONAL ANALGESIA FOR PAIN CONTROL

Regional analgesia techniques alone are of limited value during pediatric surgical procedures; the overall nonacceptance and lack of cooperation in the awake young child results in the need for such large doses of sedatives that general anesthesia usually becomes preferable. However, in the management of postoperative pain, regional analgesic techniques have become an indispensable part of our pediatric anesthesia practice (see later discussion).

Regional analgesia may provide acceptable pain control intraoperatively for some selected children:

1. Spinal and/or epidural anesthesia is useful for small infants, especially for the preterm infant with or without lung disease for herniotomy, circumcision, or lower abdominal surgery. This is a means of reducing, but not eliminating the probability of postoperative apnea.
2. Epidural analgesia may be a suitable alternative to general anesthesia in some older children (e.g., those with cystic fibrosis), and it may then be continued into the postoperative period.
3. Some older children (5 years of age and older) can be charmed into cooperation and have their upper limb fractures reduced under a regional block.
4. Intravenous regional analgesia (Bier block) can be used for some older children having superficial surgery to lesions on the distal limbs or for some fracture reductions. (Extreme caution must be exercised if a plaster cast is applied to an exsanguinated limb).
5. The possibility of using regional or local infiltration analgesia (see Table 5-1) should also be considered for any minor procedure in a high-risk patient (e.g., skeletal muscle biopsy in a child with cardiomyopathy, lymph node biopsy in a child with a mediastinal mass).

Rarely, regional blocks are also indicated for chronic pain therapy and/or diagnostic purposes.

Basic rules for regional analgesia are as follows:

1. Calculate the allowable weight-based dose of the local analgesic agent for each child and do not exceed that dose.
2. Use as much of the allowable dose of agent as is necessary to ensure a good block.
3. Use careful aseptic technique; beware of intravascular injection. Test by aspirating frequently.
4. Plan ahead; allow a generous period for the block to become well established before allowing the surgeon to approach the child.

5. Remember the special considerations for the use of local analgesic drugs in infants and young children (see previous discussion).

6. Always be prepared to deal with the complications of regional analgesia. Drugs and equipment to induce general anesthesia, secure the airway, and ventilate the lungs must be immediately available. Establish IV access before the block. A source of Intralipid should be immediately available to treat an intravascular injection of local anesthetic (see Toxicity).

7. Be prepared; unsatisfactory regional analgesia may require administration of general anesthesia to permit completion of the surgical procedure.

8. If possible, apply topical anesthetic cream over the site of the proposed initial needle insertion point (see page 634).

9. Children are generally upset by paresthesias; techniques that do not rely on eliciting these effects are preferred.

10. The use of ultrasound has been demonstrated to be very effective in accurately placing the local analgesic solution. This technique should be applied whenever possible.

11. Supplement your regional technique with age-appropriate sedation (e.g., oral midazolam), systemic analgesics (e.g., fentanyl intravenously), and distraction (i.e., video or transistor radio and earphones).

12. The consensus of pediatric anesthesiologists is that it is acceptable standard practice to perform a caudal or lumbar epidural block including passing an indwelling catheter in an anesthetized child. Children will not lie still to have the catheter inserted while they are awake or sedated. The risks of inserting the block under general anesthesia are considered less than the risks of inserting it in a distressed and mobile awake child.

13. When a choice exists, peripheral nerve blocks are generally safer than neuraxial blocks in infants and children.

14. Do not use epinephrine for blocks of areas with inadequate collateral blood supply (digits, penis).

15. Do not administer sedatives to former preterm infants with a spinal or epidural as this will markedly increase the potential for apnea.

Suggested Reading

Suresh S, Wheeler M: Practical pediatric regional anesthesia, Anes Clin N Am 20:83–113, 2002.

Eck JB, Ross AK: Paediatric regional anaesthesia—what makes a difference? Best practice and research, Clin Anaesthesiol 16:159–174, 2002.

AN OUTLINE OF PROCEDURES FOR REGIONAL BLOCKS IN INFANTS AND CHILDREN

For more detailed descriptions of the anatomic considerations and techniques of regional nerve blocks, the reader is referred to standard textbooks.

Awake Spinal Analgesia for Infants

In infants, awake spinal analgesia is most commonly indicated for surgery at or below the umbilicus, but it has also been used for upper abdominal surgery in small infants with a history of respiratory disease. It avoids the necessity to intubate and ventilate the lungs and therefore reduces the risk of additional airway damage or ventilator dependence. Very little change in blood pressure occurs in infants or children after spinal block. Postoperative apnea of the former preterm infant is less common after spinal analgesia but is still a risk. Supplemental sedation will increase the potential for apnea.

Special Considerations

1. The spinal cord may extend to as low as L3 in the infant (compared with L1–2 in the older child or adult), so perform the lumbar puncture at L4–5.
2. The dural space extends to S3–4 in the neonate.
3. The volume of cerebrospinal fluid (CSF) in infants (4 ml/kg) is relatively greater than in adults (2 ml/kg).

Contraindications

1. Sepsis or infected lumbar puncture site.
2. Coagulopathy.
3. Lack of enthusiastic parental consent.

Anesthetic Management

Preoperative

1. The child should be fasted as for general anesthesia.
2. No premedication is necessary for small infants.

Perioperative

1. Observe all special precautions for infants, both term and preterm. Prepare the anesthesia machine, endotracheal tubes, and all ancillary equipment.
2. A brandy-and-sugar soother is often useful to settle the infant. (Glucose may have analgesic properties of its own in neonates.) Sedatives such as ketamine or midazolam that supplement a spinal will cause a similar incidence of apnea as general anesthesia.

3. Establish a reliable intravenous infusion using local analgesia in the lower extremity.
4. Scrub, glove, and sterilize the skin.
5. Instruct your assistant to gently but firmly restrain the child in the chosen lateral or sitting position, but avoid neck flexion, which may compromise the airway.
6. Prepare and drape the child. Infiltrate the skin over the L4–5 interspace with 1% lidocaine.
7. Prepare a neonatal spinal needle (e.g., 22 or 25-gauge, 1 inch [26 mm] long) and measure the dead space of this needle with the use of a tuberculin syringe.
8. Prepare a syringe containing 0.4 to 1.0 mg/kg of 1% tetracaine mixed with an equal volume of 10% dextrose, plus a volume of this mixture equal to the dead space of the needle (approximately 0.2 ml). For upper abdominal/thoracic surgery, 1 mg/kg of tetracaine (1%) or bupivacaine (0.5% to 0.75%) in preterm infants (<4 kg).
9. Insert the needle at L4–5 with the bevel facing laterally until CSF is obtained.
10. Slowly inject the local analgesic solution; rapid injection may result in a high or total spinal.
11. Carefully return the infant to the supine position and place the pulse oximeter and blood pressure cuff on the lower extremity. Motor function in lower limbs usually ceases immediately. Do not allow the child's legs to be raised (e.g., to apply the cautery pad) or an excessively high level block may result.
12. Duration of anesthesia is usually about 1.5 hours.
13. **N.B.** Total spinal anesthesia in infants is heralded by apnea with little change in blood pressure. Treat with controlled ventilation until recovery occurs.

Perioperative

1. Continue to nurse the child in the horizontal position until motor function in the legs returns.
2. Monitor the infant born prematurely carefully for apnea; it is less common than after general anesthesia but may occur.

Suggested Reading

Williams RK, Adams DC, Aladjem EV, et al: The safety and efficacy of spinal anesthesia for surgery in infants: the Vermont Infant Spinal Registry, Anesth Analg 102(1):67–71, 2006.

Caudal Block

The caudal block is very useful in infants and children; it provides good postoperative analgesia after abdominal, lower limb, or perineal surgery. Caudal analgesia has also been used as an alternative to spinal analgesia for lower abdominal surgery in infants. In young infants, the contents of the epidural space offer little resistance to the spread of local analgesic solutions. In this age group, epidural analgesia is accompanied by very little change in blood pressure or cardiac output. Continuous caudal catheters have been used intraoperatively for more prolonged surgery, and they may safely be threaded to a surprising distance cephalad (T6). Local infection has not been a problem when catheters have been left in situ for 3 days.

Caudal morphine provides analgesia for thoracic and abdominal procedures and reduces the need for systemic analgesic drugs. However, caudal opioids are associated with side effects that include nausea, vomiting, and rarely respiratory depression; hence this regime is unsuitable for outpatients and for infants.

Preferred Technique

For postoperative analgesia, the block should be performed after general anesthesia has been induced but before the surgery commences. This allows for the block to become well established during surgery, offers the potential for preemptive analgesia, permits a reduction in general anesthetic agents, and allows a more rapid awakening.

The child is placed in the lateral decubitus position with the upper knee and hip well flexed. The landmarks are then identified (Figure 5-1): the tip of the coccyx to fix the midline and the sacral cornua bounding the sacral hiatus. These lie at the apex of an inverted equilateral triangle, the base of which is a line drawn between the posterior superior iliac spines. The child is carefully prepared and draped, and the operator wears gloves and a mask. The skin over the sacral hiatus is nicked with an 18-gauge needle (to avoid tracking epidermal tissues into the caudal canal), after which an IV catheter (22 gauge for children <2 yr, 20 gauge for those >2 yr) is advanced cephalad at an angle of 45° to the skin with the bevel facing anteriorly. A distinctive sudden "give" is felt as the needle passes through the sacrococcygeal ligament. At this point, the angle of the needle is reduced and the catheter only is advanced into the caudal canal (Figure 5-2). The needle is then withdrawn, leaving the intravenous catheter in the caudal/epidural space. The catheter should be observed for passive reflux of blood or CSF. If there is no evidence of

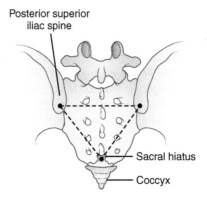

Figure 5-1 Caudal block: landmarks.

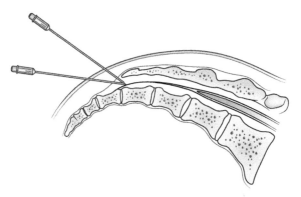

Figure 5-2 Caudal block: direction of needle insertion.

blood or CSF, the local anesthetic may be injected slowly in incremental doses (there should be no resistance to injection; if there is resistance, then the catheter is either kinked or misplaced) while the electrocardiogram is observed. Changes in QRS pattern and/or peaked T waves may be an early sign of intravascular injection. A finger should be placed over the sacrum to detect inadvertent subcutaneous injection. Advancing an intravenous catheter rather than a needle diminishes the risk of an intravascular or intraosseous injection, even if the child moves. Some advocate listening over the lower lumbar spine with a stethoscope during the injection of local anesthetic to auscultate a "Swoosh" with a successful caudal insertion.

Drugs, Concentrations, and Volumes

For single-shot caudal analgesia in outpatients, 0.125% to 0.175% bupivacaine with epinephrine provides analgesia as effective as that of 0.25% bupivacaine with less motor block. (The 0.175% bupivacaine can be prepared by adding 3 ml of preservative-free saline to 7 ml of 0.25% bupivacaine with epinephrine [total volume 10 ml] whereas the 0.125% solution is prepared with equal volumes of 0.25% bupivacaine and preservative free saline.) Ropivacaine 0.2% appears to provide similar analgesia and duration of action to bupivacaine and may be less cardiotoxic.

The addition of clonidine [1 to 2 μg/ml] to bupivacaine (where 1 ml/kg local anesthetic solution is instilled) has been reported in a systematic review to extend its duration of action approximately 3 hours. Other drugs that have been used to prolong caudal analgesia include preservative-free midazolam and preservative-free ketamine; however, approved preparations are not currently available in the United States. The following are volumes to be injected via the caudal route:

Perineal surgery (e.g., hypospadias repair): 0.5 ml/kg

Lower abdominal surgery (e.g., orchidopexy): 1.0 ml/kg

Caudal Morphine. Caudal morphine in a dose of 30 μg/kg, diluted in preservative-free saline to a volume of 0.5 ml/kg and administered as a single shot preoperatively, provides analgesia for up to 12 hours and reduces the need for other analgesic drugs. The evidence suggests that maximum analgesia (and duration) is achieved with 30 μg/kg caudal morphine and that greater doses only increase the complication rate. The child must be monitored continuously as respiratory depression may occur remote from the injection time.

Suggested Reading

Krane EJ, Tyler DC, Jacobson LE: The dose response of caudal morphine in children, Anesthesiology 71:48–52, 1989.

Orme RM, Berg SJ: The 'swoosh' test—an evaluation of a modified 'whoosh' test in children, Br J Anaesth 90:62–65, 2003.

Awake Single-Shot Caudal Analgesia for Lower Abdominal Surgery in Small Infants

As an alternative to awake spinal analgesia for lower abdominal surgery, bupivacaine 1 ml/kg of a 0.375% or 1 to 1.25 ml of a 0.25% solution produces very effective caudal analgesia plus a motor block lasting up to 90 minutes for surgery in awake infants. In small infants, a caudal block may also be readily performed while an assistant supports the infant over a shoulder ("burping" position). This is a very easy method to ensure a patent airway while performing the block. The dose of bupivacaine given when this technique is used may reach 3.75 mg/kg (to prevent leg movement), but has been considered acceptable because it is a single dose, the volume of distribution of the drug in the very small infant is large and it has proven safe in practice. A sugar-coated soother may help to calm the infant during the surgery; if sedation is administered to supplement the caudal block in an infant born preterm, the incidence of apnea may be as great as after general anesthesia.

Suggested Reading

Gunter JB, Watcha MF, Watcha JE, et al: Caudal epidural anesthesia in conscious premature and high risk infants, J Pediatr Surg 26:9–14, 1991.
Spear RM, Despande JK, Maxwell LG: Caudal anesthesia in the awake, high risk infant, Anesthesiology 69:407–409, 1988.

Continuous Caudal Analgesia

In neonates, infants, and children up to 5 years of age, prolonged intraoperative and postoperative analgesia can be provided by means of continuous caudal block. With the use of careful aseptic precautions, a 20-gauge epidural catheter may be threaded through an 18-gauge IV cannula and advanced to the desired level. (**N.B.** At epidural infusion rates, only one orifice of the multiorifice catheter is perfused.) In most infants, it is possible to pass the catheter to the thoracic level. If resistance is felt and is not relieved by rolling the catheter or slight flexion or extension of the child's spine, no attempt should be made to advance the catheter further. Threading the catheter to the lumbar and thoracic levels may not always be possible (particularly with catheters smaller than 20 gauge). However, the use of a nerve stimulator connected to a wire styletted catheter allows observation of muscle contraction as the catheter is advanced (<0.6 mA stimulation). Once the catheter is placed, tincture of benzoin is applied to the skin around the puncture site and a transparent occlusive dressing applied that should be regularly inspected. A second barrier drape is applied with benzoin to isolate the rectal area from the catheter insertion site.

Although the risk of fecal contamination is very small, some tunnel the catheter subcutaneously to further reduce the risk of contamination. This is achieved by inserting the Tuohy needle into the skin several centimeters lateral and cephalad to the catheter insertion site and tunneling it subcutaneously such that the tip of the needle emerges at the catheter insertion site. Care must be taken to avoid severing the catheter with the tip of the Tuohy needle as it passes through the catheter site. The catheter is then passed retrograde through the tip of the Tuohy needle emerging from the upper end of the needle. The Tuohy is removed, both sites are covered and the catheter is secured.

A continuous infusion of bupivacaine may be given at 0.3 ml/kg/hr (to ensure adequate spread of anesthetic) in a concentration that is calculated to deliver a safe dose (see Table 7-5, page 230).

Continuous caudal (and epidural) infusions of local anesthetics require ongoing vigilance. Trained ward nurses experienced in managing infants and children with caudal blocks is essential. If this is not available, the children should be monitored in an ICU or similar setting. The addition of fentanyl to a caudal/lumbar epidural infusion does not substantively increase the risk of perioperative apnea, but may increase the risk of urinary retention, pruritus and vomiting, depending on the dose. The addition of morphine requires increased monitoring, particularly in those infants who have multisystem diseases, who have respiratory disease and who are neurologically impaired.

Neonates and small infants metabolize bupivacaine much more slowly than do adults; hence a much smaller infusion rate is needed to preclude toxicity (see Table 7-5, page 230). Be very cautious if the infusion is continued for more than 48 hours in this age group.

Some centers use continuous infusions of lidocaine for continuous epidural analgesia. This technique has the advantage that blood levels of lidocaine can easily be measured thus avoiding toxic levels.

Suggested Reading

Bosenberg AT, Bland BAR, Schulte-Steinberg O, et al: Thoracic epidural analgesia via the caudal route in infants and children, Anesthesiology 69:265, 1988.

Peutrell JM, Holder K, Gregory M: Plasma bupivacaine concentrations associated with continuous extradural infusions in babies, Br J Anaesth 78:160–162, 1997.

Tsui BC, Wagner A, Cave D, et al: Thoracic and lumbar epidural analgesia via the caudal approach using electrical stimulation guidance in pediatric patients: a review of 289 patients, Anesthesiology 100:683–689, 2004.

Lumbar Epidural Blocks

Lumbar epidural block has been widely used for postoperative pain relief in children and occasionally for surgery in older patients with special indications. The technique used is similar to that for adults; the "loss of resistance method" using saline is recommended to identify the epidural space. Air should not be used to test for loss of resistance because an intravascular injection may occur.

Thoracic epidural block may be performed in children using a technique similar to that used in adults. A midline approach is preferred, and the needle must be advanced at an angle determined by the configuration of the vertebral spine at the level selected. (Examination of the lateral chest radiograph is helpful before performing this block.) Thoracic epidural catheters are generally used in teenagers who may be sedated but not anesthetized during catheter placement so that paresthesia will be identified.

Special Considerations

In children weighing more than 10 kg, the distance from skin to lumbar epidural space in millimeters is approximately numerically similar to the child's weight in kilograms (i.e., the distance in a 20-kg child is about 20 mm).

A 19-gauge (5 cm) Tuohy needle and a 21-gauge catheter are usually used in children younger than 5 years of age. In older children, an 18-gauge Tuohy needle and a 20-gauge epidural catheter are used.

Dose requirements for local analgesic solutions are less predictable when the lumbar (or thoracic) route is used, as opposed to the caudal route.

Epidural block is associated with little change in hemodynamic parameters in children.

Initial Volume to Be Injected

For a lumbar epidural block, bupivacaine 0.25% with 1:200,000 epinephrine or 0.2% ropivacaine is used in a dose of 0.5 ml/kg (0.75 ml/kg for infants), supplemented with a dose of 0.2 ml/kg to achieve the level of block required. For a thoracic epidural, a loading dose of 0.1 ml/kg followed by an infusion of 0.1 ml/kg/hr of 0.125% bupivacaine or 0.2% ropivacaine appears to be effective.

Continuous Infusion Epidural Analgesia

A solution of 0.1% to 0.125% bupivacaine (the former reserved for neonates and infants up to 6 months of age) or 0.2% ropivacaine are widely used, to which fentanyl (0 to 2 μg/ml) may be added (see Table 7-5, page 230). The infusion may be administered at a rate of 0.3 ml/kg/hr and adjusted to provide optimal analgesia. The maximum rate of bupivacaine administration should not exceed 0.4 mg/kg/hr in children and 0.2 mg/kg/hr in neonates.

Patient controlled epidural analgesia (PCEA) has been effective in children as young as 5 years with both bupivacaine (0.1% with fentanyl

5 µg/ml) and ropivacaine (0.2%). The optimal dosing for PCEA in children has not been determined (see Suggested reading).

Beware of toxic effects of local analgesics when children are receiving continuous infusions, especially when the duration of the infusion exceeds 48 hours. Recognize that children may not report the early symptoms of tinnitus, lightheadedness, and visual effects. Children may find common side effects such as numbness (pins and needles) or weakness in their legs upsetting and disturbing but should be reassured. The concentration of bupivacaine may be reduced to attenuate the side effects. Some hold intermittent "top-up" doses to be safer than continuous infusions in young children.

The opioids, morphine and fentanyl, have been used to provide epidural analgesia without motor block. For children, morphine may be given in a loading dose of 30-µg/kg (to a maximum of 3 mg), followed by a daily bolus of a similar dose. Fentanyl may be administered in an initial dose of 2 µg/kg (maximum, 100 µg), followed by an infusion of 5 µg/kg/day (maximum, 300 µg/day). Both regimens resulted in similar analgesia, but the side effects of nausea, vomiting, and pruritus are less frequent with fentanyl. The only way to avoid these opioid side effects is to avoid opioids in the epidural solution. Urinary retention, pruritus, and vomiting may be more common after epidural opioids in children than in adults. Children receiving extradural morphine should be closely monitored for ventilatory depression during and for 24 hours after therapy.

Suggested Reading

Antok E, Bordet F, Duflo F, et al: Patient-controlled epidural analgesia versus continuous epidural infusion with ropivacaine for postoperative analgesia in children, Anesth Analg 97:1608–1611, 2003.

Birmingham PK, Wheeler M, Suresh S, et al: Patient-controlled epidural analgesia in children: can they do it?, Anesth Analg 96:686–691, 2003.

Intercostal Nerve Blocks

Intercostal nerve blocks may be performed to relieve pain after thoracotomy or some upper abdominal procedures. For example, a bilateral T10 block provides good pain relief after umbilical hernia repair.

Special Considerations

1. Systemic absorption of local analgesics from the very vascular intercostal space can be extremely rapid, with a commensurate risk of toxic effects; take care not to exceed a total dose of 2 mg/kg of bupivacaine.

To limit this absorption, epinephrine must be added to the bupivacaine when applied for intercostal blocks.

N.B. The order of local anesthetic absorption with different blocks is easily remembered by the acronym "ICE Blocks," where I,C,E represents the speed of absorption: (i.e. intercostal > caudal > epidural blocks.

2. The risk of pneumothorax is high, especially in small children, in whom the distance from nerve to pleura is very small.

3. The intercostal nerves are sheathed in a dural layer posteriorly; injection near their origin can result in a total spinal block.

Preferred Technique

In infants and small children, the nerve in the intercostal space can be more precisely approached by angling the needle posteromedially, so that it lies almost parallel to the rib, rather than at right angles to it (Figure 5-3). Palpate the lower margin of the rib, pull the skin upward, and advance until contacting the rib. The skin is released and the needle "walked" off the rib margin. The chosen volume is then injected with only a 1 to 3 mm advancement and frequent aspiration for blood.

Ilioinguinal and Iliohypogastric Nerve Block

The ilioinguinal and iliohypogastric nerve block provides skin analgesia over the inguinal region and is useful for providing postoperative

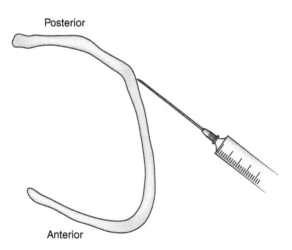

Posterior

Anterior

Figure 5-3 Intercostal nerve block: direction of needle insertion in relation to rib.

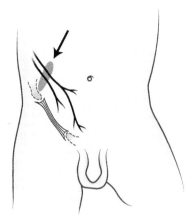

Figure 5-4 Ilioinguinal-iliohypogastric nerve block: area to be infiltrated with local anesthetic solution.

analgesia after herniotomy. (This block is inadequate for orchidopexy; a caudal block is preferred). The block should preferably be performed immediately after induction of general anesthesia, before the operation commences. The nerves run beneath the internal oblique muscle just medial to the anterior superior iliac spine and may be blocked by a fan-shaped infiltration of the abdominal wall in this region (Figure 5-4). If available, ultrasound guidance may improve success, decrease the volume of drug required, and reduce the potential for intraabdominal puncture. Bupivacaine 0.25% or 0.5% (up to 2 mg/kg) with epinephrine (1:200,000) may be used; more complete analgesia may be obtained with the use of the 0.5% solution, but very occasionally this concentration produces a transient motor block of the femoral nerve, with leg weakness.

Penile Block

The paired dorsal nerves pass inferior to the pubic bones on either side of the midline and supply the dorsal aspect of the penis and foreskin. A block of these nerves provides good pain relief after circumcision but does not provide adequate analgesia after hypospadias repair. Epinephrine-containing solutions should not be used because vasoconstriction might result in damaging ischemia to the penis. Complications have been very rare after properly performed penile block; however, it has been suggested that a subcutaneous ring block at the base of the penis is safer.

Volume to Be Injected

Up to 2 mg/kg of 0.5% bupivacaine *without epinephrine* is injected, to a maximum volume of 1 ml in the small infant or 6 ml in the large child. *Ropivacaine should not be used for penile blocks as this drug may have vasoconstrictive properties.*

Preferred Technique

With careful aseptic technique, bilateral injections are made beneath the pubis at the base of the penis at the 11 o'clock and 1 o'clock positions (Figure 5-5). The needle should be felt to pass through Buck's fascia to deposit an equal volume adjacent to each nerve. In infants, it is possible to anesthetize both nerves by inserting the needle in the midline of the dorsal surface of the penis. Alternatively, a ring block at the base of the penis may be performed (Figure 5-6).

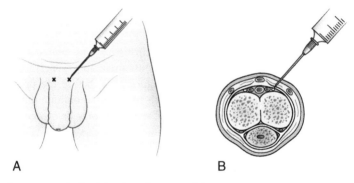

A   **B**

Figure 5-5 Block of the dorsal nerves of the penis. **A,** Injection sites. **B,** Position of nerves at base of penis.

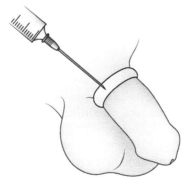

Figure 5-6 Ring block of the penis.

Head and Neck and Upper Limb Blocks

Supraorbital and Supratrochlear Nerve Blocks

These nerves are easy to block in children; the supraorbital nerve exits the supraorbital notch, which is easily palpated in children as one palpates the orbital rim from medial to lateral. The supratrochlear nerve exits the orbital rim several millimeters medial to the supraorbital notch.

Preferred technique. For both blocks, a 27-gauge needle is positioned as described previously and 1 ml bupivacaine 0.25% with epinephrine or 0.2% ropivacaine is injected. These blocks anesthetize the ipsilateral frontal region of the scalp for superficial surgery in this region (e.g., a frontal ventriculoperitoneal shunt).

Infraorbital Nerve Block

The infraorbital nerve block is simple to perform and provides good analgesia for infants and children after cleft lip repairs or for children undergoing endoscopic sinus procedures.

In older children, the site of the infraorbital foramen can be palpated 1 to 1.5 cm below the infraorbital rim in line with the supraorbital notch and the pupil. A needle can be inserted at this point and 1 to 1.5 ml of local analgesic injected.

In infants the foramen cannot be palpated, and its position must be estimated by using the following landmarks: The infraorbital nerve lies approximately under the midpoint of a line drawn between the middle of the palpebral fissure and the angle of the mouth.

Preferred Technique. Once the estimated position of the infraorbital foramen has been identified, a needle is passed vertically through the skin and gently advanced until bony resistance is felt. The needle is then withdrawn very slightly, an aspiration test is performed, and 1 ml of 0.25% bupivacaine with epinephrine or ropivacaine 0.2% is injected. A skin puncture may be avoided by lifting the upper lip and passing a 27-gauge needle via the buccal sulcus while palpating the infraorbital foramen so as to avoid entering the orbit.

Greater Occipital Nerve Block

A greater occipital nerve block may be performed by injecting 1 to 3 ml of 0.25% bupivacaine with epinephrine 1:200,000 or 0.2% ropivacaine as the nerves exit the skull next to the medial occipital artery at the level of the superior nuchal line. This will provide analgesia for superficial surgery involving the back of the head (e.g., a posterior ventricular peritoneal shunt).

Superficial Cervical Plexus Block

The nerves of the superficial cervical plexus may be readily blocked at the posterior aspect of the sternocleidomastoid muscle. A block of the greater auricular nerve and the lesser occipital nerve, which is posterior may be very useful in the child who has an incision behind the ear for mastoid surgery or tympanoplasty (Figure 5-7).

Brachial Plexus Blocks

There are several possible approaches to block the brachial plexus in children; the most commonly used are the axillary, supraclavicular, and infraclavicular routes.

Axillary Approach. The axillary approach is often recommended because of its simplicity and lack of serious complications (e.g., pneumothorax); it is easy to perform if the child can abduct the arm and is further simplified when possible by placing the hand behind the head. It is useful for forearm fractures, plastic surgery procedures, and insertion of shunts for dialysis, but the block does not include the area of the upper arm and sometimes not the area supplied by musculocutaneous nerves.

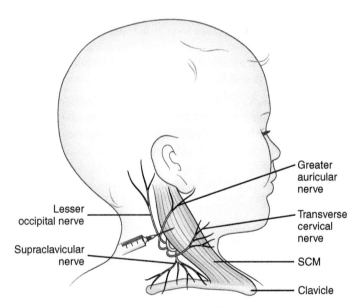

Figure 5-7 Superficial cervical plexus block along the posterior aspect of the sternocleidomastoid muscle (SCM)

Preferred Technique. With careful asepsis, after skin analgesia, a short-beveled needle is advanced cephalad, at a 45° angle to skin, alongside and parallel to the axillary artery (Figure 5-8). A slight "give" or "pop" should be felt as the neurovascular sheath is entered, and the arterial pulsations will be seen rocking the needle. With a nerve stimulator, a motor response should be detected in the ulnar, radial, or median nerve with 0.2 mA stimulation. The needle is supported gently, the plastic extension is connected to the syringe, and after aspiration the drug is carefully injected, with periodic aspiration. Pressure distally over the axillary artery may encourage proximal spread of the local analgesic solution and a more complete block.

Volume to Be Injected. Use 0.2 to 0.3 ml/kg of any local anesthetic (Table 5-1 for maximum dose). For the older child, a maximum volume of 20 ml is usually satisfactory.

Lateral Infraclavicular Approach. This block may have advantages over the axillary block, providing more reliable analgesia in the musculocutaneous nerve distribution; however, pneumothorax is a potential complication. Ultrasound guidance is strongly encouraged to reduce the risk of pneumothorax.

Preferred Technique. The block is performed inferior to the clavicle adjacent to the coracoid process of the scapula, which can readily be palpated in the child. The needle is inserted slightly caudal and slightly medial to the coracoid process and advanced vertically in a posterior direction. The use of ultrasound permits a high success rate and facili-

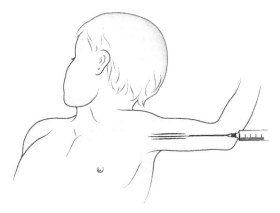

Figure 5-8 Brachial plexus block, axillary route: direction of needle in relation to artery.

tates catheter insertion if a continuous brachial plexus block is indicated. A nerve stimulator may be used when ultrasound is not available in the anesthetized child to position the tip of the needle adjacent to the cords of the plexus. Wrist or forearm extensor movements (i.e., from posterior cord stimulation) when stimulated with 0.5 mA are predictive of success.

Volume to Be Injected. Local anesthetic 0.2 to 0.3 ml/kg may then be injected (Table 5-1 for maximum dose).

Suggested Reading

Fisher P, Wilson SE, Brown M, et al: Continuous infraclavicular brachial plexus block in a child, Paediatr Anaesth 16(8):884–886, 2006.

Supraclavicular Approach. This block can be performed in children for surgery involving the upper arm and forearm. With ultrasound guidance, there are few complications but if nerve stimulation is used, there is a risk of vertebral artery injection and pneumothorax.

Preferred Technique. The use of ultrasound is preferred. If stimulation is used, the plexus is located above the clavicle using a short bevel stimulating needle (1 mA). After piercing the skin, movement of any muscles of the upper extremity is accepted as correct placement and the local anesthetic is deposited.

Volume to Be Injected. Volumes of local anesthetic for this block are 0.15 to 0.2 ml/kg (Table 5-1 for maximum dose).

Lower Limb Blocks

Femoral Nerve Block

The femoral nerve block is useful for fractures of the shaft of the femur and for muscle biopsy in patients with suspected myopathy (in which case it should be combined with a lateral femoral cutaneous nerve block).

For children with fracture of the femur, a continuous femoral nerve block may give very good continuing analgesia and also relieves the muscle spasm in the thigh.

Preferred Technique. The femoral artery is identified by palpation just below the inguinal ligament. After skin analgesia has been established, a 1-inch-long, 22-gauge short bevel needle is advanced slowly just lateral to the artery at an angle of 45° to skin (Figure 5-9). Slight resistance should be felt at two separate levels, the fascia lata and the fascia iliaca, after which the needle lies within the femoral sheath. The needle should then be gently supported, aspirated, and injected, with periodic aspiration.

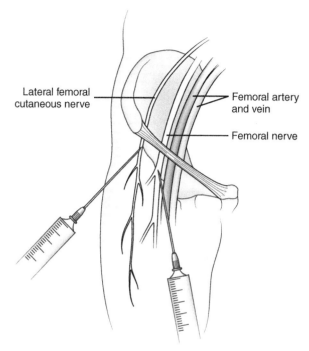

Lateral femoral cutaneous nerve

Femoral artery and vein

Femoral nerve

Figure 5-9 Femoral nerve block and block of the lateral femoral cutaneous nerve of the thigh.

Volume to be Injected. Use 0.2 to 0.3 ml/kg of 1% lidocaine with 1:200,000 epinephrine or 0.5% bupivacaine.

Continuous Femoral Nerve Block

With careful asepsis, after skin analgesia, a Tuohy needle with obturator is advanced, as outlined previously, through the two identified layers of resistance. The needle is positioned with the opening facing cephalad, and a standard epidural catheter is advanced proximally for 5 to 10 cm within the femoral sheath. When the Tuohy needle is correctly placed, the catheter should advance very easily with very little resistance. The Tuohy needle can then be withdrawn and the catheter left in situ, as when inserting an epidural catheter. Never attempt to withdraw the catheter through the needle because the tip may be sheared off and remain in the child.

Volume to be Injected. Intermittent top-up doses of bupivacaine 0.25% (0.4 ml/kg) may be given every 8 to 12 hours as required, or a continuous infusion may be used at a rate of 0.1 ml/kg/hr.

Suggested Reading

Chu RSL, Browne GJ, Cheng NG, et al: Femoral nerve block for femoral shaft fractures in a paediatric emergency department: can it be done better? Euro J Emerg Med 10:258–263, 2003.

Lateral Femoral Cutaneous Nerve Block

Block of the lateral femoral cutaneous nerve provides analgesia over the lateral aspect of the thigh.

Preferred Technique. The needle is inserted medial and inferior to the anterior superior iliac spine, just superior to the inguinal ligament, and advanced superiorly and laterally until it impinges on the iliac bone (see Figure 5-9). The local analgesic solution is injected as the needle is slowly withdrawn.

Volume to Be Injected. Use 2 to 5 ml of 1% lidocaine with 1:200,000 epinephrine or 0.5% bupivacaine injected in a fanlike manner.

Sciatic Nerve Block

The sciatic nerve in children may be blocked via an anterior, lateral or posterior approach: the latter approach is considered to be the easiest and likely to be the most successful.

Preferred Technique. The child should be anesthetized and placed in a semiprone position, with the side of the nerve to be blocked elevated. The needle should be inserted at right angles to the skin at the midpoint of a line between the sacrococcygeal membrane and the greater trochanter of the femur. The needle should be advanced at right angles to the skin (i.e., just lateral to the ischial tuberosity, until it is adjacent to the sciatic nerve. Confirm by ultrasonography or by electrical stimulation (0.5 mA) via the needle. (In this case, a sheathed insulated needle* should be used).

If a catheter is needed for a continuous infusion, insert the needle just inferior to the gluteal fold and angle the needle slightly cephalad to approach the same site. The catheter will then be easier to secure and protect while in situ.

Volume to Be Injected. For a single dose, 0.2 to 0.3 ml/kg of 1% lidocaine with epinephrine or 0.5% bupivacaine. For a continuous block, use 0.1 ml/kg/hr of local anesthetic.

---

* Stimuplex, Braun Medical, Bethlehem, Pa.

Suggested Reading

Dalens B, Tanguy A, Vanneuville G, et al: Sciatic nerve blocks in children: comparison of the posterior, anterior, and lateral approaches in 180 pediatric patients, Anesth Analg 70(2):131–137, 1990.

Popliteal Fossa Block of the Sciatic Nerve

The sciatic nerve may also be blocked as it approaches the popliteal fossa. This block is useful to provide analgesia for foot surgery. Just proximal to the popliteal fossa, the nerve divides into the tibial nerve, which innervates the posterior calf and plantar area, and the peroneal nerve, which supplies sensation to the anterior leg. To be successful, the block must be performed above the division site; this is 3 to 7 cm above the popliteal crease in children under 8 years but slightly higher (within 3.5 to 8 cm) in older children. The approximate site to make the injection is 1 cm proximal to the popliteal crease for each 10 kg body weight, the needle should be angled at 45° to the skin surface pointing cephalad. The injection is made just lateral to the midline to avoid vascular structures. The block may be performed with the child in a lateral, supine, or prone position. Successful block can be achieved using a nerve stimulator (0.2 to 0.5 mA) to locate the main sciatic nerve or preferably by ultrasound. Continuous popliteal nerve blocks are becoming increasingly popular to replace caudal/epidural blocks for lower extremity surgery; a single dose of 5 to 10 ml of local anesthetic or a 20-gauge catheter is threaded 3 to 5 cm into the fossa and local anesthetic is infused at 0.1 ml/kg/hr.

Suggested Reading

Konrad C, Johr M: Blockade of the sciatic nerve in the popliteal fossa: a system for standardization in children, Anesth Analg 87(6):1256–1258, 1998.

Berniere J, Schrayer S, Piana F, et al: A new formula of age-related anatomical landmarks for blockade of the sciatic nerve in the popliteal fossa in children using the posterior approach, Paediatr Anaesth 18(7):602–605, 2008.

Ankle Block

Blocks of the branches of the sciatic nerve at the level of the ankle are very easy to perform and require only small doses of local analgesics. An ankle block may provide good analgesia following club foot repair. It is necessary to block the deep peroneal nerve alongside the anterior tibial artery, the saphenous nerve which lies alongside the saphenous vein, the posterior tibial nerve alongside the posterior tibial artery, and the sural nerve, which is just lateral to the Achilles tendon. Infiltration of the skin over the lateral aspect of the anterior tibia will block any branches of the superficial peroneal nerve supplying the dorsum of the foot.

Intravenous Regional Analgesia

The "Bier" (intravenous) block may be useful in older children having excision of lesions on either of the limbs (e.g., ganglion). Intravenous blocks are not generally suitable for reduction of fractures because it is difficult to apply an optimally tight cast to an ischemic limb.

Preferred Technique

Insert a small intravenous cannula in the hand or foot. Use a reliable *double* pneumatic tourniquet. The success of the block varies with the degree of limb exsanguination, which can be achieved before injection of the local analgesic; use an elastic bandage, air splint, or lifting the arm if possible. Inflate the proximal cuff and inject the local analgesic solution. Do not exceed 5 mg/kg of 0.25% lidocaine or 3 mg/kg of prilocaine. Bupivacaine should never be used for an intravenous block. The addition of a very small dose of an intermediate acting muscle relaxant ($1/10$ the usual intubating dose) will provide paralysis and perhaps improve surgical conditions by eliminating movements. When the block is established (5 minutes), inflate the distal cuff and then deflate the proximal cuff. Do not release the remaining cuff until at least 30 minutes have elapsed, even if the operation is finished sooner.

Medical Conditions Influencing Anesthetic Management

6

UPPER RESPIRATORY TRACT INFECTION

Infants and children often have or are recovering from a runny nose or other manifestations of upper respiratory tract infection (URTI) when they are seen for evaluation before general anesthesia. Indiscriminate cancellation of children with any symptom of URTI is unwarranted and causes emotional and financial problems for children and their families; each case needs to be carefully evaluated. Some children seem to have a runny nose most of the time, possibly because of allergies or a chronic nasal infection; these children should be distinguished from those with an acute URTI.

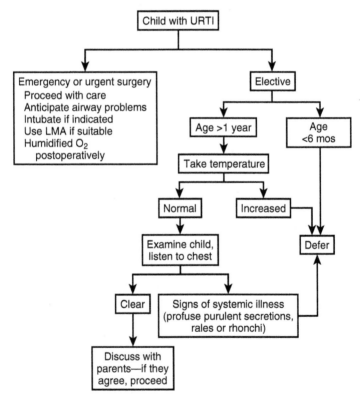

ALGORITHM FOR MANAGEMENT
OF UPPER RESPIRATORY TRACT INFECTION

Figure 6-1 Algorithm for management of upper respiratory tract infection. (Fever is > 38.5C)

Children with an uncomplicated URTI who are otherwise healthy have a greater incidence of intraoperative desaturation, bronchospasm, and laryngospasm. Although these complications can be disturbing, most are easily managed (see Laryngospasm, Chapter 4). It should be noted that airway irritability after a URTI may last for 6 to 8 weeks, thus delaying the procedure 2 weeks will not reduce the incidence of these complications. Infants less than 1 year of age, infants who were born premature, children exposed to second-hand smoke, and children with reactive airways disease with a concomitant URTI may have more serious airway problems during and after anesthesia. Children with any history of URTI should be carefully monitored en route to the PACU; postoperative desaturation is more common. Pulmonary complications in children having major (i.e., cardiac) surgery may be more common if there has been a recent (within 2 weeks) history of URTI. This may result from the fact that viral infections alter the reactivity of the airway for such a period and may also predispose to other infections.

Recent evidence suggests anticholinergics do not affect the incidence of perioperative airway complications in children with URTI. Children with chronic rhinorrhea may receive one to two drops of either Neo-Synephrine (0.25%) or oxymetazoline per nostril to dry up secretions during anesthesia.

Children with bronchospasm (i.e., asthma) that complicates a URTI may benefit from their usual dose of bronchodilators in the preoperative period. Preoperative bronchodilators and a vital capacity cough may resolve bronchospasm and airways plugged with mucus. Intraoperatively, albuterol or the more recent, levoalbuterol, may be delivered through an ETT by first agitating the canister for 30 seconds, and then second, inserting it stem down into a 60 ml syringe (after the barrel is removed) and then reinserting the barrel. The syringe should be screwed onto the capnography port of the elbow of the breathing circuit and the barrel compressed. Evidence indicates that 3% to 8% of the aerosol delivered into the ETT using this technique reaches the trachea. The remainder layers out on the wall of the tracheal tube. To deliver most of the content of each puff to the tip of the tube, a long narrow gauge (e.g., 19 gauge) catheter may be inserted to the distal third of the tracheal tube. In this manner, the majority of the aerosol reaches the tracheal mucosa. Most avoid tracheal intubation in these children if the airway can be managed with an LMA; this reduces the incidence of bronchospasm. However, evidence also suggests that the incidence of laryngospasm increases when LMAs are used in children with recent URTIs.

The following plan of action is suggested (Figure 6-1):

1. Elective surgery
   a. The child should be carefully assessed. A history of the URTI should be obtained along with a detailed history of any other illnesses. A careful physical examination should be performed, looking particularly for any evidence of systemic illness, purulent nasal secretions, or lower respiratory tract disease.
   b. Children with mild URTI but without pyrexia or any other evidence of disease may be accepted for minor surgical procedures because evidence indicates little increased risk of complications. The decision to proceed should be discussed with the parents and the surgeon. Anesthesia via a facemask or LMA, avoidance of endotracheal intubation when practical, administration of atropine, and the use of sevoflurane may reduce airway complications.
   c. Children who present for elective surgery with any one of the following should be rescheduled after 4 weeks: 1. Pyrexia greater than 38.5°C; 2. Change in behavior/diet/activity; 3. Purulent secretions; or 4. Signs of lower respiratory tract involvement (e.g., wheezing) that do not clear with a forced cough.
   d. Children with a history of asthma and a URTI demand special attention; nonurgent surgery should be deferred for 4 weeks whenever possible.
2. Emergency or urgent surgery: Children who require emergency surgery cannot be deferred because of a URTI. The anesthetic prescription should account for the presence of a full stomach and the type of surgery but the presence of a URTI requires no special modifications. Sevoflurane is an acceptable anesthetic for children with mild URTI. Airway problems and laryngospasm must be anticipated, and all necessities for their treatment should be immediately at hand. When suitable, the laryngeal mask airway (LMA) should be used as an alternative to tracheal intubation; it may result in fewer airway complications. Postoperatively, the child should be carefully observed.

Suggested Reading

Tait AR, Malviya S: Anesthesia for the child with upper respiratory tract infection: still a dilemma? Anesth Analg 100:59–65, 2005.

ASTHMA

Asthma affects 4% to 13% of children in various parts of North America. The disease is characterized by variable cough, wheezing, and breathlessness and is episodic and seasonal in many. The symptoms result from bronchoconstriction, mucosal edema, and tenacious secretions in the small airways. Severe attacks may occur throughout childhood and may be life threatening. Acute exacerbations may be associated with URTIs, allergens, irritants, exercise, or emotional stress. The treatment for mild asthma is inhaled β-adrenergics for bronchodilation and improved mucociliary clearance. For more severe asthma, inhaled corticosteroids may be added to control inflammation. Theophylline, which has been relegated to third-line asthma therapy, is sometimes used to prevent nocturnal bronchospasm. Severe asthmatic attacks may require systemic corticosteroid therapy and ICU admission. The disease often improves as the child ages. The severity of the disease is usually judged by the therapy, which is required to control the symptoms; mild asthma is controlled by inhaled β-adrenergics with increasing severity suggested by the addition of inhaled corticosteroids. Rarely, oral steroids are prescribed for asthma but if they are, it suggests a recent exacerbation.

When a child with asthma presents for elective surgery, it is most important to determine whether the child's current status is optimal. The following are important considerations.

1. If possible, surgery should be delayed for at least 1 month after the last acute attack; during this period, airway reactivity may be increased and residual mucosal edema and secretions may impair pulmonary function.
2. Elective surgery should be deferred if there is any evidence of an active viral URTI. A URTI can precipitate an exacerbation of symptoms.
3. The frequency of the asthma attacks, and the symptoms between attacks should be documented. Has admission to an intensive care unit or ventilator therapy ever been needed? If so, repeat severe attacks are likely.
4. What medications is the child taking, and are they controlling the child's symptoms? Have systemic corticosteroids been necessary? If so, in what dose? Has the child taken any of the usual asthma medications today? If the child is receiving theophylline therapy, the blood level of the drug should be measured preoperatively.
5. Physical examination of the chest is important to detect bronchospasm and exclude any other current pulmonary pathology. If wheezing is present, the child should be encouraged to cough deeply. If the wheezing is unresolved, a trial of bronchodilator therapy should be administered. If the signs do not resolve, then elective surgery should be deferred.
6. The results of recent pulmonary function tests and especially any response to bronchodilator therapy should be noted.

7. A chest radiograph should be ordered for any child with significant symptoms.

Anesthesia Management

Preoperative

1. Ensure that the child receives routine asthma medications up to the time of surgery. Oral medications can be taken with a sip of water; inhalations may be repeated, if necessary, just before transfer to the operating room.

2. A stress-dose of steroids (IV hydrocortisone [1 to 1.5 mg/kg]) should be administered at induction of anesthesia to those taking the equivalent of greater than 5 mg prednisone per day (adult dose), oral steroids within 3 months or high-dose inhaled steroids. Nonetheless, testing for adrenal suppression is uncommon, which leads prevailing opinion to suggest that a single dose of steroids is unlikely to do harm and may prevent an adrenal crisis in the perioperative period.

3. Order appropriate sedation to calm the child. Oral midazolam is the most widely used premedication for children in North America. Atropine, if considered necessary, may be given orally or intravenously at induction; it decreases secretions and causes some bronchodilation.

Perioperative

1. For intravenous induction, propofol is the preferred induction agent as thiopental may release histamine and possibly cause bronchoconstriction. Alternatively, ketamine may be used since it is a bronchodilator and may protect against bronchospasm; however, atropine should be given to limit secretions.

2. Inhalation induction with sevoflurane is preferred. Halothane may precipitate arrhythmias in children also receiving theophylline.

3. Avoid agents known to release histamine and cause bronchospasm (e.g., atracurium, morphine). Desflurane increases airway resistance in asthmatic children. Nitrous oxide, halothane, sevoflurane, fentanyl, pancuronium, rocuronium, and vecuronium are preferred drugs.

4. If tracheal intubation is necessary, it should be performed gently when the child is deeply anesthetized; otherwise, the procedure may trigger bronchospasm. Alternatively, lidocaine 1.5 mg/kg IV may be administered 3 to 4 minutes before intubation. If possible, avoid tracheal intubation for minor or brief procedures. The LMA may be a very useful alternative.

5. The anesthetic gases should be warmed and humidified—this is less essential if a circle circuit is used.

6. Intraoperative wheezing should be treated by deepening the level of anesthesia and by giving bronchodilator aerosols via the endotracheal tube (e.g., albuterol) (see URTI). Be careful to exclude nonasthmatic causes for wheezing (e.g., a partially obstructed endotracheal tube, endobronchial intubation, pneumothorax, etc.).
7. At the end of surgery, atropine and neostigmine may be administered to antagonize the muscle relaxants as necessary. Neostigmine may increase bronchomotor tone, but this effect is counteracted by the atropine. Extubation is preferably performed with the child deeply anesthetized and breathing spontaneously so as to minimize the risk of precipitating bronchospasm. If awake extubation is planned, intravenous lidocaine or propofol may be administered beforehand to reduce laryngeal reflexes.

Postoperative

1. Humidified oxygen should be administered.
2. When practical, regional analgesia is ideal for pain relief; for major surgery, continuous regional analgesia may be planned. Otherwise, use intravenous fentanyl or PCA morphine (see Chapter 7).
3. Postoperative wheezing may require additional doses of an aerosol bronchodilator and appropriate adjustment of other medications.

Suggested Reading

Doherty GM, Chisakuta A, Crean P, et al: Anesthesia and the child with asthma, Paediatr Anaesth 15:446–454, 2005.

CYSTIC FIBROSIS

Cystic fibrosis (CF) is an inherited disorder that results from a genetic defect on chromosome 9. Abnormal chloride and sodium transport result in increased electrolyte content and increased viscosity of secretions. This disorder affects many body systems and may present in the neonate as meconium ileus. During childhood, malabsorption due to pancreatic insufficiency predominates. In the second decade, however, malabsorption is superseded by increasing pulmonary problems because of abnormally viscous secretions. Respiratory failure usually develops by the second or third decade of life, secondary to retained secretions and chronic infection. Even if they appear fairly well, many of these children have severe pulmonary ventilation-perfusion ($\dot{V}/\dot{Q}$) inequality. However with intensive therapy many children are now surviving to adulthood.

Surgery for children with this condition is most commonly for nasal polypectomy (in many cases repeated), functional endoscopic sinus surgery (FESS), antral lavage, or bronchoscopy for removal of retained secretions and treatment of atelectasis. Some children with advanced disease may present for lung transplantation. Transplanted lungs do not appear to be affected by this otherwise generalized disease.

Special Anesthesia Problems

1. Copious, extremely viscous secretions are present in the respiratory tract. Violent coughing and laryngospasm may occur during induction.
2. Because of the $\dot{V}/\dot{Q}$ disturbances:
   a. Hypoxia may develop rapidly during anesthesia.
   b. Induction of anesthesia with inhalational agents is prolonged because of $\dot{V}/\dot{Q}$ mismatch; this is exacerbated with less soluble anesthetics such as sevoflurane.
3. Lung compliance is reduced. In severe late cases, very high airway pressures may be required to adequately ventilate the lungs and prevent hypoxemia. Therefore a cuffed endotracheal tube should always be used.
4. Malnutrition and underweight for age is a result of malabsorption and chronic infection. Liver function may be reduced in older children. In such cases, drug dosages should be adjusted accordingly. (In younger children metabolism of some drugs is enhanced.)
5. Many children with advanced CF suffer all the emotional upset of those with chronic disease; all of them require very careful and considerate handling and much reassurance.

Anesthesia Management

Preoperative

1. Assess the child's condition carefully; ensure that the pulmonary status is optimized before surgery by means of postural drainage, physiotherapy, and inhalation therapy. These should be continued until the immediate preoperative period.
2. Pulmonary function is usually at its worst early in the morning. If possible, schedule the surgery at a time that allows for chest physiotherapy and clearing of secretions preoperatively.
3. Do not give opioid premedication as oxygenation may be compromised. Give midazolam for anxiolysis.
4. Ensure optimal hydration; fluids must not be withheld for prolonged periods. The child should be offered clear fluids until 2 hours preoperatively.

Perioperative

N.B. Whenever possible, use local or regional analgesia.

1. Establish intravenous access for hydration and emergency drug administration.
   If general anesthesia is required:
2. Give 100% O_2 by mask for at least 5 minutes in children with pulmonary involvement; these children are very used to having IV access, so if indwelling IV is not present, start an IV and induce anesthesia intravenously with propofol and a muscle relaxant. Inhalational inductions in children with serious $\dot{V}/\dot{Q}$ mismatch will be protracted and delayed.
3. Intubate the trachea using a cuffed endotracheal tube.
4. Suction the trachea and remove secretions frequently.
5. Use humidified gases with sufficient oxygen added to maintain an adequate SaO_2 (100% O_2 may be necessary for children with severe CF).
6. Do not give long-acting medications; use a technique that ensures the child's rapid recovery.

Postoperative

1. Give fluids intravenously until the child is drinking well.
2. Nurse the child with humidified oxygen. Whenever possible place the child in a semirecumbant position that increases respiratory comfort.
3. Provide optimal analgesia. Use regional analgesia and NSAIDs for postoperative pain whenever possible.
4. Encourage early chest physiotherapy and ambulation.

Suggested Reading

Della Rocca G: Anaesthesia in patients with cystic fibrosis, Curr Opin Anaesthesiol 15:95–101, 2002.

HEMATOLOGIC DISORDERS

Anemia

Children requiring surgery may be anemic. Remember that the hemoglobin (Hb) concentration, normally 18 to 20 g/dl at birth, decreases to a nidus of about 10 to 11 g/dl by 3 months of age and thereafter increases gradually to 12 to 14 g/dl by 6 years of age (see Table 4-10).

In the preterm infant, the Hb often decreases to lower concentrations because of a reduced red blood cell mass at birth, brief survival time of fetal red blood cells, and poor erythropoietin response. Frequent blood sampling may exacerbate the anemia. In children, Hb levels below normal for age are most frequently caused by poor diet. Anemia discovered before elective surgery should be fully investigated and corrected before surgery. Most children with a chronic Hb level of 7 to 9 g/dl (i.e., renal failure) can be safely anesthetized provided no further blood loss takes place. If, however, the Hb is less than 7 g/dl, the physiologic consequences of anemia may significantly compromise the margin of safety during anesthesia, particularly if substantial surgical bleeding is expected.

The following considerations are relevant for children with anemia:

1. Transport of oxygen to the tissues can be maintained only by increased cardiac output or increased oxygen extraction from the blood. The major compensation is the increase in cardiac output; shift of the Hb-O$_2$ dissociation curve, caused by increased 2,3-diphosphoglycerate (2,3-DPG), contributes relatively little. At a Hb level less than 8 g/dl, the cardiac output must increase to compensate for the decreased oxygen-carrying capacity.
2. Coronary sinus blood is normally very desaturated; therefore, in anemia, oxygen transport to the heart muscle can be maintained only by increased coronary blood flow. At Hb levels less than 5 g/dl, the ability of the myocardium to meet its own needs is compromised resulting in subendocardial ischemia and high-output congestive cardiac failure may occur.
3. Anemic children may be at increased risk for cardiac arrest during anesthesia. The factual data to support this hypothesis are scant, but it seems reasonable to suppose that children with severe anemia have a reduced margin of safety.
4. Children with significant cardiac or respiratory disease require a greater concentration of Hb than normal children: 14 g/dl should be considered the minimum acceptable, and some children need greater concentrations.
5. Preterm infants who are anemic are more prone to perioperative apnea.

The following plan of action is suggested for routine elective surgery:

1. If a significant anemia is discovered, delay elective surgery until the anemia has been diagnosed and corrected. In children with iron-deficiency anemia, the Hb level increases significantly after 3 to 4 weeks of oral iron therapy.

2. If surgery cannot be delayed, a decision must be made whether to proceed despite the anemic state or to transfuse packed cells to correct the severe anemia. This decision depends on many factors, such as the age and health of the child and the expected surgical blood loss.
3. For the anemic child, use an anesthetic technique that is optimal for the anemic state:
    a. Avoid excessive preoperative sedation.
    b. Oxygenate the child before induction.
    c. Use increased concentrations of inspired oxygen during anesthesia.
    d. Always use an endotracheal tube.
    e. Use controlled ventilation and maintain normocapnia.
    f. Be cautious with myocardial depressant drugs.
    g. Carefully replace fluids to maintain the intravascular volume; hypovolemia must be avoided if the cardiac output is to be maintained.
    h. Do not extubate until the child is fully awake.
    i. Give additional oxygen continuously during transport to and in the postanesthesia care unit (PACU).
    j. Keep the child normothermic throughout.

Suggested Reading

Gunawardana RH, Gunasekara SW, Weerasinghe JU: Anesthesia and surgery in pediatric patients with low hemoglobin values, Ind J Ped 66(4):523–526, 1999.

Sickle Cell States

In sickle cell states, an abnormal Hb (known as sickle cell hemoglobin [HbS]) is present. When deoxygenated, sickle hemoglobin forms a gel, distorting the shape of erythrocytes, which then occlude vessels, causing infarction in lungs (acute chest syndrome), bones and brain. In addition, the erythrocyte life span is reduced and there is increased hemolysis with consequent anemia and increased bilirubin level. The course of the disease is one of many crises: sickling, hemolytic, or aplastic. Sickling crises result in ischemic pain, hemolytic crises result in further anemia, and aplastic crises may cause death. Ischemia due to sickling may involve many different organs hence the disease is multifaceted. The disease is mainly confined to persons of African and Mediterranean descent. The anesthesiologist may meet these children when they require a surgical procedure or when they are experiencing a painful crisis and require analgesia.

In the United States, all neonates are screened at birth for sickle cell; however, those born outside the United States may not have been screened. Sickle cell disease may become evident during infancy (after 6 months of age) as HbS replaces fetal hemoglobin (HbF); the latter offers some protection against sickling. Hence, performing a Sickledex test in the first 6 months of life may not detect the presence of HbS. Infants with HbSS should receive pneumococcal vaccine and penicillin prophylaxis up to 6 years of age.

The severity of the disease depends on the percentage of HbS present and the presence or absence of other abnormal forms of Hb.

1. Sickle cell trait (mild form, i.e., Hb AS-heterozygous): small concentrations of HbS (less than 50%). Sickling is unlikely to occur without very severe hypoxemia. Trait is unlikely to cause sickling during anesthesia except possibly during cardiopulmonary bypass. The incidence of sickle cell trait is approximately 8% in the African American population.

2. Sickle cell disease (severe form, i.e., Hb SS-homozygous): large concentrations of HbS (more than 75%). This may cause serious complications in the perioperative period. Sickle cell disease occurs in 0.3% to 1.3% of the Africa American population.

3. The presence of another abnormal Hb may modify the disease. For example HbC, the second most common abnormal Hb, also promotes sickling. Children with HbSC have a normal Hb concentration but an increased risk of sickling. Similarly, HbD, promotes sickling when combined with HbS. On the other hand, HbF, if it is present (i.e., in thalassemia), may protect by reducing hemolysis and sickling. It is therefore most important to know the results of the Hb electrophoresis.

4. Neonates who have a large percent of HbF are not usually anemic or considered at risk for sickling. However, sickle cell crises have been reported in severely stressed neonates. Usually, the clinical signs appear by the time the child is a few months old.

5. Splenic function is impaired, serious infections may occur, and prophylactic antibiotics are indicated. Later, autosplenectomy may occur as a result of vaso-occlusive events.

6. Renal impairment (hyposthenuria) may occur in young children, leading to increased obligatory urine output and consequent increased risk of dehydration.

7. Acute chest syndrome, consisting of chest pain, respiratory distress, fever, and multilobe lung infiltrates, is common in children with sickle cell (SS) disease and may lead to severe hypoxemia. Therapy includes antibiotics, fluid therapy, transfusion, and pain control (PCA, NSAIDs, and possibly epidural analgesia).

8. In later life, pulmonary infarction leads to pulmonary fibrosis, pulmonary hypertension, and cor pulmonale Stroke may develop in 10% of children.

Special Anesthesia Problems

1. A sickling crisis may be precipitated by general or local hypoxemia.
2. Sickling is more likely if the child is anemic, acidotic, hypotensive, dehydrated, septic, and/or hypothermic or if the child's blood contains Hb C or D.
3. If the child has sickle cell disease, previous vascular occlusive crises may have permanently impaired cardiac, hepatic, and/or renal function.
4. Serum cholinesterase activity may be reduced.

Anesthesia Management

Perioperative management of the sickle cell diseases is evolving as more experience with these conditions is gained. The assistance of a hematologist may be helpful in deciding which measures are appropriate for each child. Do not be surprised if some previously held concepts change.

Preoperative

1. All children of African American descent who require anesthesia must be screened for sickle cells:
   a. Neonatal screening using Hb electrophoresis is routine in the United States and other countries.
   b. Results of solubility tests (Sickledex, Sickleprep) are available in 5 minutes but do not differentiate sickle disease from trait.
   c. Screening tests are unreliable in infants less than 6 months of age because HbF masks the results; Hb electrophoresis provides an accurate diagnosis.
   d. Optimally, all children at risk should have a Hb electrophoresis to establish the exact diagnosis.
2. In general, a severe form of the disease is less likely if anemia is absent, but a Hb electrophoresis is still essential to exclude any other abnormal Hb (i.e., Hb C and D) and to assess the severity of the condition (Table 6-1). Children with Hb SC disease may have a normal Hb concentration but are still at risk of sickling.
3. If the child has sickle cell trait (less than 50% HbS):
   a. Avoid preoperative dehydration; encourage clear fluids until 2 hours before surgery if appropriate, or start intravenous fluids during the fasting period.
   b. Avoid excessive preoperative sedation.

TABLE 6–1   Hemoglobin Electrophoresis in Older Children

Syndrome	HbA (%)	HbS (%)	HbF (%)	HbC (%)
Sickle cell anemia	0	80–95	2–20	0
Sickle C disease	0	45–50	1–5	45–50
Sickle β-Thalassemia	0–30	65–90	2–15	0
Sickle cell trait	50–60	35–45	1–2	0
Normal	95–98	0	1–2	0

4. If the child has sickle cell disease (70% to 90% HbS):
   a. Assess the child carefully, particularly for sequelae of previous sickling crises (i.e., CNS, cardiac, pulmonary, or renal infarction).
   b. Preoperative transfusions may be given. One of two approaches may be taken:
      i. *Traditional approach:* Packed cells are infused over several days; this suppresses erythropoiesis, as evidenced by a decrease in the reticulocyte count. The HbS concentration may then be reduced to less than 40%, which has been considered safe for most surgeries.
      ii. *Conservative approach:* A blood transfusion is given as necessary to increase the Hb concentration to 10 g/dl or greater. This has been shown to be as effective as the traditional approach in preventing complications and is more conservative in the use (and hence the dangers) of transfusion. A noted sequela of either approach to blood transfusion is the development of new antibodies in the recipient, which could make it difficult to find compatible blood in the future.
   c. Those who require cardiopulmonary bypass with hypothermia should have packed cell infusions or exchange transfusion to reduce the HbS level to less than 5%.
   d. In an acute emergency, exchange transfusion may be performed.

Perioperative

1. Use high concentrations of inspired oxygen (at least 50%) to maintain 100% saturation and control ventilation.
2. Maintain normal acid-base status
3. Maintain normal body temperature.
4. Maintain fluid balance to avoid dehydration or excessive fluid administration.

5. Beware of regional ischemia:
   a. Position and pad the child carefully to avoid any regional vascular stasis.
   b. Do not use a tourniquet unless it is essential. If one is used, exsanguinate the limb well and use the tourniquet for a minimal time.
   c. Check the blood pressure cuff and other equipment frequently to see that no locally constricting effects are produced.

Postoperative

1. The child must be awake before extubation.
2. Give additional oxygen and monitor SpO_2 continuously during transport to and in the postanesthesia care unit (PACU).
3. Hydration and warmth must be maintained.
4. Be alert for the possibility of pulmonary complications; they are common in children with sickle cell disease.

Suggested Reading

Marchant WA, Walker I: Anaesthetic management of the child with sickle cell disease, Paediatr Anaesth 13(6):473–489, 2003.

Hemophilia

Factor VIII Deficiency (Classic Hemophilia Type A)

Classic hemophilia is inherited as an X-linked recessive disorder (1:10,000 incidence) and is characterized by episodes of bleeding, either spontaneous or after minimal injury. The presenting sign may be bleeding from the umbilical cord in neonates or after circumcision in infants. The diagnosis can be confirmed by factor VIII assay. During childhood, many sites may be involved, hemarthrosis is common, and retroperitoneal bleeding may occur. Hemophilic children require special care during any operation, including (most frequently) dental extractions.

Owing to the use of factor VIII concentrates from multiple donors, a high percentage of children with hemophilia have become infected with human immunodeficiency virus (HIV). Recombinant factor VIII is now available; it is as effective as that obtained from blood, and should ensure viral safety.

Surgical Management. Children with hemophilia should undergo elective surgery only in hospitals with facilities to care for this condition. Team care by a hematologist, a surgeon, and an anesthesiologist is essential. If an emergency operation is essential but the facilities of a hematology department are not available, give fresh-frozen plasma (20 ml/kg) preoperatively and consult with a pediatric hematologist as needed.

Preoperative

1. If there is any doubt about the diagnosis, the child's blood must be tested for factor concentrations. Preoperative investigation should include screening for factor VIII inhibitors (found in 5% to 10% of children), even if inhibitors were not detected previously.
2. One hour before surgery, an infusion of factor VIII concentrate (25 to 50 U/kg) should be given, followed by an assay for plasma factor VIII activity (1 U/kg factor VIII increases plasma level by 2%, $t_{1/2}$ is 12 hours). Surgery can proceed if factor VIII activity is greater than 50%.

Perioperative

1. Exercise great care during instrumentation of the airway. Avoid trauma that might provoke submucosal hemorrhage.
2. A continuous infusion of factor VIII (3 to 4 units/kg/hr) may be advisable during major surgery.

Postoperative

1. Depending on the nature of the surgery, the factor VIII levels in the blood should be maintained at 50% for several days. This is achieved by giving factor VIII, as dictated by repeated assay, preferably by continuous infusion.
2. After dental extraction, ε-aminocaproic acid (Amicar) may help to inhibit fibrinolysis of formed blood clot.

N.B. When factor VIII inhibitors are present, therapy presents a major challenge. Various methods have been used, including very large doses of factor VIII combined with immunosuppressive therapy, porcine factor VIII, and recombinant factor VIIa.

Factor IX Deficiency (Christmas Disease, Hemophilia Type B)

The disease is essentially similar to Hemophilia A. Children with factor IX deficiency are treated as for factor VIII deficiency except that factor IX levels are assayed and factor IX infusions are given. Problems with inhibitors are common in this condition as well.

Suggested Reading

Dunn AL, Abshire TC: Recent advances in the management of the child who has hemophilia, Hematol Oncol Clin N Am 18:1249–1276, 2004.

Rodriguez NI, Hoots WK: Advances in hemophilia: experimental aspects and therapy, Pediatr Clin N Am 55:357–376, 2008.

Von Willebrand Disease

Von Willebrand disease is the most common congenital bleeding disorder; it may affect 1% of children. There are many forms of the disease, both congenital and acquired, and its incidence varies widely among different ethnic groups. It may occur secondary to another disease (e.g., congenital heart disease, Wilms tumor) and may resolve with treatment of that disease. The basic defect present in von Willebrand disease is the lack of a plasma cofactor that is a carrier protein for factor VIII and is necessary for normal platelet function. There are three general types of the disease:

Type 1: Common (90% of cases) and mild—the bleeding time is prolonged, but the prothrombin time (PT) and partial thromboplastin time (PTT) are often normal.

Type 2: (a) With normal platelet count and (b) with thrombocytopenia.

Type 3: Most severe form (fewer than 1% of cases)—von Willebrand factor and factor VIII are undetectable.

The clinical manifestations depend on the severity of the disease. Cutaneous and mucous membrane bleeding are common, but deep tissue bleeding may also occur. A history of easy bleeding or failure to clot after dental extraction should alert the anesthesiologist. In type 1 and type 2a disease, 1-deamino-8-D-arginine vasopressin (DDAVP) is effective, but it may exacerbate type 2b and is ineffective in type 3 disease. The latter types must be treated with cryoprecipitate or fresh-frozen plasma.

If the type of disease is unknown preoperatively, it may be appropriate to assess the effect on coagulation studies of an infusion of DDAVP. If the bleeding time is shortened, DDAVP may be useful perioperatively. If not, blood products will be necessary.

Suggested Reading

Blanchette VS, Manco-Johnson M, Santagostino E, et al: Optimizing factor prophylaxis for the haemophilia population: where do we stand? Haemophilia 10(Suppl 4):97–104, 2004.

Dunn AL, Abshire TC: Recent advances in the management of the child who has hemophilia, Hematol Oncol Clin N Am 18:1249–1276, 2004.

ATYPICAL PLASMA CHOLINESTERASES

The genetically determined abnormal cholinesterases may result in prolonged apnea after the administration of muscle relaxants (e.g., succinylcholine). Five alleles of pseudocholinesterase found on chromosome 3 comprise the majority of phenotypes: normal, atypical, fluoride resistant, silent gene, and E Cynthiana (or Neitlich or C5 variant). More recent evidence added the H, J, and K variants. Atypical, fluoride resistant, and silent gene may significantly prolong recovery after succinylcholine in the homozygote state. The E Cynthiana variant rapid degrades succinylcholine. In the homozygote atypical state (incidence 1:2500 children), recovery of muscle strength may be delayed for 5 to 6 hours; in the heterozygous state (incidence 1:30), the delay may be unrecognized, 5 to 25 minutes (Table 6-2).

Management of Prolonged Apnea

If muscle activity fails to recover after administration of succinylcholine:

1. Continue to ventilate the lungs and provide sedation/anesthesia.
2. Confirm persistence of the neuromuscular block, using a nerve stimulator.
3. Allow the child to recover completely before ventilation and sedation/ anesthesia are discontinued (this may take up to 3 to 6 hours).

N.B. Prolonged apnea after succinylcholine due to an atypical cholinesterase is not serious provided the above steps are followed. Do not attempt to modify the neuromuscular block by giving drugs, infusing fresh blood, and so on, because further complications may arise. Ventilate the lungs and be patient.

Blood samples for cholinesterase studies should be obtained:

1. Cholinesterase activity (normal range is 60 to 200 units but varies with the individual laboratory)
2. Dibucaine number (DN; normal range, 75 to 85)
3. Fluoride number (FN; normal range, 55 to 65)

Characteristically, children with the atypical enzyme have a low DN (15 to 25) and a low FN (20 to 25) (see Table 6-2). Those heterozygous for the condition have intermediate values (DN, 50 to 70; FN, 40 to 50). The results of these tests may not be available for some days and hence are of no value in the immediate management of the child.

Other Considerations

When the diagnosis is confirmed, the child's family should have blood tests and be informed of their status. Those having homozygous atypical states should be advised to carry a warning card or wear a Medical Alert bracelet.

TABLE 6–2   Plasma Cholinesterases: Variation in Response to Succinylcholine

Genotype	Incidence	Response to Succinylcholine	Dubucaine No.	Fluoride No.
Homozygous				
E1^{u}E1^u		Normal	70	50
E1^{a}E1^a	1:2,800	Grossly prolonged	15–25	20–25
E1^{s}E1^s	1:140,000	Grossly prolonged	—	—
E1^{f}E1^f	1:300,000	Moderately prolonged	60–70	30–40
Heterozygous				
E1^{u}E1^a	1:25	Almost normal	50–70	40–50
E1^{u}E1^f	1:280	Almost normal	70–80	50–55
E1^{u}E1^s	1:190	Almost normal	70	50
E1^{a}E1^f	1:29,000	Grossly prolonged	45–50	30–40
E1^{a}E1^a	1:20,000	Grossly prolonged	15–25	20–25
E1^{f}E1^s	1:200,000	Grossly prolonged	60–70	30–35

Suggested Reading

Davis L, Britten JJ, Morgan M: Cholinesterase; its significance in anaesthetic practice, Anaesthesia 52:244–252, 1997.

DIABETES MELLITUS

Diabetes mellitus is the most common endocrine disorder of childhood. Children with symptomatic diabetes are all insulin dependent; type 2 diabetes can occur in children and adolescents, but it is asymptomatic and usually undiagnosed.

Young children typically have weight loss, polydipsia, and polyuria. However, the onset may be very abrupt, and the child may have ketoacidosis. The presentation may be accompanied by abdominal pain, leukocytosis, and mimic appendicitis. Vascular complications seldom occur in diabetic children, so the renal, cardiac, or peripheral vascular effects of the disease need not be sought.

The current approach to juvenile diabetes is to maintain blood glucose levels as close to normal as possible throughout the day by the use of twice- or thrice-daily insulin doses; some children may be using an insulin infusion pump. In some cases control is difficult, and childhood diabetes is often unstable; the anesthesiologist should consult closely with the medical team in planning the management of these cases.

Anesthesia Management

Perioperative management must be designed to achieve as close control of the blood glucose level as is possible. Hyperglycemia (>200 mg/dl) in the perioperative period is associated with increased wound infection rates in adults, similar data are not available in children.

Preoperative

1. Close monitoring of blood glucose should be instituted several days before elective major surgery to permit stabilization of the diabetes.
2. Minor elective surgery for the child with well-controlled diabetes may be planned on an outpatient basis.
3. Severe hyperglycemia and ketosis should be treated with appropriate insulin adjustments before surgery is scheduled. HbA1c should be followed to assess metabolic stability. Defer emergency surgery, if possible, until the diabetic ketoacidosis is corrected.
4. Brief procedures (less than 1 hour):
   a. Schedule as early as possible in the morning.
   b. Determine the preoperative blood glucose level.

c. Give one half to two thirds the usual dose of insulin as intermediate-acting insulin only (NPH or Lente). No short-acting insulin should be given.

d. Start an intravenous infusion of 5% glucose-containing solution and infuse at a maintenance rate (3 to 4 ml/kg/hr) unless the blood glucose is less than 5 mmol/L (90 mg/dl), in which case the rate should be increased and the blood glucose rechecked.

e. Determine the blood glucose concentration hourly during surgery and immediately after the procedure.

f. Use an anesthesia technique that will minimize PONV and permit early return to normal oral intake.

5. Prolonged procedures (>1 hour): The preferred technique is to give an infusion of insulin plus an infusion of dextrose and monitor blood glucose levels frequently (every hour) preferably using a glucometer.

a. Add 50 units of regular insulin to 500 ml of isotonic saline. (Each milliliter contains 0.1 unit of regular insulin.) Saturate the insulin-binding sites of the intravenous tubing by running 50 to 100 ml of the solution through the tubing.

b. Use a Y-tube or piggyback connection to the maintenance intravenous line, and control the rate with an infusion pump.

c. Infuse 1 ml/kg/hr to deliver 0.1 units of insulin per kilogram per hour.

d. Infuse a 5% glucose solution at a rate to maintain blood glucose at 5 to 10 mmol/L (90 to 180 mg/dl).

e. Blood glucose levels should be determined hourly during the surgery.

f. Postoperatively, the insulin infusion may be continued as long as necessary, depending on the circumstances. The child's pediatrician should control the rate and amount of the infusion based on the blood glucose concentration.

Postoperative

1. Brief procedures:
    a. If the child is receiving subcutaneous insulin, give appropriate doses of short-acting insulin as required based on blood glucose levels. Continue intravenous hydration until the child is taking fluids orally.
    b. The child's usual insulin regimen can be resumed the next day if the child is able to tolerate fluids or food.

2. Prolonged procedures:
    a. Change to subcutaneous insulin when the child's condition allows (e.g., when the child is taking fluids orally and intravenous hydration has been discontinued).
    b. Pediatricians should follow up and manage the child's diabetes.

Children Using an Insulin Pump

1. Ensure that the subcutaneous injection site is well protected and that the infusion needle does not become dislodged.
2. Plan management in consultation with the medical team. Generally the basal rate will be maintained, omitting bolus doses as meals are missed. Boluses may be administered depending upon the results of blood glucose determinations.

Emergency Surgery

Diabetic ketoacidosis may result from the physiologic stresses of the surgical disease, but remember also that the symptoms of ketoacidosis may mimic those of the acute abdomen.

1. Attempt to stabilize the child before proceeding to the operating room. Stabilization should be undertaken in cooperation with the medical team. Ketoacidosis must be corrected, intravascular volume restored, and electrolyte defects normalized.
2. Insert monitoring lines for central venous pressure (CVP) and arterial pressure to assist in correcting hypovolemia and hyperglycemia.
3. Infuse warmed fluids to correct hypovolemia; normal saline 10 to 20 ml/kg over 1 hour may be required, as indicated by CVP.
4. Intravenous regular insulin will be required. A bolus dose of 0.1 U/kg followed by an infusion of 0.1 U/kg/hr may be used.
5. Monitor blood glucose frequently; the objective is to decrease the concentration by a maximum of 100 mg/dl each hour. More rapid declines may result in detrimental osmotic shifts.
6. When the blood glucose concentration is less than 300 mg/dl, continue rehydration with 0.45% saline and 5% dextrose solution.
7. Monitor serum electrolytes frequently; hypokalemia is to be expected. Potassium must be added to the infusion provided that renal function is satisfactory.
8. Metabolic acidosis corrects spontaneously as hypovolemia is corrected and insulin administered. Ketones are metabolized, and their production is halted. Sodium bicarbonate is unnecessary and may be deleterious except when very severe acidosis (pH less than 7.0) is present.
9. Subclinical brain swelling occurs during the treatment of diabetic ketoacidosis and, rarely, dangerous cerebral edema may develop. It is recommended that children be closely monitored and that total fluid administration be limited to 4 L/m^2/24 hr.

Suggested Reading

Betts P, Brink SJ, Swift PG, et al: ISPAD. Management of children with diabetes requiring surgery, Pediatr Diabetes 8(4):242–247, 2007.

Rhodes ET, Ferrari LR, Wolfsdorf JI: Perioperative management of pediatric surgical patients with diabetes mellitus, Anesth Analg 101:986–999, 2005.

MALIGNANT DISEASES

The anesthesiologist frequently has to care for children with malignant disease. Special problems may arise depending on the site and type of the disease, but all of these children require special attention to their emotional status. Extreme care must be taken to ensure a minimum of discomfort and upset for both child and parents.

Children require special care during painful diagnostic and therapeutic procedures (e.g., lumbar puncture, bone marrow aspiration), and these should be carefully planned as described elsewhere.

Special Anesthesia Problems

The child with a malignancy may present special problems:

1. Abnormal anatomy, including the airway, may cause problems. Be especially aware of the child with enlarged hilar lymph nodes.
2. Hematologic disease may result in anemia, coagulopathy, and immune deficiency. Check laboratory results preoperatively. Coagulopathy may lead to intraoperative pulmonary hemorrhage and difficulty with ventilation. Urgent bronchoscopy is required in such cases to remove clots.
3. Increased susceptibility to infection means that care in asepsis is vital to these children.
4. A history of long-term steroid therapy necessitates consideration of preoperative corticosteroids.
5. Nausea and vomiting may complicate radiotherapy and/or drug therapy and lead to dehydration and electrolyte disturbance. Check the biochemistry levels. Do not administer dexamethasone without consulting with the oncologist—tumor lysis syndrome may result.
6. Cardiomyopathy may follow total body irradiation, cyclophosphamide, and doxorubicin or daunomycin (see later discussion).
7. Hypercalcemia may accompany malignant tumors of bone.
8. Nephropathy may lead to impaired renal function.
9. Increased intracranial pressure may occur with involvement of the central nervous system.

10. Peripheral neuropathy may occur.
11. Muscle weakness and hypotonia occur in advanced malignant disease.
12. Toxic effects of chemotherapy may be present (see later discussion).
13. Tumor lysis syndrome is a metabolic disorder that accompanies treatment of hematologic cancers. Characterized by hyperkalemia, hypocalcemia, acute renal failure, and several other metabolic derangements.

Adverse Effects of Commonly Used Drugs

All antineoplastic drugs can cause the following effects:

1. Bone marrow suppression, with anemia, leukopenia, and thrombocytopenia
2. Anorexia, nausea, and vomiting
3. Stomatitis and alopecia
4. Decreased resistance to infection

Some of these agents produce additional adverse effects:

1. Hepatotoxicity (i.e., methotrexate, cyclophosphamide), check liver function indices.
2. Renal toxic effects (i.e., cisplatin, ifosfamide), which may be increased by the use of aminoglycoside antibiotics or diuretics (furosemide).

Furthermore, specific drugs have effects of special importance to anesthesiologists:

1. Cardiotoxic effects
ECG changes are nonspecific, but prolongation of the Q-T interval suggests toxicity. Echocardiography is the most useful index of cardiac function, and recent studies should be reviewed before proceeding with anesthesia.
   a. Both *daunomycin*, used in leukemia therapy, and *doxorubicin* (Adriamycin), used in therapy for solid tumors and leukemias, affect the heart, causing
      i. Nonspecific electrocardiographic (ECG) changes, with any dose.
      ii. Disturbances of conduction, including supraventricular tachycardia, atrial and ventricular extrasystoles, and ventricular fibrillation.
      iii. Drug-induced cardiomyopathy in 1% to 2% of children, leading to congestive heart failure.

iv. The cardiac effects of doxorubicin are dose-related. A total cumulative dose of 250 mg/m^2, or 150 mg/m^2 if combined with mediastinal radiation, must alert the anesthesiologist and is an indication for a full cardiologic assessment particularly an echocardiogram to assess cardiac contractility. Children with a history of congestive heart failure are particularly likely to experience perioperative complications.

v. Myocardial depressant drugs (e.g., halothane) should be used with caution or avoided and cardiac parameters should be closely monitored.

vi. Beta blockers and calcium channel-blocking drugs may dangerously increase the cardiotoxic effects and should be avoided.

b. *Mitoxantrone* may cause cardiotoxicity, especially if given after previous anthracycline therapy and with cumulative doses greater than 120 mg/m^2.

c. *Cyclophosphamide, cisplatin, 5-fluorouracil, amsacrine, mithramycin, mitomycin, vincristine,* and *actinomycin D* may all be cardiotoxic or contribute to cardiotoxicity at large doses.

2. Pulmonary toxicity

a. *Bleomycin,* used in therapy for testicular tumors and Hodgkin disease, causes pulmonary fibrosis in approximately 10% of patients and may result in death (1%). *The effects on the lung are accelerated by hyperoxia, and oxygen therapy should be carefully controlled at all times. Fluid therapy should be strictly limited since overload may further compromise lung function by causing pulmonary edema.*

b. *Busulfan, carmustine, methotrexate,* and *mitomycin* may cause pulmonary fibrosis with large doses.

c. *Cytosine arabinoside, vinblastine,* and *mitomycin* have been associated with noncardiac pulmonary edema.

3. Anticholinesterase inhibition

a. *Cyclophosphamide* and other alkylating agents—used for lymphomas, Hodgkin disease, and leukemias—inhibit serum cholinesterase; prolonged apnea with succinylcholine may occur.

Suggested Reading

Huettemann E, Junker T, Chatzinikolaou KP, et al: The influence of anthracycline therapy on cardiac function during anesthesia, Anesth Analg 98(4):941–947, 2004.

McDowall RH: Anesthesia considerations for pediatric cancer, Semin Surg Oncol 9(6):478–488, 1993.

DOWN SYNDROME

Down syndrome (trisomy 21; T21) is common (1.5 cases per 1000 live births). Developmental delay is invariably present but varies in severity from child to child; many children with this syndrome are quite cooperative and capable of relatively independent function in a protected environment.

Associated Conditions

1. Congenital heart disease occurs in approximately 40% to 50% of children, particularly atrioventricular canal, ventricular septal defect, patent ductus arteriosus, and tetralogy of Fallot. Pulmonary hypertension may accompany CHD and chronic airway obstruction.
2. Respiratory infections are common. This may be related to the genetic anomaly, an immune deficiency, and/or the social and institutional implications of the syndrome. Chronic sinus and ear infections are also common.
3. Generalized hypotonia and joint laxity are present. Atlantoaxial joint instability occurs in 12% of afflicted children and may lead to cervical spinal cord injury. The neck is particularly unstable in the flexed position, but caution should be exercised to minimize excessive motion. Great care should be taken during positioning, particularly for ear surgery; avoid excessive rotation of the neck.
4. Congenital subglottic stenosis is common. Ensure that the endotracheal tube selected is not too large and that there is an audible leak when positive pressure is applied.
5. Adenotonsillar hypertrophy is often present and obstructive sleep apnea is common.
6. Thyroid hypofunction is common as the child ages (15% to 20% of young children) and diabetes may develop.
7. Polycythemia is a frequent finding in neonates and may necessitate phlebotomy to relieve circulatory failure. Leukemia develops in 0.7% of children with Down syndrome.
8. Duodenal atresia is common in the neonate, as is umbilical hernia, renal malformations, undescended testis, and hypospadias.
9. Radial artery abnormalities (i.e., single median artery) are common and may make percutaneous cannulation difficult or impossible.

Special Anesthesia Problems

1. Airway: The large tongue and small nasopharynx predispose to respiratory obstruction, particularly during mask anesthesia and recovery stages. Have an oropharyngeal airway and LMA ready. Congenital subglottic stenosis predisposes to postoperative stridor.

2. Lungs: Is there any acute infection present that requires therapy before surgery? Is there a history suggestive of OSA?
3. Problems of associated cardiac disease: endocarditis prophylaxis may be required (see Chapter 14, page 462).
4. Atlantoaxial joint instability may predispose to injury during laryngos-copy and tracheal intubation. Inquire preoperatively for any signs or symptoms suggestive of C-spine compression (pain, gait disturbances, hand dysfunction, dizziness, bowel and bladder function). Gently examine the neck and perform CNS examination. Routine neck x-rays are not warranted in the absence of signs or symptoms. Any excessive neck movement should be avoided (especially flexion). Position the head very carefully, especially for ENT procedures.
5. Cognitively challenged children are more difficult to manage during induction of anesthesia. Often the parents can be of great help.

N.B. Children with Down syndrome have been reported to be espe-cially sensitive to the effects of atropine. This is not true; in practice, we have used the same dosage schedule for these as for other children with-out any problems.

Suggested Reading

Steward DJ: Anesthesia considerations in children with Down Syndrome, Semin Anesth Periop Med Pain 25:136–141, 2006.

MALIGNANT HYPERTHERMIA

Malignant hyperthermia (MH), a potentially fatal abnormal response to inhaled anesthetic agents and succinylcholine, is a pharmacogenetic disor-der of skeletal muscles. All potent inhalational anesthetics including sevo-flurane and desflurane, but not nitrous oxide, may trigger MH. No other drugs have been identified as triggers of MH. It is characterized by a rapid increase in $PetCO_2$, heart rate and respiratory rate, and the rapid onset of generalized muscle rigidity. Subsequently, body temperature increases. If untreated, profound biochemical changes occur later.

MH is a rare condition, probably occurring in fewer than 1 in 100,000 cases in which general anesthetics are given, although the quoted inci-dence in children is 1 in 15,000. Children and young adults have most frequently been affected, and it has been reported in an infant as young as 2 months of age. Increased awareness of MH, leading to earlier diagno-sis and prompt institution of treatment, plus the availability of a specific therapy (dantrolene), has reduced the mortality rate from more than 70% to less than 10%.

Knowledge of the pathophysiology of MH has progressively increased. It is now clear that the disease process is associated with altered calcium homeostasis in skeletal muscle. Malignant hyperthermia-susceptible (MHS) patients demonstrate an increased calcium ion concentration in skeletal muscle, and studies in MHS swine show a marked increase in the intracellular calcium concentration on exposure to triggering agents. This increased calcium level has been linked with a potential defect in the "calcium-induced calcium release" mechanism within the cell, now further linked with a defect in the calcium release channel of the sarcoplasmic reticulum. The mechanism of the disease process in the cell produces a sustained contracture of skeletal muscle, causing increased muscle metabolism with associated heat production. The further manifestations of the acute syndrome are secondary to the acceleration of metabolic processes within skeletal muscle, which is accompanied by large increases in oxygen consumption and CO_2 production. If the acute reaction persists, cellular energy substrates become depleted, with consequent failure of cellular functions, including those regulating the intracellular and extracellular chemical composition. Substances released by damaged cells (potassium, CK, myoglobin, etc.) trigger the continuing manifestations of the acute crisis, including coagulopathy and renal failure.

Detection of Susceptibility

There are still no simple, reliable screening tests to identify MHS individuals preoperatively. Creatine phosphokinase (CPK) levels may be increased, but this test is nonspecific. Many MHS children do have local or generalized muscular disease; however, most with a muscle disease are not MHS. Although a positive family anesthetic history of MH is the most reliable clue, its absence does not guarantee an individual's nonsusceptibility to triggering agents. Even uneventful previous anesthesia does not preclude an MH crisis during a subsequent anesthesia.

At present, MHS patients can be identified with reasonable certainty only by in vitro study of fresh living muscle tissue obtained at biopsy. Caffeine- and halothane-induced contracture of the biopsy specimen is usually diagnostic; this is presently the "gold standard." Up to the present time a relatively large biopsy specimen has been required, so the test is not usually recommended for small children (younger than 10 years of age). In recent years, much progress has been made toward standardizing contracture testing for MHS and establishing uniform criteria for a positive diagnosis to be made.

Less invasive tests to determine MH susceptibility have been disappointing. MRI has been used to identify abnormalities of skeletal muscle energy substrates in MHS subjects, but a reliable, specific marker for the disease has not been identified. Several genetic permutations have been identified in MHS patients (chromosome 1q, 3q, 5p, 7q, 17q, and 19q with the defect on chromosome 19 accounting for 40% of the genetic defects). Therefore, at the present time, there are no noninvasive methods to diagnose the MH susceptibility with certainty.

Clinical Manifestations

Nonspecific, early signs include:
1. Increased $PetCO_2$, unexplained tachycardia, tachypnea (or attempts to breathe against the ventilator), sweating, desaturation, cyanosis, and overheating of the CO_2 absorbent
2. Hypertonus of skeletal muscles, particularly large muscle groups
   a. It may occur immediately after the administration of succinylcholine.
      i. Failure of skeletal muscle to relax. This is an indication to postpone surgery and reevaluate.
      ii. Abnormally severe muscle fasciculations or intense masseter muscle spasm. This should arouse suspicion.
   b. It may also occur later during anesthesia, after the use of potent inhalational anesthetics.
3. A rapid increase in body temperature (more than 1 °C) is a late sign.
   The prognosis is much more favorable if the reaction is recognized early and dantrolene is administered before a significant increase in the body temperature occurs.

Confirmatory evidence of an MH crisis consists of biochemical changes: severe metabolic acidosis (base deficit >25 mEq/L) and severe respiratory acidosis (partial pressure of carbon dioxide [Pco_2] >60 mm Hg). Venous desaturation may occur. Serum potassium may be increased. Generalized muscle rigidity, ventricular arrhythmias, cyanosis, and increasing body temperature are predictive of an impending MH crisis.

Therapeutic Regimen*

1. Discontinue all inhalational anesthetics; inform the surgeon of the diagnosis; insist that surgery be urgently terminated. **Send for help!**
2. Hyperventilate with 100% O_2 using a high flow. A T-piece type circuit (e.g., Bain) may not provide adequate ventilation for large children even at large fresh gas flows; therefore, change to a new circle absorber system as soon as possible.

---

* Further advice can be obtained in North America from the MHAUS hotline telephone number: 209–634–4917.

3. Immediately give the following:
   a. *Dantrolene*: The initial dose is 2.5 mg/kg, given as a rapid IV infusion. If necessary, repeat at 1 mg/kg IV every 5 minutes until the end-tidal carbon dioxide decreases, the heart rate begins to slow and become regular, muscle tone decreases, and the child's fever abates. Then withhold the dantrolene and observe the heart rate, muscle tone, and temperature. If these deteriorate again, then repeat IV dantrolene until clinical improvement is apparent.
   b. If intravenous dantrolene is not available or if arrhythmias persist, infuse *procainamide* intravenously (1 mg/kg/min, up to a maximum of 15 mg/kg) and monitor the results with the ECG. This infusion may relieve muscle contracture promptly and prevent further increase in body temperature.
   c. *Sodium bicarbonate (7.5%)*: 4 ml/kg IV immediately; repeat in accordance with blood gas analyses to reverse the metabolic acidosis if dantrolene is not available. However, if alveolar ventilation is already maximized, bicarbonate may cause a respiratory acidosis.
   d. *Mannitol*: 0.5 g/kg; mannitol is present in the dantrolene mixture (150 mg for each milligram of dantrolene), but supplementation may be needed to maintain an adequate urine output (more than 1 ml/kg/hr). A urinary catheter will prevent bladder distention.
4. If dantrolene is not available, commence active cooling. Symptomatic cooling should occur in cool/tepid water; iced temperature immersion may cause cutaneous vasoconstriction preventing heat loss. Place the child on a rubber sheet and use fans. Intragastric cooling and cold enemas may also be necessary. Infuse refrigerated saline solution intravenously at 10 ml/kg/hr as necessary.
5. Continue monitoring the child closely:
   a. Monitor by stethoscope, pulse oximeter, and ECG.
   b. If an arterial line is not already present, insert one to measure pressure and obtain blood samples.
   c. Insert a CVP line to monitor volume status and oxygen extraction.
   d. Insert a urinary catheter and monitor urine output.
   e. Attach a multichannel thermometer (rectal, esophageal, skin, and muscle leads). Beware of overtreatment leading to hypothermia.
6. Obtain frequent arterial blood samples for the following studies:
   a. Blood gas and acid/base determinations (repeat every 10 minutes)
   b. Serum electrolytes (Na, K, Cl, Ca, inorganic phosphate)
   c. CPK (obtain immediately at the onset of a reaction (normal value), peak concentration occurs at 12 to 18 hours.

    d. Serum enzymes: serum glutamic oxaloacetic transaminase (SGOT), lactate dehydrogenase (LDH), creatine kinase (CK), 3-hydroxybutyrate dehydrogenase (3-HBDH).

    e. Coagulation studies

8. Correct any electrolyte imbalance on the basis of biochemical indices. To treat hyperkalemia, give 0.15 units/kg of regular insulin with 0.5 g/kg of glucose.

9. Continue to measure urine output, and maintain it at 1 ml/kg/hr or greater, using diuretics as necessary to prevent rhabdomyolysis-induced renal failure.

10. Coagulopathy must be expected to develop later and may necessitate therapy on the basis of demonstrated factor deficiencies.

11. Avoid the administration of drugs that might complicate matters: calcium, digitalis, and adrenergic agents have previously been considered contraindicated. In fact they may not cause further problems, but they are probably best avoided unless definitely indicated. *Calcium channel-blocking agents are considered contraindicated; they may interact with dantrolene to produce profound myocardial depression and do not have a therapeutic role in MH.*

12. Monitor the child in the intensive care unit with the same aggressive monitoring as in the operating room; MH may recur within the first 24 hours. Sequelae of the episode may also demand aggressive therapy. Depending on the severity of the reaction, the airway may require ongoing intubation and hyperventilation. For example:

    a. Recrudescence may occur in up to 20% of those who have had MH reactions, IV dantrolene may be repeated as required to treat recrudescence.

    b. Cerebral edema may appear because of hypoxic insult.

    c. Pulmonary edema may present because of fluid overload or myocardial dysfunction.

    d. Coagulopathy and renal failure may require continued care.

Anesthesia Regimen for Patients With Known Susceptibility to Malignant Hyperthermia

All personnel who may be concerned in the care of an MHS patient in the operating room (OR) and PACU must be fully acquainted with a suitable protocol that describes the location of drugs, equipment, etc., and the procedures to be implemented if MH develops.

Children at Risk

1. Survivors of an MH crisis
2. Children with a positive muscle biopsy
3. A first-degree relative of anyone known to be MHS (i.e., positive muscle biopsy or survivor of an MH crisis)
4. Those with muscle abnormalities and/or an increased serum CPK level, in whom MH may be suspected
5. Children with central core disease

In the management of children, the clinician must frequently assume possible MH susceptibility on questionable evidence (i.e., a family history of anesthetic difficulties but no positive muscle biopsy in the family). The simple course then is to provide a trigger-free anesthetic.

Preoperative Investigation

A preoperative investigation should be done for children with a positive or strongly suggestive family or personal history.

1. Review the family and personal history carefully, noting especially muscle disease, cardiac abnormality, and drug- or anesthesia-induced reactions.
2. Order laboratory investigations: serum enzymes (SGOT, LDH, CK, 3-HBDH).
3. Order an ECG and an echocardiogram.
4. If the findings indicate a strong possibility of MH susceptibility and the child is older than 12 years of age, it may be advisable to arrange for muscle biopsy at a suitably equipped center. Younger children and infants must be presumed to be at risk for MH and treated accordingly until they are old enough for testing (or until an improved, less invasive diagnostic test becomes available). A medic alert bracelet should be sought with any documented family history of MH.

Preoperative Preparation

1. For anxious children, a sedative may be ordered the night before surgery. For minor surgery, oral midazolam may be administered 15 to 30 minutes before surgery. If excessive anxiety and muscle cramps have been present, the child should be admitted to the hospital 24 hours preoperatively for preoperative sedation.
2. Routine dantrolene pretreatment is not recommended for MHS children. However, in very high risk MHS children or those undergoing

emergency or trauma surgery (who are stressed) preoperative dantrolene, 2 to 4 mg/kg IV, should be considered.
3. If diagnostic muscle biopsy is to be performed, dantrolene must not be given (it affects the test results).
4. Ensure that all necessary drugs and equipment have been prepared:
    a. Drugs for anesthesia—All intravenous induction agents, nondepolarizing relaxants, opioids, nitrous oxide, ketamine, atropine, and anticholinesterases are safe.
    b. Drugs for emergency use if MH develops, including refrigerated lactated Ringer's solution, normal saline, 7.5% sodium bicarbonate, warmed 20% mannitol and 50% glucose solutions, dantrolene, procainamide, hydrocortisone, furosemide, potassium chloride, soluble (Regular) insulin, heparin, chlorpromazine, and propranolol.
    c. Equipment: vapor-free anesthetic machine, plastic disposable circuit and reservoir bag, ventilator, hypothermia blankets, multichannel thermometer, and probes. (If dantrolene is not available, ice and ice bags should be available to the OR suite.) Remove all triggering anesthetics from the operating room (to prevent any possibility of accidental use).

Induction of Anesthesia

1. Induce and maintain anesthesia using only nontriggering agents; these include propofol, thiopental, nitrous oxide, opioids, benzodiazepines, nondepolarizing muscle relaxants, and local analgesics.
2. For all major procedures, insert arterial and CVP lines and bladder catheter.
3. Monitor closely for early signs of an MH crisis (PetCO$_2$, heart rate, and respiratory rate [if breathing spontaneously]).

Postoperative (After Uneventful Anesthesia)

1. Transfer the patient to the PACU, with monitoring equipment and intravenous cannulas in place.
2. Ensure that *all* PACU staff are aware of the possibility of a delayed MH reaction and know what to do if one occurs.
3. Vital signs are recorded at 5-minute intervals initially.
4. Do not transfer the child to the ward or home until vital signs have been stable for 4 hours and the results of any laboratory tests are satisfactory.
5. After the child is returned to the ward, vital signs are recorded hourly for 4 hours and then every 4 hours for 1 day.

6. Dantrolene should be administered to any child who exhibits any untoward signs (e.g., persistent tachycardia or dysrhythmia, temperature rise) and the child transferred to ICU for monitoring.

Suggested Reading

Hopkins PM: Malignant hyperthermia: advances in clinical management and diagnosis, Br J Anaesth 85(1):118–128, 2000.

Yentis SM, Levine MF, Hartley EJ: Should all children with suspected or confirmed malignant hyperthermia susceptibility be admitted after surgery? A 10 year review, Anesth Analg 75:345–350, 1992.

Masseter Spasm

Masseter spasm is sometimes observed when succinylcholine is administered intravenously to a child, most commonly one who is anesthetized with halothane. This phenomenon has caused much confusion in the past, and it has been suggested that this form of masseter spasm might commonly be associated with MH trait. It is now recognized that many children respond with transient increased masseter tone if the "halothane followed by succinylcholine" sequence is used. This is probably a normal response that varies in intensity. We suggest that the whole problem can be prevented by avoiding the use of succinylcholine during halothane anesthesia.

If masseter spasm occurs in isolation or in combination with other signs of MH, various courses of action have been suggested, ranging from discontinuing the anesthesia and recommending a muscle biopsy to continuing the anesthesia with known MH-triggering agents. We suggest that a conservative approach is to continue with anesthesia, monitor the child carefully, and avoid known triggering agents. Isolated masseter spasm after the thiopental plus succinylcholine sequence is very rare and must be considered a possible early sign of MH trait (see previous discussion).

Suggested Reading

Lazzell VA, Carr AS, Lerman J: The incidence of masseter muscle rigidity after succinylcholine in infants and children, Can J Anaesth 41:475–479, 1994.

O'Flynn RP, Shutack JG, Rosenberg H, et al: Masseter muscle rigidity and malignant hyperthermia susceptibility in pediatric patients: an update on management and diagnosis, Anesthesiology 80:1228–1233, 1994.

Neuroleptic Malignant Syndrome

Neuroleptic malignant syndrome is a disorder characterized by the insidious onset of fever, muscle rigidity, tachycardia, and autonomic instability in patients receiving antipsychotic medication. It is rare but has been reported in children, in whom the diagnosis may be missed or may be confused with MH. The disease can progress to hepatic and renal failure. Treatment is by withdrawal of the antipsychotic medication. The likelihood that this syndrome is associated closely with MH susceptibility is considered remote.

Suggested Reading

Levine MF, Lerman J: Neuroleptic malignant syndrome in a child, Paediatr Anaesth 3:47–50, 1993.

LATEX ALLERGY

Latex allergy can cause a severe, life-threatening intraoperative immunoglobulin E-mediated anaphylactic reaction. Urticaria, bronchospasm, and/or circulatory collapse may occur. A history of repeated exposure to latex (e.g., frequent catheterization for neurogenic bladder, repeated surgery) and/or reactions to rubber balloons or dental dams may be elicited. Up to 40% of children with spina bifida have latex allergy. The risk of developing allergy may be related to the number of surgeries (>5 surgeries) and the presence of atopy; hence, older children are more likely to have developed allergy. Cross-reactivity to bananas, avocado, kiwi fruit, and chestnuts may be found. Skin-prick testing or radioallergosorbent testing (RAST) to latex may confirm the allergy, though there is some controversy as to the use of such tests.

Latex allergy should be considered if signs of an anaphylactic reaction occur during surgery and cannot be related to drug administration. The initial signs usually develop 30 to 200 minutes after induction of anesthesia while the surgeon is handling large surface areas of mesentery or tissue; the signs include increased airway pressure, decreased oxygen saturation, flushing and/or urticaria, hypotension, and tachycardia. One author has observed an urticaria the shape of a hand indicating the cutaneous contact with a latex glove.

The condition demands rapid, aggressive intervention including ventilation with oxygen, rapid infusion of warmed intravenous fluids to expand the blood volume, and epinephrine 1 to 5 µg/kg IV bolus followed by an infusion of 0.1 to 0.3 µg/kg/min. Other drugs that should be used include antihistamines (diphenhydramine, 1 mg/kg); histamine$_2$ (H$_2$) receptor-blocking drugs (cimetidine, 4 µg/kg); and corticosteroids (hydrocortisone 2 mg/kg).

Children at risk should be carefully reviewed; those with a history suggestive of latex allergy should be skin tested if possible. Those who are positive or those with a history suggestive of latex allergy may be pretreated before surgery to minimize the risk of an anaphylactic reaction, although reactions have occurred despite pretreatment. A regimen of corticosteroids (prednisone, 1 mg/kg) and H_1- and H_2-blocking drugs (diphenhydramine, 1 mg/kg, and cimetidine, 5 mg/kg) has been suggested. The child may then be anesthetized and carefully monitored. It is most important that all members of the surgical team use nonlatex gloves and that all latex materials be excluded from the surgical and anesthesia equipment (Table 6-3).

It is practical and important to eliminate latex from all items that may come into close contact with the child (e.g., syringes, masks). It may be less practical and less important to change remote items (i.e., ventilator bellows) than to substitute latex gloves. All items of equipment that are latex free should be clearly labeled as such in the storage area. All items containing latex should be clearly marked with a warning label.

It is strongly recommended that all children who are at risk for development of latex allergy (i.e., those with myelomeningocele) should be treated in a latex-free environment from the outset.

In summary:

1. All parents and older children should be questioned about a history of lips swelling after touching toy balloons, tongue swelling after dental

TABLE 6–3   Anesthesia Equipment That May Contain Latex

Intravenous bag
Anesthesia circuit and bag
Airway or bite block
Plastic syringes
Vials
Intravenous bag
IV set (ports)
Catheters
Adhesive tape
Tourniquets
Face mask
Endotracheal tube
Anesthesia circuit and bag
Ventilator bellows
Blood pressure cuff
Gloves

rubber dams in the mouth, and allergy to bananas, avocado, kiwi fruit, and chestnuts.

2. Children in high-risk groups should be identified and offered skin tests.
3. All equipment should be clearly labeled as to its latex content.
4. All procedures on children who have a positive history or are at high risk for development of latex allergy should be performed in a latex-free environment.

Suggested Reading

Holzman RS: Clinical management of latex-allergic children, Anesth Analg 85(3):529–533, 1997.

THE CHILD WITH CEREBRAL PALSY

Children with cerebral palsy (CP) frequently present for anesthesia and the increased survival of very-low-birth-weight infants may further increase their numbers. CP is a collective term for a variety of clinical conditions resulting from a nonprogressive neurologic insult early in life (possibly intrauterine or interuterine). The clinical state varies from mild local weakness with normal intelligence to severe spastic quadriplegia with gross mental retardation.

Special Anesthesia Problems

1. Communication with the child may be very difficult or impossible, compromising the assessment of pain and eliminating the potential for any rapport with the anesthesiologist and explanation of threatening procedures. In these circumstances the parents or other caregivers should be co-opted and relied upon for their assistance.
2. Many children have undergone repeated procedures and are extremely sensitized to the hospital environment. Careful planning is required to prevent further stresses.
3. The nutritional state may be suboptimal and may compromise anesthesia care and recovery from surgery. Preoperative hyperalimentation should be considered before extensive surgery; a feeding gastrostomy may lead to improved wound healing and decreased postoperative infections.
4. Gastroesophageal reflux disease (GERD) is common and together with increased salivation may predispose to chronic pulmonary aspiration and recurrent pneumonia. Drugs administered to treat GERD may have significant implications during anesthesia:

    a. Cisapride is associated with prolonged Q-T interval and serious ventricular arrhythmia. (No longer available for use in children in United States and Europe.)

    b. Sodium valproate affects platelet function and may increase bleeding.

5. Spasticity and contractures may make intravenous access and positioning for surgery very difficult. Great care must be taken to prevent skin damage or nerve injury by using effective padding and/or a soft air mattress.

6. Baclofen (an agonist at $GABA_\beta$ receptors in the dorsal horn) is commonly used to treat pain and contractures in CP. It is poorly absorbed via the GI tract and hence is given by an intrathecal pump. Overdose leads to drowsiness, respiratory depression, eventual coma, and has been a cause of delayed anesthesia recovery. Mild side effects may be treated by IV physostigmine or flumazenil; severe symptoms require decreased pump infusion rates. Sudden cessation of baclofen may lead to seizures.

7. Antiseizure medication is frequently required (30% of CP children). It should be continued perioperatively and may affect the actions of anesthesia drugs. Postoperatively, after extensive surgery, it is important to check anticonvulsant drug levels and restore these promptly. If the child remains NPO, fosphenytoin may be administered IV to prevent seizures.

8. Latex allergy is common in children with CP; the history should be carefully evaluated for evidence of this and appropriate precautions taken.

Anesthesia Management

1. Very careful preoperative evaluation is required to assess comorbidities and to determine whether acute disease is present, which requires preoperative treatment. In particular the pulmonary status should be carefully evaluated.

2. The parents or other caregiver should be questioned about previous anesthesia experiences and their child's responses. Sedative premedication should be considered for all of these children except for those who are severely obtunded or have a suspected difficult airway. A reduced dose may be appropriate in some cases. Anticholinergic premedication may be useful to decrease hypersalivation and airway secretions.

3. If intravenous induction is proposed, a suitable site should be selected and a topical local anesthetic (see page 634) applied at the appropriate time. If the child is vasoconstricted, application of local warming may produce venodilation and improve success.

4. Intravenous propofol may be advantageous as an induction agent as it tends to decrease airway and bronchial reactivity. Otherwise, use sevoflurane to induce anesthesia.

5. The need for a RSI must be assessed for each child. Succinylcholine does not induce hyperkalemia in children with CP; the ED_{50} for succinylcholine may be slightly less than in nonaffected children. Children with excessive secretions should have the endotracheal tube suctioned after insertion. Sputum should be sent for culture in those with pulmonary disease.

6. The MAC of the inhalational anesthetics in children with CP is 20% less than it is in unaffected children. BIS values for children with CP were found to be less than in unaffected children, both awake and at similar end-tidal levels of sevoflurane anesthesia. Reduced doses of propofol are required to achieve reduced BIS values in children with CP.

7. Resistance to vecuronium has been observed in some children with CP and might be a result of interaction with anticonvulsant drug therapy or alterations in the neuromuscular acetylcholine receptors. Increased doses of neuromuscular blocking drugs may be required, a NM block monitor should be used.

8. Children with CP are prone to hypothermia, great care should be taken to monitor and maintain body temperature intraoperatively.

9. Endoscopic surgery for GER procedures is preferred; children with CP tolerate the physiologic stresses imposed by pneumoperitoneum, and postoperative pain and complications are reduced.

10. Blood losses with extensive surgery (i.e., spinal instrumentation) may be greater than in normal children. This may be related to changes in vasomotor control and to platelet and clotting factor deficiencies. Appropriate supplies of blood and clotting factors should be available and used as indicated.

Postoperative Care

1. Regional analgesia is ideal for the control of postoperative pain; continuous infusion of local analgesics or opioids produces good analgesia, which can be readily monitored. The addition of clonidine to the infusion may reduce spasticity. Placement of an epidural or peripheral nerve(s) catheter during anesthesia is indicated whenever possible.

2. The parents or other caregiver should be present in the postoperative area to assist in the assessment of the child's discomfort.

3. After major spinal surgery in the child with CP, a stormy postoperative course must be anticipated and the full resources of a pediatric intensive care unit are essential.

4. Antiseizure medications should be carefully continued. After major surgery blood levels of these drugs should be obtained to guide therapy.

Fosphenytoin may be administered to those who remain NPO for any length of time.

5. Children with casts should be carefully monitored especially when epidural analgesia is employed. Compartment syndrome may follow osteotomies and is difficult to detect. Close cooperation with the orthopedic surgeon is essential.

Suggested Reading

Nolan J, Chalkiadis GA, Low J, et al: Anaesthesia and pain management in cerebral palsy, Anaesth 55(1):32–41, 2000.

Choudhry DK, Brenn BR: Bispectral index monitoring: a comparison between normal children and children with quadriplegic cerebral palsy, Anesth Analg 95(6):1582–1585, 2002.

Wongprasartsuk P, Stevens J: Cerebral palsy and anaesthesia, Paediatr Anaesth 12(4):296–303, 2002.

Saricaoglu F, Celebi N, Celik M, et al: The evaluation of propofol dosage for anesthesia induction in children with cerebral palsy with bispectral index (BIS) monitoring, Paediatr Anaest 15:1048–1052, 2005.

THE CHILD WITH A TRANSPLANT

There are now numerous children living with transplanted organs; these children require special considerations.

1. These children and their families have survived extensive medical and surgical interventions; they require very considerate emotional care.
2. All of them receive a regimen of antirejection drugs, which may have important side effects.
   a. All of the antirejection drugs cause reduced resistance to infection. *Take extreme care with aseptic technique.* Insert only those intravenous and monitoring lines that are really needed, and remove them as soon as possible.
   b. Cyclosporine can cause hypertension, hyperkalemia, and nephrotoxicity; therefore check renal function tests. In addition, it may interact with and potentiate barbiturates, fentanyl, and muscle relaxants, especially vecuronium and atracurium.
   c. Azathioprine can cause bone marrow depression and hepatotoxicity; check liver function. It also has anticholinesterase effects and may prolong the action of succinylcholine and antagonize nondepolarizing relaxants.
   d. Prolonged steroid therapy demands the usual considerations and appropriate supplementation.

e. OKT3, usually used to treat rejection crises, can cause anaphylaxis and acute pulmonary edema, especially if fluid overload is present. It may also cause psychiatric disturbances.

3. Children have a relatively high rate of noncompliance with their anti-rejection therapy. This may lead to problems with graft rejection.

Special Considerations for the Child with a Transplanted Heart

Children with a denervated transplanted heart have altered cardiac function.

1. Effects normally mediated via the autonomic nervous system are absent (i.e., vagal slowing, baroreceptor responses to blood pressure changes). Changes in heart rate as an index of light anesthesia or hypovolemia are unreliable.

2. Indirect drug effects that depend on autonomic pathways are absent (i.e., the chronotropic effects of atropine, pancuronium, or opioids).

3. Compensation for changes in blood volume and cardiac filling pressure is limited and delayed.

4. Coronary atherosclerosis is accelerated in transplanted hearts and may occur in children. In the denervated heart, ischemia may occur without pain and coronary angiography is required for diagnosis. Careful intraoperative ECG monitoring is essential.

The following are considerations for anesthesia in the child with a heart transplant:

1. The child should be carefully screened for signs of rejection, which if present may increase the risks of anesthesia and surgery. Signs include:
   a. Poor appetite, irritability, fluid retention
   b. Decreased cardiac function on echocardiogram
   c. Low-voltage ECG

2. Practice meticulous asepsis. Avoid unnecessary cannulation; use only essential invasive monitoring lines, and remove these as soon as is safe.

3. Maintain normovolemia; ensure adequate fluid replacement.

4. Avoid high doses of drugs that have a direct cardiac depressant effect (e.g., halothane, lidocaine).

5. Maintain afterload; avoid agents and techniques that cause rapid changes in vascular tone.

6. If cardiotonic drugs are indicated, use direct-acting agents (e.g., isoproterenol, dopamine).

Most children have been successfully managed using a opioid- and relaxant-based anesthetic technique. Despite theoretic considerations of interaction between muscle relaxants and immunosuppressive therapy, the usual doses are often required (but neuromuscular blockade must be monitored).

Special Considerations for the Patient With a Transplanted Lung

Heart and lung transplantation may be performed for children with cardiac disease complicated by pulmonary hypertension. Lung transplantation is performed in children with end-stage CF, primary pulmonary hypertension, or idiopathic pulmonary fibrosis. The transplanted lungs are prone to infection and also to obliterative bronchiolitis that progresses to respiratory failure.

Regular bronchial alveolar lavage with transbronchial biopsy is performed to monitor for infection or signs of rejection. General anesthesia usually is required. A technique using a propofol infusion and *cis*-atracurium with controlled ventilation has been found to be most satisfactory. The largest endotracheal tube that can easily be passed should be used. Many of these children experience considerable dyspnea on emergence from anesthesia and are more comfortable if placed in a sitting position as they awaken. Secretions may also be troublesome.

Special Considerations for the Patient With a Transplanted Liver

After a successful liver transplantation, children can be expected to have normal metabolic functions and drug metabolism. Therefore any suitable anesthesia regimen can be used, and no agents are contraindicated. However, these children are prone to infections, particularly by viral agents (cytomegalovirus, Epstein-Barr virus, hepatitis virus), and require very careful aseptic precautions.

Those children with abnormal liver function may have abnormal drug distribution, protein binding, metabolism, and clearance. In addition they may have a coagulopathy. The PT is considered one of the most useful tests of hepatic function because it becomes prolonged before most other tests are abnormal. In these children, anesthesia regimens should be carefully chosen; inhalational agents may be used cautiously, but the response to opioids can be unpredictable. *Cis*-atracurium is the relaxant of choice.

Suggested Reading

Williams GD, Ramamoorthy C: Anesthesia considerations for pediatric thoracic solid organ transplant, Anesthesiol Clin N Am 23(4):709–731, 2005.

Kostopanagiotou G, Smyrniotis V, Arkadopoulos N, et al: Anaesthetic and perioperative management of paediatric organ recipients in nontransplant surgery, Paediatr Anaesth 13(9):754–763, 2003.

THE POSTANESTHESIA CARE UNIT

General Management

All children should be transported to the postanesthesia care unit (PACU) in the lateral decubitus position with the head extended so as to provide an unobstructed airway; all children—other than absolutely healthy children having minor surgery—should receive oxygen and be monitored with SpO_2 during transport to PACU. The anesthesiologist walks at the head of the bed facing forward so as to be in the optimal position to observe the child and then monitors the child continuously. During transfer to the PACU, there is a danger of respiratory obstruction, so be alert to this possibility. If the airway is in doubt, do not leave the operating room (OR). If the airway becomes precarious while on route to the PACU, apply digital pressure to the condyle of the mandible behind the pinna to open the upper airway. There is evidence that decreases in SpO_2 during transport are most likely due to airway obstruction. Children with a history of upper respiratory tract infections (URTI) are particularly at risk.

In the PACU, the anesthesiologist:

1. Transfers the child to the care of the PACU nurses (see later discussion); summarizes the child's underlying medical and surgical conditions, the operative procedure and any associated issues (e.g., bleeding, vascular compromise); provides the timing and doses of antibiotics and analgesics, intravenous fluid therapy, and blood loss and replacement; and describes the anesthesia technique including any complications and their management.
2. Completes the anesthesia record with the initial vital signs in PACU.
3. Writes postoperative (PACU) orders, including pain and antiemesis orders, intravenous fluids, and respiratory therapy.
4. Confirms the child's vital signs on arrival are recorded by the receiving nurse.
5. Remains with the child until it is safe to transfer the care to the PACU nurses.

In the PACU, every child receives humidified oxygen via face mask or nasal prongs as tolerated. The anesthesiologist should not transfer the care of a child to the PACU nursing staff if there is any doubt about the airway, that ventilation is inadequate, and requires an oropharyngeal airway or tracheal tube. *A child who still requires an oropharyngeal airway may still need an anesthesiologist.*

Remember that small infants (younger than 3 months of age) may not rapidly convert to mouth-breathing if the nasal passages are blocked (i.e., after cleft lip or palate repair). If such obstruction occurs, insert an oropharyngeal or nasopharyngeal airway for patency until the child is fully awake. Also, an orogastric tube may be inserted before emergence to decompress the stomach (and may also serve to open the oral airway).

The progress of recovery should be documented with a postanesthesia scoring system along with regular recording of the vital signs. All children should receive oxygen initially until they awaken and can maintain an adequate SpO_2 in room air. SpO_2 should be continuously monitored until the child is fully awake and ready for discharge.

As soon as the child begins to awaken, with stable vital signs and good pain control, the parents should be brought to the bedside. This decreases the child's anxiety in the PACU, reduces crying, and reduces the need for sedation. It also clarifies whether the child is crying because of pain or because of separation from parents.

After ketamine anesthesia, recovery should take place in a quiet dimly lit area with minimal tactile and auditory stimulation. If, despite these precautions, delirium and/or hallucinations develop, midazolam 0.05 to 0.1 mg/kg IV or diazepam (0.1 to 0.2 mg/kg IV) may be administered.

Complications in the Postanesthesia Care Unit

Laryngospasm

Laryngospasm occurs most commonly during emergence from anesthesia. During anesthesia, it may be treated as outlined below and possibly by deepening the level of anesthesia. During extubation and recovery, it is more likely to occur in children with blood or secretions in the pharynx or in those with a history of URTI (see Chapter 4). It should be managed by bag-mask ventilation with oxygen, maintaining positive pressure, and subluxation of the TMJ. Be prepared to administer a short-acting muscle relaxant; reintubate the trachea if necessary and do not delay reintubation if desaturation progresses. Often a very low dose of succinylcholine (0.2 mg/kg) will relieve the laryngospasm. Noncardiogenic pulmonary edema may follow immediately upon relief of severe laryngospasm. If it occurs, treat with continued positive pressure ventilation, furosemide, fluid restriction, and supplemental oxygen as indicated.

Postoperative Stridor

Postoperative stridor caused by subglottic edema may occur especially after endoscopy, children with a history of croup, those who were intubated as neonates, or after the unwise use of too large an endotracheal tube. Stridor is also more common in children with Down syndrome and after surgery during which head movement occurred. Stridor usually appears within 30 to 60 minutes after extubation. The use of humidified oxygen and intravenous dexamethasone may reduce subglottic edema. If stridor persists, administer racemic epinephrine by spontaneous respirations or preferably intermittent positive-pressure breathing for 15 minutes; this is usually efficacious. Very rarely, it may be necessary to reintubate the airway in the PACU for persistent severe stridor. In such cases a smaller-diameter tube that is accompanied by an audible leak is preferred. If racemic epinephrine is used, then the child should be observed for an extended period of time for possible rebound edema.

Emergence Agitation

Agitation occurs most commonly but not exclusively in children 2 to 6 years of age after sevoflurane anesthesia, with a reported incidence up to 80%. Agitation has also been reported after desflurane, halothane, and isoflurane. It is characterized by the presence of restless, thrashing, and inconsolable behaviors; disorientation; failure to establish eye contact; and a lack of purposeful movement and awareness of their surroundings.

The agitation is usually transient, dissipating spontaneously within 10 to 20 minutes, without sequelae. The incidence may be attenuated by pretreatment with propofol, fentanyl, dexmedetomidine, clonidine, or NSAIDs (ketorolac). Difficulty differentiating emergence agitation from postoperative pain has been addressed in part, with the introduction of a validated scale to measure agitation in children. Treatment in the PACU may require small doses of fentanyl.

Suggested Reading

Cravero J, Surgenor S, Whalen K: Emergence agitation in paediatric patients after sevoflurane anaesthesia and no surgery: a comparison with halothane, Paediatr Anaesth 10:419–424, 2000.

Sikich N, Lerman J: Development and psychometric evaluation of the pediatric anesthesia emergence delirium scale, Anesthesiology 100:1138–1145, 2004.

Shivering and Rigidity

Shivering and rigidity may occur during recovery from anesthesia, sometimes associated with hypothermia and other times, in normothermic children. As this may increase the metabolic rate and oxygen requirement, it should be treated. If halothane is used for anesthesia, shivering may become so severe that it compromises the surgical results (e.g., in a child with a recently reduced fracture). Intravenous meperidine (Demerol) (0.25 mg/kg IV) or dexmedetomidine (0.5 µg/kg IV slowly) may eliminate the shivering.

Suggested Reading

Akin A, Esmaoglu A, Boyaci A: Postoperative shivering in children and causative factors, Paediatr Anaesth 15(12):1089–1093, 2005.

Nausea and Vomiting

Postoperative nausea and vomiting may be troublesome in the recovery period; it is a leading cause of delayed discharge from the PACU or, more rarely, of unplanned admission of the day surgery patient. The incidence of PONV can be significantly reduced by some general measures:

1. Avoid the indiscriminate use of opioids; a single dose dramatically increases PONV. Use alternative analgesic drugs (e.g., nonsteroidal antiinflammatory drugs [NSAIDs]) or regional analgesia whenever possible. However, pain itself may cause PONV—so ensure analgesia.
2. Do not "push" oral fluids postoperatively; wait until the child asks for them or is thirsty.
3. Do not rush to mobilize the child, especially after eye surgery.

TABLE 7-1   Antiemetic Drug Doses for Children

Dexamethasone	100–150 µg/kg (Maximum 8 mg)
Ondansetron	50–100 µg/kg (Maximum 4 mg)
Granisetron	40 µg/kg (Maximum 0.6 mg)
Dimenhydrinate	0.5 mg/kg (Maximum 25 mg)
Droperidol	10–15 µg/kg (Maximum 1.25 mg)

When nausea and vomiting can be anticipated (e.g., eye surgery, tonsillectomy), the incidence can be reduced by the choice of the anesthetic regimen (e.g., propofol), by avoiding nitrous oxide (in emetogenic surgery), by administering large volumes of intravenous fluids (20 to 30 ml/kg) and by prophylactic multimodal antiemetic therapy (dexamethasone and a serotonin-receptor antagonist, such as ondansetron). In children with unexpected nausea and vomiting, rescue medication with an antiemetic drug is necessary (Table 7-1).

Dimenhydrinate and metoclopramide are both moderately effective antiemetics and cause little sedation. Droperidol in doses adequate to combat nausea and vomiting may cause sedation, with delayed recovery and discharge. Ondansetron, dolasetron, and granisetron are probably the most effective agents for PONV. (**NB**. Dolasetron has been associated with rare fatal arrhythmias in children.) Dexamethasone is very effective for PONV, particularly in children undergoing tonsillectomy and adenoidectomy and strabismus surgery. The combination of ondansetron (0.05 to 0.1 mg/kg) and dexamethasone (0.0625 to 0.15 mg/kg) is currently the optimal PONV prophylactic regimen.

Suggested Reading

Gan TJ, Meyer TA, Apfel CC, et al: Society for ambulatory anesthesia. Society for ambulatory anesthesia guidelines for the management of postoperative nausea and vomiting, Anesth Analg 105(6):1615–1628, 2007.

Kim MS, Coté CJ, Cristoloveanu C, et al: There is no dose-escalation response to dexamethasone (0.0625–1.0 mg/kg) in pediatric tonsillectomy or adenotonsillectomy patients for preventing vomiting, reducing pain, shortening time to first liquid intake, or the incidence of voice change, Anesth Analg 104:1052–1058, 2007.

Duration of Stay in the Postanesthesia Care Unit

Children remain in the PACU until they are fully awake and have recovered from the effects of anesthesia. As a general rule, a minimum stay of

30 minutes or two sets of vital signs is required. Infants weighing less than 5 kg are usually kept in the PACU for a more prolonged period or transferred to a monitored bed. Be alert for possible postoperative complications (e.g., stridor after surgery of or near the airway or after endoscopy; bleeding after a kidney or liver biopsy, tonsillectomy), and specify a longer stay in the PACU for such children.

Children who remain more than 1 hour in PACU must have deep-breathing and coughing exercises and be turned hourly. Each child should be signed out of the PACU by an anesthesiologist except for the most simple of cases (e.g., myringotomy). If the discharge order from the PACU is delegated to the nurse, specific written clinical criteria should be documented. If an anesthetic complication occurs, the child must be reevaluated by the anesthesia team before discharge from PACU.

MANAGEMENT OF PAIN

The ability of infants and children to feel pain was misunderstood in the past, and this led to its undertreatment. It is now recognized that the biochemical and nervous components of the pain perception pathways are completely formed during fetal life and that even the preterm infant can feel pain. Furthermore, the adverse effects of unmodified pain have been documented even in very young infants. Studies suggest that inadequate treatment of pain in infants may lead to increased sensitivity to pain later in life.

There are many reasons why pain in children was undertreated in the past and why even today it is inadequately treated:

1. Infants cannot tell us when they feel pain, and it is sometimes difficult to determine whether they are crying because they are in pain or for another reason.
2. The older child's response to pain differs from that of the adult; often these children are quiet and withdrawn, failing to announce their discomfort.
3. In the days when intramuscular injection of an opioid was the standard therapy for postoperative pain, children often feared the injection more than the pain and preferred to suffer in silence. This tended to perpetuate the myth that children do not feel pain as much as adults.
4. Physicians have been uncertain of the safety of the analgesic drugs given to infants. It was stated that infants are "exquisitely sensitive" to the respiratory depressant effects of morphine; this led to an ultraconservative approach in prescribing opioids.

5. Many physicians, and especially those junior staff to whom the responsibility for pain management was customarily delegated, were unsure of the correct dosage of analgesics for infants and children.
6. Nurses have tended to underestimate pain in children; many healthcare providers have overestimated the danger of the child's becoming addicted to opioids.
7. If an opioid is administered, then the child must be observed for an extended period to assure that there is no respiratory compromise.

More recently, a much greater understanding of childhood pain has been acquired. We know that all children can experience pain, we are better equipped to assess the severity of the pain, and we have better means to control pain. Postoperative pain management should be planned when the preoperative evaluation is performed, and it should be discussed with the child and parents.

For outpatients it is most important that the parents are well instructed on the management of pain when the child arrives home:

1. Analgesic drugs must be administered before pain becomes significant and repeated regularly by schedule rather than waiting for pain to be a problem.
2. The "analgesic gap" as regional analgesia wears off must be anticipated (most often manifest by the child becoming irritable) and suitable analgesics administered in advance.
3. Parents should be instructed to look for signs of pain, to use assessment tools (e.g., visual analog scales [VAS]) and to administer effective analgesics appropriately. A standard VAS may be sent home with the child for the parent's use.

Assessment of Pain

It is essential for optimal pain management to establish regular, objective pain level assessments recorded on the medical record. For infants, the level of pain is assessed by physiologic or behavioral indices. Indices of pain include tachycardia, tachypnea, increased blood pressure, sweating, facial expressions, posture, and crying. Of the behavioral indices, facial expression may be most reliable, but cry characteristics and body movement (especially flexion of the limbs) are also useful. The opinion of the parent and of the child's nurse in interpretation of these behavioral signs is very useful. These indices are incorporated into a numeric scale that can be scored and recorded (Table 7-2).

Older children may be asked to report their pain level using one of a variety of visual analog scales, such as the Wong-Baker FACES Pain Rating

TABLE 7-2 A Pain Scale for Preverbal and Nonverbal Infants (FLACC Scale)

	Score		
Category	0	1	2
Face	No particular expression or smile	Occasional grimace or frown, withdrawn, disinterested	Frequent to constant quivering chin, clenched jaw
Legs	Normal position or relaxed	Uneasy, restless, tense	Kicking or legs drawn up
Activity	Lying quietly, normal position, moves easily	Squirming, shifting back and forth, tense	Arched, rigid or jerking
Cry	No cry (awake or asleep)	Moans or whimpers, occasional complaint	Crying steadily, screams or sobs, frequent complaints
Consolability	Content, relaxed	Reassured by occasional touching, hugging, or being talked to; distractable	Difficult to console or comfort

Reproduced with permission of Merkel SI et al: The FLACC: A behavioral scale for scoring postoperative pain in young children. Pediatr Nurs 23:392, 1997.

Scale (Figure 7-1). They may also be asked to rate their pain on a color scale or to report it by coloring their pain on a body outline.

Adolescents can be assessed with the use of standard adult self-report scales. Note, however, that at this age psychological and emotional factors may influence the response much more than in younger children.

When treating pain at any age, it is essential to monitor the response to therapy with an objective scoring system. Pain scores should be regularly recorded on the patient's vital signs chart.

POSTOPERATIVE PAIN

Postoperative pain has adverse physiologic and psychological effects. Optimal postoperative pain relief minimizes the metabolic rate for oxygen, reduces cardiorespiratory demands, promotes early ambulation, and speeds recovery. In addition, postoperative emotional disturbance is reduced if pain is well controlled. Plan for optimal postoperative pain

WONG-BAKER FACES PAIN RATING SCALE

	0	1	2	3	4	5
	No hurt	Hurts little bit	Hurts little more	Hurts even more	Hurts whole lot	Hurts worst
Alternate coding	0	2	4	6	8	10

Figure 7-1 Wong-Baker FACES pain rating scale. (*© Reproduced with permission of Dr. Donna L. Wong and Mosby Inc. Wong DL, et al. (eds): Nursing Care of Infants and Children, 6th ed. St. Louis, Mosby-Year Book, 1999.*)

control when the child is first seen preoperatively; some of the methods that might be chosen require informed consent and advance planning (e.g., an intraoperative nerve block or placement of an epidural catheter). Discuss the plans for postoperative pain management with the parents and with those children who are old enough to understand.

Suggested Reading

Maxwell LG, Yaster M: Perioperative management issues in pediatric patients, Anesthesiol Clin North Am 18:601–632, 2000.

Systemic Analgesic Drugs

After minor procedures, when no regional or local analgesia regimen is possible, the use of a systemic analgesic is indicated. Dosages in common use are listed in Table 7-3. Meperidine is no longer recommended for perioperative analgesia in children because of the potential for seizures associated with its metabolite normeperidine; its only indication is to treat shivering.

The appropriate drug should be chosen for the magnitude of the pain, and a satisfactory effect should be confirmed. It is preferable to administer the first dose of the analgesic drug before the child emerges from general anesthesia—for example, for tonsillectomy give 0.05 to 0.1 mg/kg IV morphine during surgery (if no OSA is present), and for minor superficial surgery give 30 to 40 mg/kg acetaminophen PR after induction of anesthesia. *Do not* cut suppositories of acetaminophen (or any other drug) as the acetaminophen may not be evenly distributed throughout

TABLE 7-3   Common Dosages for Systemic Analgesics

For minor procedures:
Acetaminophen, 10-20 mg/kg PO or 30-40 mg/kg PR (maximum 90-100 mg/kg/24 hr)
Codeine,* 1-1.5 mg/kg IM or PO q4h
Ibuprofen, 5-10 mg/kg PO
Ketorolac,* 1 mg/kg IM
For major procedures:
Morphine,* 0.1-0.2 mg/kg IM/IV q2-4h
Hydromorphone, 0.005-0.015 mg/kg IV q4h
* NB: only use IM analgesics while anesthetized.

the suppository. Remember that peak blood levels by this route are not achieved for 60 to 180 minutes, so the suppository must be administered immediately after induction and this route is not appropriate for brief procedures; multiple suppositories with several strengths may be simultaneously administered to achieve the desired 30 to 40 mg/kg PR dose. Avoid intramuscular injections in awake children; give analgesics by the intravenous, rectal, or oral route.

Mild Analgesics and NSAIDS

Acetaminophen. Acetaminophen is a mild analgesic and antipyretic drug, but it provides good analgesia and antipyresis after minor procedures, especially if given before the surgery. It is considered safe in neonates, but metabolism and elimination are delayed in neonates compared with adults, so repeat doses should be given at 6- rather than 4-hour intervals. Excessive doses can cause hepatic failure; the total daily dose should not exceed 90 to 100 mg/kg. Make sure that clear instructions are given to parents about dosage after the child is discharged. Hepatic damage has been reported after reduced doses of acetaminophen when it was given to debilitated children; it is wise to avoid the drug in such cases. After major surgery, acetaminophen combined with opioids reduces the dose of the latter, thereby reducing the risk of respiratory depression. Acetaminophen does not affect surgical bleeding. Proparacetamol, an IV formulation available in some countries, is not currently available in North America. The dose for proparacetamol in children is 30 mg/kg IV.

Diclofenac. Diclofenac has been widely used in children and may be administered orally or rectally; it is reported to be effective for pain control after minor surgical procedures. After tonsillectomy, it reduces the need for opioids and hence reduces PONV. A rectal dose of 2 mg/kg is commonly administered after induction of anesthesia yielding a greater bioavailability than the enteric-coated formulation and at peak blood levels by 50 minutes. It does not significantly affect bleeding or clot strength in children after tonsillectomy. The smallest suppository available in the United States is 50 mg.

Ibuprofen. Ibuprofen, an NSAID, may be given by either the oral or rectal route, 5 to 10 mg/kg every 6 hours. It reduces the child's opioid requirements postoperatively. However, ibuprofen can cause gastrointestinal upset (nausea, vomiting, diarrhea), and decrease platelet aggregation, which could result in increased bleeding. Ibuprofen may not be indicated for treating tonsillectomy pain.

Ketorolac. Ketorolac is another NSAID; its potent analgesic effects may rival those of morphine without the respiratory depressant effects of the latter. When given before surgery, ketorolac 1 mg/kg IV appears to provide postoperative analgesia comparable to 0.1 mg/kg of morphine; however, this dose is now considered excessive. In common with other NSAIDs, ketorolac inhibits platelet aggregation and is not recommended when bleeding may be a problem. Impaired bone healing after ketorolac remains controversial. Other serious but uncommon potential side effects include gastrointestinal hemorrhage, interstitial nephritis, and acute renal failure. The recommended IV dose is 0.5 mg/kg to a maximum of 15 mg in children less than 50 kg and 30 mg in children greater than 50 kg. Once hemostasis has been achieved, it is our practice to ask the surgeon if ketorolac can be administered given its potential negative effects on platelet function and bone healing.

Opioid Drugs

Morphine. Morphine remains a most useful drug in the management of postoperative pain. It produces effective analgesia together with sedation and a useful degree of euphoria. For children, it is preferably administered intravenously in a dose of 0.05 to 0.1 mg/kg every 7 to 10 minutes until comfortable or for ongoing pain, by continuous infusion/PCA (see later discussion).

Codeine. Codeine has been used to treat moderate pain. It may be given intramuscularly or orally, but must not be given intravenously; severe hypotension may result. Codeine has been considered a safe drug for infants and children, but respiratory depression similar to that associated with morphine may occur, especially after repeated doses. There are some populations that carry polymorphisms of CYP2D6 that may either prevent or reduce the pain relief from codeine or convert codeine to morphine so rapidly that respiratory depression may suddenly occur (see Chapter 3 for details). For most children, the usual dose of codeine is 1 to 1.5 mg/kg IM or PO (maximum, 60 mg).

Hydromorphone (Dilaudid). Hydromorphone is a long-acting opioid analgesic that is 5 to 8.5 times more potent than morphine in the IV form. Thus the IV analgesic dose in children is between 0.005 and 0.015 mg/kg. Its elimination half-life is 2.5 hours. Hydromorphone may be given as an alternative postoperative analgesic to morphine.

Oxycodone. Oxycodone is an opioid that is derived from the opiate alkaloid, thebaine. Oxycodone is most commonly prescribed as an oral analgesic, but is also approved for IV, IM, and sublingual routes in some countries. For chronic pain, a sustained release oral preparation is also available. Single doses of oxycodone via all routes are 0.1 to 0.2 mg/kg every 6 hours. It has been used in older children to transition from PCA to oral analgesics. Its side effect profile is similar to that of morphine.

Tramadol. Tramadol is a synthetic opioid that has an elimination half-life of 6 to 7 hours in adults. In North America, it is only available in an oral formulation and indicated only for adults. There are limited dosing recommendations in children (from studies outside of North America) but a dose of 1 to 2 mg/kg IV has provided good pain relief in children after adenotonsillectomy and may be particularly useful in children with OSA.

Continuous Opioid Infusions

A continuous infusion of morphine, using a dilute solution administered by a specially designed patient controlled analgesia (PCA) pump provides for a constant level of analgesia with good sedation and is appropriate for many children after major surgery. The child must have close nursing supervision and be monitored by pulse oximetry. The dose administered should be frequently titrated against the observed and recorded pain level.

Recommended doses:

Children older than 1 year: Loading dose, 0.1 mg/kg IV; infusion,* 10 to 30 µg/kg/hr

---

* An infusion can be prepared by adding 1 mg morphine/kg to 100 ml of fluid. Infuse at 1 ml/hr to yield 10 µg/kg/hr. For some children, the loading dose may have to be repeated to establish an initial satisfactory level of analgesia.

Infants younger than 1 year: Loading dose, 0.05 mg/kg; infusion, 5 to 15 µg/kg/hr

Reduced infusion rates may be adequate after cardiac surgery, especially in children who are receiving vasopressors, when the clearance rates for morphine are reduced.

Infants receiving a morphine infusion should be carefully monitored during the infusion and for 24 hours after the infusion is discontinued to detect respiratory depression.

Patient-Controlled Analgesia

Children older than 5 or 6 years of age are capable of using a PCA system to obtain excellent pain relief. Children may especially benefit from PCA; they do not have to ask for pain relief and can be "in control." Most children are familiar with computer games and have no problem mastering the principles of PCA. It is important that a safe regimen be established and that both child and parents be reassured that the system has an appropriate lockout time and total dosage safeguards. The parents (and other adults) should be warned not to trigger the PCA for the child. Recent evidence, however, suggests that parents or nurses can effectively and safely manage PCA for a child who is unable to do so for age, cognitive, or physical reasons. If such an approach is used, an educational program for the surrogate user must be delivered successfully before they are allowed to participate. *Always be aware that overdose is a potential complication when well meaning parents are allowed to push the PCA button.*

All children being treated with opioids should have a loading dose. Whether a background infusion is used to supplement boluses is controversial, but in children a continuous infusion of a small dose of morphine complemented with PCA supplements may give the best results in terms of both pain control and sleep pattern. However, these children should be closely supervised and have continuous pulse oximetry.

The regimen used should be tailored to the type of surgery; after orthopedic surgery, children have greater morphine requirements than after general surgery, and after spinal surgery, the requirements are even greater. It is convenient to adjust the background infusion rate to suit the type of surgery (Table 7-4).

Side effects of PCA include the following:

1. *Nausea and vomiting:* This may be troublesome and may require a reduction in the opioid dosage and administration of promethazine (0.25 to 0.5 mg/kg), ondansetron (0.1 mg/kg up to 4 mg), or other antiemetics. Be aware that promethazine may cause sedation. Low-dose

TABLE 7-4 Dosages for Patient-Controlled Analgesia With Morphine

For orthopedic surgery	
0.1–0.2 mg/kg IV until settled	
Initial bolus doses	0.1–0.2 mg/kg IV until settled
PCA bolus dose	10 µg/kg
Lockout period	7–10 min
Background infusion	
For general surgery	0–20 µg/kg/hr
For orthopedic surgery	0–25 µg/kg/hr
For spinal surgery	0–40 µg/kg/hr
Maximum hourly dose	0–100 µg/kg

naloxone infusions (0.25 µg/kg/hr) have attenuated opioid-associated side effects.

2. *Excessive sedation:* Monitor children carefully and have naloxone ready to treat excessive narcosis and respiratory depression. It may be prudent to keep naloxone and a bag-mask oxygen source at the bedside. Be alert to the possibility that someone who is unaware that the child is receiving a PCA may order a "stat dose" of another analgesic or sedative drug and thereby produce respiratory depression. Write specific orders on the charts of children with PCA pumps that they are to have no additional drugs without the knowledge of the PCA team.

Suggested Reading

Brislin RP, Rose JB: Pediatric acute pain management, Anesthesiol Clin North Am 23(4):789–814, 2005.

Lonnqvist PA, Morton NS: Postoperative analgesia in infants and children, Br J Anaesth 95(1):59–68, 2005.

Regional Analgesia for Postoperative Pain

The pain that occurs after many procedures can be effectively treated by regional analgesia and this should be used whenever possible. Frequently, no additional drugs, or at the most, only mild analgesics (e.g., acetaminophen) will be required. Thus the side effects of opioids are avoided and the child rapidly returns to full activity after minor surgery. These blocks are performed using surface landmarks (caudal epidural block), nerve stimulation, or ultrasound. Provision should be made, however, for transition to systemic analgesics after the block dissipates. Studies have shown that significant pain may occur at this time, especially in outpatients. The parent should be carefully instructed to administer an analgesic drug (e.g., acetaminophen or other analgesic) in anticipation of this need.

After major surgery, appropriate nerve blocks (e.g., intercostal nerve block) using local analgesic drugs may permit a reduction in the dosage of opioids and earlier mobilization.

The possibility that a regional block established before the surgical incision (preemptive analgesia) may modulate total postoperative pain by preventing biochemical changes ("windup") within the central nervous system is appealing, but the results of well-designed studies have been disappointing. Regional blocks performed before the surgical incision do provide intraoperative analgesia, thus reducing the dose of general anesthetic drugs required. This reduction in anesthetic requirement indicates that the block is well-established before emergence.

Studies of complications after pediatric regional analgesia procedures strongly suggest that peripheral nerve blocks are associated with fewer complications than neuraxial blocks. Hence, whenever there is a choice, a peripheral nerve block should be performed.

Peripheral Nerve Block or Local Infiltration

The following blocks are commonly used in children; for details of technique, see Chapter 5. Bupivacaine or ropivacaine up to a maximum dose of 2.5 or 3 mg/kg, respectively, is commonly used.

1. For thoracotomy or flank incisions (e.g., renal), block the appropriate intercostal nerves using 1 to 2 ml of 0.25% bupivacaine with epinephrine several dermatomes above and below level of desired block.
2. For inguinal hernia surgery, block the ilioinguinal and iliohypogastric nerves just medial to the anterior superior iliac spine.
3. For umbilical surgery, block the tenth intercostal nerve bilaterally or infiltrate along each wound edge.
4. For circumcision, perform a penile nerve block or use topical lidocaine gel, which may also be very effective.
5. Local infiltration of the incision site before surgery, using 0.125% or 0.25% bupivacaine, may provide pain relief when there is no suitable nerve to block.

Caudal Analgesia

Caudal analgesia is useful for many abdominal, perineal, and lower limb procedures. Insertion of a catheter provides for continued pain relief (see Chapter 5).

Lumbar and Thoracic Epidural Analgesia

Continuous epidural analgesia has been used to provide pain relief after thoracic, abdominal, perineal, and lower limb surgery. Bupivacaine, ropivacaine, or levobupivacaine (the last only outside North America) is commonly used and may be delivered by continuous infusion via an epidural catheter or by intermittent doses. Infusion rates for bupivacaine in infants should be reduced because they metabolize bupivacaine less rapidly (Table 7-5); it has been suggested that intermittent top-up doses may be safer than continuous infusions in small infants.

All children must have constant nursing observation. The level of analgesia should be monitored and the child should be observed for early signs of toxicity (e.g., restlessness, twitching, tinnitus, lightheadedness).

Suggested Reading

Suresh S, Wheeler M: Practical pediatric regional anesthesia, Anesthesiol Clin North Am 20(1):83–113, 2002.

Lerman J, Nolan J, Eyres R, et al: Efficacy, safety and pharmacokinetics of levobupivacaine with and without fentanyl after continuous epidural infusion in children: a multicenter study, Anesthesiology 99:1166–1174, 2003.

Ecoffey C: Pediatric regional anesthesia—update, Curr Opin Anaesth 20:232–235, 2007.

Epidural Opioids

Epidural opioids via the lumbar or caudal epidural route have been shown to be effective after major cardiac, general, urologic, or orthopedic surgery in children. Some investigators claim that more effective pain relief may be obtained if the opioid is administered before surgery. A single dose of epidural morphine (33 µg/kg) provides analgesia for up to 12 hours, at which time the dose can be repeated if necessary.

Fentanyl administered via the lumbar or caudal epidural route is less likely to cause respiratory depression because of its increased lipid solubility and consequently more limited distribution and decreased rostral spread. When administered via the epidural space, fentanyl likely acts by systemic absorption. It may be added to continuous epidural infusions of local anesthetic or given alone or by PCEA (patient controlled epidural analgesia) in older children (see Table 7-5).

The side effects after regional blocks with opioids in children are similar to those observed in adults, with pruritus, urinary retention, and nausea/vomiting being the most common. Intestinal ileus may complicate epidural morphine and may be prolonged. Ventilatory depression may occur, and the ventilatory response to carbon dioxide may be depressed for up to 24 hours.

TABLE 7-5   **Suggested Dosages for Epidural/Caudal Blocks**

Bupivacaine:		
Loading dose (0.25%)		0.5 ml/kg
Infusions*	Children:	0.4-0.5 mg/kg/hr for (0.125% at 0.3 ml/kg/hr)
	Infants:	0.25 mg/kg/hr for (0.125% at 0.3 ml/kg/hr)
	Neonates:[†]	0.2 mg/kg/hr (0.1% at 0.2 ml/kg/hr)
Ropivacaine:		
Loading dose (0.2%):		0.5 ml/kg
Infusion:		0.4 mg/kg/hr
PCEA (0.2%):		
Bolus dose:		2 ml bolus
Lockout interval:		10 min
Background infusion:		1.6 ml/hr
Levobupivacaine:		
Loading dose (0.25%)		0.0625%-0.125% @ 0.3 ml/kg/hr[‡]
Morphine:		
Single dose:		0.030[§] (range of 0.01- 0.10) mg/kg preservative-free morphine in up to 15 ml preservative-free saline
Fentanyl:		
Infusion:		1-2 µg/ml @ 0.3 ml/kg/hr without local anesthetic
PCEA:		
Loading dose:		1.4 µg/kg;
Bolus dose:		0.5 µg/kg
Lockout interval:		15 min
Background infusion:		0.5 µg/kg/hr

* Start infusion immediately after the loading dose.
[†] Limit infusions to 48 hr.
[‡] No benefit adding fentanyl to this solution.
[§] Most effective and commonly used dose; larger doses generally increase side effects.

All children should receive appropriate nursing observation and should be monitored by a pulse oximeter. Nurses should be instructed to check the child's level of consciousness frequently; increased somnolence and bradypnea are the most reliable early signs of impending respiratory depression. The child should be observed for at least 24 hours after the last administration of epidural morphine.

Common complications after neuraxial opioids include:

1. *Pruritus:* This may be controlled without loss of analgesia by the use of small bolus doses of naloxone (1 to 2 μg/kg) or by a naloxone infusion (1 to 2 μg/kg/hr). A very small dose of propofol (10 mg in adults) has also been reported to relieve pruritus.
2. *Urinary retention:* This may require catheterization; for this reason, epidural opioids may be contraindicated if it is necessary to avoid catheterization.
3. *Nausea and vomiting:* This may be improved by the use of antiemetics, metoclopramide, naloxone, or a scopolamine patch.
4. *Respiratory depression:* This effect is infrequent but may be delayed (up to 24 hours) after neuraxial morphine. Risk is increased if systemic opioids or other sedating medications are concurrently administered. It is reversed by IV naloxone.

Epidural Clonidine

Clonidine 1 to 2 μg/kg added to epidural local anesthetic or opioids improves the quality and duration of analgesia (by ~3 hours). The incidence of nausea and vomiting may also be reduced. The analgesia outlasts the duration of sedation produced by clonidine.

Suggested Reading

Cucchiaro G, Dagher C, Baujard C, et al: Side-effects of postoperative epidural analgesia in children: a randomized study comparing morphine and clonidine, Paediatr Anaesth 13:318–323, 2003.

Anesthesia for Specific Procedures

Neurosurgery and Invasive Neuroradiology 8

GENERAL PRINCIPLES

1. Perioperative management must be planned to minimize the possibility of increasing the intracranial pressure (ICP) and to ensure optimal operating conditions for the neurosurgeon.
2. Light general anesthesia is adequate for most neurosurgical operations; additional techniques may be required to prevent or treat increased ICP. All anesthetic drugs used should be short-acting and rapidly eliminated thus assuring that the child speedily emerges from anesthesia, permitting accurate, continuous postoperative neurosurgical assessment.
3. Prior infiltration of the scalp incision site with local anesthetic with epinephrine by the surgeon reduces blood loss, blunts responses to the initial incision, reduces the need for anesthetic drugs, and possibly minimizes postoperative pain.
4. Postoperative pain after intracranial surgery must be effectively treated, but respiratory depression must be avoided. For major procedures such as a craniofacial reconstruction, a morphine infusion may be titrated to achieve satisfactory analgesia. For minor procedures, oral codeine, ketorolac, or acetaminophen may suffice.
5. Some children may benefit from a period of postoperative controlled ventilation after major intracranial surgery. This is usually determined after consultation with the neurosurgeon.

Intracranial Physiology and Pathophysiology

1. Normally, cerebrovascular autoregulation ensures maintenance of constant blood flow to the brain during alterations in mean arterial blood pressure (BP). This system operates over a wide range of mean arterial pressures from 50 to 150 in adults, and as low as 20 to 60 mm Hg in the supine infant.
2. Cerebral blood flow (CBF) in infants and children (90 to 100 ml per 100 g/min) is greater than in adults (50 to 60 ml per 100 g/min). CBF varies directly with changes in $PaCO_2$ between 20 and 80 mm Hg. CBF changes approximately 4% per mm Hg change in $PaCO_2$.
3. Vasodilation of normal reactive cerebral vessels reduces blood flow in areas that have lost autoregulation (e.g., AVMs, vascular tumors or areas of infection or trauma). This has been termed intracerebral steal.
4. Vasoconstriction of normal reactive cerebral vessels has the opposite effect (i.e., inverse intracerebral steal). Hence, hyperventilation as a

means for rapidly reducing cerebral blood volume (ICP) is generally reserved for acute increases in ICP and not recommended for prolonged periods of time.

5. In older children, the total volume of the intracranial contents is fixed. However, any of its three constituents—blood, CSF, and brain tissue—can increase or decrease if compensated by an equal and opposite change in the volumes of the others (revised Munro-Kelly hypothesis).

6. Infants have a less rigid skull than older children; an increase in the contents may be accommodated to some extent by stretching of the dura, expansion of the fontanels, and separation of the suture lines. The ICP may be estimated by palpation of the fontanel.

7. The effect of a space-occupying lesion on ICP depends on its volume and rate of expansion and the rigidity of the skull. Initially, the lesion displaces CSF and/or venous blood from the skull, the sutures may separate in infants, and ICP increases slowly if at all. As expansion continues, compensation is no longer possible, and small increases in volume result in progressively larger increases in ICP. With a rapidly expanding lesion (i.e., intracranial bleeding), pressure increases rapidly from the outset.

Effects of Specific Anesthetic Drugs on Intracranial Physiology

1. All inhalation agents increase CBF and may increase ICP unless accompanied by mild hyperventilation ($PaCO_2 \sim 30$ to 35 mm Hg):

   a. N_2O may cause a very small increase in CBF but has been used successfully in pediatric neurosurgery for many years. It may increase ICP if air is present within the cranium and in these circumstances is contraindicated.

   b. The increase in CBF follows the order: desflurane > halothane > isoflurane > sevoflurane.

   c. Cerebral autoregulation during changes in arterial BP is blunted as the concentrations of inhalational agents increase, but appears to be preserved at 1 MAC isoflurane and sevoflurane anesthesia. This emphasizes the importance of using moderate concentrations of potent inhalation agents; the CBF responses to changes in $PaCO_2$ is retained. Moderate hypocarbia tends to modify or reverse the effects of agents that increase CBF (e.g., halothane, isoflurane, sevoflurane). Prior hypocapnia minimizes the increase in ICP with halothane. During isoflurane anesthesia, the CBF returns to control levels more rapidly with mild hyperventilation.

    d. The $CMRO_2$ is reduced by halothane, isoflurane, and sevoflurane. Isoflurane and sevoflurane at greater concentrations may even provide some cerebral protection against hypoxia/ischemia.

2. Intravenous anesthetic agents (with the notable exception of ketamine) either have no effect on CBF or decrease it, but if hypercarbia is present, these effects are reversed:

    a. Thiopental reduces ICP and therefore is an ideal induction agent in neurosurgery. It does not prevent an increase in BP and ICP during laryngoscopy and intubation; these may, however, be attenuated by prior administration of lidocaine (1 to 1.5 mg/kg IV) and an opioid (e.g., fentanyl 2 to 5 µg/kg).

    b. Propofol reduces CBF and $CMRO_2$, preserves autoregulation, and may offer some cerebral protection. Induction doses (3 mg/kg) may cause mild hypotension but also more effectively blunt the cardiovascular responses to laryngoscopy and intubation.

    c. Remifentanil, fentanyl and sufentanil have little effect on CBF provided that ventilation is maintained. Autoregulation and the cerebrovascular response to $PaCO_2$ are also maintained. Alfentanil has been demonstrated to increase CSF pressure in children with cerebral tumors.

    d. Ketamine increases CBF and $CMRO_2$; CSF pressure is increased. This drug should not be used in neurosurgical patients with raised ICP.

    e. Midazolam and diazepam decrease CBF, $CMRO_2$, and ICP and may control seizures. Flumazenil, which antagonizes benzodiazepines, also antagonizes their effects on CBF and ICP. The latter should be used with caution.

3. Nondepolarizing muscle relaxants have no direct effect on CBF. (Vasodilation resulting from histamine release after atracurium is a possible exception.) The duration of action of vecuronium and rocuronium may be reduced in children taking chronic anti-seizure medications.

4. Succinylcholine may transiently and very slightly increase CBF and ICP in children with space-occupying lesions; this response may be attenuated by prior administration of a small dose of a nondepolarizing muscle relaxant. Hyperkalemia has been reported after succinylcholine was given to children with cerebral trauma and other central nervous system diseases, including paraplegia, encephalitis, and subarachnoid hemorrhage.

5. Sodium nitroprusside, nitroglycerin, adenosine, and the calcium channel-blocking drugs impair cerebral autoregulation and may increase CBF and ICP.

6. Dexamethasone (0.15 mg/kg IV to a maximum of 8 mg) may decrease focal cerebral edema in response to surgical trauma of brain tissue.

7. If an independent vasodilator effect is absent, drugs that decrease neuronal function decrease CBF (such as thiopental).

8. Drugs that increase neuronal function increase CBF (such as ketamine).

9. Somatosensory evoked potentials (SSEPs), to monitor brain or spinal cord function, are attenuated by inhalational anesthetics if these agents are given in more than minimal concentrations. Nitrous oxide, propofol, opioids, and muscle relaxants have little effect on SSEPs.

10. Motor evoked potentials (MEPs), to monitor brain and spinal cord function, are much more sensitive to the presence of inhalational anesthetics than SSEPs. Although the requirements for MEP monitoring varies among neurophysiology groups, in general nitrous oxide is completely avoided, as are muscle relaxants; inhalational agents are limited to 0.5 MAC. Propofol, alpha-2 agonists, benzodiazepines and opioids do not significantly compromise MEP monitoring.

ANESTHESIA MANAGEMENT

Premedication

Children with increased ICP should not receive excessive doses of drugs that depress ventilation, prolong recovery, or hamper postoperative assessment. Therefore, with one exception (see later discussion), do not give heavy sedative premedication to those undergoing craniotomy. If IV access has not been established, topical local anesthetic will facilitate pain-free insertion. Some children may benefit from a small dose of midazolam to calm them before surgery, but they should be closely observed. Children with normal ICP who are undergoing elective or noncranial surgery (e.g., laminectomy) may be given the usual dose of oral midazolam before anesthesia.

Exception. Children with a vascular aneurysm or AVM, especially if there is a history of hemorrhage, may benefit from effective preoperative sedation so as to minimize changes in venous and arterial pressures with crying or stress at induction of anesthesia or tracheal intubation.

Induction of Anesthesia

Management during induction of anesthesia should aim to minimize changes in ICP and fluctuations in arterial and venous pressures.

Gentle preoxygenation followed by an intravenous induction using thiopental or propofol, and then a muscle relaxant to facilitate tracheal intubation and ensure optimal ventilation, is preferred. Lidocaine (1 to 1.5 mg/kg IV) and fentanyl (2 to 5 µg/kg) may be given 3 minutes before intubation to minimize changes in ICP associated with laryngoscopy and tracheal intubation.

Anesthesia for children with vascular anomalies should be induced as above but should then be deepened with an inhalation agent using gentle controlled ventilation to prevent hypercapnia. The blood pressure during induction is carefully monitored to prevent hypertension.

Some children undergoing emergency surgery have a full stomach and should have a rapid sequence induction using succinylcholine or high-dose rocuronium (1.2 mg/kg) with all precautions to prevent regurgitation and aspiration.

For surgery in the prone position, for small infants, and for any procedure that entails changes in position, a nasotracheal tube is preferred. (An orotracheal tube may kink in the prone patient or become dislodged if saliva loosens the adhesive tape; a nasotracheal tube is easier to secure firmly and accurately in the infant). Alternately, in older children use a reinforced oral tube, secure this firmly using tape and benzoin, and limit drooling with glycopyrrolate and a soft throat pack in the mouth. Be alert and always check ventilation bilaterally after the child is positioned; remember that flexion of the head (as in posterior fossa surgery) pushes the tip of the tracheal tube towards the carina whereas extension pulls the tracheal tube cephalad. (**N.B.** To prevent an endobronchial intubation after positioning prone, flex the neck after the tube is taped but while the child is still supine. If wheezing or an endobronchial intubation is detected, withdraw the tube and retape.)

Sudden preoperative apnea may occur in neurosurgical patients awaiting operation and may indicate acutely increased ICP. If this occurs, hyperventilate the lungs with 100% oxygen and advise the surgeon to tap the CSF immediately.

Maintenance

Inhalational anesthetics may increase CBF; therefore they should be used in the smallest concentrations compatible with adequate anesthesia and should be accompanied by muscle relaxant drugs and mild-moderate hyperventilation. Otherwise, N_2O together with short-acting opioids (e.g., fentanyl, remifentanil, sufentanil), which ensure rapid postoperative recovery, may be preferred. Deep anesthesia is unnecessary. Propofol infusions may be a useful alternative in some children, particularly toward the end of a prolonged procedure when other drugs have been discontinued to provide for rapid emergence.

Ventilation

Controlled hyperventilation is used to decrease brain bulk and ICP during intracranial surgery and to improve the quality of cerebral arteriograms during neuroradiology. A $PaCO_2$ approximately 30 to 35 mm Hg is preferred during controlled ventilation.

Monitoring

The child should be monitored as follows:

1. Esophageal stethoscope, pulse oximeter, automated BP cuff.
2. Continuous recording of body temperature (esophageal or rectal).
3. ECG.
4. $PetCO_2$ monitor; this is useful both as a guide to the adequacy of ventilation and as a means of detecting air embolism.
5. For major neurosurgery, arterial and central venous access should be considered. Arterial access is useful to assess rapid fluctuations in blood pressure because of traction on neural tissues, blood loss or air embolism and for laboratory testing. Central venous access will help assure a stable circulating blood volume, provide a means for administering vasoactive drugs (dilator or inotrope) and provide a possible means for aspirating embolized air. Central venous access is best sited in the subclavian (or femoral) vein to prevent misleading readings and occluding neck/intracranial veins. Rapid blood transfusions should not be given into CVP lines in small infants as cold, hyperkalemic blood may lead to cardiac arrest.
6. Measurement of urinary output via catheter, during all major neurosurgery and if diuretics will be given.
7. A precordial Doppler flowmeter should be used for operations when air embolism is a danger. This includes those performed with the child in the sitting or head-up position and all major cranial reconstructions (including cranioplasty for craniosynostosis). The Doppler probe should be placed over the right atrium (second right interspace adjacent to the sternum).
8. If neurophysiologic monitoring is planned (SSEPs, MEPs), or EEGs, ensure that the anesthetic prescription is consistent with producing optimal signals. Important considerations are:
   a. The depth of anesthesia should remain constant if sequential recordings are to be compared. Ventilation ($PaCO_2$) and oxygenation should remain constant.
   b. Body temperature should remain constant.

   c. Opioids do not affect neurophysiologic monitoring.

   d. Nitrous oxide has little effect on latency of SSEPs but depresses the amplitude; it is contraindicated for MEPs.

   e. Inhalational anesthetics generally increase latency and depress amplitude of SSEPs; they are limited to ≤ 0.5 MAC for MEPs.

   f. Propofol, ketamine, midazolam, and α_2-agonists exert little effect.

In practice, a prescription using 0.5 MAC of an inhalational agent in an oxygen/air mixture, an opioid infusion (remifentanil or sufentanil), midazolam, and a propofol infusion provides acceptable conditions for monitoring both SSEPs and MEPs. For SSEPs, muscle relaxants may also be used, whereas for MEPs, muscle relaxants must be avoided after tracheal intubation. We prefer succinylcholine, or cis-atracurium for tracheal intubation when MEPs are planned. If remifentanil is used, be certain to administer a long-acting opioid to control postoperative pain before discontinuing the remifentanil.

Suggested Reading

Pajewski TN, Arlet V, Phillips LH: Current approach on spinal cord monitoring: the point of view of the neurologist, the anesthesiologist and the spine surgeon, Euro Spine J 16(Suppl 2):S115–S129, 2007.

INTRAVENOUS THERAPY AND CONTROL OF INTRACRANIAL PRESSURE

Strategies for Intravenous Fluid Therapy

A very reliable intravenous cannula is essential for children undergoing neurosurgery; at least 22- or 20-gauge cannulas for infants and 18-gauge or larger cannulas for older children. Small infants undergoing major surgery should have at least two large and well-secured IV routes. (Exsanguination during neurosurgery in small infants happens!)

General Rules for Intravenous Therapy

1. Avoid giving hypo-osmolar fluids because they increase brain edema; use normal saline. SIADH may follow neurosurgical procedures and may result in hyponatremia; the use of hypotonic solutions increases this danger.

2. Avoid dextrose-containing solutions except for documented hypoglycemia. Dextrose administration may increase the risk of neurologic damage secondary to local ischemia, including that caused by surgical retraction. If there is concern that hypoglycemia might result (i.e., in infants), regular blood glucose determinations should be performed and glucose solutions administered by rate limiting devices (i.e., an infusion pump).

3. Maintain the intravascular volume but avoid excessive fluid administration; third-space losses are very small in neurosurgical patients.
4. Blood losses are difficult to measure; therefore replace volumes, using cardiovascular indices (heart rate, BP, contour of the arterial wave form, and CVP) as guides. Colloid solutions or blood should be administered as required for extensive losses (see later discussion).

Control of ICP and Reduction of Brain Volume

Most important in the conduct of neuroanesthesia is to ensure that the surgeon has absolutely optimal intracranial operating conditions. This can be ensured as follows:

1. Prevent any episodes of hypoventilation or hypoxemia, coughing or straining, during induction of anesthesia.
2. Provide a clear, unobstructed airway at all times as increases in intrathoracic and airway pressures are directly transmitted to the CNS. The largest tracheal tube that will pass easily should be used. It should be positioned so that there is no possibility of kinking or compression. Reinforced tubes should be used where applicable. Monitor airway pressures.
3. Provide mild hyperventilation to a $PaCO_2$ of approximately 30 to 35 mm Hg.
4. A slight head-up tilt is preferred (15°). The veins in the neck should be totally unobstructed, avoid significant neck rotation.
5. Administer furosemide 0.5 mg/kg IV followed by mannitol 20% (0.5 to 1 g/kg) infused over 20 to 30 minutes as the skull is being opened (or as requested by the neurosurgeon).

After administering a diuretic, the schedule of fluid therapy also depends on the urine output. When urine volume equals 10% of the estimated blood volume (EBV), further urine losses are replaced (volume for volume) with normal saline. Alternatively, fluid administration can be guided by the CVP; maintaining a constant CVP generally indicates a stable circulating blood volume. Subsequently, serum electrolyte determinations should be made to exclude abnormalities and guide replacement.

Blood Replacement

Because blood loss during neurosurgery cannot be measured accurately, it must be gauged clinically from observation of the amount of bleeding and measurement of the child's cardiovascular indices. The systolic BP must be monitored as it is the most valuable guide to volume status; fluid replacement should maintain it at 60 mm Hg in infants and 70 to 80 mm Hg in older children. (**N.B.** The latter may lose up to 20% of EBV without a significant decrease in blood pressure). When surgery is complete but before the dura is closed, sufficient colloid or crystalloid are given to return the arterial pressure to the preblood loss level. The decision to transfuse blood is based on determination of the hematocrit together with clinical judgment of the blood losses occurring in relation to the allowable blood loss.

If a major blood transfusion has occurred, particularly in small infants, serum Ca^{++} may decrease. Hypotension unresponsive to further volume replacement should be treated with parenteral calcium gluconate or chloride. Assess coagulation indices and replace clotting factors as indicated.

Controlled Hypotensive Techniques

Controlled hypotensive anesthesia is rarely used in children but may be indicated for resection of a large AVM or aneurysm. An arterial line is essential if controlled hypotension is planned. A safe range of mean arterial pressure in the supine position is 50 to 65 mm Hg in children up to 10 years of age and 70 to 75 mm Hg in older children. If the child is positioned head-up, the arterial transducer must be zeroed at the level of the head so as to accurately reflect cerebral perfusion pressure.

Drugs to Induce Hypotension

1. *Isoflurane.* The inspired concentration can be increased progressively until the desired pressure is obtained. This method is easy to apply and results in very stable BP levels but is not readily reversed.
2. *Sodium nitroprusside* (SNP) has been widely used to induce hypotension but may result in tachyphylaxis, often results in wide swings in pressure, and in large doses may cause toxic effects. Because SNP interferes with cerebral autoregulation and may increase ICP, its infusion should not be commenced until the skull is opened.
3. Remifentanil offers an excellent alternative since high doses generally result in moderate reductions in blood pressure, it is not associated with toxicity, and it is readily reversed by simply slowing or stopping the infusion. However, its onset of effect is slower than occurs with SNP.

Air Embolism

Air embolism is a particular hazard when surgery is performed with the child in the sitting position, but it may also occur when the child is prone or supine if the head is elevated. It is relatively common during cranio-synostosis surgery and has also occurred during laminectomy. Air may be drawn in rapidly if a venous sinus is entered, or it may trickle in through veins within the bone. Air embolism detected by Doppler ultrasonography has a similar incidence in children and in adults, but is more likely to produce cardiovascular instability in children.

Embolism most often occurs during opening of the skull, but may also occur at the time of skin closure when the skin clips are removed. The signs, in order of decreasing sensitivity, include:

1. Changes in Doppler ultrasound over the precordium or appearance on transesophageal echocardiogram
2. Sudden decrease in $EtCO_2$ (or increase in end-tidal nitrogen level)
3. Hypotension
4. Change in heart sounds (windmill murmur or muffled/muted heart tones)

Early diagnosis and rapid therapy are required to prevent a serious outcome.

1. Inform the surgeon, who will compress and/or flood the wound with saline to prevent the entrainment of further air.
2. Lower the head; this increases the venous pressure at the wound and augments venous return from the legs. If the child is prone but in a head holding device thought should be given to covering the wound, releasing the head and turning the child supine so as to be able to perform chest compressions if needed.
3. Compress the jugular veins in the neck.
4. Ventilate with 100% O_2, discontinue N_2O to prevent further expansion of air emboli within the bloodstream, and add 5 to 10 cm H_2O PEEP.
5. Attempt to aspirate air via the central venous catheter; this is successful in fewer than 60% of cases.
6. Initiate cardiopulmonary resuscitation and other measures (e.g., inotropes) as required. **N.B.** measureable expired carbon dioxide indicates the adequacy of chest compressions.

Postoperative Considerations

All children should be fully recovered from the effects of anesthetic drugs and awake at completion of the procedure. Extubation should be smooth, without coughing or bucking; this can be facilitated by giving lidocaine 1.5 mg/kg IV. If the child remains unresponsive or respirations are depressed, leave the endotracheal tube in place and control ventilation until the cause is determined. After some major neurosurgery, it may be preferable to continue controlled ventilation into the postoperative period and extubate the trachea later, particularly if the surgery was in proximity to structures that control ventilation.

Postoperative nursing care should include routine monitoring of neurologic signs. The fluid status should be carefully monitored because regulatory mechanisms (i.e., antidiuretic hormone levels) may be altered after craniotomy. Often a brief CT scan is performed immediately postoperatively to assess the success of the surgical procedure.

Suggested Reading

Soriano SG, McCann ME, Laussen PC: Neuroanesthesia. Innovative techniques and monitoring, Anesthesiol Clin N Am 20(1):137–151, 2002.

HYDROCEPHALUS

Hydrocephalus may be caused by a congenital defect (e.g., Arnold-Chiari malformation, aqueduct stenosis) or by acquired disease (e.g., hemorrhage, infection, tumor). In the neonate, hydrocephalus may be secondary to the Arnold-Chiari malformation. (In many cases it is accompanied by meningomyelocele; this combined defect is present in 1 to 3 of every 1000 live births), although the latter defect has dramatically decreased with the use of prenatal folic acid vitamin supplements.

Surgical Procedures: Creation of Cerebrospinal Fluid Shunts

For noncommunicating hydrocephalus (see Chapter 2), the following procedures are performed:

1. Ventriculo-peritoneal shunt (lateral ventricle to peritoneum)—most common and preferred, because it allows the most room for growth
2. Ventriculo-atrial shunt (lateral ventricle to right atrium)—still used occasionally but may lead to long-term complications, particularly pulmonary thromboembolism and cor pulmonale because of pulmonary hypertension.
3. Ventriculo-pleural shunt (lateral ventricle to pleural cavity)—rare
4. Fourth ventriculostomy

For communicating hydrocephalus (see Chapter 2), a lumboperitoneal shunt (lumbar subarachnoid space to peritoneum) is performed.

Endoscopic instruments are often used to position shunts in the lateral ventricles, for fourth ventriculostomy, and for making a connection between ventricles. Very occasionally, these endoscopic procedures may be accompanied by considerable bleeding. Alternatively, shunts may be positioned under ultrasound guidance.

Special Anesthesia Problems

1. Increased ICP may occur and is sometimes severe. In such cases, the child may have been vomiting and become dehydrated; check fluid and electrolyte status preoperatively. Occasionally, acute symptoms of raised ICP demand immediate surgery.
2. Children may have had repeated anesthesia for shunt revisions; check the old records for problems with venous access, intubation, technical problems with successful shunt positioning, and latex allergy.
3. Blood loss is usually minimal, but very occasionally bleeding occurs from a large vessel. Always be prepared with large and secure intravenous access.
4. The child should be fully awake at the end of the procedure to permit rapid neurologic assessment.
5. Latex precautions should always be used in these children.

Anesthesia Management

Preoperative

1. Exercise special care if the ICP is increased. The child should be monitored carefully until surgery because the child's condition can deteriorate suddenly, necessitating immediate ventricular tap or lumbar puncture (depending on whether the hydrocephalus is non-communicating or communicating).
2. If the child becomes apneic, intubate, hyperventilate, and arrange for an immediate ventricular tap.
3. Assess fluid status. Intravenous fluids should be given to correct hydration in those with inadequate oral intake.

Perioperative

1. Exercise special care during induction of anesthesia to prevent hypoventilation, hypoxia, and systemic hypertension.
   a. An intravenous induction with propofol or thiopental plus a muscle relaxant is preferred, so that the airway can be secured rapidly and excellent ventilation ensured.
   b. Lidocaine (1.5 mg/kg IV) and fentanyl (2 to 5 µg/kg) may be given approximately 3 minutes before induction to attenuate the hypertensive response to laryngoscopy and intubation.
2. During surgery, maintain anesthesia with N_2O and low concentrations of isoflurane or sevoflurane. The addition of a nondepolarizing

relaxant drug (*cis*-atracurium preferred for short cases) permits the use of minimal inhalational agent, with rapid recovery when antagonized. Controlled ventilation is preferred for all children.

3. Pay special attention to the following situations:

   a. Hypotension at the time of CSF tap. If the arterial BP was increased secondary to increased ICP and if inhalational agents have been given, the BP may decrease precipitously as the ICP returns to normal (i.e., at the time of CSF tap). Discontinue all anesthetic agents, ventilate with 100% O_2, and give a fluid bolus to restore the BP to a normal level.

   b. Bradycardia and other arrhythmias may occur after or during placement of the intraventricular catheter, probably as a result of shifts in intracranial contents.

   c. Ventriculo-atrial shunts. Apply controlled positive-pressure ventilation to prevent air embolism while the vein is open for insertion of the cardiac end of the ventriculo-atrial shunt. The ECG may be used as a guide for positioning the atrial end of the shunt. Fill the shunt tubing with hypertonic saline and attach it by a sterile extension wire to the left-arm ECG lead. Switch the ECG to lead III. Advance the tubing; as the tip approaches the right atrium the height of the P waves increase, and when it reaches its correct position in the atrium, they become small and biphasic (Figure 8-1).

4. Blood loss is usually minimal but a secure and large-bore intravenous line should always be placed.

5. Inject local anesthetic to block the supraorbital nerve for a frontal shunt and a block of the posterior auricular nerve for posterior shunts.

6. Discontinue inhalational anesthetic agents before the end of surgery so that the child is completely awake and responsive before leaving the OR.

Postoperative

1. Order routine postcraniotomy nursing care.

2. Order analgesics as required. NSAIDS or codeine are often optimal; if local analgesic drugs have been injected at the surgical sites, the need for systemic analgesics is usually minimal.

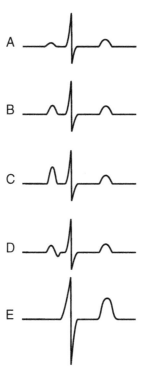

Figure 8-1 Drawing of ECG tracings obtained as a VA shunt catheter is advanced toward the heart. (**A**), When the catheter tip is in the SVC, P waves become large as the tip approaches the right atrium (**B** and **C**), then smaller and biphasic as the atrium is entered (**D**). If the catheter is advanced too far into the ventricle, the QRS complexes become very large and the P waves disappear (**E**).

CRANIOSYNOSTOSIS

Premature fusion of a suture between bones of the cranial vault leads to deformity. Most frequently only the sagittal suture is involved, leading to cosmetic deformity. Fusion of more than one suture may lead to increased ICP and later to developmental delay and possibly optic atrophy. Early surgical repair (at < 6 months of age) gives improved cosmetic results with less blood loss than repair at an older age.

Associated Conditions

1. Craniofacial abnormalities such as Crouzon disease and Apert syndrome

Surgical Procedure

1. Craniectomy—division of skull along suture lines

Special Anesthetic Problems

1. Possible increased ICP.
2. Sudden massive blood loss from damaged cerebral venous sinuses. Continued bleeding owing to the vascularity of the scalp and other membranes.
3. Difficult airway in children with craniofacial syndromes.
4. Venous air embolism (VAE) is a very real potential intraoperative danger.

Anesthetic Management

Preoperative

1. Check that blood is available in the OR for transfusion.
2. Use caution with premedication if the ICP is increased.

Perioperative

1. Intravenous induction with propofol (or thiopentone) and a muscle relaxant is optimal to rapidly secure the airway and prevent hypoventilation in infants with increased ICP but a standard inhalation induction may be used in infants without an increased ICP. A nasotracheal tube is preferred for infants; otherwise, use an armored oral or RAE (if supine) tube. (Choanal atresia is occasionally associated with craniosynostosis.)
2. Maintain anesthesia with N_2O/O_2, low concentrations of sevoflurane or isoflurane, and a relaxant; control ventilation.
3. Establish a secure large-bore intravenous line and have checked blood ready in the OR. Monitor blood loss carefully. An arterial line should be inserted if extensive surgery is planned (always discuss the surgical plan and the potential for rapid massive blood loss with the surgeon).
4. Mild hyperventilation and possibly diuresis may be needed to ensure that the volume of the intracranial contents is not increased.
5. Position a precordial Doppler probe and monitor carefully for air embolism as the skull is opened. Treat VAE as outlined above.
6. Administer low dose opioids for postoperative analgesia (e.g., 50 µg/kg morphine IV).
7. Discontinue inhalational anesthetics before the end of surgery so that the child is wide awake and responsive before leaving the OR.

Postoperative

1. Order routine postcraniotomy nursing care.
2. Exercise caution when prescribing opioids since this procedure is not as painful as it seems.
3. Assure that the open cranium is appropriately protected.

MYELODYSPLASIA: MENINGOMYELOCELE AND ENCEPHALOCELE

Meningomyelocele and encephalocele result from failure of the neural tube to fuse in the fetus. The incidence of meningomyelocele is approximately 1 to 4 per 1000 live births, with a large geographic variation. Encephalocele is much less common. Early operation should be performed because of the risk of infection and to prevent further damage to nerve tissue. Extensive skin dissection to mobilize flaps may be needed in some cases, and this may result in considerable blood loss.

Associated Conditions

Hydrocephalus, in many cases with Arnold-Chiari malformation and aqueductal stenosis, occurs in 80% of infants with meningomyelocele or encephalocele.

Short trachea has been described in association with meningomyelocele. Inspiratory stridor may be present secondary to cranial nerve dysfunction.

Surgical Procedures

Excision of the sac and repair of the defect is usually performed as soon as possible after birth.

Special Anesthesia Problems

1. Potential difficulty in positioning the child for intubation; placing the defect in the middle of a "doughnut" will prevent pressure on the open defect but also necessitates additional padding beneath the shoulders and head. Beware that children with meningomyelocele may also have a short trachea. *Ensure that the endotracheal tube is not in an endobronchial location.*
2. Blood loss is difficult to measure and may be considerable.
3. Difficulty maintaining body temperature during surgery.
4. Possibility of postoperative stridor, ventilatory depression or apnea, or cranial nerve palsy;ventilatory control may be abnormal in infants with meningomyelocele.

N.B. Succinylcholine does not cause hyperkalemia in infants and children with myelomeningocele.

Anesthesia Management

Observe all special precautions for the neonate.

Preoperative

1. The lesion is kept covered with sterile dressing.
2. Ensure that cross-matched blood is available in the OR.
3. Ensure that the OR has been warmed to at least 24°C.

Perioperative

1. Use all modalities for thermal homeostasis (see Chapter 4).
2. Do not give neuromuscular blocking agents until it has been ascertained whether the surgeon wishes to use a nerve stimulator to identify nerve roots. Alternatively, intubation may be facilitated with low dose rocuronium (0.3 mg/kg), which will wear off by the time the nerve stimulator is needed. Induce anesthesia and intubate. In cases of encephalocele, laryngoscopy and intubation are easier if the child is positioned in the left lateral decubitus, with an assistant applying forward pressure at the back of the head and backward pressure on the shoulders to prevent neck extension. If intubation cannot be performed in this position, place the infant supine, supported on a ring cushion to protect the spinal cord defect. Check the position of the tube carefully.
3. Continue anesthesia with N_2O and isoflurane or sevoflurane, with controlled ventilation. An arterial line should be inserted if an extensive procedure is necessary.
4. For surgery, the infant is positioned prone on bolsters. Assure that all pressure points are adequately padded and the eyes are protected.
5. Blood loss cannot be measured accurately. Estimate the amount of bleeding and monitor the arterial systolic pressure and the hematocrit as a guide to replacement.

Postoperative

1. Return the infant to a warm incubator, to be nursed prone on a frame.
2. Instruct the nursing staff to observe closely for signs of increased ICP, especially in cases of encephalocele. Monitor the adequacy of ventilation and for the development of stridor.
3. Do not give opioids until it is determined that there is sensory innervation of the surgical site.
4. Check hemoglobin and hematocrit on arrival in the postanesthesia care unit.

ARNOLD-CHIARI MALFORMATION

The Arnold-Chiari malformation consists of an elongated cerebellar vermis that herniates through the foramen magnum with associated compression of the brain stem. Infants with this disease may have difficulty swallowing, recurrent aspiration, stridor, and possible apneic episodes. The gag reflex may be depressed or absent.

Associated Conditions

Syringomyelia is often associated and leads to arm weakness and possible sensory deficit.

Surgical Procedure

The surgical procedure consists of decompression of the posterior fossa, enlargement of the foramen magnum with upper cervical laminectomy, opening of the dura, and lysis of adhesions. If syringomyelia is present, it is treated by drainage of the hydromyelia.

Special Anesthesia Problems

1. Control of ventilation is abnormal; stridor may require preoperative intubation and postoperative apnea may occur.
2. Recurrent aspiration frequently results in impaired pulmonary function, complicating the ventilatory status.
3. Stridor may not always improve immediately after surgery.
4. The child must be positioned prone and with the neck flexed for surgery; position the nasotracheal tube carefully (see previous discussion).

Anesthetic Management

Anesthesia management is the same as for posterior fossa exploration. The child should be very carefully monitored postoperatively. Rarely, the endotracheal tube must be left in place if the child cannot protect the airway; later, tracheostomy may rarely be required.

CRANIOTOMY FOR TUMORS AND VASCULAR ANOMALIES

Intracerebral tumors are relatively common during childhood, with a peak incidence at the age of 5 to 8 years; about 60% are in the posterior fossa. Benign vascular lesions may also be indications for craniotomy.

Surgical Procedures

1. Exploratory biopsy and/or excision of lesion.

Special Anesthetic Problems

1. Increased ICP and/or hydrocephalus may be present and may result in nausea, vomiting, and electrolyte disturbance.
2. Anesthesia techniques must be designed to provide optimal intracranial conditions for surgery.
3. Blood loss may be rapid, massive, and difficult to measure accurately. Appropriate invasive monitoring and peripheral venous access will be required.
4. Small infants with AVMs may have associated high-output congestive heart failure. These infants have a low diastolic blood pressure and do not tolerate further reduction in blood pressure intraoperatively (cardiac arrest may occur). Anesthesia in older children with an aneurysm or AVM must be very carefully managed to prevent intraoperative hypertension; controlled hypotension may be required to facilitate the surgery.
5. Postoperatively, the child must be free of residual effects of anesthesia to permit accurate neurologic assessment and monitoring. Hypertension is avoided to prevent bleeding.
6. In a few cases, it may be necessary to perform intraoperative neurophysiologic studies. In others, it may be necessary to record cortical SSEPs intraoperatively. The use of 0.5% isoflurane in N_2O provides satisfactory SSEP readings. Greater concentrations of inhalational agents may interfere with the recording.
7. In very few cases, the child remains awake and cooperative during surgery (i.e., to map the speech area) after a brief period of deep sedation during the craniotomy.

Anesthesia Management

Preoperative

1. Assess the child carefully. Review and understand the pathology and the surgical procedures that will be required. Check laboratory results.
2. Check that blood is available for transfusion (at least 1000 ml for craniotomy and more for removal of vascular anomalies).
3. Do not give sedative premedications except to children with vascular lesions (see previous discussion). Establish rapport with older children; reassure them, and explain the planned procedures.

Perioperative

1. Induce anesthesia, preferably using intravenous propofol (2 to 3 mg/kg) (or thiopental 5 to 7 mg/kg), lidocaine 1.5 mg/kg, fentanyl (2 to 5 µg/kg), and a full dose of a muscle relaxant; this prescription permits the airway to be secured rapidly and prevents hypoventilation, hypoxia, coughing, or straining, and adverse hemodynamic responses associated with tracheal intubation.

2. Intubate using the largest endotracheal tube that passes the larynx easily. A nasotracheal tube may be preferred for small infants and for those in whom postoperative ventilation may be required.

3. Light general anesthesia is adequate for neurosurgery (i.e., N_2O and isoflurane 0.5% to 0.75% plus a muscle relaxant); little further opioid analgesia is required once the skull is open. Control ventilation with intermittent doses of *cis*-atracurium, vecuronium, or rocuronium while monitoring neuromuscular block; antagonism should be readily accomplished. Alternatively, an infusion of muscle relaxant while monitoring the train-of-four response can maintain a stable degree of neuromuscular blockade (1 to 2 twitches) for many hours and simplifies management. That is start at 10 µg/kg/min rocuronium and increase or decrease by 2 to 3 µg/kg/min until the desired steady state is achieved.

4. For vascular tumors and vascular anomalies, an arterial line should be inserted and possibly CVP access (see previous discussion). A urinary catheter should be inserted.

5. Encourage the surgeon to infiltrate the area for the proposed scalp incision with 0.125% bupivacaine with epinephrine 1:200,000 (maximum volume, 2.0 ml/kg).

6. Give a diuretic to reduce brain edema when requested by the surgeon.

7. Give dexamethasone 0.15 mg/kg IV (maximum dose, 8 mg) to minimize focal cerebral edema).

8. If extubation is planned at the end of surgery, discontinue inhalational anesthetics before the end of surgery so that the child is fully awake and responsive before leaving the operating room.

Special Considerations: Anterior and Middle Fossa Surgery

1. Use an armored orotracheal tube or a nasotracheal tube.

2. Position child with a 15° head-up tilt.

3. Maintain anesthesia and monitor as previously described.

4. Watch for arrhythmias or changes in BP, especially during dissections in the region of the pituitary gland and hypothalamus. If these occur, alert the surgeon to discontinue surgery until the situation resolves. Intravenous atropine may be required for bradycardia.

Special Considerations: Posterior Fossa Surgery (Prone Position)

1. Use a nasotracheal tube in small children. It can be precisely secured at the nostril, it is less likely to kink than an oral tube, and its taping is unlikely to be loosened by saliva.
2. The child should lie prone on a frame (e.g., Relton frame) or bolsters, with a 15° head-up tilt and with the thorax and abdomen hanging free.
3. Anesthetize as for anterior or middle fossa surgery (see previous discussion). Monitor vital signs very carefully during manipulations in the region of the brain stem.

Special Considerations: Posterior Fossa Surgery (Sitting Position)

Many pediatric neurosurgeons use the prone or park-bench position, but unfortunately some still prefer the sitting position.

1. Air embolism is a prime concern; monitor carefully with a precordial Doppler probe and capnograph and place a CVP line at the junction of the superior vena cava and right atrium using ECG guidance. The CVP line can be used to aspirate air in case of embolism and also as a guide to fluid therapy.
2. Zero the arterial transducer at the level of the ear and the CVP transducer at the level of the heart. Cardiovascular stability is the next problem; the lower limbs should be bandaged to promote venous return, and the child positioned carefully and gradually while continuously monitoring the blood pressure.

Postoperative

1. The child must be fully recovered from the effects of anesthesia before leaving the OR.
2. Order routine postcraniotomy nursing monitoring and care.
3. Be very cautious with opioids to prevent respiratory depression; a morphine infusion at an appropriately low rate is usually very effective. **N.B.** The child is often also given an antiseizure medication.
4. Body temperature may increase; measures to restore normothermia may then be required.
5. SIADH may occur with resulting oliguria and electrolyte disturbance.

CRANIOPHARYNGIOMA

This is the most common pituitary tumor in children. It may become very large and compress adjacent structures (e.g., the optic chiasm), may cause a considerable increase in ICP, and may result in significant endocrine disturbance. Even after aggressive removal of the tumor under microscopic guidance, recurrence is common (10%).

Special Problems

1. Children with this disease often have growth retardation because of growth hormone deficiency, and they tend to be obese. They may also have behavior disturbances.
2. Adrenal insufficiency must be anticipated postoperatively; corticosteroid replacement therapy should be commenced before operation.
3. Diabetes insipidus may be present preoperatively and almost certainly will appear intraoperatively or postoperatively. Monitor CVP, urine output, and serum electrolytes during the operation. Be prepared to replace excessive urine losses and to administer DDAVP if necessary.
4. The surgical approach via a frontal craniotomy requires optimal reduction in brain mass (i.e., perfect neurosurgical anesthesia) if good access to the tumor is to be obtained.
5. The procedure may be prolonged; the child must be very carefully positioned and padded.
6. After excision of a craniopharyngioma, children require thyroid and growth hormone replacement therapy.

ANEURYSM OF THE VEIN OF GALEN

This uncommon disease, an AVM involving the great cerebral vein of Galen, is a considerable challenge to the pediatric neuroanesthesiologist. The disease may manifest in the neonate, evidenced by severe congestive cardiac failure and a cerebral bruit; the operative risk is greatest in lesions that appear at this age. Current management usually is by initial transcatheter coil occlusion of the feeding vessels. When lesions of the vein of Galen manifest later in life, the course is more benign, and the lesion may be managed like other AVMs.

Special Anesthesia Problems

1. Neonates and very young infants are likely to have severe congestive cardiac failure preoperatively. This condition can sometimes be improved by embolization of some of the aberrant vessels. Staged closed embolization may represent the safest therapeutic approach to this disease.
2. The surgical mortality rate is high, usually because of uncontrollable bleeding or intraoperative cardiac arrest. The use of profound hypothermia with circulatory arrest has been attempted, but the results

were poor. Current management is by transcatheter embolization of feeding vessels in the neuroradiology suite, possibly followed by surgical excision. Careful intraoperative management of the cardiovascular parameters may improve the outlook.

Anesthetic Management

1. It is important that hypovolemia or hypotension be avoided before the vessels are clipped. The AV shunt through the lesion places a great stress on the heart; failure is common, and myocardial perfusion is threatened by the low diastolic pressure. If the diastolic pressure decreases, myocardial perfusion will be inadequate and cardiac arrest will occur. Hypotensive techniques are contraindicated, and the blood pressure should be maintained until the aneurysm can be clipped or embolized. Aggressive cardiovascular monitoring is recommended for accurate monitoring of the intraoperative status and replacement of blood as needed.

2. When the aneurysm is clipped, the ventricular afterload suddenly increases and decompensation may occur. Vasodilators and inotropic agents should be prepared to compensate for this development if necessary.

3. A "cardiac anesthetic" (i.e., high-dose fentanyl analgesia or a remifentanil infusion) may be indicated for those in CHF.

4. If general anesthesia is employed during closed embolization, careful attention to the volume of contrast medium used is essential; excessive doses may lead to further volume overload or renal toxicity.

Suggested Reading

Ashida Y, Miyahara H, Sawada H, et al: Anesthetic management of a neonate with vein of Galen aneurysmal malformations and severe pulmonary hypertension, Paediatr Anaesth 15(6):525–528, 2005.

ELECTROCORTICOGRAPHY AND OPERATIONS FOR EPILEPSY

Many older children (beyond 8 years of age) cooperate adequately during awake/sedated craniotomy for electrocorticography and operations for epilepsy (i.e., temporal lobectomy).

Special Anesthesia Problems

1. Drugs that modify the EEG significantly (e.g., barbiturates) must not be given. A propofol or dexmedetomidine infusion, supplemented with a short-acting opioid is preferred.

2. The child must be awake and cooperative (including being able to speak).
3. Anesthetic techniques must be designed to provide optimal intracranial conditions for surgery.
4. Blood losses are difficult to measure and may be considerable.
5. Postoperatively, the child must be free of residual effects of anesthesia, to permit accurate neurologic assessment and monitoring.

Anesthesia Management

Preoperative

1. At the preoperative visit, assess the child and judge the likelihood that the child is able and motivated to cooperate.
2. Explain to the child the anesthetic technique proposed and the reasons for it. Encourage enthusiastic cooperation in the procedure (i.e., explain that in this procedure children experience a dreamy state and feel no pain, but they themselves must help make the operation a success).
3. Do not give premedication.
4. Omit anticonvulsant drugs the morning of the surgery.
5. Check that blood is available.

Perioperative

1. Ensure that equipment is at hand for emergency intubation and ventilation.
2. Insert a large-bore intravenous catheter and arterial line (use local anesthesia as needed).
3. The anesthetic technique must provide an initial period of sedation/ anesthesia to prepare the child and perform craniotomy after which the child is allowed to awaken to permit the child to respond to commands.
4. For the initial period of sedation/anesthesia, dexmedetomidine ± propofol may be used: dexmedetomidine may begin as a slow bolus of 1 to 2 µg/kg over 10 minutes followed by or simply begin with an infusion of 0.2 to 0.7 µg/kg/hr. Alternately a bolus of propofol 1 to 2 mg/kg IV followed by an infusion of 100 to 300 µg/kg/min may be used. A combination of propofol and dexmedetomidine has also been used. Titrate these to effect. Fentanyl 1 to 2 µg/kg IV should be titrated intermittently or a remifentanil infusion commenced until the skull is open. Low concentrations of N_2O may also be delivered via nasal cannulas while continuously monitoring $EtCO_2$ and SaO_2.

5. With the onset of sedation, surgeons shave the child's head and then insert a urinary catheter (ensure that lidocaine jelly is used).
6. A scalp block is performed on the side of the surgery using 1% lidocaine with 0.25% bupivacaine, with 1:200,000 epinephrine. Effective scalp analgesia is the key to success.
7. Continuously monitor the BP and frequent arterial blood gases.
8. Although the skull is being opened, give mannitol 1 to 2 g/kg or furosemide 0.5–1.0 mg/kg and dexamethasone 0.2 mg/kg as needed.
9. If excessive respiratory depression occurs, titrate very small incremental doses of IV naloxone (0.05 to 0.25 μg/kg).
10. After the skull is open, the infusion rates of the sedative drugs should be reduced until the child recovers, is able to respond to commands or speak, but remains still. Encourage deep respiration.
11. Management of children for awake craniotomy is not a procedure that you can master by reading a book. It requires considerable attention to detail that can only be gained by observing the procedure being performed.

Postoperative

1. If the child remains excessively drowsy, repeat small doses of naloxone.
2. Order routine postcraniotomy nursing care.

Suggested Reading

Soriano SG, Bozza P: Anesthesia for epilepsy surgery in children, Childs Nerv Syst 22(8):834–843, 2006.
Everett LL, Van Rooyen IF, Warner MH, et al: Use of dexmedetomidine in awake craniotomy in adolescents: report of two cases, Pediatr Anesth 16:338–342, 2006.

SPINAL CORD TUMORS AND TETHERED CORD

Spinal cord tumors are less common in children than in adults, but they can occur at any site in the spinal cord.

Tethered cord causes bladder and bowel symptoms and weakness of one or both lower limbs. This syndrome is confirmed by myelography and computed tomography, which demonstrate a low conus, a thickened filum, and a transverse orientation of nerve roots.

Surgical Procedure

Surgical division of the filum terminale is the treatment.

Special Anesthesia Considerations

1. Muscle relaxants should not be used if the surgeon wishes to use nerve stimulation intraoperatively to identify peripheral nerves. Anorectal manometry or SSEPs from the pudendal nerve may also be used to monitor neurologic function intraoperatively.
2. The child must be carefully positioned on a frame or bolsters to avoid pressure on the abdomen. Such pressure diverts blood from the abdominal veins to the vertebral venous plexus and increases bleeding at the surgical site.
3. General endotracheal anesthesia with N_2O, low concentrations of isoflurane, and small doses of fentanyl with controlled ventilation is very satisfactory.

SELECTIVE POSTERIOR RHIZOTOMY FOR SPASTICITY

Some children with spasticity secondary to CP may benefit from rhizotomy of some of the fascicles of the posterior roots of L2 to S1 bilaterally. Intraoperative EMG monitoring is used to determine which fascicles demonstrate a normal response to stimulation (brief local contraction) and which give an abnormal response (a sustained or diffuse contracture). The latter are then divided. Many children benefit significantly, with a generalized reduction of spasticity, improved limb function, and even improved speech function. Sensation is not significantly affected.

Management of anesthesia should be as for tethered cord (see previous discussion) *and with all considerations for the child with CP* (See Chapter 6, page 207). Nondepolarizing muscle relaxants should not be administered because the resulting neuromuscular block compromises interpretation of the EMG findings. Succinylcholine may be given for intubation if required; it is safe to use in the child with CP. Alternatively, low doses of nondepolarizing muscle relaxants will wear off before the need to interpret the EMG.

Intrathecal morphine (10 to 30 µg/kg), placed by the surgeon, has been successfully used for postoperative analgesia in these children.

Suggested Reading

Dews TE, Schubert A, Fried A, et al: Intrathecal morphine for analgesia in children undergoing selective dorsal rhizotomy, J Pain Symptom Manage 11(3):188–194, 1996.

ANESTHESIA FOR PEDIATRIC INVASIVE NEURORADIOLOGY

The development of microcatheters and occlusive materials that can be delivered via microcatheters has altered the management of pediatric neurovascular lesions. Neuroradiologists are currently treating AVMs and vein of Galen and other intracranial aneurysms using endovascular techniques. Therapeutic materials include particulate and nonparticulate embolic substances and microcoils.

Although morbidity after the use of these methods may be generally less than after open surgery, providing anesthesia to these children in the radiology suite introduces some problems for the anesthesiologist.

Special Anesthesia Problems

1. The radiology suite may be at a distance from the OR and anesthesia support services; ensure that all equipment and supplies that might be needed are available before commencing anesthesia. Make sure that communications to the OR are readily available so that additional equipment or help can be obtained if needed.
2. General endotracheal anesthesia with neuromuscular block (using a nerve stimulator) is always required for infants and young children; it is crucial that children do not move, especially during injections of embolizing materials. Brief periods of apnea may be requested.
3. Access to the children may be limited by the radiologic equipment; check ventilation carefully after tracheal intubation, and secure the endotracheal tube firmly. A RAE tube® may be suitable for some cases, but usually a standard tracheal tube is preferred because it can be used if postoperative ventilation is required. Ensure that ventilator circuits and monitoring lines can be routed so that they are absolutely secure throughout the procedure.
4. Maintenance of normal body temperature may be difficult when the child is on the x-ray table. Use humidified, warmed gases and forced-air warming mattresses. Keep the child covered as much as possible.
5. SSEPs may be monitored to guide the procedure; for this reason, inhalational anesthetics must be limited to small concentrations. In some cases, an amobarbital (Amytal) infusion may be used together with SSEPs to map cortical areas before embolization.

6. After the procedure, the child's neurologic status must be assessed and monitored. Therefore, a technique should be used that permits rapid and complete awakening.

7. Potential complications of the procedure include perforation of a vessel or aneurysm, accidental closure of normal vessels or draining veins, and adhesion of catheters. Some cases might need to proceed to craniotomy.

Anesthetic Management

1. No preoperative sedation is routinely administered, but it may be preferred for some children with intracranial aneurysm or AVM.

2. Induction and intubation should be planned as for craniotomy for AVM to minimize changes in ICP and hemodynamic parameters.

3. N_2O with sevoflurane (up to 1%) may be used for maintenance and does not significantly affect SSEP monitoring. Opioids (e.g., fentanyl 1 to 2 µg/kg or remifentanil infusion) may minimize postoperative headache and pain. Midazolam (0.1 mg/kg IV) at induction of anesthesia may confer amnesia.

4. A nondepolarizing muscle relaxant should be used (vecuronium or rocuronium), and the degree of neuromuscular block should be carefully monitored.

5. The child should be carefully positioned and padded to avoid pressure injuries. Means to maintain body temperature should be provided (see previous discussion).

Postoperative Care

1. It is desirable for the child to rest quietly but to not be obtunded, so that an accurate early postoperative neurologic assessment can be made.

2. The catheterization sites and the distal circulation should be regularly checked.

3. Suitable sedation and gentle restraint may be necessary to prevent movement that might result in bleeding or hematoma at the catheterization sites.

Suggested Reading

Steward ML: Anesthesia and interventional neuroradiology, Pediatrics Semin Anesth Periop Med Pain 19:304–308, 2000.

9 Ophthalmology

GENERAL PRINCIPLES

1. General anesthesia is almost always required because children do not tolerate sedation and local analgesia for eye surgery.

2. Intraocular surgery and surgery of the nasolacrimal duct and eyelids require a bloodless field. Although induced hypotension is seldom indicated for these operations, all measures should be taken to ensure that the anesthetic does not increase bleeding. Smooth, general anesthesia—with optimal airway, good positioning of the child, and quiet emergence without coughing or straining—is important.

3. The oculocardiac reflex (OCR) is powerful in children but is readily blocked by intravenous atropine (0.01 to 0.02 mg/kg) at induction of anesthesia. Do not rely on atropine given intramuscularly or on local anesthetic (retrobulbar) blocks to prevent this reflex. *Monitor the heart rate carefully during manipulation of the eyes and extraocular muscles.* In the rare event that atropine is contraindicated, remember that the oculocardiac reflex is more likely to be triggered by a sudden pull than by a gradually applied progressive traction on the extraocular muscles. The reflex usually fatigues rapidly; that is, a second pull does not elicit the same powerful effect.

4. Some children may be taking medications that have significant side effects (Table 9-1).

TABLE 9-1   Ophthalmic Eye Drops That May Cause Systemic Side Effects

Ophthalmic Medication	Indication	Side Effects
Echothiophate iodide (phospholine iodide), (long-acting plasma cholinesterase inhibitor)	Glaucoma, esotropia	Nausea, vomiting, abdominal pain, prolonged apnea after administration of succinylcholine
Timolol maleate topical (ß-blocking agent)	Glaucoma	Bradycardia refractory to atropine, bronchospasm, Exacerbation of the disease in asthmatics
Acetazolamide (Diamox) (Carbonic anhydrase inhibitor)	Glaucoma	Metabolic acidosis, and depletion of sodium, potassium, and water. It may also rarely trigger anaphylaxis, Stevens-Johnson syndrome, and bone marrow depression.
Dorzolamine (Carbonic anhydrase inhibitor)	Glaucoma	Bradycardia

5. Medications that are applied to the conjunctivas or injected into the eye during surgery may have important systemic effects or significant implications (Table 9-2).
6. The effects of anesthetic drugs and techniques on IOP must be remembered:
   a. Atropine (by any route) causes only a very slight increase in IOP. Its use as a premedicant is not contraindicated in children with glaucoma.
   b. All potent inhalation anesthetic agents, intravenous agents (i.e., propofol, thiopental) and nondepolarizing relaxants decrease IOP; effect may be dose related.
   c. Intravenous succinylcholine may cause a transient increase in IOP that is not reliably prevented by pretreatment with a nondepolarizing relaxant drug. The increase in IOP occurs within 30 seconds after administration but abates quickly, returning to normal within 6 minutes. Succinylcholine is usually avoided in children undergoing intraocular surgery. The increase in IOP may be less in those in whom the IOP is already increased (i.e., glaucoma), but it seems prudent to omit succinylcholine in such children, especially if IOP is to be measured. The use of succinylcholine in children

TABLE 9-2   Ophthalmic Medications That May Have Significant Effects During Anesthesia

Medication	Potential Adverse Effects and Implications
Epinephrine, phenylephrine	Hypertension and arrhythmias (especially dangerous during halothane anesthesia). Epinephrine eye drops are specifically contraindicated in children with tetralogy of Fallot because they may precipitate a cyanotic "tet" spell. Phenylephrine drops cause fewer problems, especially if the concentration is limited to 2.5%; but if instilled on a hyperemic conjunctiva, they may cause severe hypertension. Monitor the heart rate and blood pressure carefully after drug instillation. Ensure that you know what is being instilled: 10% phenylephrine drops should not be used in children; cardiac arrest may occur.
Cyclopentolate (Cyclogyl)	Ataxia, disorientation, psychosis, and convulsions, especially if a 2% solution is used. A 0.5% solution should be used for infants, and a 1% solution for children
Tropicamide (Mydriacyl)	Behavior disturbance, psychotic reactions, and rarely, vasomotor collapse.
Scopolamine eye drops	Excitation, disorientation, possible psychosis; may be treated with physostigmine 0.01 mg/kg IV.
Pilocarpine	Hypertension, tachycardia, bronchospasm, nausea, vomiting, and diarrhea.
Intraocular injection of acetylcholine	Increased secretions, salivation, bronchospasm, and bradycardia. Treat with IV atropine (to produce miosis after lens extraction).
Sulfur hexafluoride gas or air injection to globe (to assist in retinal reattachment surgery)	Discontinue N_2O 20 minutes beforehand to prevent an increase in intraocular pressure (IOP) followed by an even more dangerous decrease in IOP as the N_2O is withdrawn; this could damage the retinal reattachment

with penetrating eye trauma has been controversial. Although it was originally contraindicated, it has been shown to be safe in at least one very large series. Indeed, when given after thiopental in a rapid sequence induction, succinylcholine does not increase in IOP. However, with the intermediate duration, relatively rapid-acting nondepolarizing relaxants (i.e., rocuronium), there are alternatives to succinylcholine for RSI in children with penetrating eye injury.

  d. Ketamine, originally thought to increase IOP, probably has little effect.

  e. Diuretic drugs decrease IOP, and chronic diuretic therapy may reduce the increase in IOP after succinylcholine administration.

  f. Pressure on the globe from a facemask increases IOP, avoid compressing the eyes; use of a contoured mask (i.e., Rendell-Baker-Soucek mask) in small children makes it easier to do this. Laryngoscopy and endotracheal intubation may increase IOP; this effect can be modified by the administration of lidocaine 1 mg/kg IV, preferably 3 minutes before intubation. The insertion of a LMA causes a smaller increase in IOP than tracheal intubation, and its removal may be associated with less coughing and straining. Therefore, the LMA may be useful for children undergoing elective eye surgery.

  g. Coughing, bucking, crying, and straining all markedly increase IOP. Smooth extubation with reduced risk of coughing can be effected by prior administration of lidocaine 1 to 2 mg IV, a small dose of propofol (1 mg/kg) immediately before removal of the tracheal tube, or by deep extubation (contraindicated in the presence of a full stomach).

  h. Hypercapnia increases IOP, and hypocapnia decreases it.

7. Succinylcholine causes contracture of the extraocular smooth muscles and interferes with forced duction testing that is performed within 15 minutes after its administration.

8. The depth of anesthesia for ophthalmology surgery must be sufficient to ensure that the eyes are immobile and fixed centrally; during light anesthesia the eyes often "roll up" cephalad. Ketamine is generally unsatisfactory for ophthalmic surgery because of the associated nystagmus.

9. Postoperative pain may be troublesome after eye operations, but nonsteroidal antiinflammatory drugs such as rectal acetaminophen (35 to 45 mg/kg administered postinduction) may be sufficient after minor surgery. Immediately after intraocular surgery or trauma repair a retrobulbar block placed during anesthesia may be very effective. Topical analgesics (i.e., tetracaine ophthalmic drops) may significantly reduce postoperative discomfort.

10. Postoperative nausea and vomiting are common. It may be reduced by the use of propofol as the primary anesthetic, and it may be further reduced by the intraoperative administration of intravenous ondansetron (0.1 mg/kg), dexamethasone (0.0625 to 0.15 mg/kg), dimenhydrinate (0.5 mg/kg), or metoclopramide (0.15 mg/kg). Avoid dimenhydrinate which produces sedation if adjustable sutures are being used.

11. Be very cautious when using facemask anesthesia for surgery of the eyelids and similar operations (e.g., chalazion excision). Do not use high concentrations of oxygen, which might leak around the mask when the surgeon uses cautery; serious facial burns may occur if the drapes catch fire. An air or helium/oxygen mixture is preferred. Avoid N_2O.

CORRECTION OF STRABISMUS

Correction of strabismus is the most common eye operation in children.

Associated Conditions

Malignant hyperthermia is very rare, but strabismus may be an associated condition.

Special Anesthesia Problems

1. Oculocardiac reflex—Severe bradycardia and even cardiac arrest can occur as a result of traction on the extraocular muscles (see previous discussion).
2. "Oculogastric reflex"—vomiting after eye muscle surgery is very common and should be prevented as outlined previously. Vomiting may also be precipitated by "pushing" oral fluids postoperatively and by early ambulation. It is our recommendation that children only ingest clear fluids when they express the desire to drink.
3. Postoperative pain after strabismus may be considerable in older children.
4. If adjustable sutures are used, the child must be assessable postoperatively; excessive sedation should not be ordered. If a second anesthetic might be required to adjust the sutures, an intravenous line or a heparin lock should be left in place to facilitate induction of a second anesthetic. Do not use droperidol as an antiemetic in such children because they may be too drowsy to cooperate; the combination of ondansetron and dexamethasone is preferred (see later discussion).

Anesthesia Management

Preoperative

1. Do not give heavy sedation.
   a. The surgeon may wish to examine the child immediately before the operation.
   b. Oral midazolam (0.5 to 0.75 mg/kg for children 1 to 6 years of age) is an effective premedication with rapid onset.

   c. Clonidine (4 µg/kg PO) is effective as a premedication although it must be given 60 to 90 minutes before surgery. The latter may cause bradycardia, hypotension, and postoperative sedation but does provide postoperative analgesia.

2. Give atropine, preferably intravenously, at induction. If not administered it must be readily available, drawn up in a syringe, in case the OCR is elicited.

Perioperative

1. Induction is accomplished either by inhalation of sevoflurane or halothane in nitrous oxide or by intravenous propofol or thiopental followed by a relaxant.

2. If induction includes halothane, consider IV atropine before the start of surgery.

3. After a sevoflurane induction, a dose of propofol (up to 3 mg/kg IV) facilitates tracheal intubation and permits spontaneous respiration during surgery. After an intravenous induction and a muscle relaxant, maintain anesthesia with an inhaled agent and spray the larynx well with lidocaine before tracheal intubation. In both instances, intubate with an oral RAE tube. Alternatively, in suitable children, use a well-lubricated LMA.

4. Maintain anesthesia with N_2O/O_2/isoflurane or sevoflurane; allow spontaneous ventilation (provided the duration of surgery is not excessive).

5. From the start of surgery, listen to the child's heart sounds continuously via a precordial stethoscope and monitor the electrocardiogram. If bradycardia occurs, ask the surgeon to discontinue traction, additional intravenous atropine may be given; alternatively repeated gentle traction on the muscle may fatigue the reflex.

6. Give ondansetron (0.1 mg/kg) plus dexamethasone or dimenhydrinate (0.5 mg/kg) intravenously to reduce postoperative vomiting, or metoclopramide (0.15 mg/kg) immediately after the operation. Avoid opioids intraoperatively.

7. Provide for postoperative analgesia. IV ketorolac decreases postoperative pain and is associated with less PONV than opioids. Tetracaine eye drops instilled by the surgeon provide analgesia as does subtenon injection of bupivacaine or ropivacaine.

Postoperative

1. To prevent subconjunctival hemorrhage, the trachea must be extubated or the LMA removed without causing coughing and straining by the child. Extubate while the child is still deeply anesthetized, and allow the child to awaken smoothly while supporting the airway and administering oxygen by mask. Intravenous lidocaine (1.5 mg/kg) or low-dose propofol (0.5 to 1 mg/kg) administered before extubation may reduce coughing during emergence.

2. Provide analgesics for pain as indicated, avoid opioids where possible.
3. Intravenous rehydration during surgery should obviate the need for early oral ingestion in the postanesthesia care unit. Delaying ingestion of oral fluids decreases the incidence of poststrabismus vomiting. Do not attempt to mobilize the child rapidly; there is a motion sickness component to PONV after strabismus surgery. Beware that vomiting may occur en route to home in outpatients. These children tend to sleep more than most in part because they have double vision in the immediate postoperative period. It is reasonable to inform parents that their child will be quite sleepy the rest of the day.
4. If nausea and/or vomiting occur, order additional antiemetic therapy and continue with intravenous fluids.

Suggested Reading

Gayer S, Tutiven J: Anesthesia for pediatric ocular surgery, Ophthalmol Clin N Am 19:269–278, 2006.

Anninger W, Forbes B, Quinn G, et al: The effect of topical tetracaine eye drops on emergence behavior and pain relief after strabismus surgery, J Am Assoc Ped Ophthalmol Strab 11:273–276, 2007.

INTRAOCULAR SURGERY AND EXAMINATION UNDER ANESTHESIA FOR GLAUCOMA OR TUMOR

Children most commonly require general anesthesia for cataract or glaucoma surgery, treatment of detached retina, or examination under anesthesia (EUA) for glaucoma or tumor.

Special Anesthesia Problems

1. The oculocardiac reflex (see previous discussion).
2. Intraocular pressure—may be affected by anesthesia drugs and techniques (see previous discussion).
3. Coughing and straining—*may elevate the intraocular pressure.* (Induction of and emergence from anesthesia should be as quiet and smooth as possible.)

Anesthesia Management

Preoperative

1. Give adequate sedation to prevent coughing and straining.
2. It is safe to give atropine to children with congenital open-angle glaucoma.

3. Explain to older children that their eye will probably be covered with an eye patch after surgery.

Perioperative

1. Induce anesthesia as smoothly as possible, by inhalation of sevoflurane and N_2O or intravenously with propofol or thiopental.
2. *Do not administer succinylcholine.*
3. For brief EUA procedures use a facemask, but prevent pressure on the globe as it may increase IOP. Otherwise, either deepen anesthesia using a single dose of propofol (up to 3 mg/kg IV) or spray the larynx with lidocaine before intubating the trachea or inserting a well-lubricated LMA. For prolonged surgeries, a nondepolarizing muscle relaxant may be administered.
4. Maintain anesthesia with N_2O/O_2 and isoflurane, sevoflurane, or desflurane. Allow spontaneous ventilation for brief EUA procedures; otherwise, control ventilation to prevent hypercapnia. Alternatively, use a propofol infusion to maintain anesthesia because it may be advantageous in reducing postoperative vomiting.
5. Discontinue N_2O early if sulfur hexafluoride or air is to be injected into the eye.
6. A retrobulbar block with bupivacaine or ropivacaine may be useful to reduce postoperative pain.
7. At the end of surgery, suction the pharynx carefully and extubate the trachea, or remove the LMA, while the child is still deeply anesthetized. Lidocaine 1.5 mg/kg IV, administered before extubation decreases the risk of coughing or straining during emergence.
8. Reapply the facemask, support the airway, and give oxygen until the child awakens.

Postoperative

1. Order adequate sedation and analgesics.
2. Order an antiemetic as required.

PROBING OF THE NASOLACRIMAL DUCT AND CHALAZION EXCISION

These minor procedures are performed on an outpatient basis and usually give rise to no special problems. Tracheal intubation is usually unnecessary, and the procedure can often be carried out with facemask or LMA anesthesia. Nasolacrimal duct surgery is usually performed in infants (less than 12 months of age) and while it is usually brief, if a silicon Crawford tube must be inserted, this may take additional time. Patency of the duct is confirmed by either injecting a dilute fluorescein solution into the ducts and detecting it on a pipe cleaner in the nose or by the touch of metal to metal in the nose. Either fluorescein or blood from unblocking the duct may drain into the nasopharynx and trigger laryngospasm. To prevent such an occurrence, we place a roll under the shoulders and position the infant in Trendelenburg position (head down). In this position, pharyngeal fluids drain away from the glottis. Beware of oxygen leaks under the mask if cautery (for chalazion surgery) is used (see previous discussion). If it appears that the procedure may be more difficult and prolonged, intubate the trachea or insert an LMA.

PENETRATING EYE TRAUMA

Penetrating eye trauma is a relatively common injury in children.

Special Anesthesia Problems

1. Any increase in IOP in the presence of an open eye injury may cause extrusion of anterior chamber structures and/or vitreous humor. Crying, coughing, and straining should be prevented as much as possible. Although one may be tempted to sedate the child preoperatively, in most cases a full stomach is present and sedation is relatively contraindicated. Whenever a foreign body is lodged in the eye, the ophthalmologist prescribes IV antibiotics immediately to prevent endophthalmitis, hence intravenous access will be established in the emergency room. If a rapid sequence induction is indicated, an intermediate-acting, nondepolarizing relaxant such as rocuronium may be used. Succinylcholine has traditionally been contraindicated in children with open eye injuries, although it has been used in a large series without serious sequelae. The increase in IOP after succinylcholine is minimal compared with that caused by coughing, crying, or struggling. Hence, many would consider it justified if other indications exist for its use. Intravenous propofol or lidocaine minimizes the increase in IOP caused by laryngoscopy.
2. It may be difficult to position a mask if the eye is covered with a dressing.
3. The child usually has a full stomach.

Anesthesia Management

Preoperative

1. Give light sedation and analgesics as required provided a full stomach is not present; avoid upsetting the child.
2. If indicated, as early as possible before induction, give metoclopramide (Reglan) 0.1 mg/kg IV to expedite gastric emptying.
3. Give intravenous atropine at induction. (**N.B.** Atropine blocks the effect of metoclopramide and therefore should not be given earlier.)

Perioperative

1. Most children require a rapid sequence induction; give 100% O_2 by mask for 2 minutes if possible before inducing anesthesia.
2. Inject lidocaine 1 mg/kg IV slowly, followed 3 minutes later by propofol (or thiopental), and rocuronium (1.2 mg/kg).
3. Have an assistant apply cricoid pressure as needed.
4. Intubate the trachea before inflating the lungs. Aspirate the stomach.
5. Control ventilation and maintain anesthesia with N_2O/O_2 and isoflurane, sevoflurane, desflurane, or a propofol infusion.

Postoperative

1. Administer IV lidocaine before extubation to decrease coughing.
2. Extubate the trachea when the child is fully awake and in the lateral position.

Suggested Reading

Seidel J, Dorman T: Anesthetic management of preschool children with penetrating eye injuries: postal survey of pediatric anesthetists and review of the available evidence, Pediatr Anesth 16:769–776, 2006.

THE PRETERM INFANT FOR LASER TREATMENT OF DETACHED RETINA

Improved management of very-low-birth-weight infants has led to an increase in the incidence of retinopathy of prematurity. The outcome of this disease is improved if cryotherapy or laser treatment of detached retina is performed when the disease is at threshold level. Attempts to treat this condition using local analgesia are often unsuccessful and are accompanied by major complications. Therefore, general anesthesia is often indicated for very small infants for this procedure.

Special Anesthesia Problems

1. The infant is usually still very small and subject to all the problems of the preterm infant in the perioperative period. All precautions for the preterm must be observed (see page 136).
2. The infant may lose heat and become hypothermic during transport to the operating area. Preterm infants who are transported in an open infant bed invariably become hypothermic even if well covered. A proper heated transport incubator must be used.
3. Access to the infant during treatment is limited. Airway, ventilation, and comprehensive monitoring must be assured before the procedure commences. Thermal environment must be optimized (i.e., heated operating room and forced air warmer).
4. Postoperatively the infant's trachea should remain intubated and the lungs ventilated until judged stable by the neonatal team. A period of ventilation for 24 to 36 hours is commonly required even if the infant had been weaned before the eye treatment. A period of ventilatory instability is common postoperatively.

Suggested Reading

Allegaert K, Van de Velde M, Casteels I, et al: Cryotherapy for threshold retinopathy: perioperative management in a single center, Am J Perinatol 20:219–226, 2003.

ANESTHESIA FOR RADIOTHERAPY

Infants and children with retinoblastoma may require daily repeated radiotherapy for which they must remain absolutely still; hence, general anesthesia is required.

The challenge is to administer short-acting anesthetics and return the child to normal activity and feeding as soon as possible. A lens-sparing radiotherapy technique may be used, which means that the head must be firmly and accurately restrained; this may compromise the airway. Various techniques have been used including inhaled sevoflurane and intravenous propofol with or without an LMA. This avoids repeated risk of laryngeal trauma and should maintain a good airway despite positioning of the head. Nasal oxygen and capnometry combined with pulse oximetry help to assure adequate ventilation and oxygenation during the procedures.

More recently, the use of the Head/Fix Immobilization Device,* which uses suction to a mold of the palate, firmly supports the head and also generally maintains a very good airway without further instrumentation. Our experience is that a propofol infusion is safe and effective in these children.

An intravenous cannula may be placed at the first anesthetic and maintained in place with a heparin lock for use on subsequent occasions. Alternatively, many children will have an indwelling venous port or PICC line for the duration of their radiation therapy treatments.

Photoradiation therapy using a hematoporphyrin derivative (HpD) to mark tumor (ie., retinoblastoma) cells for subsequent argon laser therapy is sometimes used. Children undergoing HpD therapy are nursed in total darkness to prevent skin pigmentation and burns. General anesthesia in darkness is required; pulse oximetry is safe and reliable in the presence of HpD. It is suggested that, if necessary, tracheal intubation and other procedures can be performed with the use of a night vision scope.

Suggested Reading

Uchida I, Kinouchi K, Tashiro C: A new photoradiation therapy and anesthesia, Anesth Analg 70:222–223, 1990.

ANESTHESIA FOR VISUAL EVOKED POTENTIALS OR ELECTRORETINOGRAPHY

Visual evoked potentials (VEPs) are exquisitely sensitive to the effects of sedative and anesthetic agents because of the complex cortical pathways involved. Hence, the anesthesia technique must be carefully planned if meaningful results are to be obtained.

1. Nitrous oxide significantly depresses the amplitude of VEPs.
2. Potent inhaled agents decrease amplitude and increase the latency of VEPs. At 1.5 MAC VEPs are unrecordable.
3. Thiopental decreases amplitude and increases latency of VEPs. An induction dose of etomidate has less effect, only a slight increase in latency and no change in amplitude.
4. Propofol has a dose-related affect on amplitude and latency—hence low doses may be acceptable.

---

* Medical Intelligence, Schwabmünchen, Germany.

5. Ketamine has a negligible effect on latency and a dose-related effect on amplitude of VEPs.
6. Fentanyl significantly decreases the amplitude.

In summary, it is difficult to provide anesthesia care for infants and small children for VEPs. A technique based on low-dose ketamine or propofol is recommended.

The results of electroretinography (ERG) are less affected by anesthesia and sedative agents. Suitable conditions for these studies have been obtained using a barbiturate (i.e., IV pentobarbital [see page 525] or rectal methohexital [see page 60]).

Suggested Reading

Banoub M, Tetzlaff JE, Schubert A: Pharmacologic and physiologic influences affecting sensory evoked potentials: implications for perioperative monitoring, Anesthesiology 99:716–737, 2003.

Gayer S, Tutiven J: Anesthesia for pediatric ocular surgery, Ophthalmol Clin N Am 19:269–278, 2006.

Otorhinolaryngology 10

GENERAL PRINCIPLES

Although much of it is simple and commonplace, ear, nose, and throat surgery has a disproportionately large potential for anesthetic and surgical complications. It demands meticulous attention to all aspects of the child's perioperative care.

277

1. Because many of these operations involve the airway, the anesthesiologist must be prepared to provide good surgical access while maintaining a safe ventilatory pathway for the child.
2. The advent of the surgical microscope has permitted development of delicate and precise surgery for the middle ear. Anesthesia for such procedures must provide quiet operating conditions with minimal bleeding, smooth emergence from anesthesia, and minimal disturbance postoperatively.
3. After surgery involving the airway, skilled nursing care in the postanesthesia care unit (PACU) is essential, so that signs of impending complications can be detected early and appropriate therapy instituted.
4. The use of the laser to treat lesions of the larynx creates additional potential problems for anesthesia management.
5. When topical vasoconstrictors are used, the anesthesiologist must be aware of the drugs and doses that will be used because significant systemic absorption may cause dangerous effects. A maximum initial dose of 20 μg/kg of phenylephrine has been recommended for children, but this is considerably less than has been commonly used. Monitor the child carefully when topical vasoconstrictors are applied. Topical phenylephrine may lead to hypertension, which resolves rapidly and requires no treatment. Occasionally, severe hypertension may occur; this should be treated with direct vasodilators (e.g., sodium nitroprusside) or α-adrenergic receptor antagonists (e.g., phentolamine). Do not use β-blockers or calcium channel blockers in the presence of hypertension; these may cause a disastrous decrease in cardiac output and the severe hypertension may cause pulmonary edema.

Suggested Reading

Groudine SB, Hollinger I, Jones J, et al: New York State guidelines on the topical use of phenylephrine in the operating room, Anesthesiology 92:859–864, 2000.

CHOANAL ATRESIA

If it is a complete obstruction, as in 90% of cases, choanal atresia (membranous or bony occlusion of the posterior nares) causes respiratory distress immediately after birth. The distress is intermittent; being relieved whenever the infant cries because neonates are primarily nose-breathers. The diagnosis can be easily confirmed by listening for air exchange over each nostril with a stethoscope. Once the diagnosis is established the obstruction can be relieved with an oropharyngeal airway. The passage of an orogastric tube may open the oral airway in some infants and also facilitates feeding of the infant. Early endonasal puncture and stenting may be performed in the neonate, but is usually delayed in the preterm infant. It is now recognized that even incomplete choanal atresia may lead to chronic nasal problems; therefore early repair is common.

Associated Conditions

The "CHARGE" association consists of **C**oloboma, congenital **H**eart disease, choanal **A**tresia, growth and mental **R**etardation, **G**enitourinary abnormalities with genital hypoplasia, and **E**ar anomalies.

Surgical Procedures

1. Endoscopic transnasal puncture may be preferred, especially in preterm infants or in those with associated significant disease (e.g., the CHARGE association).
2. Transpalatal repair if indicated is usually performed at age 1 to 2 days in the healthy, full-term infant. Stents are left in postoperatively for varying periods.

Special Anesthesia Problems

The primary problem is maintenance of the airway until completion of surgery.

Anesthesia Management

Preoperative

1. Adequate ventilation requires continued use of an oropharyngeal airway.

Perioperative

1. Observe all special precautions for neonates (see Chapter 4).
2. Leave the oropharyngeal airway in place: give 100% O_2 by mask.
3. Induce anesthesia by inhalation of sevoflurane or halothane. Confirm that manual ventilation via the mask and oropharyngeal airway is successful and, if so, administer a short-acting muscle relaxant; intubate using an oral RAE tube®.
4. Maintain anesthesia with N_2O and small concentrations of sevoflurane or isoflurane with controlled ventilation.
5. Suction the pharynx very carefully at the end of the operation and ensure that the stents are clean and patent.
6. Do not extubate the trachea until the child is fully awake.

Postoperative

1. Order humidified oxygen. The stents must be regularly suctioned with a fine catheter to keep them clear.
2. Constant observation is essential because aspiration during feeding commonly occurs after repair of choanal atresia.
3. Subsequent repairs may be necessary later in childhood for restenosis, but these operations present no other special anesthetic problems.
4. Order appropriate analgesia.

Suggested Reading

Thevasagayam M, El-Hakin H: Diagnosing choanal atresia—a simple approach, Acta Paediatrica 96:1238–1244, 2007.

NASOPHARYNGEAL TUMORS

Teratomas, dermoid cysts, nasal encephaloceles, and other tumors require surgical excision. Juvenile nasal angiofibroma is a rare benign but very vascular tumor that may involve the nose. Biopsy of these tumors may result in extensive bleeding that is very difficult to control; therefore diagnosis is usually made on the basis of imaging studies. An operation to remove the tumor may result in massive blood loss and should be prepared for accordingly. Postoperatively, there may be persistent nasal obstruction and continued bleeding; the endotracheal tube should be left in place until the child is fully awake.

SURGERY OF THE NOSE

The most common procedures for nasal surgery are reduction of nasal fractures, septoplasty, rhinoplasty, and excision of nasal polyps.

Special Anesthesia Problems

1. The nasal airway may be blocked. The surgeon may wish to pack the nose with gauze and a vasoconstrictor (e.g., cocaine) preoperatively.
2. Children with nasal polyps usually have cystic fibrosis.
3. Functional endoscopic sinus surgery (FESS) may precipitate special problems (see later discussion).

Anesthesia Management

Preoperative

1. Assess the nasal airway.
2. If the child has cystic fibrosis, order appropriate preoperative care (see Chapter 6, page 177).

Perioperative

1. Induce anesthesia by inhalation or intravenously with propofol or thiopental, followed by a muscle relaxant.
2. If the nose is blocked, insert an oropharyngeal airway before attempting mask ventilation.
3. Perform orotracheal intubation, with a cuffed tube.
4. Insert a throat pack to prevent blood pooling in the pharynx and esophagus.
5. Position the child with a slight head-up tilt.
6. Extubate the trachea when the child is fully awake; premature extubation may lead to laryngospasm or airway obstruction.

Postoperative

1. Order analgesics as required.
2. Administer humidified oxygen by mask.
3. Postoperative airway obstruction may occur and may require reintubation. If prolonged, obstruction may predispose to postobstructive pulmonary edema. This requires therapy with oxygen, a diuretic, and morphine. If pulmonary edema is severe, tracheal intubation and positive-pressure ventilation may be required.

FUNCTIONAL ENDOSCOPIC SINUS SURGERY (FESS)

FESS has become a standard surgical treatment for chronic sinus disease. Precise endoscopic resection of diseased tissue and relief of obstruction while preserving normal mucosa is the objective to restore normal sinus function.

Special Anesthesia Problems

1. Many of these children have chronic diseases (e.g., cystic fibrosis).
2. Successful endoscopic surgery requires extensive use of vasoconstrictors. Ensure that maximal permissible doses are not exceeded so as to prevent severe hypertension: 2 to 3 mg/kg cocaine or 10 μg/kg epinephrine. If hypertension ensues, treat it by deepening

anesthesia or using vasodilators; do not use β-blockers or calcium channel-blocking agents.

3. Bleeding may be considerable and may require that packing remain in place postoperatively. Because this is likely to cause complete nasal obstruction, have the child fully awake before extubation.

4. Rarely, the surgery may encroach on the orbit or intracranial space. In the latter case intracranial bleeding may occur. There is also a danger of pneumocephalus if positive pressure is applied via a facemask.

TONSILLECTOMY AND ADENOIDECTOMY (T&A)

Chronic inflammation and hypertrophy of lymphoid tissues in the pharynx may necessitate surgery to relieve obstruction or to remove the focus of infection. Repeated middle ear infections may be improved by adenoidectomy. Obstructive sleep apnea (OSA) is now the commonest indication for T&A in North America. Rarely, acute tonsillitis leads to a peritonsillar abscess (quinsy tonsil).

T&A surgery is now often performed in the ambulatory unit; this demands special considerations in the selection of suitable children and in their postoperative evaluation before discharge home. An efficient follow-up service must be provided to deal with unexpected complications. Some children may not be suitable for outpatient T&A.

The following criteria are indications for admission after T&A:

1. Age less than 3 years
2. Those with abnormal coagulation studies or a history suggestive of increased bleeding tendency
3. Those with evidence of significant OSA (see later discussion)
4. Those with other systemic diseases that place them at additional perioperative risk (e.g., congenital heart disease, endocrine or neuromuscular disease, chromosomal abnormalities, obesity)
5. Those with craniofacial or airway abnormalities, including Down syndrome
6. Those with a history of peritonsillar abscess
7. Those who live at an excessive distance from the medical facility or whose home, social, or parental situation might preclude safe postoperative care.

T&A is still one of the most common procedures in children and should be very safe. However, T&A-related deaths still occur: the usual cause is excessive sedation of children with airway compromise, OSA, or mismanagement of postoperative bleeding. Postoperative nausea and vomiting are common after T&A but may be significantly reduced by withholding postoperative oral fluids until the child requests them, rehydration during anesthesia (20 to 25 ml/kg lactated Ringer's solution or equivalent), and the administration of dexamethasone and a serotonin-receptor antagonist.

Obstructive Sleep Apnea (OSA)

Chronic obstruction due to lymphoid hyperplasia may result in OSA, and this is now a most common indication for T&A. Affected children may be obese (or asthenic), show difficulty arousing in the morning or daytime somnolence, nocturnal enuresis and behavior problems (attention deficit disorder and limited attention span), nocturnal apnea and sweat profusely.

If such a history is obtained preoperatively, ideally a sleep study (polysomnography) should be performed; if the results are significantly abnormal, admission after tonsillectomy is advised. Polysomnographic indications for admission after tonsillectomy for the T&A with a history of OSA include:

1. A baseline value for partial pressure of carbon dioxide ($PaCO_2$) ≥ 50 mm Hg
2. A baseline awake oxygen saturation value $\leq 92\%$
3. Episodes of oxygen desaturation $\leq 80\%$
4. Apnea/hypopnea index greater than 1

If polysomnography is unavailable, overnight oxygen saturation monitoring has been suggested as a valuable screening tool; resting saturations less than 90% and episodes less than 80% are strongly predictive of severe OSA. Although the positive predictive value of overnight SpO_2 monitoring is very high, a negative test is less helpful and should be interpreted cautiously.

Children with OSA have reduced responses to rebreathing CO_2 and may be exceedingly sensitive to opioids, requiring dramatically reduced doses of opioids.

Children with mild OSA are reported to have few complications after T&A. Those with moderate/severe apnea require careful postoperative care.

The child with OSA should be closely monitored before and after surgery; supervised mild sedation (oral midazolam) is safe preoperatively but is often omitted. In all children with diagnosed OSA, spontaneous respiration is indicated after tracheal intubation and small incremental doses of opioid should be administered (i.e., IV fentanyl 0.5 µg/kg or morphine 0.025 mg/kg). Children with upregulated opioid sensitivity may develop apnea after these small opioid doses despite surgical stimulation. In such cases, no further opioids should be administered and postoperative opioid doses should be markedly reduced. Rectal acetaminophen (35 to 45 mg/kg) may be administered after induction of anesthesia, with subsequent rectal doses of 20 mg/kg q6h (maximum daily dose 90 to 100 mg/kg/day). Alternatively oral acetaminophen (10 to 15 mg/kg) may be administered. Posttonsillectomy ketorolac has been criticized because of the risk of bleeding and reoperation, although the data are controversial. There may be roles for diclofenac, tramadol, and ketamine for posttonsillectomy analgesia, although experience with these analgesics in children with OSA is limited. Postoperative sleep studies show that 90% or more improve by 6 months (fewer improve if obesity or moderate/severe OSA is present). Those who do not improve (usually severe OSA), should be investigated for residual soft tissue obstruction and evaluated for uvulopalatopharyngoplasty. Children generally do not tolerate CPAP or BiPAP devices.

Suggested Reading

Clinical Practice Guideline: Diagnosis and management of childhood sleep apnea syndrome. section on pediatric pulmonology, subcommittee on obstructive sleep apnea syndrome, Pediatrics 109:704–712, 2002.

Cardiorespiratory Syndrome

In very rare instances, severe chronic airway obstruction by adenoidal tissue may lead to pulmonary hypertension and right-sided heart failure (cardiorespiratory syndrome). This condition usually occurs in boys and is more common in African American children. There is usually a history of symptoms lasting 1 year or longer. The child is usually febrile (due to associated adenoid or pulmonary infection) with tachycardia and tachypnea. Chest radiography may reveal cardiomegaly, and the electrocardiogram indicates right ventricular hypertrophy. Children with cardiorespiratory syndrome may be critically ill and may require emergency intubation to relieve the obstruction. Once this is done and the heart failure is controlled with digitalis and diuretics, T&A should be performed. They may need to remain intubated postoperatively and should be admitted to the ICU for further treatment.

Suggested Reading

Sie KC, Perkins JA, Clarke WR: Acute right heart failure due to adenotonsillar hypertrophy, Intl J Ped Otorhinolaryngol 41(1):53–58, 1997.

Special Anesthesia Problems for T&A *surgery*

1. Sharing the airway with the surgeon
2. Danger of postoperative bleeding
3. A history of bleeding tendency or recent salicylate therapy. Salicylate ingestion during the days before operation increases blood loss during T&A. If such a history is obtained, a test of bleeding time should be performed; if the time is prolonged (more than 10 minutes), the operation is deferred.
4. A history suggestive of OSA; such children may be at risk for perioperative apnea and demonstrated increased sensitivity to opioids (see previous discussion).

Anesthesia Management

1. For children with a history of chronic infections, anesthesia may be induced intravenously or by inhalation and supplemented with an intermediate relaxant to facilitate intubation. For children with a history of OSA, after induction of anesthesia, we advocate tracheal intubation without the use of a muscle relaxant to assess the respiratory responses to small incremental doses of intravenous opioids during surgery.
2. Perform tracheal intubation with a RAE tube that is positioned under a slotted tongue blade of the mouth gag. Check the airway patency carefully after the gag is positioned. Check for bilateral ventilation because the tip of the RAE tube may become endobronchial after insertion of the mouth gag or if the neck is flexed. Some advocate an LMA in place of a tracheal tube; however, in our opinion the low morbidity and additional security of an endotracheal tube does not justify substituting an LMA.
3. Administer standard antiemetic therapy to all children: ondansetron (0.10 to 0.15 mg/kg) and dexamethasone 0.0625 to 0.15 mg/kg IV (maximum 8 mg), and lactated Ringer's solution (20 to 25 ml/kg) to reduce nausea and vomiting and improve postoperative comfort.
4. When the indication for surgery is for chronic infection, maintain anesthesia with N_2O and sevoflurane or isoflurane, assist ventilation (with or without a relaxant) and supplement with opioids. Plan for postoperative analgesia morphine 0.05 to 0.1 mg/kg IV for postoperative

analgesia. When the indication is for OSA, an inhalational anesthetic with spontaneous respiration should be supplemented with small incremental doses of opioids while their respiratory responses are monitored. If apnea or hypopnea develops, no further opioids are administered. In addition, some surgeons infiltrate the tonsil fossae with bupivacaine *before* surgery to reduce postoperative pain, although this is unproven and presents a significant risk for intravascular injection. Ketamine 0.5 mg/kg IV during surgery reduces the need for other analgesics and may be particularly useful in children with OSA.

5. Measure and chart blood losses carefully.
6. Carefully suction the pharynx; the presence of small amounts of blood in the pharynx may lead to laryngospasm. Extubate the trachea when the child is fully awake and airway reflexes are fully restored (especially with OSA). Do not pass suction catheters through the nose because doing so may make the adenoidal area bleed.

Postoperative

1. Order morphine (0.05 to 0.1 mg/kg) IV in the PACU q5-10 min until comfortable in children without OSA. Acetaminophen (10 to 20 mg/kg PO) with or without codeine is often adequate if an opioid has been given and/or bupivacaine has been infiltrated intraoperatively, although early administration of any PO medications may trigger emesis. Children with OSA should be carefully monitored (pulse oximetry) in PACU; morphine in doses 10% to 50% of the usual dose should be titrated to ventilations. Caution: pulse oximetry is a poor measure of adequacy of ventilation if supplemental oxygen is being administered.
2. An intravenous infusion should be maintained until the child is ready for discharge. It is particularly important to ensure that children undergoing T&A on an outpatient basis are well hydrated before discharge.
3. Do not push oral fluids; order fluids by mouth as requested by the child (i.e., cola beverages, Popsicles) when the child is awake. If PONV occurs and further antiemetic therapy is required (e.g., ondansetron), be aware that this might prevent the child who is continuing to bleed from vomiting and thus conceal the hemorrhage.
4. Closely monitor those children with a history of OSA; such children may become apneic with sedation and/or airway obstruction. Constant nursing attention should be provided (i.e., admit to a monitored unit). Some children (especially the obese) may benefit from nasal CPAP therapy or nasal oxygen.

5. Be cautious when ordering opioids for the restless child, especially if there is any evidence of airway compromise. Restlessness may be a symptom of hypoxia secondary to obstruction, and opioids may produce apnea.

6. The outpatient should be evaluated directly by the surgeon for bleeding and the anesthesiologist for adequacy of ventilation before discharge. In general, we recommend observing children for at least 4 hours before discharge.

7. A telephone consultation service should be provided for follow-up of outpatients on the evening after surgery.

8. Complaints of abdominal pain after T&A are suggestive of swallowed blood from ongoing bleeding, especially after potent antiemetic therapy. Suspicion of tonsil/adenoidal bleeding should be raised.

Reoperation for Bleeding After Tonsillectomy

Special Anesthesia Problems

1. The stomach contains blood that may be regurgitated during induction.

2. Hypovolemia may be present and is easily underestimated. There may be little blood to be seen, but much may have been swallowed.

3. The child may have a bleeding disorder that has been not been identified.

Anesthesia Management

Preoperative

1. Ensure that sufficient fluids have been administered to restore the blood volume, correct severe anemia, and produce normal cardiovascular indices. Bleeding is rarely so brisk that complete restoration of blood volume cannot be achieved before operation.

2. Check that further blood is available in case of need.

3. Check coagulation indices.

4. In some instances, gentle restraint permits examination, insertion of packing, cautery or ligation of bleeding vessels without the need for general anesthesia.

Perioperative

1. Prepare all equipment for a rapid sequence induction (2 suctions, 2 functioning laryngoscope blades, and 2 functioning handles).

2. Check again that the child has been adequately fluid resuscitated.

3. Give 100% O$_2$ by mask.
4. Rapidly inject propofol (or ketamine or etomidate) with atropine added, followed immediately by succinylcholine (2 mg/kg). If there is a contraindication to succinylcholine, then give high-dose rocuronium (1.2 mg/kg) but anticipate a prolonged recovery from neuromuscular blockade after control of bleeding (~75 minutes).
5. Have an assistant immediately apply cricoid pressure (see page 99).
6. Intubate the trachea as rapidly as possible with a styletted tracheal tube.
7. Maintain anesthesia as for T&A (see previous discussion), although surgery for tonsil rebleeding is much less painful compared with the original T&A surgery.
8. Extubate the trachea when any residual neuromuscular blockade has been adequately antagonized and the child is fully awake.

Postoperative

1. Check the hemoglobin level to confirm adequacy of blood replacement.
2. Be alert to the possibility of further bleeding.
3. Monitor oxygen saturation and vital signs closely.
4. Order suitable doses of analgesic as needed (not acetylsalicylic acid).
   a. Oversedation could result in complete obstruction of the airway.
   b. Restlessness may indicate hypoxia rather than a need for sedation.

Peritonsillar Abscess (Quinsy)

Special Considerations

1. Trismus and swollen tissues in the pharynx may make tracheal intubation difficult.
2. There is a danger that the abscess may burst and flood the pharynx with pus that leads to pulmonary aspiration.

Anesthesia Management

Preoperative

1. Children with tonsillar abscess should be closely observed for impending airway obstruction. Check the extent to which the mouth can be opened; significant trismus may be present.
2. Avoid sedative premedications if possible, particularly in children with any degree of airway obstruction.

Perioperative

1. Check that the child can open the mouth. Ensure that strong suction is available. Give atropine 0.02 mg/kg IV.
2. Induce anesthesia by inhalation of N_2O with sevoflurane or halothane. Maintain spontaneous ventilation. Position the head slightly down and turned to the affected side.
3. Do not give muscle relaxants (airway obstruction may occur).
4. When the child is *deeply* anesthetized, discontinue N_2O and continue with sevoflurane in 100% O_2; give 1 mg/kg lidocaine IV to reduce the risk of coughing or breath holding during laryngoscopy and endotracheal intubation. Be careful not to rupture the abscess during airway instrumentation.
5. Maintenance is the same as for T&A for chronic infection (see previous discussion).
6. Suction carefully and extubate the fully awake child in a lateral position.

N.B. Sometimes the inflammatory swelling involves the supraglottic structures, and postextubation obstruction may occur. Dexamethasone (0.1 mg/kg up to 8 mg) IV should be considered. Close observation is essential.

Suggested Reading

Clinical Practice Guideline: Diagnosis and management of childhood sleep apnea syndrome. section on pediatric pulmonology, subcommittee on obstructive sleep apnea syndrome, Pediatrics 109:704–712, 2002.

OTOLOGIC CONDITIONS

Surgery for ear conditions ranges from (minor surgery) simple myrin-gotomy and tubes to (major) prolonged surgery for tympanomastoidec-tomy and cochlear implants. Myringotomy and tube surgery is the briefest surgery performed in the operating room (OR) (as brief as <5 min) but is not without risk because these infants and children often have or had recent URTIs. In contrast, tympanomastoidectomy and cochlear implan-tation require considerations for prolonged surgery, require tracheal intu-bation and are associated with PONV.

Special Anesthesia Problems

1. The child may have had repeated procedures and may be very apprehensive.
2. The child's hearing may be impaired, making communication difficult.

3. During middle ear procedures, even a small amount of bleeding may interfere with surgery. Position the child carefully and avoid anesthetic causes of bleeding (e.g., hypoventilation, coughing, NSAIDs). However, induced hypotension is not usually warranted for this type of surgery in children.

4. The surgeon may wish to use vasoconstrictor drugs (e.g., epinephrine, cocaine). In such cases the dose should not exceed the maximum (see previous discussion).

5. Otologic procedures can be lengthy; if this is the case, ventilation should be controlled and careful attention should be paid to positioning, padding, and maintenance of body temperature.

6. In rare cases, the child's cooperation is required during surgery (see Chapter 8, page 258, Awake Craniotomy).

7. If the surgeon uses a nerve stimulator, relaxants are limited to induction of anesthesia.

8. Postoperative PONV secondary to labyrinthine disturbance is common. Prior therapy with antiemetics (e.g., ondansetron) may be useful.

9. Use of a postauricular nerve block before surgical incision and repeated at the end of surgery has been demonstrated to reduce vomiting compared with opioids.

Minor Otologic Procedures

Minor otologic procedures are usually performed in the outpatient department. N_2O has been shown to pass into the middle ear cavity if air is present and may modify findings at operation, but in general its use is not contraindicated. N_2O does not increase the incidence of postoperative vomiting.

Special Anesthesia Problems

1. Some children who require repeated minor otologic procedures have associated congenital deformities of the upper airway that predispose to their ear disease (e.g., cleft palate, Treacher Collins). Check previous anesthetic records carefully for potential airway problems.

2. Many of these children present for anesthesia with signs of an upper respiratory tract infection (URTI). In such instances, the decision to proceed must be based on the urgency of surgery (i.e., acute middle ear infection) compared with the severity of the URTI. If the child's temperature is normal, behavior and eating habits have been normal and there are no mucopurulent secretions or chest wheezing/rales, then surgery should proceed (see Chapter 6, page 172).

Anesthesia Management

Preoperative

1. Sedation is often unnecessary, but oral midazolam is useful for the very upset child, though it delays recovery after very brief surgery. Parental presence at induction of anesthesia may provide adequate anxiolysis.

Perioperative

1. Induce anesthesia by inhalation of sevoflurane or intravenously with propofol or thiopental.
2. Maintain anesthesia with N_2O and sevoflurane or isoflurane by facemask.
3. Tracheal intubation is not required, but a laryngoscope and suitable endotracheal tubes should be immediately available in case of unexpected difficulties. Likewise an IV infusion is not usually required.
4. Ensure that you can comfortably hold the child's head very still during the procedure— resting your elbow on the table will help with this.
5. Analgesics are not usually required, especially if the surgeon inserts local analgesic drops. Oral (10-15 mg/kg preoperatively) or rectal acetaminophen (35 to 45 mg/kg intraoperatively) may be administered. A 0.25 injection of 0.125% bupivacaine without epinephrine of the nerve of Arnold (interior surface of the tragus) provides analgesia and reduces the incidence of vomiting. Others have also administered intranasal or IM fentanyl for perioperative pain control.

Postoperative

1. Oral codeine may be administered for ongoing pain.
2. Resume PO fluids when the child is awake.

Major Otologic Procedures

Anesthesia Management

Preoperative

1. Order adequate sedation, especially for children who have had surgery previously.
2. Hearing aids may be worn until induction of anesthesia after which time they should be removed, turned off and stored until the child recovers.
3. If the child communicates by sign language, then either a parent or healthcare professional who can sign should accompany the child to

the OR. If the child can lip-read, do not cover your lips until the child is anesthetized.

Perioperative

1. Induce anesthesia by inhalation or intravenously with propofol (or thiopental), followed by a suitable relaxant. If nerve stimulation (usually for facial nerve) is required during surgery, only use a single dose of short (succinylcholine) or intermediate-acting relaxant (rocuronium or cis-atracurium) for intubation.
2. Spray the larynx with lidocaine; then insert an orotracheal (regular or RAE®) tube. Extended breathing circuit tubing is usually required as the anesthetic machine is located at the foot of the OR table. Ensure adequate ventilation for the increased breathing circuit compliance.
3. Maintain anesthesia with N_2O/O_2 and an inhalational anesthetic; anesthesia must be deep enough to prevent any possibility of bucking on the tube, which increases bleeding. Supplement with opioids as needed, but beware that this may increase PONV (consider remifentanil)
4. Position the child with a 15° head-up tilt to minimize bleeding.
5. If epinephrine is to be infiltrated, ensure that the dose does not exceed the maximum.
6. Prophylactic antiemetic therapy should be given. IV balanced salt solution should include 20 to 25 ml/kg to decrease postoperative pain and emesis.
7. For tympanoplasty, discontinue N_2O from the inspired mixture before the graft is positioned. (N_2O bubbles might float the graft off the desired position.)
8. Smooth tracheal extubation, without coughing, is essential. Therefore, administer intravenous lidocaine 1 mg/kg or propofol 0.5 to 1 mg/kg and remove the tube while the child is still deeply anesthetized and breathing spontaneously. Maintain the airway and allow the child to awaken while administering oxygen by mask.

Postoperative

1. Order analgesics and antiemetics as required.

Awake Ear Surgery

For certain operations (e.g., ossicular reconstruction), the surgeon may wish to assess hearing during the surgical procedure. Most older children cooperate well if such operations are performed under a combination of sedation and local analgesia.

Anesthesia Management

Preoperative

1. Explain in detail what will happen during the operation and reassure the child that there will be no pain.
2. Order PO midazolam in a sufficient dose to ensure adequate sedation preoperatively.

Perioperative

1. Establish an intravenous line using a local analgesic.
2. Titrate propofol ± dexmedetomidine infusions until an adequate degree of sedation is achieved (see Chapter 8, page 258, Awake Craniotomy, for dosing regimen). Titrate small doses of fentanyl (1 to 2 µg/kg) or a remifentanil infusion until the child is comfortable.
3. Ensure that the child is positioned comfortably, and warn the child not to cough or move the head.
4. Talk with the child periodically to assess the effects of the drugs, but allow the child to sleep when cooperation is not required.
5. Monitor ventilation via nasal capnometry, administer supplemental oxygen and, if necessary, remind the child to breathe deeply periodically.

Postoperative

1. Smaller than usual doses of analgesics are effective in most cases.
2. Antiemetic medications may be required.

ENDOSCOPY

Endoscopy is often indicated in infants and children for diagnosis (e.g., stridor) or for therapy (e.g., removal of a foreign body).

Procedures

1. Laryngoscopy
2. Bronchoscopy
3. Esophagoscopy

Special Anesthesia Problems

1. Existing airway problem or tracheotomy
2. Difficulty maintaining optimal ventilation during endoscopy, particularly in a child with a very small airway
3. Possibility of complete airway obstruction during some procedures (i.e., removal of foreign body)

4. Danger of airway fire if cautery or laser is used
5. Danger of postoperative reduction in airway lumen by subglottic edema

N.B. Many conditions for which endoscopy is performed can progress to complete obstruction under anesthesia. Always have a selection of laryngoscopes and endotracheal tubes prepared; from the start of anesthesia, ensure that the endoscopist is at hand in case surgical intervention with either a rigid bronchoscope or tracheotomy become urgently necessary.

General Anesthesia Management

1. *Spontaneous ventilation* is usually preferred during endoscopy in children. It may be safer than controlled ventilation if there is airway compromise, and it allows the endoscopist to examine the dynamic structure of the airway under normal physiologic conditions. Maintaining spontaneous respirations is particularly important when evaluating the child for airway compression, laryngeal, tracheal, or bronchomalacia. Abnormal airway compression or collapse may not be adequately detected during controlled ventilation.
2. *Controlled assisted ventilation* is necessary for children who are in respiratory failure and for those who cannot maintain effective ventilation when anesthetized.

Laryngoscopy

Anesthesia Management

Preoperative

1. Do not give heavy sedation to children with airway problems. Oral midazolam is useful for some older children having repeated endoscopy, but beware of sedating any child with a dubious airway. Children with laryngeal papillomata present a particular risk because of the possibility of ball-valve obstruction, airway fire, or embolism of tumor fragments distally. These cases require complete discussion with the surgeon so that the anesthetic prescription needed for that particular child is clear (i.e., spontaneous ventilation with insufflation, intermittent intubation, or paralysis with apneic oxygenation).

Perioperative

1. Apply monitors, including pulse oximeter, and induce anesthesia by inhalation of N_2O and O_2 with sevoflurane and insert an appropriate size intravenous catheter.
2. Hydration with 20 ml/kg of lactated Ringer's solution will support the circulation during deep inhalation anesthesia.

3. When the child is deeply anesthetized, discontinue the N_2O, continue with sevoflurane in O_2, perform laryngoscopy and spray the larynx and supraglottic structures with lidocaine (maximum dose, 4.5 mg/kg).

4. Replace the mask until the lidocaine becomes effective (2 to 3 minutes). The duration of the procedure may be brief in some cases but prolonged in others. Anesthesia may be continued with an infusion of propofol (± remifentanil).

5. Monitor ventilation visually, with a precordial stethoscope and by capnometry.

Postoperative

1. Observe the child closely until awake.
2. Order humidified oxygen postoperatively.
3. Maintain NPO status until 2 hours after application of the lidocaine spray.

N.B. The previous method of anesthesia, employing topical analgesia and propofol with spontaneous ventilation is considered overall the safest and most satisfactory method. Endotracheal tubes get into the surgeon's field of vision, and all other methods are cumbersome and complicated and therefore may fail. "Jet ventilation" methods can be dangerous in children, especially if the high pressure jet migrates distal to an obstructing lesion; fatal pneumothorax and pneumomediastinum may occur.

Special Considerations

Laryngomalacia. A common cause of inspiratory stridor in the neonate, laryngomalacia can be diagnosed during laryngoscopy while the infant is awake or is awakening from anesthesia. The stridor usually disappears during deeper levels of anesthesia and with small amounts of positive end expiratory pressure (PEEP); PEEP is especially useful in maintaining a patent airway during the initial phases of induction. In this condition, there is incomplete maturation of the cartilages of the larynx and a tendency for the epiglottis or one of the arytenoid cartilages to prolapse into the glottis during inspiration, causing marked inspiratory stridor. The condition is self-limited and disappears as the child ages; no special therapy is usually required. However, laryngoscopy is indicated to rule out other causes of stridor (e.g., cysts).

Congenital Cysts. Congenital cysts may occur in the region of the epiglottis and aryepiglottic folds. There may be inspiratory and expiratory stridor and a poor cry. The diagnosis is usually confirmed by radiologic imaging. Therapy is by excision or marsupialization.

Congenital Webs. Subglottic webs reduce the cross-sectional diameter of the upper airway lumen to 2 to 4 mm in neonates. These webs usually have a single central perforation through which the neonate ventilates. Because of the limited diameter of the perforation and the oxygen requirements of the neonate, respiratory distress often occurs soon after birth. Laryngoscopy may reveal the presence of a web, otherwise, an appropriate sized tracheal tube may not pass below the vocal cords. When the diagnosis is confirmed by bronchoscopy, laser resection of these webs effectively restores the lumen of the upper airway.

Subglottic Hemangioma. Subglottic hemangioma may manifest with crouplike symptoms and a barking cough, usually commencing at a few months of age. The child frequently has other visible hemangiomas, especially on the face. The symptoms persist or recur, and diagnosis is confirmed with endoscopy. Commonly therapy is by laser ablation; however, this is sometimes followed by subglottic stenosis. Open resection of the hemangioma is now advocated by some.

Anesthesia Management

For laser resection:

1. Manage as for laryngeal papillomata (see later discussion)
2. Humidified oxygen should be administered postoperatively after laser therapy

For open excision:

1. An initial laryngoscopy and bronchoscopy will be performed to assess the lesion. This may be managed with inhalational anesthesia plus topical lidocaine (see later discussion).
2. Following the endoscopic examination, an oral endotracheal tube is inserted and general anesthesia continued.
3. An anterior incision in the neck is made to display and open the larynx.
4. At this stage the oral endotracheal tube is withdrawn and a second sterile tracheal tube passed by the surgical team via the lower end of the incision into the trachea.
5. The hemangioma on the posterior aspect of the larynx is now resected.
6. On completion of the operation a nasotracheal tube is passed through the glottis and larynx into the trachea and left in situ.

7. The child is returned to the ICU for continued ventilation, sedation, and paralysis for the initial postoperative days. Immobility of the laryngeal structures is important during the early healing period.
8. The child is returned to the OR for examination before extubation several days later. Dexamethasone is administered before removing the tube. Close observation is required for a further period of 2 to 3 days.

Suggested Reading

O-Lee TJ, Messner A: Open excision of subglottic hemangioma with microscopic dissection, Intl J Ped Otorhinol 71(9):1371–1376, 2007.

Laryngeal Papillomas. These rare lesions are caused by a virus, and the cauliflower-like papillomas can cause serious airway obstruction. Various therapies have been tried, including cryoprobing, ultrasound, and immune sera. Currently, the preferred therapy is resection by laser. Children with this condition usually present at 2 to 4 years of age and return for repeated laryngoscopy and resection. Recurrences are almost certain until adolescence, when the lesions usually regress spontaneously. Increasing hoarseness and dyspnea are the usual indications for reoperation, and on each occasion the extent of regrowth is impossible to determine before laryngoscopy. Sometimes extensive papillomas completely obscure the glottis. A cautious approach is indicated in all cases since ball-valve obstruction is always a risk. Provide humidified gases postoperatively.

Special Anesthesia Problems

1. Acute airway obstruction may occur during induction of anesthesia, therefore spontaneous ventilation is preferred.
2. The glottic opening may be difficult to visualize, therefore barbiturates and relaxants are contraindicated.
3. Surgical therapy by laser demands an unobstructed view of the larynx and immobile vocal cords.
4. Instrumentation of the trachea below the glottis should be avoided because it may "seed" papillomas into the lower airways. Therefore, endotracheal tubes should be avoided if possible, and tracheostomy is usually considered to be contraindicated.

Anesthesia Management for Laser Surgery

The safest plan is as outlined previously: no premedication, careful inhalation induction followed by laryngoscopy, and lidocaine spray to the larynx. If obstruction develops during induction, an endotracheal tube must be inserted to establish the airway. The tube can be removed when deep plane of anesthesia is achieved and most of the papillomas have been resected. Usually tracheal intubation is unnecessary, and laser resection can proceed once topical analgesia has been applied. Extremely rarely, critical airway obstruction may occur necessitating an urgent rigid bronchoscopy. Inhaled sevoflurane anesthesia may be supplemented or replaced with a propofol or propofol/remifentanil infusion.

Alternatively, a nonflammable endotracheal tube* (or foil-wrapped tube) may be inserted. In this case ventilation can be controlled, but the surgeon must work around the tube.

N.B. Jet ventilation can be very dangerous in cases of obstructing lesions of the airway. Laryngeal obstruction during jet ventilation may lead to pneumomediastinum and pneumothorax. If jet ventilation is used, extreme care must be taken to avoid barotrauma: the jet must not be advanced beyond the lumen of the laryngoscope, and distal airway pressure should be monitored and restricted (15 mm Hg).

Special Precautions for Use of the Laser

1. Cover the child's eyes.
2. All personnel in the OR should wear eyeglasses for protection in case the laser beam is accidentally reflected in their direction. Post a warning sign on all doors that the laser is in use.
3. Special facemasks may be worn to protect against inhalation of vaporized viral tissue.
4. Airway fires are a real danger during laser therapy. Use the minimal FiO_2 in either air or helium. Avoid N_2O. If a tracheal tube should ignite, it must be immediately disconnected from the anesthetic circuit and removed from the airway. Injury results both from the burn and from the products of tube combustion.

Bronchoscopy

Bronchoscopy may be performed for various indications (e.g., removal of a foreign body, diagnosis of respiratory disease, removal of secretions, treatment of atelectasis, evaluation for tracheomalacia, bronchomalacia, or airway compression by vascular structure or mediastinal tumors).

Special Anesthesia Problems

1. Difficulty maintaining adequate ventilation during the procedure, when the airway must be shared with the endoscopist

---

* Phycon laser shielding tube, Fuji Systems Corp., Tokyo.

2. Existing impairment of ventilation in some cases

Anesthesia Management

Preoperative

1. Assess the airway and the respiratory status carefully.
2. Do not give heavy premedication if there is any doubt about the airway or ventilation.

Perioperative

Spontaneous ventilation is preferred for all children except those with respiratory insufficiency.

1. Induce anesthesia by inhalation of N_2O and sevoflurane in O_2 and establish adequate venous access.
2. Discontinue the N_2O and deepen anesthesia with sevoflurane in 100% O_2.
3. When the child is adequately anesthetized, remove the mask and perform laryngoscopy. Spray the larynx and trachea with lidocaine (maximum 4.5 mg/kg).
4. Replace the mask; continue anesthesia with O_2 and sevoflurane until the lidocaine takes effect (2 to 3 minutes), at which time the bronchoscope can be inserted.
5. Supply O_2 and sevoflurane to the side arm and allow spontaneous ventilation, but remember that when a telescope is in use through a small bronchoscope (3.5 mm or smaller), the resistance to ventilation is high. At such times, ventilation should be assisted or controlled and the telescope may have to be removed periodically. Sevoflurane anesthesia may be supplemented with a propofol or remifentanil/propofol infusion or bolus doses of propofol IV. Be aware that the dead space of the bronchoscope may not allow for detection of expired carbon dioxide. It is important to assess the adequacy of ventilation by observing chest expansion.
6. Monitor oxygen saturation closely; set the sound at an adequate level so that the surgeon is immediately aware if the saturation begins to fall. During bronchoscopy it is useful to have a precordial stethoscope in place, and also sometimes to listen over other areas of the lungs.
7. Be alert to the possibility of pneumothorax, a rare complication of pediatric bronchoscopy.
8. When controlled ventilation is essential, as for children in respiratory failure, a Venturi device (e.g., Sanders injector) may be used, but remember that children whose severe chronic respiratory disease has reduced lung compliance may not ventilate well with this method. For such children, control ventilation using the anesthetic circuit connected to the side arm of the bronchoscope, as described previously (Figure 10-1).

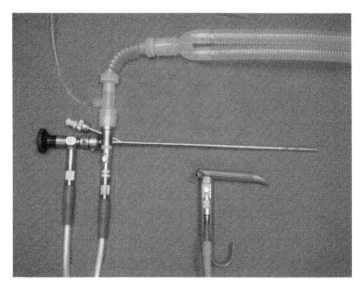

Figure 10-1 Pediatric rigid bronchoscope with anesthesia circuit attached for controlled/assisted ventilation. Right is anterior commissure laryngoscope.

Postoperative

1. Order nothing by mouth for at least 2 hours (after lidocaine spray).
2. Order humidified O_2.
3. Watch for signs of stridor.
4. Check the postoperative x-ray for possible pneumothorax.

Flexible Bronchoscopy

Small-diameter flexible fiberoptic bronchoscopes permit diagnostic bronchoscopy to be performed with the child awake or with minimal sedation and topical analgesia. In young children, however, general anesthesia is preferred. In such cases the bronchoscope may be passed through an adapter into the facemask and via the mouth or nose of the anesthetized child. The use of an LMA is particularly useful as it assures adequate airway patency and a means for continuing to deliver anesthesia. Alternatively, an endotracheal tube can be inserted as a conduit for the bronchoscope. In all cases, topical anesthesia with lidocaine spray as described for rigid bronchoscopy is indicated.

Rigid Esophagoscopy

In children, rigid esophagoscopy is usually performed to dilate a stricture or for removal of a foreign body.

Special Anesthesia Problems

1. The child may have undergone esophagoscopy repeatedly and therefore may be very apprehensive.
2. In small infants, passage of an esophagoscope may compress the trachea and obstruct ventilation, even when an endotracheal tube is in place.
3. Coughing, straining, or other movements can result in esophageal perforation during the procedure. Children must be anesthetized adequately to maintain complete immobility.
4. Lower esophageal strictures or achalasia may result in esophageal dilation more cephalad. Food and secretions accumulated in the dilated segment may be aspirated during anesthesia.
5. Rarely, a sharp or potentially damaging foreign body may lodge in the hypopharynx, possibly to be displaced into the airway if the child coughs or strains.
6. Special attention to securing the endotracheal tube and manually holding the tracheal tube during movement of the esophagoscope will help to prevent unintended extubation of the trachea.

Anesthesia Management

Preoperative

1. Order adequate sedation, especially for children who have undergone esophagoscopy previously.
2. Check whether the radiographs show esophageal dilation and/or retained material.
3. Discuss with the surgeon any special considerations he/she may have and alter the anesthetic prescription accordingly.

Perioperative

1. Give 100% O_2 by mask.
2. Induce anesthesia intravenously and intubate the trachea rapidly. (Use cricoid pressure whenever there is a risk of regurgitation and aspiration—except in the case of a sharp object in the upper esophagus or in the presence of Zenker diverticulum)

3. In the case of a sharp foreign body in the hypopharynx, a gentle, smooth inhalation induction of deep anesthesia is indicated.
4. Deepen the anesthesia before permitting the endoscopist to proceed.
5. Monitor ventilation, oxygenation, and hemodynamics using standard monitors.

Postoperative

1. Observe the child until fully awake.
2. Be alert for signs of esophageal perforation, especially if difficulty was encountered. These signs include
   a. Tachycardia
   b. Fever
   c. Signs of pneumothorax
   d. Radiographic evidence of pneumothorax or mediastinal air
3. Order nothing by mouth until 2 hours after application of the lidocaine spray.

AIRWAY INFECTIONS

Epiglottitis

Supraglottic infections (epiglottitis) used to be most commonly caused by *Haemophilus influenzae* B (*HiB*) bacterial infection and less frequently by staphylococcus and fungae in severely immunocompromised children. Since the introduction of a *HiB* vaccine, epiglottitis has become a rare disorder in children, but still does occur in adults. As the disease becomes rarer, there is an increased danger that the diagnosis may be missed. However, epiglottitis does still occur and there is recent evidence of a resurgence in *HiB* epiglottitis because of nonimmunized immigrant children and ineffective/failed vaccinations.

Epiglottitis is most common in children 3 to 7 years old but also occurs in infants or adults. It is accompanied by severe systemic illness with pyrexia and leukocytosis. In addition to the epiglottitis, all the supraglottic structures are swollen and inflamed, contributing to the obstruction. Blood cultures are almost always positive for the infective agent, which is typically *HiB,* although other bacteria and fungal infections are possible, but rare. The common symptoms are sore throat, dysphagia, and drooling; severe airway obstruction may develop rapidly. Typically, the child appears toxic and anxious and sits in a tripod position with chin extended and mouth open. In infants the presentation is less typical, occurring with sudden apnea during investigation of a high fever. Therefore, epiglottitis should be considered in the differential diagnosis of the infant with pyrexia and any respiratory difficulty.

Extraepiglottic infection may occur: pneumonia, cervical adenitis, otitis media, septic arthritis, and meningitis are described in association with epiglottitis.

Anesthesia Management

Preoperative

1. Once the diagnosis is suspected, the child should be disturbed as little as possible. Avoid venipunctures or painful injections because the child may cry and become acutely obstructed. Do not try to visualize the pharynx because acute obstruction may result. Gently apply a face-mask and give O_2.
2. The child must be attended constantly by a physician capable of establishing an emergency airway and equipped to do so.
3. Assemble the team and transfer the child rapidly to the OR; administer O_2, allowing the child to remain in the chosen posture.
4. Soft-tissue radiographs of the neck may be misleading and are unnecessary in the typical case. If x-ray studies are required to make the diagnosis, the child must be accompanied to the radiology department by a physician in case the airway becomes obstructed during the examination. The child should not be made to lie down for the x-ray examination. The lateral neck film will reveal a dilated hypopharynx, thickened aryepiglottic folds, a thumblike epiglottis obstructing the laryngeal inlet, and loss of the vallecula because of swelling of the tongue surface of the epiglottis.
5. The OR should be prepared for emergency bronchoscopy and possible tracheotomy (surgeon present, scrubbed, and ready to intervene if needed).

If Apnea Occurs (At Any Time)

1. Try to ventilate the lungs with O_2 by bag and mask. This is usually successful.
2. If unsuccessful, proceed to an immediate attempt at laryngoscopy and intubation. Also prepare for an emergency tracheotomy if intubation proves impossible.

Perioperative

1. Gently apply a precordial stethoscope, pulse oximeter, BP cuff, and EKG electrodes.
2. Do not place the child supine. Induce anesthesia with O_2 and sevoflurane (or halothane) by placing the mask gently over the child's face while the child remains seated, either on the OR table or on the anesthesiologist's or parent's knee. Having a parent present may

reduce the child's upset and therefore minimize dynamic tracheal collapse with crying against an obstructed upper airway.

3. When anesthesia is induced, gently place the child in the supine position. Assisted ventilation may be necessary at this time.

4. Apply other monitors and establish an intravenous infusion; administer intravenous atropine and 20 to 30 ml/kg of lactated Ringer's solution. These children are febrile and usually dehydrated since swallowing is painful.

5. Remember that anesthetic induction is likely to be very prolonged because of the shallow respirations and possible V̇/Q̇ mismatch should the child also have pneumonia. If the airway is satisfactory there is no urgency to rush the process. Our rule of thumb is that when you think the child is deep enough to perform laryngoscopy, wait 1 more full minute because it is quite easy to underestimate the depth of anesthesia.

6. Administer lidocaine 1 mg/kg IV to minimize the risk of coughing and laryngospasm; then perform laryngoscopy and orotracheal intubation with a styletted tracheal tube. In the rare event that the glottis is obscured by swelling and distortion of the supraglottic structures, compress the chest with one brisk compression. This usually expels a bubble through the larynx, providing a guide to the location of the glottis. Another useful trick is to insert the laryngoscope blade down the center of the tongue until the swollen epiglottis is observed. At this point the tip of the blade is forced into the vallecula (which has been obliterated by the swollen tongue surface of the epiglottis). This will then apply pressure at the base of the tongue and force the epiglottis into a more favorable position for visualization of the laryngeal inlet.

7. Obtain a blood culture once the airway is secured.

8. When the child is anesthetized and well oxygenated, the tube may be changed from an oral to a nasotracheal tube (one size smaller than predicted for age) as follows:

   a. Move the oral tracheal tube to the left side of the mouth and allow an assistant to hold that tube while gently assisting respirations.

   b. Pass a well-lubricated nasal tracheal tube into the hypopharynx.

   c. Perform laryngoscopy and ascertain the location of the nasal tube.

   d. With "baby McGill" forceps, position the tip of the nasal tube in the laryngeal inlet immediately next to the orotracheal tube.

   e. Remove the oral tube and insert the nasal tube (secure this very firmly—accidental extubation must be avoided). (Once the airway has been established with an oral tube, the subsequent passage of a nasal tube through the glottis is easy.)

9. Very rarely, pulmonary edema occurs immediately after intubation for epiglottitis. This is thought to be caused by sudden release of the negative pressure caused by breathing against an obstructed upper airway, hypoxia, elevated catecholamines, and disturbed alveolar-capillary pressure gradient. Treatment is with controlled ventilation, positive end-expiratory pressure (PEEP), and diuretics.

Postoperative

1. Constant (24 hr/day) nursing care in an intensive care unit is essential. Accidental extubation is a serious early complication and must be prevented by suitable restraints and adequate sedation.
2. Ensure adequate humidification of inspired gases and regular suctioning of the nasotracheal tube. Blockage of the tube may result from tracheal secretions.
3. Commence antibiotic therapy. Cefuroxime, a cephalosporin with a high margin of safety and good penetration of the cerebrospinal fluid, is considered the drug of choice for *HiB* infections.
4. Extubate the trachea after the pyrexia has resolved (usually within 12 to 36 hours). Flexible laryngoscopy may be performed before extubation to examine the state of the supraglottic structures.
5. Observe the child after extubation for several hours. Very rarely does the trachea require reintubation for recurrent obstruction. It is reasonable to perform the extubation in the operating room so that if the child fails extubation, reintubation is greatly facilitated.

Suggested Reading

Rafei K, Lichenstein R: Airway infectious disease emergencies, Pediatr Clin North Am 53(2):215–242, 2006.

Croup or Laryngotracheobronchitis

"Acute infectious croup" or laryngotracheobronchitis, is most commonly caused by a virus and occurs most often in children 2 to 5 years of age. Do not overlook other causes including a foreign body. Inspiratory stridor is the principal symptom caused by swelling of the loose tracheal mucosa at the level of the cricoid cartilage. Symptoms are frequently worse at night.

Therapy varies according to the severity of the disease:

1. In mild to moderate cases, conservative measures (oral dexamethasone) is usually effective.

2. In more severe cases, epinephrine inhalations in addition to oral dexamethasone usually result in improvement.
3. Very rarely, nasotracheal intubation is required.

Epinephrine Inhalations

Inhalations of epinephrine are widely reported to be efficacious in cases that fail to respond to conservative measures.

1. Prepare the nebulizer solution of epinephrine: add 0.5 ml of 2.25% racemic epinephrine to 3.0 ml distilled water.
2. Attach a suitable pediatric-size face mask, and hold this gently on the face while the child is held comfortably by the mother or father.
3. These children are hypoxic. Add at least 40% O_2 to the inspired gases; children usually then settle well and accept the mask quietly. Closely monitor oxygen saturation.
4. Monitor ventilation and heart rate via a precordial stethoscope. Some increase in heart rate may occur, but other arrhythmias are very rare.
5. Give the therapy for 20 minutes, by which time considerable improvement is usually apparent. (If not, the diagnosis of croup should be reconsidered.)
6. After inhalations, observe the child carefully. Rarely, the stridor increases rapidly, necessitating immediate establishment of an artificial airway.
7. Some children require more than one therapy. Total failure to respond with any improvement is an indication to review and question the diagnosis. The use of racemic epinephrine is contraindicated in infants with tetralogy of Fallot because a severe "tet" spell may be precipitated.

Nasotracheal Intubation

If conservative measures and epinephrine inhalations with IPPB fail to relieve symptoms, an artificial airway may be required. Nasotracheal intubation has been used successfully in many centers, with only a small incidence of complications reported. The critical factor seems to be the diameter of the endotracheal tube, which should be sufficiently small as to provide a leak at approximately 20 cm H_2O peak inflation pressure. The tube is carefully secured as described above for epiglottitis and left in place for 7 to 10 days. Constant (24 hr/day) expert respiratory care is essential; the presence of a small tube and thick secretions renders accidental blockage very likely.

On the rare occasion, a child does not respond as favorably to nasotracheal intubation and cannot be successfully extubated after the standard time. This occurs most commonly in infants, less than 1 year of age, in those with branchial arch deformities or a history of congenital subglottic stenosis, and in those with a history of repeated croup. Tracheotomy may be necessary in these children.

Tracheotomy

Tracheotomy may become necessary in the therapy of upper airway obstruction or to facilitate respiratory care in other conditions.

Anesthesia Management

Preoperative

1. Give 100% O_2 by mask, and assist ventilation manually as necessary.
2. Do not give sedatives or opioids.

Perioperative

1. Continue 100% O_2 by mask, induce anesthesia with sevoflurane or halothane and O_2, and assist ventilation as required (the intravenous line must be checked for adequacy and replaced if necessary).
2. Deepen anesthesia and spray lidocaine on the larynx. The surgeon may perform a diagnostic bronchoscopy before the tracheostomy, and allow the surgeon to pass a bronchoscope. (Tracheotomy in children is usually performed after passage of a rigid bronchoscope. This makes it easy for the surgeon to identify the trachea and also enables the anesthesiologist to see immediately that the tracheotomy tube has in fact been passed into the lumen of the trachea.)
3. In case of a "difficult airway" (i.e., Pierre Robin syndrome), anesthesia may be induced by mask and continued after insertion of a laryngeal mask airway (LMA), which may then be used as a conduit to intubate the trachea.

Postoperative

1. As soon as possible, obtain a chest radiograph. Check that the tube is positioned correctly and that pneumothorax (a rare complication of tracheotomy) is not present.
2. Be alert to the possibility of accidental extubation before the track into the trachea becomes established. If this happens, it may be very difficult to reinsert the tube. Many surgeons leave long black silk sutures

through the edges of the trachea to facilitate emergency reinsertion of the tracheotomy tube.

3. Add an appropriate concentration of oxygen to the inspired gases (to overcome the continuing danger of hypoxemia).
4. Order close, constant observation of the child.

   a. Establishment of the airway does not result in immediate return to normal pulmonary function.
   b. Respiratory arrest may occur during the postoperative period.

Suggested Reading

Bjornson CL, Johnson DW: Croup, Lancet 371:329–339, 2008.

Bacterial Tracheitis

As the incidence of epiglottis has declined in the pediatric population, bacterial tracheitis has emerged as a more common cause of acute respiratory distress. The disease usually occurs with cough, hoarseness, stridor, and chest retraction. Drooling is rare, but the child is toxic and pyrexial with leukocytosis. Emergency bronchoscopy should be managed as for epiglottitis, and reveals that the trachea is inflamed and edematous with purulent secretions and possible pseudomembranes. The responsible organism is usually a staphylococcus or streptococcus pneumonia. Treatment is by endotracheal intubation and appropriate antibiotic therapy. Repeat bronchoscopy is indicated to monitor the progress of the disease and recovery.

Suggested Reading

Hopkins A, Lahiri T, Salerno R, et al: Changing epidemiology of life-threatening upper airway infections: the reemergence of bacterial tracheitis, Pediatrics 118(4):1418–1421, 2006.

SUBGLOTTIC STENOSIS

Subglottic stenosis is one of the most common causes of chronic airway obstruction in infants and children. The stenosis may be congenital or acquired—usually as a complication of prolonged endotracheal intubation. Severe subglottic stenosis requires a tracheotomy followed by surgery to reconstruct the subglottic space. The surgical procedure generally involves division of the cricoid cartilage and insertion of a cartilage graft to increase the diameter. A stent is then left in place to maintain the lumen. After extensive repair it is often preferred to sedate, immobilize the neck, and ventilate the child for several days to optimize healing.

Subglottic stenosis, which may prevent successful extubation in neonates, may be treated by early anterior cricoid split without a preliminary tracheostomy.

Associated Conditions (Congenital Type)

1. Congenital heart disease
2. Down syndrome
3. Tracheoesophageal fistula

Anesthesia Management for Cartilage Graft to Cricoid Ring

Preoperative

1. If a tracheostomy is in place, all care and monitoring of the tracheostomy should be continued until the child arrives at the OR.

Perioperative

1. Anesthetize via the tracheotomy tube using sevoflurane in N_2O/O_2.
2. Remove the tracheotomy tube and insert an armored tube via the stoma; suture it firmly in place. (**NB:** The lumen of the trachea will take a larger tube than is expected.)
3. Check ventilation to both lungs frequently.
4. Maintain anesthesia with N_2O and sevoflurane or isoflurane, and control ventilation.
5. Blood loss is usually minimal.

Postoperative

1. Replace the tracheotomy tube.
2. Administer humidified O_2.
3. Some intravenous fluids may be required for 1 to 2 days postoperatively until a fluid diet can be taken.
4. A full diet can usually be resumed in a week.
5. The stent is removed and laryngoscopy is performed under general anesthesia 3 months later.
6. The tracheotomy is left in place until the child is able to tolerate plugging of the lumen of the tube.

Suggested Reading

Rutter MJ, Cotton RT: The use of posterior cricoid grafting in managing isolated posterior glottic stenosis in children, Arch Otolaryngol Head Neck Surg 130(6):737–739, 2004.

For Anterior Cricoid Split (Without tracheostomy)

This procedure is performed for neonates who cannot be extubated as a result of narrowing at the cricoid.

1. The child is anesthetized via the existing endotracheal tube.
2. When the child is anesthetized the tube may be removed and a bronchoscope inserted to examine the remainder of the airway.
3. The trachea is reintubated and the cricoid cartilage divided anteriorly.
4. An age appropriate size nasotracheal tube is inserted into the trachea and left in place for 5 to 7 days.

Suggested Reading

Eze NN, Wyatt ME, Hartley BE, et al: The role of the anterior cricoid split in facilitating extubation in infants, Intl J Ped Otorhinol 69(6):843–846, 2005.

Dental Surgery

GENERAL PRINCIPLES

1. Children do not usually cooperate very well under moderate sedation (so called "conscious sedation") unless they are very motivated and specially prepared and therefore require general anesthesia more frequently than adults for dental procedures.

2. Many children who present for general anesthesia for dentistry have had previous failed attempts at dental treatment under local anesthesia and sedation and consequently are very apprehensive.

3. Some have behavior disorders or developmental delay and require special consideration, especially those with autism.

4. Others have medical conditions that require special consideration (e.g., congenital heart disease).

5. Nasotracheal intubation is preferable for children having dental surgery in hospital. Nasal intubation per se is associated with bacteremia and is an indication for prophylactic antibiotics for endocarditis prophylaxis if heart disease is present (see later discussion). Children with extensive caries show positive blood cultures after dental procedures.

6. Special care must be taken to ensure that no foreign bodies remain in the airway at the end of the procedure (especially throat packs). Counting throat packs is essential. Direct laryngoscopy must be performed before extubation to ensure that the airway is clear.

7. Dental procedures may be prolonged when extensive disease is present. In such instances recovery to a normal appetite is not as brisk as after short operations. Therefore, children should receive intraoperative intravenous fluids to restore their calculated deficit and provide maintenance fluids. It is preferred to limit the duration of general anesthesia for the outpatient to a maximum of 4 hours and to schedule surgery for such children to commence in the morning.

8. For procedures to be carried out under sedation plus local analgesia, monitoring should be applied as for general anesthesia.

9. Rarely the use of air turbine dental drills has been a cause of intraoperative subcutaneous and mediastinal emphysema, leading to airway obstruction and possible pneumothorax. If facial swelling occurs, discontinue nitrous oxide (N_2O), check for pneumothorax, and be prepared to support ventilation. Very rarely these complications may present in the postoperative period after tooth extractions.

MANAGEMENT FOR GENERAL ANESTHESIA

Preoperative

1. A careful preoperative history and physical examination should be performed as dentists are not authorized to perform "medical assessments" of patient conditions in most jurisdictions. Previously unrecognized significant disease is often discovered in children presenting for dental surgery.

2. Special investigations and treatments, as appropriate, should be ordered for children with other comorbid diseases.

3. Some children do not require premedication. Upset children may benefit from a suitable dose of oral midazolam premedication (0.75 mg/kg for children younger than 6 years of age, 0.3 to 0.5 mg/kg for older children). Every effort should be made to reassure and gain the confidence of the upset child.

4. Make sure that all special drugs have been ordered and are administered at the right time (e.g., antibiotics for children with heart disease).

5. For very upset or uncooperative children who may have behavior disorders or developmental delay it may be helpful to have the parent accompany the child to the induction area or to insert an intravenous line with the parents present before admission to surgery.

Perioperative

1. Apply standard monitors.

2. Induce anesthesia by inhalation or with propofol (or thiopental) intravenously.

3. If an inhalation induction is performed, establish IV access before attempting nasotracheal intubation.

4. Nasotracheal intubation is documented to cause a bacteremia. We recommend endocarditis prophylaxis for those at risk (see later discussion).

5. Instill a vasoconstrictor to reduce bleeding. Warming the tip of the nasotracheal tube has not been shown to reduce bleeding.

6. Give a dose of IV propofol (up to 3 mg/kg) and/or a nondepolarizing muscle relaxant, oxygenate, and perform nasotracheal intubation. To reduce the incidence and severity of bleeding, we telescope the nasal tube into a red rubber catheter and drop the lubricated catheter tip along the floor of the nose until it reaches the nasopharynx. Using the laryngoscope light to illuminate the oropharynx, we extract the catheter from the mouth (with McGill forceps) and with a snap on the catheter, dislodge it from the tip of the tube. Laryngoscopy is then performed and the tube is directed into the glottis. Since this technique involves extra steps, oxygen desaturation is more likely if the child is already cyanotic, has intrinsic lung disease, and when this technique is practiced by less experienced anesthesiologists.

7. Maintain anesthesia with N_2O and isoflurane or sevoflurane in O_2. For short procedures allow spontaneous ventilation. For more prolonged procedures, controlled ventilation may be more appropriate; if so, decrease the inspired anesthetic concentration and monitor blood pressure carefully.

8. Administer maintenance fluids during the surgery including those calculated to replace deficits caused by fasting. After all but very minor dental surgery, a delay in resuming oral intake can be anticipated; therefore any deficit should be corrected.

9. At the end of the procedure, when all dental instrumentation has been removed, a gentle laryngoscopy should be performed to ensure that the airway is free of debris or foreign material before extubation. Beware of throat packs that may have been placed by an oral surgeon.

Postoperative

1. Order analgesics as required. (Dental nerve blocks with local anesthetic reduce the requirement.) Acetaminophen is usually sufficient after dental restorations. Primary teeth often have short roots and do not cause pain when extracted. However, if major extractions occurred, IV morphine or ketorolac is usually required. Ensure that the child is provided with analgesic drugs for use after discharge.

2. Antiemetics may be required, although dental surgery is not associated with a high incidence of PONV.

3. Continue intravenous fluids until the child is ready for discharge.

MANAGEMENT FOR DEEP SEDATION

1. Barbiturates, benzodiazepines, chloral hydrate, and opioids have been used. Today, in the hands of an anesthesiologist, propofol is probably the most useful drug, allowing good moment-to-moment control of sedation and ensuring a rapid recovery.
2. Preoperative care and intraoperative monitoring should be as for general anesthesia.
3. Preoperative medication with midazolam 0.5 to 0.75 mg/kg and prior application of a topical anesthetic cream facilitate insertion of an intravenous catheter.
4. Drugs and equipment for intubation and ventilation with O_2 should be at hand.
5. Deep sedation should be commenced with a bolus dose of propofol (2.5 to 3.5 mg/kg) followed by a continuous infusion, beginning with as much as 300 µg/kg/min as required and reducing the rate progressively to 75 to 100 µg/kg/min as the local anesthetic blocks become effective. The exact dose requirement for continued anesthesia varies from child to child.
6. Oxygen may be given and end-tidal carbon dioxide sampled by a septate nasal catheter. The airway is usually well maintained, but continuous close monitoring is essential.

THE CHILD WITH CONGENITAL HEART DISEASE

The child should be managed for anesthesia with all the necessary considerations for his or her cardiac disease (See Noncardiac Surgery in Children With Congenital Heart Disease in Chapter 14, page 459).

Recommendations for prophylactic antibiotics in children with CHD having dental procedures:

The recommendations of the American Heart Association in 2007 contained some substantive changes that are listed below (see Table 11-1).

1. Patients who should receive prophylactic antibiotics include those with:
   a. Prosthetic cardiac valve or prosthetic material used for cardiac valve repair
   b. Previous infective endocarditis
   c. Congenital heart disease (CHD)
      i. Unrepaired cyanotic CHD, including palliative shunts and conduits

    ii. Completely repaired CHD with prosthetic material or device, whether placed by surgery or catheter intervention, during the first 6 months after the procedure

    iii. Repaired CHD with residual defects at the site or adjacent to the site of a prosthetic patch or prosthetic device (which inhibit endothelialization)

  d. Cardiac transplantation and cardiac valvulopathy

2. *Dental procedures that require prophylactic antibiotics* include all dental procedures that involve manipulation of gingival tissues or the periapical region of teeth or perforation of the oral mucosa. Specifically, extractions, periodontal procedures including surgery, scaling and root planning, probing, dental implant placement, reimplantation of avulsed teeth, subgingival placements, intraligamentary local

TABLE 11-1   **Endocarditis Prophylaxis**

Regimen: Single Dose 30 to 60 Minutes Before Procedure		
Considerations	**Antibiotic**	
Able to take oral medication	Amoxicillin	50 mg/kg
Unable to take oral medication	Ampicillin	50 mg/kg IM or IV
	or	
	Cefazolin or ceftriaxone	50 mg/kg IM or IV
Allergy to penicillins or ampicillin—able to take oral medication	Cephalexin	50 mg/kg
	or	
	Clindamycin or azithromycin	20 mg/kg
	or	
	Clarithromycin	15 mg/kg
Allergy to penicillins or ampicillin *and* unable to take oral medication	Cefazolin	50 mg/kg IM or IV
	or	
	Ceftriaxone	50 mg/kg IM or IV
	or	
	Clindamycin	20 mg/kg IM or IV

anesthetic injections, placement of orthodontic bands, endodontic instrumentation, surgery beyond the apex of the tooth, and prophylactic cleaning of teeth or implants (where bleeding may occur)

3. Dental procedures that do *not* require prophylactic antibiotics include routine anesthetic injections through noninfected tissue, taking dental radiographs, placement of removable prosthodontic or orthodontic appliances, adjustment of orthodontic appliances, placement of orthodontic brackets, shedding of deciduous teeth, and bleeding from trauma to the lips or oral mucosa.

Suggested Reading

Oncag O, Aydemir S, Ersin N, et al: Bacteremia incidence in pediatric patients under dental general anesthesia, Cong Heart Dis 1(5):224–228, 2006.

Childers EL, Brown RS: The 2007 AHA guidelines: issues and discussion concerning clinical dental practice, Alpha Omegan 100(4):177–181, 2007.

Satilmis A, Dursun O, Velipasaoglu S, et al: Severe subcutaneous emphysema, pneumomediastinum, and pneumopericardium after central incisor extraction in a child, Ped Emerg Care 22(10):771–773, 2006.

Dorman ML, Wilson K, Stone K, et al: Is intravenous conscious sedation for surgical orthodontics in children a viable alternative to general anaesthesia? A case review, Br Dental J 202(11):E30, 2007.

Plastic and Reconstructive Surgery

12

Many children require plastic surgery to correct congenital deformities. The head and neck are commonly affected, which may introduce special problems for the anesthesiologist. In addition, some children undergo plastic surgery for acquired lesions, such as burn scars and contractures or dog bites.

GENERAL PRINCIPLES

1. Many of these children have psychological upsets stemming from both the deformity and multiple surgical procedures. A careful, considerate approach by the anesthesiologist is essential. Review of prior anesthetic records is essential so as to adequately assess approaches to premedication, airway management, venous access, and other associated medical or surgical issues.
2. Smooth general anesthesia with quiet emergence lessens the risk of damage to grafted areas and delicately sutured repairs.
3. Many children undergoing plastic surgery have potentially serious airway problems that require careful assessment and special management.

4. Congenital structural anomalies commonly affect more than one body system. The child with defects requiring plastic surgery may also have disease affecting other systems. If congenital heart disease is present, consider the possibility that prophylactic antibiotic therapy is indicated (see Chapter 14, page 462) and carefully review the cardiac surgical history and the most recent cardiac evaluations; seek consultation with the cardiologist when indicated.

CLEFT LIP AND PALATE

Cleft lip and palate (CLP) are present in various combinations in as many as 1 of every 1000 live births. CLP defects may be isolated or occur as part of a syndrome or association of defects (Syndromic CLP). Infants with these lesions may be both malnourished and anemic as a result of feeding difficulties and may have a history of repeated respiratory infections. The treatment of CLP is optimally managed within a multidisciplinary team; the pediatric anesthesiologist is an essential member of this team.

The surgical management of CLP is evolving and debates continue about the optimal age for stages in the repair and the use of such procedures as preoperative orthodontic maneuvers to mold the bony structure of the palate. An orthodontic appliance (e.g., Latham appliance) is sometimes applied to the neonatal palate with the object of progressively molding the bony alveolar ridge into alignment before soft tissue repairs.

1. Congenital heart disease—not specifically associated with isolated cleft palate, but may be present as part of a syndrome or association.
2. Airway anomalies—for example, Pierre Robin syndrome or Treacher Collins syndrome that may make intubation extremely difficult.
3. Syndromes associated with CLP may have other specific anesthesia implications; some of these are listed in Table 12-1.

The surgical care of the patient with cleft lip/palate now comprises many possible stages, not all of which will be required by all children.

Possible Surgical Procedures

1. Application of orthodontic splints or devices to the palate.
2. Cleft lip repair—usually performed at 10 to 12 weeks sometimes earlier.
3. Cleft palate repair—usually performed at 12 to 18 months, but sometimes in younger infants.
4. Alveolar bone graft.

TABLE 12-1 Some Syndromes Associated With Cleft Palate

Syndrome Name(s) Implications	Features	Anesthesia
Arthrogryposis multiplex Congenita	Limb contractures, CHD in 10% Stiffness of joints, GU defects	Difficult intubation due to limited mouth opening, antibiotics for CHD, position and pad carefully.
Beare-Stevenson syndrome	Craniosynostosis, hydrocephalus choanal atresia, midface hypoplasia proptosis, hypertelorism, cutis gyratum	Difficult ventilation (Choanal atresia) difficult intubation, beware of tracheal stenosis, caution with neck. Cervical spine defects.
Beckwith-Wiedemann syndrome	Exomphalos, macroglossia, gigantism, hypoglycemia	Danger of hypoglycemia, infuse glucose and monitor level, tongue reduction may be required at time of palate repair.
CATCH 22	Cardiac defect, abnormal facies, thymic hypoplasia, hypocalcemia, (Di George syndrome)	Difficult airway. Antibiotics for CHD. Treat hypocalcemia.
Cornelia de Lange syndrome	Short stature, developmental delay (variable), CHD in 15%	Airway obstruction, difficult intubation, antibiotics for CHD.
Down syndrome	Short stature, developmental delay (variable), macroglossia, unstable cervical spine, narrow subglottic space. CHD in 50%	Difficult intubation, caution with neck, caution with ETT size, antibiotics for CHD, prone to airway obstruction.

(Continued)

TABLE 12-1 Some Syndromes Associated With Cleft Palate—Cont'd

Syndrome Name(s) Implications	Features	Anesthesia
EEC syndrome	Ectrodactyly, ectodermal dysplasia, hypohidrosis. Chronic respiratory infections	Malnutrition, anemia, hypohidrosis, temperature control problems. Difficult intubation, protect eyes, position and pad carefully. Caution with atropine.
Kabuki syndrome	Craniofacial and skeletal defects, hypotonia anomalies, CHD, visceral and urogenital defects, increased susceptibility to infections.	Difficult airway, caution with relaxants, antibiotics for CHD, care with asepsis.
King syndrome	Congenital myopathy, MH trait. Dysmorphic features (Noonan-like).	Malignant hyperthermia precautions.
Miller syndrome	Mandibular defects, limb anomalies, renal defects.	Difficult airway
Multiple pterygium syndrome	Webbing of skin, syngnathia, ankyloglossia, web neck.	Difficult airway—more severe with age
Nager syndrome	Malar hypoplasia, micrognathia, CHD, radial hypoplasia, absent thumbs, vertebral anomalies	Very difficult airway, limited mouth opening, cervical spine anomalies. Antibiotics for CHD.
Oto-palatal-digital syndrome	Skull deformity, hearing loss, cervical spine defect, (Arnold Chiari), limb defects, possible thoracic hypoplasia.	Possible brain-stem compression causing postoperative respiratory depression.
Patau syndrome (Trisomy 13)	Microcephaly, developmental delay, micrognathia. CHD, usually fatal in infancy.	Difficult airway, antibiotics for CHD

Pierre-Robin sequence	Micrognathia, cleft palate	Difficult airway, postoperative ventilatory obstruction.
Seckel syndrome	Birdlike facies, dwarfism microcephaly, possible glottic narrowing; post-op apnea reported.	Difficult airway, caution with ETT size. Monitor ventilation postoperative.
Smith-Lemli-Opitz syndrome	Growth failure, microcephaly, developmental delay, CHD, renal defects, hypotonia, GE reflux. Thymic hypoplasia—prone to infection.	Possible difficult airway, intraoperative muscle rigidity, temperature control problems, antibiotics for CHD.
Spondyloepiphyseal dysplasia Congenita	Dwarfism, C1-C2 instability	Caution with neck during intubation and positioning (use vacuum splint).
Stickler syndrome. (Pierre-Robin variant)	Midface hypoplasia, cleft palate, retromicrognathia, "Moon Face" one third of "Pierre Robin" patients	Difficult airway (mask ventilation and intubation)
Walker-Warburg syndrome	Micrognathia, hypotonia, hydrocephalus, developmental delay, GU anomalies.	Difficult intubation, postoperative hypoventilation.
18 trisomy	Cleft palate, lung hypoplasia, micrognathia, CHD.	Difficult airway, ventilatory failure, antibiotics for CHD.

5. Pharyngoplasty—for velopharyngeal incompetence—usually performed at 5 to 15 years.
6. Maxillary advancement (Le Fort procedure) required for some adolescent patients.

Special Anesthesia Problems

1. Airway problems, including difficulty with intubation (sometimes extreme). Intubation with isolated micrognathia tends to be difficult in the young infant and becomes easier with age. This may not apply if a syndrome is present.
2. Problems related to associated conditions (see previous discussion).
3. As plastic surgery involves soft tissue dissection, coagulopathy causes significant bleeding. Blood loss during cleft palate repair is usually insignificant but very occasionally may require transfusion.

Anesthesia Management

Preoperative

1. Carry out a very careful preoperative assessment.
   a. Direct special attention to the airway, lungs, and other systems that may be affected in congenital syndromes (see Appendix 1, page 539).
   b. Check especially carefully for upper respiratory tract infection; if such an infection is present, surgery should be postponed.
   c. Check for anemia.
2. Check for any history of bleeding tendency. Check medication history (salicylates (eg., aspirin), NSAIDs, gingko, garlic, or ginseng). If positive, determine the bleeding time; if it is prolonged, surgery should be deferred.
3. Blood is rarely needed for cleft palate surgery, but check that the child has been typed for blood and serum saved.

Perioperative

1. If there is any doubt about the ease of tracheal intubation, perform an inhalation induction and manage as for "difficult airway" see Chapter 4, page 103. Consider starting an IV before anesthesia as tolerated.
2. For inhalation induction, administer nitrous oxide (N_2O) and oxygen (O_2) with sevoflurane or halothane until the child is anesthetized adequately for laryngoscopy. Then discontinue N_2O and continue inhalational anesthesia in O_2. Establish IV access. Give lidocaine 1.5 mg/kg IV (or propofol 1 to 2 mg/kg) before insertion of the laryngoscope to minimize the risk of coughing or laryngospasm.

3. If the cleft is large or bilateral, consider packing it with moist sterile gauze to prevent trauma during laryngoscopy and intubation.

4. For orotracheal intubation, use a RAE®* preformed tracheal tube. Check carefully that bilateral ventilation of the lungs is present after the mouth gag is positioned. Insertion of the gag and flexion of the neck may advance the tip of the tube in the trachea, so that it may pass into a bronchus. Extension of the head tends to withdraw the tip of the tube and a leak may occur— especially in small infants if the tube has a "Murphy Eye."

5. For cleft lip repair, tape the tube carefully to the mandible and ensure that the upper lip is free and not distorted by the surgical tape.

6. Monitor air entry and ventilation continuously during surgery, paying special attention each time the gag is repositioned or the child is moved.

7. Maintain anesthesia with N_2O, a relaxant and controlled ventilation and a low concentration of sevoflurane or isoflurane. The inhalational agent should be discontinued before the end of the operation so that the child awakens promptly once the relaxant has been antagonized. Otherwise a TIVA regime may be used.

8. Monitor blood loss carefully and replace if indicated. The infiltration of a local anesthetic with 1:200,000 epinephrine reduces blood loss in cleft palate surgery and also provides some analgesia postoperatively.

9. Inspect the mouth and pharynx gently at the end of surgery; use a laryngoscope and remove all blood and clots. Extubate when the child is fully awake. After palate repair, acute swelling of the tongue causing obstruction has been reported as a complication of the use of the tongue blade on the mouth gag. Therefore examine the mouth carefully; if any signs of tongue swelling exist, the trachea should be left intubated.

10. A long suture is often inserted into the tongue to exert traction and facilitate immediate postoperative control of the airway in the PACU after cleft palate repair. This is usually removed when the child is fully awake but may be left in place overnight until a clear airway is assured.

Postoperative

1. Cleft lip surgery is often performed in the day surgery unit because the surgery is superficial and postoperative problems are rare. The use of an infraorbital nerve block (see Chapter 5, page 163) provides good postoperative analgesia for this type of surgery and should be routinely used.

---

* RAE = Ring-Adair-Elwyn

2. All children are admitted overnight after cleft palate surgery. Ensure constant observation for 24 hours because airway problems or bleeding may occur. A small percentage of children may have to return to the operating room for control of bleeding and some may require reintubation.

3. Order analgesics with caution to avoid excessive respiratory depression as upper airway obstruction is a particular risk in the postoperative period.

Application of Palatal Splints or Devices in the Neonate

This is sometimes performed to mold the palate and alveolar ridge and improve the aesthetic and dental results of subsequent surgery. All provisions for neonatal anesthesia should be observed. General endotracheal anesthesia is preferred; use an oral RAE tube. After the procedure the infant is usually uncomfortable and requires a mild analgesic.

Alveolar Bone Grafting

An alveolar bone graft may be required to close a gap in the bony alveolar ridge; this procedure may be performed on an ambulatory basis. The operation is preferably performed as the permanent dentition erupts so that teeth may be guided into the grafted area. Bone is often harvested at the iliac crest in which case preincisional infiltration of the donor site with bupivacaine may significantly reduce postoperative pain. For the ambulatory patient, prophylactic administration of dexamethasone and antinausea medication significantly decrease PONV and speed return to normal activity.

Pharyngoplasty

Pharyngoplasty is performed to reduce velopharyngeal incompetence and improve speech. The procedure inevitably increases resistance to ventilation. Postoperative airway problems are common. These children require close monitoring postoperatively.

Special Anesthesia Problems

1. Postoperative airway obstruction is a particular danger and may occur early in the PACU.

2. Chronic airway obstruction may persist after the operation and may lead to obstructive sleep apnea and possibly to later pulmonary hypertension.

Anesthesia Management

As for cleft palate (see previous discussion).

Postoperative

1. Observe closely in the PACU or PICU for airway obstruction and/or bleeding for at least 12 hours.
2. A nasopharyngeal airway, placed by the surgeon and left in situ for 24 hours, is effective in reducing serious postoperative respiratory complications.
3. Do not order heavy opioid sedation.
4. Continuing supervision for signs of obstruction during sleep is suggested, and a postoperative sleep study is recommended.

Suggested Reading

Robin NH, Baty H, Franklin J, et al: The multidisciplinary evaluation and management of cleft lip and palate, South Med J 99(10):1111–1120, 2006.

Fraulin FO, Valnicek SM, Zuker RM: Decreasing the perioperative complications associated with the superior pharyngeal flap operation, Plast Reconstr Surg 102:10–18, 1998.

Perry CW, Lowenstein A, Rothkopf DM: Ambulatory alveolar bone grafting, Plast Reconstr Surg 116:736–739, 2005.

FRACTURED MANDIBLE

Surgical Procedures

1. Interdental wiring
2. Open reduction and wiring

Special Anesthesia Problems

1. The child may have a full stomach.
2. Intubation may be difficult because of tissue damage, trismus, and distortion of airway anatomy.
3. Foreign bodies may be present in the airway (i.e., teeth).
4. The mouth is wired closed after the procedure; therefore postoperative vomiting is a potentially life-threatening event. Suction should be immediately available.
5. Wire cutters must be at the child's bedside at all times in case the airway must be intubated.

Anesthesia Management

Preoperative

1. Assess the child carefully. Trismus may limit mouth opening and preclude a thorough examination.
2. Determine the more patent nostril for intubation.
3. For children with a full stomach, delay surgery if possible and give metoclopramide IV.
4. Do not give heavy sedation.

Perioperative

1. For emergency surgery, use a RSI (see Chapter 4, page 98).
2. Examine the pharynx quickly but carefully during laryngoscopy to search for foreign debris. (Radio-opaque debris such as teeth may be visible on x-ray, consult radiographs before inducing anesthesia.)
3. For emergency surgery, use an orotracheal tube initially; then change to a nasotracheal tube. (If you attempt to place the nasotracheal tube initially, you may start a nosebleed—then the child has a nosebleed in addition to a full stomach. Once the oral tube is in place, insert a nasogastric tube and aspirate the gastric contents. Then pass a nasal tube through one nostril, repeat the laryngoscopy, and exchange tracheal tubes). For elective surgery, a nasotracheal tube may be inserted initially if optimal conditions for laryngoscopy are present.
4. Pack the throat with sterile gauze.
5. Maintain anesthesia with N_2O and an inhalational anesthetic and/or a propofol infusion plus relaxant using controlled ventilation. Antiemetics (dexamethasone and a 5-HT_3 receptor antagonist) should be administered. (This permits rapid reawakening and minimal PONV.)
6. Before final fixation of the jaw, remove the pack and inspect the pharynx with a laryngoscope; remove blood clots and other debris.
7. If the mandible is not wired to the maxilla, inspect the oropharynx for debris before discontinuing anesthesia in preparation for extubation. Extubate when spontaneous respirations are present, a leak is audible around the endotracheal tube and child has recovered consciousness. If the mandible is wired to the maxilla, in addition to the presence of spontaneous and sustained respirations and a leak around the endotracheal tube the child must be fully awake before extubation. With wire cutters always present, withdraw the tube to the oropharynx once suitable conditions for extubation are present. Only remove the tube completely from the nostril when you are certain the child can protect the airway and ventilation is sustainable.
8. Leave the nasogastric tube in place for use during the postoperative period.

Postoperative

1. Order close observation of the child.
2. Ensure that wire cutters remain at the bedside at all times for children whose jaws are wired closed.

Removal of Interdental Wiring

General anesthesia is usually required for removal of the wiring and arch bars when the fracture is healed. The wires holding the jaws together can be removed before induction of anesthesia. However, jaw movement remains extremely restricted because of the prolonged immobilization, rendering laryngoscopy and intubation difficult.

Ensure that the child has been fasted preoperatively. After removal of the securing wires, induce anesthesia by inhalation of N_2O and sevoflurane or halothane, or by IV propofol/remifentanil until a soft nasopharyngeal tube can be inserted for maintenance. When good ventilation is assured, allow the surgeon to proceed with removing the arch bars.

Exercise great care to maintain the airway, and have equipment for emergency intubation and/or tracheotomy immediately at hand.

RECONSTRUCTIVE SURGERY FOR BURNS

Children who suffer a burn injury require acute and chronic (reconstructive) burn care and surgery. Anesthesia for acute burn care is addressed in Chapter 17. Anesthesia for repeat reconstructive plastic surgery is addressed below.

Special Anesthesia Problems

1. Contractures that result from burns to the face and neck may make laryngoscopy and tracheal intubation and maintenance of the airway during anesthesia very difficult.
2. Extensive burns may make it difficult to obtain reliable venous access.
3. Severe emotional problems may result from the accident, the subsequent disfigurement, and from repeated surgical procedures. The last problem often gives rise to fear of the anesthesia facemask and fear of venous access.
4. Premedication with a benzodiazepine is advisable and some may benefit from the addition of oral ketamine and atropine if they have a history of inadequate response to simple benzodiazepine premedication.

5. Blood losses may be large during grafting of extensive burns.
6. Temperature homeostasis is impaired, and special measures must be taken to avoid hypothermia.
7. Emergence from anesthesia should be quiet to avoid damage to recently grafted areas.

Anesthesia Management—General Endotracheal Anesthesia

General endotracheal anesthesia may be used, but there are some special considerations:

1. A 40% larger dose of thiopental is required for children undergoing reconstructive surgery and during convalescence. Some children may require IM ketamine for induction if no IV access is available.
2. Succinylcholine is contraindicated after the first 24 hours after a burn and for 1.5 to 2 years after severe burns because it may cause cardiac arrest secondary to hyperkalemia.
3. The dose requirements for nondepolarizing muscle relaxants may be increased compared with the dose in unburned children for several years after the injury and the magnitude of the increase is in proportion to the size of the burn. This subsides once the sites have been grafted over and healed. Relaxants should be titrated to achieve the desired effect, and a neuromuscular blockade monitor should be used.
4. If the airway has been injured in the burn, subglottic stenosis may be present. Carefully select the size of the endotracheal tube, and anticipate using a smaller tube than expected. Some children may have or still have a tracheostomy in place.

Preoperative

1. Assess the child's condition carefully, and review the anesthesia history with particular emphasis on problems with inadequate premedication, difficult airway or difficult venous access. Often the child is able to tell you where "the best vein" is located.
2. Take time to talk with the child. Encourage questions, answer them honestly, and reassure the child about the planned procedure.
3. Preoperative fasting must be rigidly observed. However, many children in the chronic phase of burns are in a catabolic state often requiring close to 24 hour a day feeds (via J-tube feeds) to maintain a positive caloric intake. To that end, many institutions have reduced the fasting interval for continuous feeds to 3 hours before surgery with these feeding tubes.
4. Order adequate preoperative sedation either IV or by mouth.
5. Make sure that the operating room (OR) is warmed to 25° C.

6. Confer with the surgeon regarding any special issues such as a specific route of intubation (oral or nasal) or tracheal tube (standard or RAE), eye care, positioning, site of graft harvesting, limits on local anesthetics, and postoperative surgical concerns.

Perioperative

1. If airway problems are not present:
   a. Induce anesthesia by either IV or inhalational route.
   b. Administer nondepolarizing muscle relaxant and intubate the trachea. Note that if an LMA is appropriate, tracheal intubation is not required.
   c. Measure blood losses and be prepared to replace them when excessive.
2. If airway problems are present (i.e., microstomia or neck contractures):
   a. If the chin cannot be extended or the mouth opened, direct visual intubation may be impossible. Select from the following alternatives:
      i. Perform fiberoptic intubation, either sedated with topical analgesia or after an inhalation induction, depending on the child.
      ii. Perform a blind nasal intubation. Proficiency demands much experience, and this approach may be particularly difficult if scar tissue has distorted the airway.
      iii. Release scar tissue under local analgesia and/or ketamine, induce anesthesia and perform direct-vision tracheal intubation.
   b. Once the airway has been secured, anesthesia can be maintained as described previously.

Postoperative

1. Emergence from anesthesia should be quiet; do not disturb the patient. Order adequate analgesic drugs as required.
2. If ketamine has been used, be aware of the possibility of emergence phenomena.

MAJOR CRANIOFACIAL AND RECONSTRUCTIVE SURGERY

Extensive reconstruction is now possible for children with severe facial deformities. The improvement in appearance frequently has a major beneficial effect on the child's future life. Much of this surgery is now being performed during infancy or early childhood. The objective is to allow the child to go to school looking as normal as possible.

In recent years, the technique of external maxillary distraction osteogenesis has been applied to children requiring maxillary osteotomies.

The osteotomies are performed subperiosteally and external distraction appliances attached with which the healing bone is drawn slowly apart after a short period to allow callus formation. This technique usually results in shorter procedures and reduced blood losses. However, external appliances further limit the anesthesiologist's access to the airway.

General Principles

1. A team approach is essential for successful performance of this type of surgery.
2. Operations involving the jaws are usually delayed until dentition is complete (i.e., 13 years or older).
3. Operations not involving dentition (e.g., for craniofacial dysostosis) are usually performed at an earlier age.

Special Anesthesia Problems

1. Intubation of the airway may be difficult if the deformity is severe. In rare instances, the airway cannot be secured; in these cases, tracheotomy is performed using local analgesia and sedation preoperatively.
2. Blood loss may be very extensive from the surgical and bone graft donor sites (e.g., pelvic girdle or ribs).
3. Surgery is of long duration, and special precautions must be taken to protect the child against complications of prolonged anesthesia (i.e., pressure sores, nerve compression, eye protection).
4. Surgical manipulation involving the orbit and face may initiate the oculocardiac reflex.
5. Surgical manipulations may damage the tracheal tube intraoperatively (rare).
6. The children must awaken rapidly after surgery so that the surgeon can check cranial nerve function.
7. Extensive postoperative swelling of adjacent tissues may dictate the need for prolonged intubation after the operation.

Anesthesia Management

Preoperative

1. Examine the child very thoroughly, particularly for airway abnormalities and cardiopulmonary disease.
2. Consider the possibility of associated congenital defects or other features of a syndrome that may have implications for anesthesia (see Appendix 1). Some children (i.e., those with Apert or Crouzon

syndrome) may have sleep apnea, and this possibility should be investigated in a sleep laboratory.

3. Check all laboratory results, especially for indications of coagulopathy.
4. Order any further tests necessary to assess the child fully before surgery.
5. Ensure that adequate supplies of blood and blood products will be available and that serum has been saved for further cross-matching if necessary.
6. Reassure the child and family and explain the planned procedures, including postoperative care.
7. Order preoperative sedation: midazolam for children or lorazepam (Ativan) for adolescents.

Perioperative

1. Induce anesthesia:
   a. If there are no airway problems, either an IV or inhalational induction may be performed followed by tracheal intubation.
   b. If a difficult airway is anticipated, induce with an inhalational anesthetic and proceed to intubation via a laryngeal mask airway (LMA) or other means.
   c. In some cases of extremely difficult airway, a tracheotomy may be performed under local analgesia. This can then be used for anesthesia and as a postoperative airway until swelling subsides.
2. The endotracheal tube should be sutured in position, with due consideration being given to the movements of the facial bones that may accompany the surgery. The tube should either be sutured to a structure that will not be moved or be so positioned in the trachea as to allow for the effects of movement at its point of fixation. An armored tube should be used if possible. The SWAY tube,* which is armored only in the proximal extratracheal segment, may be useful if prolonged intubation is anticipated.
3. Maintain anesthesia with N_2O (if there is a risk of air embolism, substitute oxygen/air for oxygen/N_2O) and opioid (i.e., fentanyl 2 to 3 µg/kg/hr) and a suitable nondepolarizing muscle relaxant.
4. Control ventilation to an arterial carbon dioxide pressure ($PaCO_2$) of 30 to 35 mm Hg.
5. Position the patient with 10° to 15° head-up tilt.
6. Pad all pressure areas well, including occiput and areas compressed by the endotracheal tube (i.e., nares, lip).

---

* Phycon SWAY tube, Fuji Systems Corp., Tokyo.

7. Place protective ointment in the eyes (the surgeon will usually perform tarsorrhaphy).
8. Monitor:
   a. Standard anesthetic monitors
   b. Central venous and arterial blood pressure by direct means
   c. Acid-base, blood gas, and hematocrit by serial determinations
   d. Temperature
   e. Coagulation indices (during transfusion if massive)
   f. Urine output
   g. Precordial Doppler ultrasound/end-tidal Pco_2—for air embolism during craniectomy
9. Be prepared for massive blood replacement
10. If reduction in brain mass is required, give furosemide 1 mg/kg IV or mannitol 0.5 gm/kg.
11. When indicated, induce hypotension using either isoflurane, remifentanil, or sodium nitroprusside.
12. The child should be sufficiently awake in the OR at the end of surgery, so that the surgeon can check the child's vision and ascertain whether cranial nerve injury has occurred during surgery.

Postoperative

1. Order routine postcraniotomy nursing care when applicable.
2. Leave the tracheal tube in place until the child is fully awake *and* there is no further danger that postoperative tissue swelling might obstruct the airway. (Many children require intubation for 48 to 72 hours postoperatively.) The timing of tracheal extubation must be based on the adequacy of spontaneous ventilation, the resolution of facial swelling, presence of leak around the tube, and the level of consciousness of the child. Some children will be most safely extubated if returned to the operating room. Intravenous dexamethasone may be administered before extubation to prevent stridor.
3. Particular caution should be exercised if external distraction apparatus has been applied. In these cases and whenever in doubt; an airway exchange catheter may be inserted via the endotracheal tube and left in place after extubation to aid in reintubation should this be required. The airway exchange catheter can then be removed 1 to 2 hours later when it is apparent that reintubation will not be required.
4. Observe caution when using opioid analgesics.
5. Check hemoglobin and hematocrit to ensure adequacy of blood replacement.

Children With External Maxillary Distraction Devices

These children will require a second anesthetic for removal of the hardware. Difficulty with intubation may be anticipated; apart from limitation of access due to the devices, trismus secondary to immobilization of the jaw will be present, together with increased prominence of the maxilla. The trismus resolves over the course of a few days after removal of the wires.

Suggested Reading

Wong GB, Nargozian C, Padwa BL, et al: Anesthetic concerns of external maxillary distraction osteogenesis, J Craniofac Surg 15:78–81, 2004.
Roche J, Frawley G, Heggie A: Difficult tracheal intubation induced by maxillary distraction devices in craniosynostosis syndromes, Paediatr Anaesth 12:227–234, 2002.

TUMORS IN THE NECK—CYSTIC HYGROMA AND CONGENITAL CERVICAL TERATOMA

Cystic hygroma is a cystic lymphangioma that usually occurs in the neck and less commonly in the axilla. Intraoral extension of this benign tumor may cause airway obstruction. Three percent of cervical tumors extend into the mediastinum.

Teratomas may occur in the neonate, and though most occur in the sacral region, they may also involve the neck. Giant congenital cervical teratoma may cause life-threatening airway compromise.

Occasionally extremely large tumors in the neck are diagnosed by antenatal ultrasound and require intervention to establish an airway at the time of birth (see Exit Procedure, see page 335).

Special Anesthesia Problems

1. There may be existing airway obstruction.
2. Intubation may be difficult because of distortion of the airway.
3. Complete removal of tumor may involve extensive dissection and be accompanied by major blood loss.

Anesthesia Management

Preoperative

1. Assess the child carefully, looking especially for evidence of intrathoracic extension of the tumor.

2. Do not administer heavy sedation.
3. Ensure availability of blood and blood products for transfusion.
4. Prepare a selection of tubes and laryngoscope blades.

Perioperative

1. Induce anesthesia cautiously by inhalation of N_2O and sevoflurane or halothane. Maintain spontaneous ventilation.
2. When the child is anesthetized, establish a reliable large-bore intravenous route.
3. Before attempting intubation, discontinue N_2O and give O_2 and sevoflurane or halothane for several minutes. Coughing and breath holding and/or laryngospasm during attempts at intubation may be minimized by administering propofol (1 to 2 mg/kg) and lidocaine 1.5 mg/kg IV.
4. Intubate, preferably using an armored tube, and secure the tube firmly. For some children, if intraoral dissection is planned, a nasal tube may be preferable. In the case of a difficult intubation, insert an oral tube first, then change to a nasal tube if this is possible without further airway compromise.
5. Maintain anesthesia with N_2O and relaxant and low concentrations of isoflurane with controlled ventilation.
6. For large tumors requiring extensive dissection, an arterial line should be inserted.
7. Beware of vagal reflexes during dissection in the neck. Give atropine IV if these reflexes occur.
8. Replace blood losses carefully with appropriate fluids, guided by the blood pressure and the measured losses.
9. After the operation, extubate the airway smoothly; prevent excessive coughing and bucking, which might cause bleeding at the surgical site.
10. If extensive surgery has been performed adjacent to the airway, extubation should be delayed until the extent of postoperative swelling is determined. If swelling is significant, intubation is required until it resolves. A few children may require tracheotomy.

Postoperative

1. If extubated:
   a. Order close observation in the PICU or PACU overnight (because of the danger of bleeding into the surgical site or compression of the airway).
   b. Avoid large doses of opioid analgesics.

2. If intubated:

    a. Confirm the position of the tracheal tube by radiography.

    b. Order appropriate humidified O_2 in air and continuing care.

THE EXIT PROCEDURE—EX UTERO INTRAPARTUM TREATMENT

This procedure is designed to maintain the infant by means of the placental circulation until an airway can be established and pulmonary ventilation commenced (airway management on placental support). The essentials are as follows:

1. The position of the placenta is delineated to avoid damage at hysterotomy.

2. The mother is anesthetized using a technique predicted to cause uterine relaxation and prevent placental separation, high concentrations of inhalational anesthetics, and/or nitroglycerin. Maternal blood pressure is optimized by positioning and vasopressors as required. Massive rapid maternal blood loss is possible.

3. Hysterotomy is performed and the head of the fetus accessed. The airway is established by tracheal intubation, bronchoscopy or surgical tracheostomy.

4. Once airway and ventilation are satisfactory, the umbilical cord is clamped and the infant transferred to the NICU or another OR for further treatment as appropriate; some will require an urgent tracheostomy.

Suggested Reading

Chinnappa V, Halpern SH: The ex utero intrapartum treatment (EXIT) procedure: maternal and fetal considerations, CJA 54(3):171–175, 2007.

13 General and Thoracoabdominal Surgery

GENERAL PRINCIPLES

1. Many of the children requiring thoracoabdominal procedures are neonates and preterm infants and therefore demand special considerations.

2. In most cases, the pathophysiology of the surgical disease dictates the optimal anesthesia management. The anesthesiologist should understand the effects of the lesion on normal physiology.

3. Surgery is very rarely required immediately; usually some time is available for preoperative evaluation and resuscitation as necessary. The optimum time for surgery must be decided by consultation among anesthesiologist, neonatologist, and surgeon.

4. For emergency abdominal surgery, the problem of the full stomach must be considered. (Even if the child has not eaten for some time, secretions accumulate in the stomach, and emptying may be delayed by obstruction or ileus.) Children with gastroesophageal reflux are at increased risk.

   a. Remember the effects of drugs on the barrier pressure (i.e., lower esophageal pressure [LES] minus intragastric pressure). Barrier pressure is reduced by atropine, diazepam, inhalational anesthetics, and cricoid pressure. It is increased by metoclopramide, pancuronium, and vecuronium, and it is little changed by succinylcholine.

   b. Drugs can be used to reduce the volume and acidity of gastric contents: cimetidine (oral or rectal), ranitidine, metoclopramide, and sodium citrate.

Possible plans of action:

i. Pass a gastric tube and aspirate the stomach where appropriate. In suitable children, pretreat with medications to reduce volume and acidity of the gastric contents.

ii. Neonates and small infants at high risk: aspirate stomach contents through a vented gastric tube in the supine, right, and left decubitus position (in neonates and infants this may remove up to 95% of fluid gastric contents), preoxygenate, and perform a RSI or awake sedated intubation.

iii. Older children: aspirate stomach contents (if appropriate) and perform a RSI with cricoid pressure. Cricoid pressure must be commenced as soon as any drugs are given that may reduce LES. There is still no relaxant drug that can replace succinylcholine for speed of onset, offset, and intensity of neuromuscular block.

iv. Make sure that the child is deeply anesthetized and relaxed before tracheal intubation. Struggling during attempts at intubation in an incompletely anesthetized and relaxed child is a common precursor to vomiting and aspiration.

Remember: During RSI, succinylcholine does not increase intragastric pressure in children younger than 10 years of age, and pretreatment with a low-dose nondepolarizing relaxant is not indicated (see Chapter 3, page 70).

5. During thoraco-abdominal surgery, blood loss may be considerable; be prepared to handle a major blood transfusion (see Chapter 4, page 135).

6. For major abdominal surgery, always establish intravenous access in the upper limbs or neck. The inferior vena cava (IVC) may rarely have to be clamped or may be otherwise compressed during the operation; this renders transfusion via the lower limb veins ineffective.

7. N_2O diffuses into the lumen of gas-containing bowel, causing further distention and difficulties for the surgeon. Do not use N_2O when conditions predispose to this condition (e.g., intestinal obstruction).

8. The airways are small and, during lung surgery, bronchial secretions (often sanguinous) may accumulate and interfere with ventilation. Perform tracheobronchial toilet as indicated.

9. During thoracotomy, $\dot{V}/\dot{Q}$ ratios in the lungs are disturbed; therefore increase the inspired O_2 concentration to maintain an acceptable SaO_2.

10. In infants and small children, retracting the lungs may obstruct major airways, impairing ventilation, or it may compress the heart and great veins, leading to a precipitous decrease in cardiac output and hence in blood pressure. Constant monitoring of breath sounds via stethoscope, shape of the capnogram, and observation of SaO_2 is essential. In the event of decreasing saturation, bradycardia, hypotension, or impaired ventilation:
    a. Ask the surgeon to remove all retractors immediately.
    b. Ventilate the lungs with 100% O_2.
    c. Use large manually delivered tidal volumes with relatively high peak inflation pressures to reexpand areas of atelectasis.
11. Even children who require minor surgery (e.g., herniotomy) may be preterm and/or have other conditions (e.g., anemia) that can complicate anesthesia and require special precautions (see Chapter 6).
12. Many general surgery procedures can now be performed with the use of video-assisted endoscopic techniques. It is anticipated that additional advances in these techniques will further extend the scope of minimally invasive pediatric surgery.

SPECIAL CONSIDERATIONS FOR MINIMALLY INVASIVE/ ENDOSCOPIC SURGERY IN INFANTS AND CHILDREN

Advances in optical systems, video equipment, and surgical instrumentation over the past decade have allowed the extensive development of endoscopic surgery techniques for infants and children. The advantages are smaller scars, less postoperative pain, and earlier discharge, plus presumably less psychologic upset. In the future, robotic surgery via endoscopic access may become the optimal treatment for many surgical conditions.

Special Considerations

I. All procedures planned as endoscopic may require urgent open operation should unexpected complications arise; always be prepared for emergency laparotomy or thoracotomy.
II. Bleeding may occur and may be difficult to rapidly control until an open operation is performed; ensure that reliable large-bore intravenous routes are established.
III. Access to the child may be limited by the equipment required for minimally invasive and especially for robotic surgery: ensure that you can adequately monitor the child and rapidly intervene should this be required.

1. *Laparoscopic procedures*

    A. Physiologic changes secondary to a CO_2 pneumoperitoneum.

        i. The diaphragm is splinted with a consequent decrease in chest wall compliance. This effect is increased if the child is placed in the Trendelenburg position. Elevation of the diaphragm is followed by decreasing lung volumes, increasing the potential for airway closure to occur during tidal breathing and consequent hypoxemia.

        ii. Increased intraabdominal pressure (IAP) leads to decreased venous return, decreased cardiac output, and increased total systemic resistance. The magnitude of these effects is related to the IAP and is increased if the child is placed in the reverse Trendelenburg position. These hemodynamic effects are magnified in the volume-depleted child.

        iii. Carbon dioxide is readily absorbed into the circulation increasing the $PaCO_2$ and the requirement for increased ventilation. Positioning, pneumoperitoneum, and the requirement for increased ventilation may cause the PIP to markedly increase. Absorption of CO_2 may be greater in children than in adults owing to the physiologic properties of the peritoneum.

        iv. The extent of the above changes depend upon the pressure within the abdomen. Pressures up to 5 mm Hg cause very little effect; up to 15 mm Hg is well-tolerated by healthy children in a neutral horizontal position. Positions other than horizontal or IAP greater than 15 mm Hg may cause serious cardiorespiratory derangements that require interventions.

    B. Anesthesia management.

        i. Careful preoperative assessment of cardio-respiratory status, state of hydration, and volume replacement is necessary. Respiratory or cardiac disease and/or volume depletion could cause adverse responses to induced pneumoperitoneum. Volume status should be optimized (i.e., in infants with pyloric stenosis) and any cardio respiratory limitations considered carefully preoperatively.

Limiting the IAP and careful positioning may permit some children with cardio-respiratory disease to tolerate pneumoperitoneum but some may not be ideal candidates for this surgery (e.g., children with Fontan physiology).

        ii. Controlled ventilation with increased positive inspiratory pressure is required. Oxygenation and $EtCO_2$ should be closely monitored, though the latter may be unreliable and give false low readings in infants. Increases in FIO_2 and minute ventilation (MV) are required. MV may need to be increased by 66% to maintain near homeostasis. Up to 5 cm PEEP may be required.

iii. Nitrous oxide should not be used:
- When bowel distention is possible.
- When air embolism might occur.
- Intraabdominal cautery is used. (N_2O supports combustion.)

iv. For upper abdominal surgery, a gastric tube should be passed to empty the stomach and improve exposure. For lower abdominal surgery, either have the child empty the bladder preoperatively or pass a urinary catheter. For pyloromyotomy, a small amount of air may be injected into the stomach via the gastric tube to check the integrity of the duodenal mucosa.

v. Monitor ventilation in both lungs throughout using a stethoscope. When the pneumoperitoneum is created in small infants, the cephalad movement of the diaphragm and lungs may cause the tip of the endotracheal tube to enter a bronchus. In addition, pneumothorax is a recognized complication and should be watched for. The addition of positive end-expiratory pressure may decrease the adverse effects of high IAP and also limit the potential effects of pneumothorax.

vi. Heart rate should be monitored during all intraabdominal manipulations; brisk vagal reflexes may be observed and require immediate cessation of surgical manipulations and treatment with IV atropine.

vii. Carbon dioxide embolism is very rare, but it has occurred during laparoscopy, causing cardiovascular collapse. Monitor carefully throughout the procedure and notify the surgeon immediately if there are any unexplained physiologic changes such as a sudden decrease in $EtCO_2$ or blood pressure, or a wind-mill murmur.

2. *Video assisted thoracic surgery (VATS)*
A. Physiologic considerations.

i. Infants have a high metabolic rate for oxygen and a high Va/FRC ratio. Any compromise in ventilation rapidly leads to hypoxemia.

ii. In infants in the lateral decubitus position for intrathoracic procedures, ventilation of the uppermost lung exceeds that of the dependent lung, but perfusion favors the dependent lung. There is increased $\dot{V}/\dot{Q}$ mismatch.

iii. In order to visualize the intrathoracic structures some degree of lung collapse must occur. This may be obtained by selective one-lung ventilation or as a result of gas insufflation into one hemithorax. In the latter case, some gas transfer can occur on the operated side but $\dot{V}/\dot{Q}$ mismatch is further increased.

iv. One-lung ventilation tends to direct perfusion away from the unventilated lung because of hypoxic pulmonary vasoconstriction (this is partly attenuated by inhalational anesthetics or other drugs) and mechanical effects within the collapsed lung thus normalizing $\dot{V}/\dot{Q}$ relationships somewhat.

v. Absorption of insufflated CO_2 from the pleural cavity occurs and requires increased pulmonary ventilation for homeostasis to be achieved.

vi. In this situation PEEP is also quite helpful in preserving ventilation of the dependent lung.

In summary, oxygenation and ventilation during VATS is unpredictable, requires careful monitoring, and a high FIO_2 will likely be necessary, especially in small infants. However VATS has been very successfully employed in a variety of neonatal and pediatric thoracic procedures.

B. Anesthesia management for VATS.

i. Careful preoperative evaluation of the cardiorespiratory system and the volume status is essential.

ii. A plan for one lung ventilation must be developed, some alternatives are (also see Congenital Lobar Emphysema):

a. Plain endotracheal tube (*no* Murphy eye) guided into the contralateral main bronchus. This is the usual option for small infants. A tube one size smaller than predicted for normal use should be used. The tube can usually be inserted blindly into the (R) main bronchus. Right upper lobe atelectasis may occur in this situation. A fiberoptic bronchoscope or stylet is usually necessary to enter the (L) main bronchus. Using this technique, it is not possible to suction or inflate the operated side without withdrawing the tube.

b. A bronchial blocker may be placed on the operated side. A Fogarty catheter has been used in small infants, although there is no central channel for suction or to allow the lung to collapse completely, it has a high pressure cuff and it might cause damage to the bronchial mucosa. Low pressure cuffs are found on biliary catheters, which may also be used as a bronchial blocker. Bronchial blockers in small infants may be difficult to accurately position and may become displaced—possibly causing serious airway obstruction.

In children over 2 years, the Arndt 5 Fr pediatric bronchial blocker may be used, which has a high volume low pressure cuff. With the guide wire removed, this channel may also be used to suction or deflate the operated lung.

This blocker is inserted via a special adaptor into the endotracheal tube and guided into position using a FOB passed through the wire loop on the tip of the blocker. The use of the Arndt 5 Fr blocker passed through the trachea external to the endotracheal tube has also been described. The blocker is passed into the trachea before intubation and positioned either by fluoroscopy or with the aid of the FOB.

    c. The Univent tube may be used in children of 6 years or over and has the advantage of a channel to suction the operated side bronchus. It should be positioned with the aid of a FOB. The Univent tube is available in 2 pediatric sizes that may be suitable for older children:

3.5 mm Univent tube - external diameter 7.5 to 8 mm
(= 5.5 mm ID plain tube)

4.5 mm Univent tube - external diameter 8.5 to 9 mm
(= 6.5 mm ID plain tube)

    d. Double lumen endotracheal tubes (26 Fr) may be successfully inserted into children of 6 to 8 years of age. Correct positioning should always be confirmed with the FOB. A very small double lumen tube (designed by Marraro) for use in infants is only available as a special product from Smiths Industries (Portex) Inc.

  iii. Anesthetic agents that interfere with normal hypoxic pulmonary vasoconstriction (e.g., halothane) should be avoided to ensure that pulmonary blood flow is optimally distributed away from the collapsed lung. Low concentrations of isoflurane or intravenous agents (e.g., propofol, fentanyl) are preferred.

  iv. During one-lung ventilation (OLV) the child must be closely monitored to detect any displacement of the device used. If obstruction to ventilation should occur, the cuff of a blocker should be immediately deflated.

v. Following a period of OLV, the lung on the operated side should be carefully observed for reinflation. A postoperative chest x-ray should be obtained to exclude persistent atelectasis.

Suggested Reading

Rothenberg SS: Thoracoscopic pulmonary surgery, Semin Pediatr Surg 16(4):231–237, 2007.

Choudhry DK: Single-lung ventilation in pediatric anesthesia, Anesth Clinics N Am 23(4):693–708, 2005.

Marciniak B, Fayoux P, Hebrard A, et al: Fluoroscopic guidance of Arndt endobronchial blocker placement for single-lung ventilation in small children, Acta Anaesthesiol Scand 52:1003–1005, 2008.

Pawar DK, Marraro GA: One lung ventilation in infants and children: experience with Marraro double lumen tube, Paediatr Anaesth 15(3):204–208, 2005.

CONGENITAL DEFECTS THAT MAY NECESSITATE SURGERY DURING THE NEONATAL PERIOD

Congenital Lobar Emphysema

Abnormal distention of a lobe (usually the upper or middle lobe) compresses the remaining normal lung tissue and displaces the mediastinum; respiratory distress and cyanosis result. When severe, this condition manifests as an extreme emergency during the early neonatal period. Obstruction of the bronchus supplying the distended lobe may be extrinsic (e.g., abnormal blood vessels), intraluminal (e.g., bronchial papilloma), or it may be caused by a defect of the bronchial wall (bronchomalacia). More than one lobe may be involved and sometimes the disease may be bilateral. The chest radiograph demonstrates a hyperlucent area with sparse lung markings (differentiating it from pneumothorax) and mediastinal shift. The lesion must also be differentiated from congenital diaphragmatic hernia or cystic adenomatoid malformation, which can have a similar radiologic appearance.

Less severe forms may pass unnoticed for months or even years, and conservative management may be appropriate in some cases.

Associated Condition

1. Congenital heart disease—an incidence of up to 37% in reported series.

Surgical Procedure

1. Lobectomy (if no intraluminal or extrinsic cause can be found and corrected). This may be performed using video assisted thoracic surgery (VATS) in children other than those in extremis.

Special Anesthesia Problems

1. Severe respiratory failure may occur because of compression of normal lung tissue.
2. There is the possibility of a "ball-valve" effect, which further increases the size of the affected lobe during positive-pressure ventilation.
3. N_2O may cause further distention of the lobe and is therefore contraindicated.
4. Considerations for the use of VATS.

Anesthesia Management

1. Observe special precautions for neonates.

Preoperative

1. The child is cared for in the semiupright position.
2. Give O_2 by hood. Avoid intermittent positive-pressure ventilation (IPPV) if possible (danger of "ball-valve" effect).
3. Insert a gastric tube and apply continuous suction. This prevents gastric distention from further compromising ventilation.
4. Check that blood is available for transfusion.
5. Sudden serious deterioration of the child's condition may demand immediate emergency thoracotomy to exteriorize the affected lobe and allow the normal lung tissue to ventilate.

Perioperative

1. Bronchoscopy to exclude intraluminal obstruction may be performed before thoracotomy or VATS.
2. Give atropine intravenously and preoxygenate.
3. If a bronchoscopy is planned, induce anesthesia with sevoflurane in O_2. Otherwise, induce anesthesia with either sevoflurane or ketamine in O_2. Spray the vocal cords with lidocaine while maintaining spontaneous ventilation. Perform laryngoscopy and intubate the trachea or pass the bronchoscope. After bronchoscopy, change to a tracheal tube.
4. Maintain anesthesia with either sevoflurane or ketamine in O_2 with spontaneous ventilation. If assisted ventilation is required this should be applied very gently.

5. VATS can usually be managed with a tracheal tube and gentle positive pressure ventilation during inflation of the thorax with CO_2. Rarely is there a need to isolate the lung. In such instances consider:

   a. Selective endobronchial intubation by advancing the tracheal tube into the bronchus of the contralateral lung. FOB should be used to verify the location of the tip of the tube while the neonate is supine. Intubation of the right bronchus may occlude the right upper lobe bronchus causing desaturation. Advancing the tube into the left bronchus may be accomplished by rotating the tube 180° before advancing it. The tube position should always be verified after the neonate is in the decubitus position.

   b. Bronchial blockers may be inserted into the affected bronchus either endoscopically or radiographically. The blocker should be small, high compliant, and its position verified. Blockers are inserted outside the tracheal tube lumen and positioned by passing a FOB through the tracheal tube and verifying the blocker location after inflation. These blockers may dislodge easily during surgery and suddenly obstruct the tracheal tube. Be prepared to deflate them should this occur.

6. Continue with spontaneous or very gently assisted ventilation until the thorax is open or accessed. In children in extremis, the affected lobe balloons out of the chest on thoracotomy and ventilation must be controlled. If VATS is used, CO_2 will be insufflated into the affected hemithorax. Careful control of ventilation and monitoring of oxygenation during one lung ventilation is required. A high FiO_2 will likely be required. Some hypercarbia may have to be accepted during this period.

7. A nondepolarizing neuromuscular blocking drug can be given to facilitate controlled ventilation and minimize the need for inhaled anesthetic vapors once the lobe has been controlled. The fraction of inspired oxygen (FiO_2) should be maintained at a level that ensures full hemoglobin saturation.

8. After the affected lobe has been excised, the remaining lung tissue will gradually expand to fill the thorax, although a pneumothorax may remain.

Postoperative

1. Discontinue all anesthetic drugs and administer 100% O_2. Antagonize muscle relaxants.

2. When the infant is wide awake, suction the tracheal tube and remove it.

3. Place the infant in a heated incubator and supply O_2 as required to maintain Sao_2.

4. A chest drain (connected to underwater drainage and suction) is required.

Anesthesia Management—Older Children

In approximately 10% of cases, a congenital emphysematous lobe is discovered at an older age. If surgery is planned, the children should be managed as outlined for younger children. A double lumen endotracheal tube may be used to facilitate surgery or VATS.

Suggested Reading

Tobias JD: Anaesthesia for neonatal thoracic surgery, Best Pract Res Clin Anaesthesiol 18(2):303–320, 2004.

Means LJ, Green MC, Bilal R: Anesthesia for minimally invasive surgery, Semin Pediatr Surg 13(3):181–187, 2004.

Iodice F, Harban F, Walker I: Anesthetic management of a child with bilateral congenital lobar emphysema, Paediatr Anaesth 18(4):340–341, 2008.

Congenital Diaphragmatic Hernia (CDH)

The incidence of congenital diaphragmatic hernia is 1 in 4000 live births. There are several types: anterior through the foramen of Morgagni, posterolateral via the foramen of Bochdalek, and at the esophageal hiatus. The most common lesion is posterolateral, through the foramen of Bochdalek, usually on the left side. Herniation of abdominal contents into the thorax is associated with respiratory distress, mediastinal displacement ("dextrocardia"), and a scaphoid abdomen. Breath sounds are absent over the affected side. Bowel sounds are very rarely heard over the thorax. The radiographic appearance is usually diagnostic but may be indistinguishable from that of congenital lobar emphysema.

In many children with CDH, both lungs may be severely hypoplastic. Currently, CDH is thought to be a primary failure of lung development associated with a failure of diaphragm development.

The infant with CDH is usually in severe respiratory distress at or soon after birth. In recent years, the diagnosis has generally been made antenatally by fetal ultrasound.

Associated Conditions

1. Malrotation of the gut (40% of cases)

2. Congenital heart disease (15%)

3. Renal abnormalities (less common)
4. Neurologic abnormalities
5. Cantrell's pentalogy (defined as CDH, omphalocele, sternal cleft, ectopia cordis, and intracardiac defect (VSD or diverticulum of left ventricle)

Surgical Procedure

1. Reduction of the hernia and repair of the diaphragmatic defect: usually a transabdominal procedure—often performed via the laparoscope.

Special Anesthesia Problems

1. Optimal preoperative preparation of the child: The trend in recent years is not to rush to surgery. Relief of compression of the lungs by reduction of the herniated abdominal viscera usually does not solve the problem; indeed, there is evidence that respiratory mechanics and hemodynamics are worse postoperatively. It is now preferred to treat the respiratory insufficiency by muscle paralysis, controlled gentle ventilation, and therapy to reduce pulmonary vasoconstriction (including surfactant, hyperventilation, oxygenation, correction of metabolic acidosis, anesthesia and paralysis, and nitric oxide). If these measures fail, ECMO may be instituted. Surgical correction is performed later, as an elective procedure, when the infant is improving and can be weaned from respiratory support.

Anesthesia Management

Preoperative
Preoperative management requires the facilities and trained staff of a specialist unit. The infant is nursed in a semiupright, semilateral position, facing toward the involved side. A gastric tube is passed and maintained on low suction to prevent further distention of intrathoracic abdominal viscera. All but the exceptionally fit older infant require intubation and ventilation: Bag-mask ventilation should be avoided because it may further distend the stomach and increase respiratory distress.

1. Muscle paralysis after intubation facilitates controlled ventilation and minimizes struggling, thereby decreasing the O_2 demand. It also reduces airway pressure, minimizes further lung damage, and diminishes the ever-present danger of pneumothorax. (Pneumothorax is a constant danger and must be watched for and immediately treated.)
2. Ventilation should be gentle—not to exceed positive inspiratory pressures of 20 cm H_2O. Some degree of hypercapnia may have to be

accepted rather than using high pressure that might cause further damage to the hypoplastic lungs.

3. High-frequency ventilation may be applied to facilitate gas exchange while minimizing pressure swings, which might cause further lung damage. Surfactant therapy may be administered to preterm infants with CDH.

4. Pulmonary vascular resistance may be reduced by general measures such as fentanyl infusion and minimal handling of the child. Nitric oxide may be administered by inhalation and may further reduce pulmonary vascular resistance in some children although the results of NO in CDH children are unimpressive.

5. When all of these measures fail, ECMO is indicated and may permit survival of some children until the pulmonary status improves.

Aggressive invasive monitoring using arterial pressure and ECHO-derived pulmonary artery pressures is required to ensure optimal treatment for the pulmonary status. The best predictors of the degree of pulmonary hypoplasia, and hence of survival, are the $PaCO_2$ and the respiratory index (the product of mean airway pressure and respiratory rate). Those children who are easy to ventilate and not grossly hypercarbic have a better prognosis. Those who are hypercarbic and hypoxic with a high mean airway pressure are less likely to survive. ECMO may increase survival of this latter group. If the child improves on ECMO, surgery is usually performed just before weaning.

Perioperative

CDH may be repaired in the NICU or in the OR. Children on ECMO and HFOV and those who have circulatory instability often undergo surgery in the NICU; most surgeons prefer to transport all other children to the OR for surgery.

1. Induce and maintain anesthesia with IV fentanyl. Ventilate with isoflurane as tolerated and O_2/air to maintain SaO_2. N_2O is avoided as it could further distend gas-containing herniated viscera.

2. Monitor airway pressure. This should *not* exceed 20 cm H_2O (greater pressures may cause further lung damage or contralateral pneumothorax).

3. Do not try to expand the lungs after reduction of the hernia (lung damage may result).

4. Monitor blood gas and acid-base status frequently and correct as indicated.

For children having surgery on ECMO:

1. Common practice has been to administer additional doses of relaxant and opioids. However, very often infants on ECMO develop tolerance to fentanyl and require very large doses to blunt the cardiovascular response to surgery. Instead, low concentrations of isoflurane may be titrated to blunt the responses by adding it to the oxygenator gas supply.
2. Ensure ECMO cannulas do not become kinked during positioning for surgery.
3. Even though the child may be heparinized, excessive bleeding usually is not a problem.

Postoperative

1. Return the child to the intensive care unit (ICU) for continued intensive respiratory care.
2. Some infants who have been salvaged by heroic intensive care measures may remain oxygen-dependent for years.

Suggested Reading

Robinson PD, Fitzgerald DA: Congenital diaphragmatic hernia, Paed Resp Rev 8(4):323–335, 2007.
Becmeur F, Reinberg O, Dimitriu C, et al: Thoracoscopic repair of congenital diaphragmatic hernia in children, Semin Pediatr Surg 16(4):238–244, 2007.

Tracheoesophageal Fistula and Esophageal Atresia

Tracheoesophageal fistula and esophageal atresia, interrelated conditions, may occur in several combinations. The overall incidence is 1 in 3000 live births. Maternal polyhydramnios is present, and premature birth is common.

The most common form (approximately 90% of cases) is esophageal atresia with a fistula between the trachea and the distal segment of the esophagus (Figure 13-1, Type 1). This condition might be detected when the neonate chokes at the first feeding, but ideally it should be diagnosed antenatally by ultrasound or at birth by the inability to pass a soft rubber catheter into the stomach. Plain radiography confirms the diagnosis, showing the catheter curled in the upper esophageal pouch and an air bubble in the stomach, indicating a fistula. Contrast medium should not be used because it may be aspirated and further damage the lungs.

Esophageal atresia without fistula is the second most common form of the disease (Figure 13-1, Type 2); there may be a large gap between the upper and lower segments of the esophagus. In such children, it is not pos-

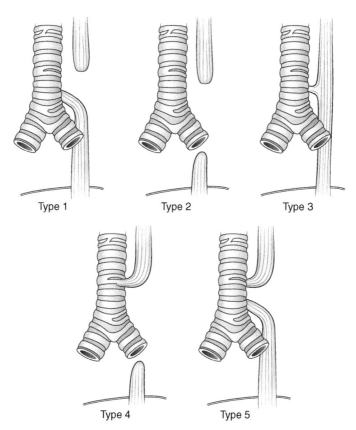

Figure 13-1. Esophageal atresia and tracheoesophageal fistula
(see text for details).

sible to pass a catheter into the stomach, and there is no gastric air bubble. Aspiration from the upper pouch is an immediate danger. Constant suctioning of the upper pouch should be instituted pending surgical repair.

The third most common form is the H-type fistula without atresia (Figure 13-1, Type 3); diagnosis of this type may be more difficult and is often delayed. In such cases, there is usually a history of repeated respiratory infections. The fistula may be difficult to locate even when contrast studies and endoscopy are used. Once the fistula is identified, surgical ligation often can be performed via a neck dissection.

There are other, rarer anatomic variants of this disease, many of which include tracheal stenosis.

Associated Conditions

1. Prematurity (30% to 40%)
2. Congenital heart disease (22%)
3. Additional gastrointestinal abnormalities (e.g., pyloric stenosis)
4. Renal and genitourinary abnormalities
5. The VACTERL association: VATER association (*V*ertebral defects, *A*nal atresia, *T*racheoesophageal fistula, *E*sophageal atresia, *R*adial and *R*enal dysplasia) with added *C*ardiac and *L*imb defects
6. Tracheomalacia and other abnormalities of the trachea (e.g., stenosis)

Surgical Procedures

The infant's general condition and the anatomy of the defect govern the choice of surgical management:

1. Primary complete repair (ligation of fistula and esophageal anastomosis), which is preferred
2. Staged repair (gastrostomy followed by division of the fistula, followed later by repair of the esophagus)

The current surgical trend is to perform early primary repair. Often the operation is preceded by bronchoscopy to define the site of the fistula and exclude other tracheal defects.

Special Anesthesia Problems

1. Prematurity and other associated diseases (congenital heart disease is common) may complicate the case.
2. Pulmonary complications secondary to aspiration may be present.
3. There is a possibility of intubating the fistula.
4. Anesthetic gases may inflate the stomach via the fistula.
5. Surgical retraction during repair may obstruct ventilation.
6. Subglottic or tracheal stenosis may be present.

Anesthesia Management—Primary Repair

1. Observe special precautions for neonates.

Preoperative

1. The infant is nursed in a semiupright position.
2. The proximal esophageal pouch is suctioned continuously to prevent aspiration of secretions.

3. Institute intensive respiratory care to reduce pulmonary complications. (Even so, the lung condition seldom improves until after ligation of the fistula; therefore surgery should not be delayed in the hope that pulmonary status will markedly improve.)

4. Examination of the infant to detect other associated lesions should be completed (i.e., echocardiography to rule out a congenital heart defect).

5. Establish a reliable intravenous route and ensure that blood is available for transfusion.

6. Give maintenance fluids intravenously, but bear in mind that dehydration is not a major problem; neonatal fluid requirements are low during the first 24 hours, and fluid and electrolyte depletion does not occur with esophageal obstruction.

7. In the preterm infant with RDS and poor lung compliance, there is a danger of massive distention of the stomach (or massive leak from a gastrostomy if present) and consequent failure to ventilate. Rupture of the stomach and pneumoperitoneum may occur. The risk of massive gastric distention in infants with RDS has disappeared since the introduction of surfactant therapy. It has been suggested that a gas leak through the fistula may be controlled by one of:
   a. A balloon catheter passed via a gastrostomy into the lower esophagus.
   b. A balloon catheter inserted into the fistula under bronchoscopic guidance.
   c. Most commonly by early simple ligation of the fistula in infants with RDS who develop high airway pressures. The operation is brief and can be followed by esophageal reconstruction after the child's respiratory function has improved.

8. Beware of the possibility of subglottic stenosis; have small tube sizes available.

9. TEF may be repaired using VATS in which case the considerations of one-lung surgery must be observed.

Perioperative

1. Suction the upper pouch. Apply lidocaine 4% to the gums and palate using a gauze sponge; this lessens the response to intubation.

2. Apply the usual monitors and prepare to monitor ventilation using a precordial stethoscope in the left midaxillary line.

3. One of two approaches may be taken to secure the airway:
   a. Induce anesthesia with sevoflurane or halothane in O_2, maintaining spontaneous ventilation. Perform laryngoscopy and spray the larynx with lidocaine (maximum dose, 5 mg/kg).

Return to the mask and continue sevoflurane anesthesia for 2 or 3 minutes.

b. Alternately, and if a bronchoscopy is *not* planned, sedate with fentanyl (0.5 to 1 µg/kg) and midazolam (25 µg/kg) and spray the larynx with lidocaine.

Then:

a. Intubate the trachea with the bevel of the tube facing posteriorly (to avoid intubating the fistula).

b. Alternately, if a rigid bronchoscopy is planned, once the surgeon passes the bronchoscope, attach the anesthesia circuit to the side arm of the bronchoscope and continue with spontaneous or gently assisted ventilation. When the bronchoscopy is completed, insert a tracheal tube with the bevel facing posteriorly, or

c. If a fiberoptic bronchoscopy is planned, insert the tracheal tube with the bevel posterior and attach a bronchoscopic adapter to accommodate the fiberoptic bronchoscope. Gently assist ventilation while the endoscopy proceeds.

4. Immediately after intubation, check ventilation throughout the lung fields. *If ventilation is unsatisfactory*, remove the tube, give O_2, and reinsert the tube. It is advantageous to place the tube with its tip just above the carina; this can be done by advancing the tube into the bronchus and then withdrawing it until bilateral ventilation is heard. This should place the tip of the tube below the fistula in most cases, although in some children the fistula lies at the level of the carina. At this time, the tube should be rotated so that the bevel faces anteriorly (to prevent inflating the fistula). More complicated methods to position the tube have been described but are unnecessary in our experience. Always check ventilation again after positioning of the child is complete. It is preferable to use a tube without a "Murphy eye," to minimize the possibility of leaks via the fistula.

5. Once the tube has been properly placed, oxygenate and perform tracheobronchial suction to remove any accumulated secretions before the surgery commences.

6. Maintain anesthesia with air, O_2, and sevoflurane or isoflurane with spontaneous or gently assisted ventilation. If the inhalational anesthetic is not tolerated, small doses of fentanyl should be substituted (up to 10 to 12 µg/kg).

7. *If spontaneous ventilation is inadequate:* assist ventilation cautiously, while observing and auscultating over the stomach for inflation. If gastric inflation occurs, allow the child to breathe spontaneously (with gentle manual assistance) until the fistula is ligated.

8. Monitor ventilation carefully during surgical manipulation: large airways may be kinked by retraction, especially as the fistula is manipulated.

9. Once the fistula is ligated, give a muscle relaxant and control the ventilation in the usual manner.

10. Reports suggest that VATS may be useful in the repair of TEF, the view on the video-screen allows very precise repair of the esophagus. In this case, it may not be necessary to advance the endotracheal tube into the bronchus to continue with one lung anesthesia. As the surgeon insufflates CO_2 under $5\,cm/H_2O$ pressure, the "up" lung is compressed and the lesion visualized, in effect, obtaining one-lung anesthesia by increasing intrathoracic pressure. During this period, ventilation may become difficult and a high FiO_2 required. Avoiding the necessity to intubate the bronchus may be advantageous as persistent upper lobe atelectasis may occur after endobronchial intubation.

Postoperative

1. The child with a clear chest who is awake and moving vigorously should be extubated in the OR. Some surgeons, however, may prefer to keep the trachea intubated and a gastroesophageal tube in place for several days to avoid reintubation and damage to the tracheal repair.

2. If there are pulmonary complications or any doubts about the adequacy of ventilation, continue controlled ventilation.

3. The pharynx is suctioned with a soft catheter that has a suitable maximum length of insertion clearly marked; it must not reach (and damage) the anastomotic site.

4. Prolonged intensive respiratory care may be required. (Swallowing is not normal postoperatively and aspiration may occur.)

5. Prognosis after the repair depends on the maturity of the infant, whether other congenital anomalies are present, and whether pulmonary complications develop. In the absence of these conditions, the prognosis is excellent.

6. Postoperative analgesia may be provided by a caudal epidural catheter inserted intraoperatively and threaded to the thoracic level; careful management of local anesthetic doses is required (see Chapter 5, page 156).

Anesthesia Management-Staged Repair

If staged repair is planned, a preliminary gastrostomy is performed under local or general anesthesia. Management of the second stage (ligation of the fistula) should follow the sequence outlined for primary repair. Further surgery (to repair the atresia) may be done later, when the child's condition is optimal.

Late Complications

1. Diverticulum of the trachea, at the site of the old fistula, is common in children who had a tracheoesophageal fistula repaired during infancy. Be aware of this possibility and the danger of intubating the diverticulum during anesthesia in later life.
2. The tracheal cartilage structure is abnormal, and tracheomalacia may cause symptoms during infancy after repair of a tracheoesophageal fistula. Episodes of stridor, dyspnea, and cyanosis ("dying spells") characteristically occur during feeding. This is caused by compression of the soft trachea between the dilated esophagus and the arch of the aorta. Severe symptoms require surgical treatment by aortopexy or tracheoplasty with an external splint. These children often have a deep barking cough much like children with croup.
3. Stricture may develop at the site of the esophageal anastomosis with episodes of esophageal obstruction with food (the hotdog in the esophagus); it may require repeated dilations and, later, possibly resection with replacement, using the colon or a gastric tube.

Suggested Reading

Goyal A, Jones MO, Couriel JM, et al: Oesophageal atresia and tracheo-oesophageal fistula, Arch Dis Child Fetal Neo Ed 91(5):F381–F384, 2006.

Naik-Mathuria B, Olutoye OO: Foregut abnormalities, Surg Clin N Am 86(2):261–284, 2006.

Krosnar S, Baxter A: Thoracoscopic repair of esophageal atresia with tracheoesophageal fistula: anesthetic and intensive care management of a series of eight neonates, Paediatr Anaesth 15(7):541–546, 2005.

Congenital Laryngotracheoesophageal Cleft

This is a very rare anomaly in which there is a cleft in the posterior wall of the larynx that communicates with the esophagus. Four types are described, depending on the extension of this cleft distally. Type 1 is confined to the larynx, type 2 extends to the trachea, type 3 extends to the carina, and type 4 extends into the bronchi.

Mild type 1 forms of this anomaly may be missed initially, and the child may later have a hoarse cry, cyanotic spells during feeding, and repeated episodes of aspiration pneumonia. Type 1 and type 2 clefts may be repaired endoscopically. These procedures are performed with the child breathing spontaneously and without an endotracheal tube, thus ensuring good surgical access to the lesion.

Severe clefts manifest early in life with severe respiratory distress, which may be relieved by passage of a gastric tube. Pulmonary damage from aspiration may be severe. Early tracheostomy and gastrostomy may be lifesaving.

Anesthesia Management

1. Careful preoperative assessment is performed to exclude other significant congenital lesions.
2. All the usual considerations for neonatal anesthesia are observed.
3. Inhalation induction of anesthesia using sevoflurane or halothane is performed.
4. A reliable IV route is established and IV atropine administered to limit secretions.
5. Topical anesthesia is thoroughly applied to the larynx and trachea (lidocaine 5 mg/kg).
6. A suspension laryngoscope is positioned.
7. Anesthesia is maintained by insufflation of sevoflurane or halothane via a nasopharyngeal tube or alternatively by a propofol infusion or a combination of the two.
8. An oxygen/air carrier gas should be used; if cautery is planned, use the minimal FIO_2 to reduce the fire risk.
9. Postoperatively biphasic BPAP may be applied to ensure ventilation as is required, and a soft feeding tube may be inserted into the stomach.

Note: This method of anesthesia (spontaneous ventilation, no endotracheal tube, inhaled anesthetic, and meticulous topical anesthesia to the airway) is extremely useful for endoscopic surgery for the larynx and upper trachea. Scavenge gases around the head. We have used it successfully in hundreds of cases. However, obsessive attention is required—the child must be maintained at a constant level of anesthesia and not allowed to awaken or move. The topical anesthesia must be thoroughly applied and for long cases may need to be repeated. Halothane is a better anesthetic than sevoflurane for this purpose as awakening is slower if the concentration decreases for any reason—if you have it, use it. Otherwise sevoflurane may be used—but maintain deep anesthesia. This is often difficult with sevoflurane alone; supplementation with propofol either intermittently or by infusion is advised. Alternatively, a TIVA technique with a propofol infusion may be used and is perhaps the better choice if halothane is unavailable.

Type 3 and 4 clefts require open surgery; definitive repair may involve a combined cervical and thoracic approach. Good intraoperative control of the airway is vital and demands close cooperation between the anesthesiologist and surgeon in planning the repair. A cuffed tube may be inserted into the esophagus to prevent ventilation of the stomach. In one report, a bifurcated endotracheal tube was used to preclude esophageal ventilation.

Suggested Reading

Sandu K, Monnier P: Endoscopic laryngotracheal cleft repair without tracheotomy or intubation, Laryngoscope 116(4):630–634, 2006.

Kubba H, Gibson D, Bailey M, et al: Techniques and outcomes of laryngeal cleft repair: an update to the Great Ormond Street Hospital series, Ann Otol Rhinol Laryng 114(4):309–313, 2005.

Miyamoto Y, Kinouchi K, Taniguchi A, et al: A bifurcated tracheal tube for a neonate with tracheoesophageal fistula, Anesthesiology 100:733–736, 2004.

Congenital Hypertrophic Pyloric Stenosis

Congenital hypertrophic pyloric stenosis, a common surgical problem of infancy, occurs in up to 1 of every 300 live births in some populations; the incidence has considerable geographic variation. First-born male infants are more commonly affected. Hypertrophy of the muscle of the pyloric sphincter causes gastric outlet obstruction, leading to persistent vomiting. Dehydration, hypochloremia, and alkalosis develop. If the diagnosis is promptly made, severe derangements are avoided.

Diagnosis is made on the basis of the history and by palpation of an olive-sized mass in the region of the pylorus. Confirmation is by abdominal ultrasound examination.

Associated Condition

1. Jaundice (2% of children), which is caused by glucuronyl transferase deficiency: No special therapy is required, and the jaundice clears after pyloromyotomy.

Surgical Procedure

1. Pyloromyotomy—commonly now performed using the laparoscope (see Special Considerations)

Special Anesthesia Problems

1. Ensure that dehydration and electrolyte imbalance are fully corrected before surgery (pyloromyotomy is never a surgical emergency).

2. There is a danger of vomiting and aspiration during anesthesia.
3. Observe considerations for laparoscopic surgery (see page 339)

Anesthesia Management

1. Observe special precautions for neonates.

Preoperative

1. Insert a gastric tube and apply continuous suction.
2. Rehydrate the child, correcting the electrolyte imbalance; this may require 24 to 48 hours.
  a. Give 2:1 dextrose-saline solution and/or normal saline as indicated by serum electrolyte values; children with greater fluid and sodium deficits may require normal saline. Add potassium chloride (KCl supplements, 3 mEq/kg/day) when urine flow is established.
  b. Delay surgery until the infant appears clinically well hydrated and has normal electrolyte levels, acid-base balance, and good urine output.
3. Immediately before surgery, reassess the child to ensure that the fluid status and electrolytes are satisfactory:
  a. Check for clinical signs of adequate hydration (alertness, skin turgor, normal anterior fontanel, normal vital signs, moist tongue, urine output).
  b. Check biochemistry: pH, 7.3 to 7.5; sodium (Na), greater than 132 mmol/L; chloride (Cl), greater than 88 mmol/L; potassium (K), greater than 3.2 mmol/L; and bicarbonate, less than 30 mmol/L.

Perioperative

1. Give atropine intravenously.
2. Insert a vented orogastric suction catheter and suction the stomach in the supine, right and left lateral decubitus positions (even if the stomach has been on continuous gastric suction).
3. Give 100% O_2 by mask.
4. Use a RSI.
5. Maintain anesthesia with N_2O and a potent inhaled anesthetic.
6. Give a muscle relaxant (or propofol) and control ventilation. (This permits the use of minimal amounts of inhalational agents.) The choice of relaxant is dictated by the probable duration of surgery (i.e., the speed of the surgeon). No relaxant, succinylcholine (2 mg/kg) and low dose rocuronium (0.3 mg/kg) or cisatracurium (0.1 mg/kg) may also be used for brief procedures.
7. Ensure that the infant is well relaxed and immobile while the pyloric tumor is being split. (Coughing or movement could result in surgical

perforation of the mucosa.) The surgeon may request that a small amount of air be insufflated into the stomach to check the integrity of the mucosa.

8. Acetaminophen (30 to 40 mg/kg PR in a single loading dose) should be administered at induction of anesthesia. Surgeons should infiltrate the wound with a long-acting local anesthetic such as 0.25% bupivacaine with epinephrine 1:200,000 to limit the perioperative pain. (Administering opioids during surgery, especially during laparoscopic pyloromyotomy, will markedly delay emergence.)

9. At the end of the operation, the infant must be wide awake and in a lateral position before extubation.

Postoperative

1. If analgesia is insufficient, administer small doses of IV morphine (0.02 to 0.03 mg/kg).

2. Maintain intravenous infusion of fluids until oral intake is adequate (usually 24 hours). Hypoglycemia has been reported when intravenous fluids containing glucose were discontinued before oral intake was adequate. Oral feeding is generally started with clear fluids 6 to 12 hours postoperatively.

3. Postoperative respiratory depression may occur as a result of the effect of preoperative alkalosis on the pH of the cerebrospinal fluid. Apnea has been reported in full-term infants after pyloromyotomy. The frequency of apnea and its causes are unclear, but infants should be carefully monitored (apnea monitor and/or pulse oximetry) for 24 hours postoperatively.

Suggested Reading

Allan C: Determinants of good outcome in pyloric stenosis, J Paed Child Health 42(3):86–88, 2006.

Aspelund G, Langer JC: Current management of hypertrophic pyloric stenosis, Semin Pediatr Surg 16(1):27–33, 2007.

Omphalocele and Gastroschisis

In omphalocele and gastroschisis, abdominal contents herniated through the anterior abdominal wall. The incidence of these conditions varies between 0.4 to 3 in 10,000 live births for gastroschisis and 1.5 to 3 in 10,000 for omphalocele.

In gastroschisis, the defect is lateral to the umbilicus (usually on the right side), the umbilical cord is situated normally, other congenital defects are rare, but the bowel is exposed to damaging effects of amniotic fluid in utero. Left sided gastroschisis has a greater incidence of associated extraintestinal defects.

In omphalocele, the umbilical cord is continuous with the apex of the sac, which is covered by peritoneum and amnion, and associated congenital defects are common (75%).

The physiologic consequences of the abdominal wall defect are, however, similar in both lesions. The treatment objective is to close the abdominal defect without exposing the contained viscera to excessive pressure. High IAP may result in cardiorespiratory failure, renal failure, decreased hepatic function, ischemic damage to the bowel, and death.

Associated Conditions (Omphalocele)

1. Prematurity incidence of 30%
2. Other gastrointestinal malformations (i.e., malrotation, diaphragmatic hernia): 25%
3. Genitourinary anomalies: 25%
4. Congenital heart disease: 10%
5. Beckwith-Wiedemann syndrome (omphalocele, macroglossia, and severe hypoglycemia). These infants are usually large and have visceromegaly of the liver, kidney, and pancreas. They may also have hyperviscosity syndrome.

Surgical Procedures

The size of the abdomen in relation to the lesion determines the surgical procedure.

1. Primary closure is preferred because there is less risk of infection and other gastrointestinal complications. However, primary closure usually increases intraabdominal pressure, which, if excessive, may lead to impaired ventilation, reduced cardiac output, hypotension, and splanchnic ischemia, with impaired hepatic, renal, and bowel function. It has been recommended that the intragastric pressure be measured and used as a guide to the safety of primary closure: pressures higher than 20 mm Hg are poorly tolerated.
2. Skin closure only may be indicated in some infants.
3. In others, the procedure is a staged procedure: This approach involves initial closure using a preformed silo and the defect progressively reduced over time without anesthesia.
4. Very large omphaloceles may simply be painted with silver sulfadiazine and allowed to epithelialize over a period of weeks or months with delayed surgical closure.

Special Anesthesia Problems

1. Heat and fluid loss from exposed viscera.
2. Severe fluid and electrolyte disturbance and hypovolemic shock from transudation of fluid into the bowel and from exposure of viscera to air (hypoproteinemia may occur).
3. Increased IAP after closure may lead to compromised ventilation, decreased cardiac output, renal failure, and hepatic impairment (including delayed clearance of drugs, notably fentanyl).
4. Possible hypoglycemia in infants with visceromegaly.

Anesthesia Management

1. Observe special precautions for neonates.

Preoperative

1. The child is nursed in a semiupright position with exposed viscera wrapped in sterile plastic film and covered by towels; this is done to prevent infection and minimize heat and fluid losses.
2. A gastric tube is usually inserted to decompress the bowel.
3. Monitor the blood glucose frequently; if the child is hypoglycemic (less than 40 mg/dl), infuse glucose continuously (6 to 8 mg/kg/min).

N.B. Children with Beckwith-Wiedemann syndrome have an increased insulin response; severe rebound hypoglycemia may occur if bolus doses of glucose are given.

4. Rehydrate the child and correct the hypovolemia and electrolyte and oncotic status. Initial fluid requirements are high (up to 140 ml/kg/24 hr); normal saline plus colloid (albumin) is required to correct the hypovolemia.
5. Order blood for possible transfusion.

Perioperative

1. Ensure that the OR is warmed to at least 24 °C and that heating lamps and forced-air warming devices are available.
2. Aspirate the gastric tube.
3. Give 100% O_2 by mask.
4. Perform a rapid-sequence induction with cricoid pressure. Note that children with Beckwith-Wiedemann syndrome are reported to have larger tracheas and may require a larger or cuffed endotracheal tube; their large tongue may interfere with normal laryngoscopy. In these children, a sedated awake intubation may be indicated.

5. Induce and maintain anesthesia with sevoflurane or halothane in O$_2$ and air.
   a. N$_2$O is contraindicated because it distends the bowel.
   b. Opioids (e.g., fentanyl) may not be metabolized as rapidly as expected because of the effect of increased intraabdominal pressure postoperatively.
6. Muscle relaxants may or may not be required to control ventilation.
7. Intragastric pressure should be measured during abdominal closure to determine whether a primary closure will be tolerated. If the intragastric pressure exceeds 20 mm Hg, hemodynamic instability, and renal insufficiency may follow. As a simple adjunct, it is suggested that monitoring SaO$_2$ at postductal sites above and below the abdomen (i.e., left hand and foot) may predict increased IAP. If the reading from the L foot decreases significantly below the L hand, or if the quality of the waveform is markedly less in the foot compared with the hand, then IAP may be excessive.

Postoperative

1. Assess spontaneous ventilation; if in doubt, change to a nasotracheal tube and continue controlled ventilation. This may be required for a considerable period.
2. Continue nasogastric suction until bowel function recovers.
3. Continue intravenous fluids and glucose. Fluid requirements may remain high in the postoperative phase. Some infants require a prolonged period of intravenous alimentation because bowel function may be impaired for a long period (even weeks or months).

Suggested Reading

Suver D, Lee SL, Shekherdimian S, et al: Left-sided gastroschisis: higher incidence of extraintestinal congenital anomalies, Am J Surg 195(5):663–666, 2008.

Kimura Y, Kamada Y, Kimura S: Anesthetic management of two cases of Beckwith-Wiedemann syndrome, J Anesth 22(1):93–95, 2008.

Ledbetter DJ: Gastroschisis and omphalocele, Surg Cl N Am 86(2):249–260, 2006.

Aizenfisz S, Dauger S, Gondon E, et al: Gastroschisis and omphalocele: retrospective study of initial postoperative management in the ICU, Euro J Ped Surg 16(2):84–89, 2006.

Hong CM, Patel A: Novel intraoperative pulse oximetry monitoring for gastroschisis: a noninvasive monitor of intraabdominal pressure, Paediatr Anaesth 18(4):344–355, 2008.

Biliary Atresia

Biliary obstruction in the neonate most commonly results from neo-natal hepatitis or biliary atresia. Atresia of the extrahepatic bile ducts may be a result of an intrauterine inflammatory process. Biliary obstruction leads to hepatocellular damage and ultimate cirrhosis, the infant becomes increasingly jaundiced. The incidence of biliary atresia is 0.5 to 1 in 10,000 live births. The problem in the persistently jaundiced neonate with direct (mixed) hyperbilirubinemia is to rule out other causes and confirm the diagnosis of atresia of the bile ducts. This is usually achieved by percutaneous liver biopsy, scintography, and endoscopic retrograde cholangiography.

Associated Anomalies

1. Polysplenia syndrome; intestinal malrotation, preduodenal portal vein, situs inversus, absent inferior vena cava, cardiac defects, and anomalous hepatic artery supply.

Surgical Procedure

1. Hepatic portoenterostomy (Kasai procedure). The extrahepatic bile ducts are resected, and the porta hepatis is dissected to a depth of 2 to 3 mm; then a Roux-en-Y jejunal anastomosis is performed. The major preoperative survival determinant seems to be the age at which the operation is performed. If the infant is older than 12 weeks of age, success is less likely. These older infants are often listed for liver transplantation.

Anesthesia Problems

1. Hepatic function is impaired, especially in the older child.
2. Hypoprothrombinemia develops and leads to impaired coagulation, especially in older infants.
3. Blood loss may be extensive, but this is unusual.
4. Intraoperative radiographs may be needed in some children.
5. The procedure may be performed using robotic surgery via laparoscope. (See previous Special Considerations)
6. Some children will have associated thrombocytopenia because of hypersplenism.

Anesthesia Management

Preoperative

1. Observe all considerations for anesthetizing the neonate.
2. Check the coagulation profile and verify that the child has received vitamin K_1.

3. Check that adequate blood, fresh-frozen plasma, and platelets if low are available for transfusion.

Perioperative

1. Administer 100% O_2 by mask and place monitors.
2. Induce anesthesia intravenously or by inhalation of sevoflurane or halothane.
3. Administer a muscle relaxant and intubate. *Cis*-atracurium is preferred in children with possibly impaired hepatic function.
4. Induce and maintain anesthesia with low concentrations of sevoflurane or isoflurane in an O_2/air mixture. Fentanyl or remifentanil may be used for analgesia.
5. Supplement relaxant drugs as necessary and continue to control the ventilation.
6. Insert large-bore intravenous lines into upper limbs or neck. Insert a gastric tube.
7. Monitor the BP carefully; be alert to the possibility of sudden hypotension because of IVC obstruction during surgical manipulation of the liver. Placing the infant in a slight head-down position may minimize falls in BP during manipulations of the liver.
8. Infuse glucose-containing solutions at maintenance rates and monitor blood glucose levels.
9. Monitor the temperature; use an overhead heater and a forced air heater (or both) in addition to all other measures to maintain normothermia.

Postoperative

1. Prolonged IV hyperalimentation may be required.
2. Ascending cholangitis is common, and portal hypertension may develop.
3. Many children develop esophageal varices and have repeated episodes of bleeding.
4. Postoperative ventilation for 24 to 48 hours may be needed.
5. If the trachea is intubated postoperatively, either IV fentanyl or morphine should be used to titrate to analgesia. If extubated, IV morphine should be used.

Suggested Reading

Green DW, Howard ER, Davenport M: Anaesthesia, perioperative management, and outcome of correction of extrahepatic biliary atresia in the infant: a review of 50 cases in the King's College Hospital series, Paediatr Anaesth 10(6):581–589, 2000.

Mariano ER, Furukawa L, Woo RK, et al: Anesthetic concerns for robot-assisted laparoscopy in an infant, Anesth Analg 99(6):1665–1667, 2004.

Intestinal Obstruction in the Neonate

Intestinal obstruction in the neonate may result from various lesions (e.g., duodenal atresia, duplication, midgut volvulus, malrotation) or from accumulation of viscid meconium ("meconium ileus").

Associated Conditions

1. Prematurity.
2. Down syndrome and hence congenital heart disease (40% to 50%).
3. Cystic fibrosis (invariably accompanies meconium ileus).
4. Subglottic stenosis with duodenal atresia.

Special Anesthesia Problems

1. Hypovolemia; acid-base and electrolyte imbalance.
2. Gross abdominal distention in some cases.
3. Risk of regurgitation and aspiration.

Anesthesia Management

1. Observe special precautions for neonates.

Preoperative

1. Check that the child has had adequate fluid volume replacement.
2. Check acid-base and electrolyte status and correct any imbalance as far as possible.
3. Ensure that the gastrointestinal tract has been decompressed as much as possible (via an indwelling gastric tube).
4. Ensure the availability of blood and blood products as indicated.

Perioperative

1. Give atropine intravenously.
2. Aspirate the stomach contents via the gastric tube.
3. Give 100% O_2 by mask.
4. Intubate the trachea with the child awake or after a RSI. Beware of the possibility of subglottic stenosis.
5. Maintain anesthesia with isoflurane or sevoflurane in an air/O_2 mixture. Avoid N_2O because it may further distend the bowel.
6. Give small doses of relaxant drugs and control ventilation.
7. Despite apparently adequate preoperative fluid resuscitation, some infants become hypotensive once the abdomen is open, especially

those with small bowel atresia or midgut volvulus. They may need surprisingly large volumes of intravenous fluid (even blood or plasma) to restore the BP. Be prepared!

Postoperative

1. Do not extubate the trachea until the infant is fully awake and vigorous. Extubate with the infant in the lateral position.
2. Prolonged intravenous or gastrostomy feeding may be required.
3. After meconium ileus, problems including prolonged bowel dysfunction, sepsis, and pneumonia must be anticipated.

Suggested Reading

Lynn HB: Duodenal obstruction: atresia, stenosis, and annular pancreas. In Ravitch MM, Welch KJ, Benson CD, et al: Pediatric Surgery, 3rd ed Chicago, 1979, Year Book.

Sears BE, Carlin J, Tunnell WP: Severe congenital subglottic stenosis in association with congenital duodenal obstruction, Anesthesiology 49:214, 1978.

Stevenson RJ: Neonatal intestinal obstruction in children, Surg Clin North Am 65:1217–1234, 1985.

Neonatal Necrotizing Enterocolitis

Neonatal necrotizing enterocolitis (NEC), a disease of low-birth-weight infants (usually less than 34 weeks gestation), is characterized by intestinal mucosal injury secondary to ischemia of the bowel. It may lead to perforation and peritonitis. Severe fluid and electrolyte disturbance, endotoxic shock, and coagulopathy because of thrombocytopenia may develop. As the disease progresses, multiple system organ failure may occur. The cause of NEC is uncertain, but the disease usually affects infants with a history of birth asphyxia, respiratory distress syndrome, and shock. Other possible causes include enteral feeding, infection, and umbilical artery catheterization.

The clinical picture is one of abdominal distention, bloody diarrhea, temperature instability, and lethargy; apnea may occur. Abdominal radiography may show intramural bowel or portal venous gas.

The medical management of NEC includes cessation of feeding and institution of continuous gastric suction, use of intravenous fluids and alimentation, IV antibiotics, and correction of anemia and/or coagulopathy. Steroids and inotropes may be used to treat shock. Bowel perforation is the usual indication for surgery.

Special Anesthesia Problems

1. Prematurity and respiratory distress.
2. Shock, hypovolemia, electrolyte disturbance, and coagulopathy.
3. Sepsis, acidosis, and congestive cardiac failure.
4. Interstitial gas in the bowel wall.
5. Interaction of antibiotics with relaxant drugs.

Anesthesia Management

Preoperative

1. Restore blood and fluid volumes: blood, plasma, platelets, and crystalloid solutions may be required; third space losses are considerable. If volume replacement does not improve the BP, inotropes are indicated. Check Hct, blood gases, electrolytes, and the blood glucose level.
2. Check coagulation: thrombocytopenia must be corrected by platelet infusions.
3. Exchange transfusion may be required for severe sepsis. Correct the acid-base status.
4. Monitor carefully for apnea.
5. Prepare infusions of dopamine and epinephrine (on pumps and at appropriate concentrations for an infant) for possible use intraoperatively.
6. Prepare syringes of epinephrine for possible resuscitation or treatment of hypotension.
7. Prepare syringes of calcium gluconate or calcium chloride for anticipated hypocalcemia during rapid infusion of blood products.

Perioperative

1. Observe all special precautions for the preterm infant. Reliable intravenous routes and an arterial line are essential. Ensure that all monitors are functioning well before surgery commences.
2. Use of fentanyl (10 to 12 µg/kg) and ventilation with appropriate concentrations of O_2 is the preferred method. (Avoid N_2O to prevent expanding intramural bowel gas.)
3. Administer muscle relaxant as required.
4. Continue fluid resuscitation throughout surgery as dictated by clinical status and laboratory studies. Warm all intravenous fluids.
5. Anticipate that major fluid infusions may be required to maintain cardiovascular homeostasis when the abdomen is opened. Carefully

monitor the BP and infuse adequate volumes of appropriate crystalloid and colloid to correct hypotension.

6. Anticipate the possibility of massive rapid blood loss. Be prepared.
7. Anticipate the possible need for vasopressors. Have them set up and in place ready for emergent use.
8. Anticipate possible severe hypocalcemia if rapid infusion of blood products (FFP or platelets) are needed.

Postoperative

1. Return the infant to the neonatal ICU for continued management of possible multisystem dysfunction (cardiac, pulmonary, renal, etc.).

Suggested Reading

Kafetzis DA, Skevaki C, Costalos C: Neonatal necrotizing enterocolitis: an overview, Curr Opin Infect Dis 16(4):349–355, 2003.
Spaeth JP, O'Hara IB, Kurth CD: Anesthesia for the micropremie, Semin Perinatol 22(5):390–401, 1998.

OTHER MAJOR THORACOABDOMINAL LESIONS AND PROCEDURES

Neuroblastoma and Ganglioneuroma

Neuroblastoma is the most common solid malignant tumor of infancy. More than 50% of such tumors appear in the retroperitoneal space, but they may occur anywhere along the sympathetic chain. Four stages of the disease are described: Stage 1, limited to the primary site; stage 2, extension from primary but not across the midline; stage 3, beyond the midline; and stage 4, beyond the midline with metastases. Metastases are present at diagnosis in more than 50% of cases.

The diagnosis is sometimes based on fetal ultrasound. In neonates and young infants, the diagnosis may be made by palpation of an abdominal mass. The older child frequently has evidence of chronic disease, including fever, weight loss, and anemia. The tumor secretes catecholamines, which may cause hypertension, and a vasoactive intestinal peptide, which may cause watery diarrhea, dehydration, and electrolyte disturbance. The tumor may also cause symptoms as a result of its extension to involve other tissues; for example, the extradural space may be involved and neurologic signs may appear. The tumor may also wrap around or compress major vessels such as the vena cava or aorta. Most children have increased levels of catecholamines and metabolites in the urine (positive VMA). Computed tomography (CT) and magnetic resonance imaging (MRI) permit localization of the tumor and identification of metastases.

Treatment of stage 1 or 2 disease is by surgical excision. Stage 3 or 4 disease is treated by initial chemotherapy or radiotherapy, or both. Children with widespread disease may be treated by total body radiation, chemotherapy, and bone marrow transplantation.

Special Anesthesia Problems

1. Massive blood loss may occur during surgery, especially in those who had preoperative radiotherapy. Major vessels (e.g., IVC) may be invaded by tumor and may be a source of rapid blood loss and clot or tumor emboli.
2. Catecholamine levels are usually increased and hypertension may be present, but cardiac arrhythmias are unusual. Those very rare children with severe hypertension should be assumed to have a contracted blood volume and may benefit from preoperative preparation as outlined for pheochromocytoma.
3. Thoracic tumors may compress the lungs and produce respiratory failure. Cervical tumors may displace the trachea and compress the airway.
4. Children with extension to the extradural space (dumb-bell tumor) may need a combined abdominal and neurosurgical approach with laminectomy.
5. Hyperthermia (*not* MH) has been reported during surgery for neuroblastoma.

Anesthesia Management

Preoperative

1. Carefully assess the systemic effects of the disease on the child. Check the hemoglobin level and serum electrolytes. Check the results of CT or MRI for evidence of major blood vessel or neurologic involvement.
2. Assess the extent of hypertension and its control by preoperative therapy.
3. Administer appropriate sedation (e.g., midazolam 0.5 mg/kg PO or 0.05 mg/kg IV).
4. Important: Adequate supplies of blood for transfusion must be available, together with facilities to measure (and replace) large blood losses. Be prepared.

5. Anticipate the need for vasopressors. Have them available for emergent use.
6. Anticipate possible severe hypocalcemia if rapid infusion of blood products (FFP or platelets) are needed.

Perioperative

1. Observe all special considerations for infants.
2. Place monitors and induce anesthesia.
3. Maintain anesthesia with N_2O and isoflurane; avoid the former in abdominal procedures and the latter can be titrated to control BP easily.
4. Rocuronium or vecuronium are preferred for relaxation; they provide cardiovascular stability and minimal histamine release.
5. Establish reliable large-bore intravenous routes in the upper limbs or neck.
6. Routine monitors should be supplemented with an arterial line and a urinary catheter. A double-lumen line via the jugular vein provides for infusions and monitoring of central venous pressure (CVP).
7. Fluctuations in BP may occur during surgical manipulation of the tumor. These can usually be treated by adjusting the inspired concentration of isoflurane. Rarely, it may be necessary to use small doses (0.2 mg/kg) of phentolamine or an infusion of sodium nitroprusside (see page 638).
8. Be prepared to provide rapid infusions of warmed blood. A decrease in BP is common as the tumor is removed. This usually responds to fluid infusions. Be aware that hypotension might also result from surgical retraction compromising IVC flow.
9. If major blood transfusion becomes necessary, check coagulation indices and prepare to correct deficiencies.
10. Anticipate possible ionized hypocalcemia due to the rapid infusion of blood products (FFP or platelets).

Postoperative

1. In most children, the trachea can be extubated at the end of surgery; however, if the child is unstable, do not extubate the trachea.
2. Plan for optimal postoperative pain management; epidural analgesia is ideal for many children.
3. Continue to monitor volume status and urine output to ensure adequate fluid replacement.

N.B. Ganglioneuromas are benign tumors arising from sympathetic ganglia. They do not invade other tissues but gradually enlarge and may produce symptoms because of their size and pressure on adjacent structures. They do not generally secrete significant amounts of catecholamines or other active peptides; however, in atypical forms this may occur. In such a case, though preoperative catecholamine levels are normal, intraoperative hypertension may occur when the tumor is handled. Surgical excision is usually simpler than for neuroblastomas, but it may be complicated by the tumor's location and size. Many may be treated by endoscopic resection.

Suggested Reading

Seefelder C, Sparks JW, Chirnomas D, et al: Perioperative management of a child with severe hypertension from a catecholamine secreting neuroblastoma, Paediatr Anaesth 15(7):606–610, 2005.

Mayhew JF: Intraoperative hyperthermia in a child with neuroblastoma, Paediatr Anaesth 16(8):890–891, 2006.

Batra YK, Rajeev S, Rao KL: Anesthesia management of a ganglioneuroma with seizures presenting as pheochromocytoma, Paediatr Anaesth 17(5):479–483, 2007.

Lung Surgery

Lung surgery may be indicated for the following conditions:

1. Lung abscess
2. Bronchiectasis
3. Lung cysts
4. Bronchogenic cysts
5. Diagnostic biopsy (in children, usually to confirm or exclude infection by a virus or other pathogen)
6. Pulmonary arteriovenous malformation
7. Sequestrated pulmonary lobe
8. Pulmonary neoplasm
9. Chronic pulmonary infection

Special Anesthesia Problems

1. Once the thorax is open, major $\dot{V}/\dot{Q}$ inequalities should be anticipated; increase the FIO_2 and monitor SaO_2. Blood and secretions within the bronchial tree may compound this problem; if so, suction the tracheal tube frequently.
2. Major hemorrhage may occur suddenly if large vessels are accidentally cut or torn. Therefore reliable large-bore infusion routes must be established and blood for transfusion must be immediately available in the OR.
3. Postoperative pain limits coughing and deep breathing, especially in older children, predisposing to atelectasis. Plan for optimal analgesia (e.g., thoracic epidural catheter).

4. Pulmonary function may be seriously impaired, resulting in respiratory failure in some children (e.g., those admitted for lung biopsy). In such children, even minor fluid overload can precipitate serious deterioration in lung function postoperatively; be extremely cautious with fluid therapy.

5. Pus from purulent lesions (e.g., lung abscess, bronchiectasis) may become dispersed during surgery unless a lobe or lung can be isolated. Preoperative bronchoscopy to remove accumulated secretions is useful for some children.

6. Pulmonary arteriovenous malformation results in a very large right-to-left shunt, with consequent arterial desaturation that cannot be corrected by increasing the FiO_2.

7. Methods for one-lung ventilation are described at the beginning of this chapter.

A further alternative in the case of unilateral purulent disease, thoracotomy may be performed with the child in the prone (Parry Brown) position with the head slightly dependent. In this position, purulent secretions tend to drain out via the endotracheal tube and do not contaminate the dependent lung.

Anesthesia Management

Preoperative

1. Assess the child carefully.
   a. Evaluate pulmonary function as fully as possible (only limited data may be obtainable for children too young or otherwise unable to cooperate in the full range of tests).
   b. Check the results of blood gas and other available studies. Ensure that the child is in the best possible condition for the planned surgery.

2. Ensure that adequate supplies of blood products are ordered and adequate serum has been saved for additional cross-matching.

3. Ensure that appropriate respiratory care is ordered. For older children, explain the value of preoperative breathing exercises and the need for postoperative respiratory care.

4. Order appropriate preoperative sedation, taking care to prevent respiratory depression in children with impaired pulmonary function. Midazolam (0.5 mg/kg PO or 0.05 to 0.1 mg/kg IV) is often ideal.

Perioperative

1. Apply monitors.
2. Give 100% O_2 by mask.

3. Induce anesthesia by inhalation of either sevoflurane or halothane; if an IV is in place then propofol or thiopental followed by an intermediate or long-acting muscle relaxant to facilitate tracheal intubation.

4. Ventilate with 100% O_2 until the child is fully relaxed, then perform a bronchoscopy if indicated. Otherwise, intubate the trachea as required for the surgery and the child's size. If lung isolation is required, use one of the techniques described (see page 342).

5. Establish a reliable wide-bore intravenous route.

6. Insert an arterial line (except for "minor" procedures in healthy children).

7. Maintain anesthesia with sevoflurane or isoflurane in oxygen/air with opioid, adding sufficient O_2 to maintain the saturation at 95% to 100%. Nitrous oxide may be used if a gas-filled cavity is not present.

8. Control the ventilation (aim for a $PaCO_2$ of 35 to 40 mm Hg).

9. After the child has been positioned for thoracotomy, recheck the ventilation of the lungs.

11. Suction the endotracheal tube as needed.

12. If one-lung anesthesia is used, administer sufficient oxygen to maintain SaO_2 greater than 95%.

13. Periodically inflate the lungs fully during thoracotomy and as the chest is being closed, give several large breaths with high peak pressures while observing reexpansion of the lung. The surgeon may also fill the chest with saline and ask for large breaths to check for possible air leaks.

14. When the chest is closed, ensure that chest drains are appropriately set.

15. At the end of surgery, before extubation, ensure that the child is awake and responding and has adequate spontaneous ventilation. If in doubt, leave the tracheal tube in place and continue assisted ventilation until it is safe to withdraw this support.

Postoperative

1. Provide analgesia: A thoracic epidural block using bupivacaine with fentanyl is ideal and may be left in place for up to 72 hours postoperatively. Otherwise, intercostal nerve blocks plus an opioid infusion or patient-controlled analgesia may be used.

2. Ensure that chest drains are patent and are connected to an underwater seal and suction.

3. Order arterial blood gas determinations as necessary to assess the adequacy of ventilation.

4. Ensure that chest radiography is performed, and check the films for residual pneumothorax or atelectasis.
5. Order hemoglobin (Hb) and hematocrit (Hct) determinations to assess the adequacy of blood replacement.

Suggested Reading

Haynes SR, Bonner S: Anesthesia for thoracic surgery in children, Paediatr Anaesth 10:237–251, 2000.

Anterior Mediastinal Masses

Anterior mediastinal masses (AMM) (bordered by the retro-sternum, pericardium, xiphoid, and angle of Louis) may press on middle mediastinal structures (trachea/bronchi or heart (pulmonary artery, right atrium) resulting in impaired or life-threatening loss of function. Four tumors that are common in the anterior mediastinum are:

1. Lymphoma, Hodgkin disease, etc.
2. Teratoma
3. Thyroid
4. Thymoma (less common)

Tumors also arise in the middle and posterior mediastinum (e.g., neuroblastoma, ganglioneuroma, and dermoid cysts) although they do not usually present substantive anesthetic challenges.

Children with AMM may need general anesthesia for cervical node biopsy, indwelling ports, radiologic investigations or excision of the tumor. Consider local anesthesia or general anesthesia.

Special Anesthesia Problems

1. Acute airway obstruction may occur during anesthesia, even in children with no history of dyspnea. Tracheal intubation may fail to relieve the obstruction, advancing the tube into a bronchus may be required to establish an airway and maintain ventilation. This is especially likely in children with massive enlargement of hilar nodes or a direct tumor effect causing tracheomalacia or extramural tracheobronchial compression. Even during simple, minor procedures, general anesthesia may be extremely dangerous.
2. The AMM mass may compress the heart (right atrium and pulmonary artery), compromise ventricular filling, and cause acute hypotension and sudden disappearance of the capnogram.
3. Major blood loss may occur during mediastinal surgery.
4. Myasthenic children require special consideration.

Anesthesia Management

Preoperative

1. Assess the child carefully, and anticipate potential airway and cardio-vascular problems. A night cough and several pillow orthopnea are classic for upper airway compromise. The latter is a sign of potential disaster. Inquire about any postural dyspnea and which position gives the easiest breathing. Look for signs of superior vena cava obstruction or upper body edema. In some cases it is best to delay surgery until the size of the tumor can be reduced by a 12-hour exposure to steroids or radiation. Discuss this with the surgeon and oncologist.
2. Examine radiologic studies and pulmonary function tests:
   a. Chest x-ray. Use the posteroanterior (PA) view to diagnose a compressed, deviated or scabbard trachea (suggesting tracheomalacia).
   b. CT scan to define the extent of airway compromise; if the area of the airway is decreased by more than 50%, extreme caution is recommended (i.e., consider preoperative steroids or operation under local anesthesia). Evidence of main stem bronchus compression is ominous. Examine the potential for heart and great vessel compression by the tumor mass.
   c. Echocardiogram to assess the heart for structural (compression of the right atrium or pulmonary artery) and pericardial (pericardial effusion or constrictive pericarditis) involvement.
   d. Flow-volume loop, although most young children cannot cooperate well enough; if expiratory flow rates are deceased by 50% or more, extreme caution is recommended (see previous discussion).
3. For mediastinal surgery, ensure that adequate blood is immediately available and that additional units can be secured.
4. If there is any danger of airway obstruction, do not premedicate.
5. If airway problems are anticipated, prepare a full range of endotracheal tubes, stylet, and laryngoscope blades and have a skilled surgeon with a rigid bronchoscope present during induction.

Perioperative

N.B. Cervical lymph node biopsy in the child with a very large AMM that prevents the child from lying flat requires special consideration. Preoperative steroids or radiation for 12 hours should be considered. Node biopsy may be accomplished with the child in the sitting position using local anesthetic. If that is not possible or if another surgery is planned, general anesthesia may be induced using inhalational anesthesia with the child in the left lateral decubitus position.

For general anesthesia:

1. Establish IV access using local anesthetic or nitrous oxide.
2. Check that the awake child can tolerate the position chosen for surgery. Anesthesia should be induced by inhalation while maintaining spontaneous ventilation.
3. Breath sounds, the shape of the capnogram, and SaO_2 should be monitored continuously and check carefully after any changes in the child's position. If the airway obstructs or the capnogram loses its trace, before tracheal intubation:
   a. Intubate the trachea and turn the child to the left lateral decubitus position. If vital signs are not restored, turn the child prone. In this position, gravity pulls the tumor off the mediastinal structures. If anesthesia was induced supine and vital signs are lost, an alternative to turning the child is to have the surgeon apply towel clips to the xiphoid and suprasternal notch and lift the sternum to release the pressure on the mediastinal structures.
   b. Advance the tube past the obstruction-endobronchial if necessary.
   c. If this fails, perform rigid bronchoscopy.
   d. In extreme cases, emergency thoracotomy may be required.
4. Maintain anesthesia with N_2O and sevoflurane or isoflurane; spontaneous ventilation is preferable.
5. Monitor the cardiac rhythm during surgical dissection.
6. At the completion of surgery, check adequacy of ventilation before extubation.
7. If ventilation is inadequate, leave the trachea intubated and transfer to the PICU.

Postoperative

1. If applicable, ensure that the nurses in the PACU are aware that airway obstruction or cardiac compromise might occur in certain positions.
2. Order maintenance fluids and appropriate analgesia.
3. If blood replacement was required, check the Hct.
4. Obtain a chest radiograph in the PACU; check for pneumothorax.
5. Admit to the PICU for more extensive observation and monitoring if there is any question.

Suggested Reading

Anghelescu DL, Burgoyne LL, Liu T, et al: Clinical and diagnostic imaging findings predict anesthetic complications in children presenting with malignant mediastinal masses, Paediatr Anaesth 17(11):1090–1098, 2007.

Hammer GB: Anaesthetic management for the child with a mediastinal mass, Paediatr Anaesth 14(1):95–97, 2004.

Myasthenia Gravis

Myasthenia presents in three forms in infants and children:

1. *Transient neonatal myasthenia* occurs in babies of myasthenic mothers. The infant presents within a few hours of birth, usually with hypotonia and difficulty feeding. Improvement occurs within a few weeks although anticholinesterases are needed.
2. *Juvenile myasthenia gravis* (autoimmune myasthenia) usually manifests in childhood or adolescence. The disease may be generalized or limited to the ocular muscles. Abnormal fatigability, limb weakness, and ptosis are the usual presenting clinical features. The diagnosis is confirmed by a decreased compound muscle action potential on repetitive nerve stimulation, or by improved muscle power after an intravenous anticholinesterase drug (edrophonium).
3. *Congenital myasthenic syndromes* due to various defects of neuromuscular transmission may cause symptoms during infancy or childhood and are difficult to distinguish from autoimmune myasthenia without complex testing.

Associated Condition

1. Hyperthyroidism may be present.

Treatment

1. Anticholinesterase therapy produces symptomatic improvement, but secretions may become a problem; pyridostigmine is the drug of choice.
2. Plasmapheresis or intravenous immunoglobulin results in temporary improvement in many children and may reduce the need for surgery.
3. Prednisone and azathioprine have been effective in some children.
4. Thymectomy may increase the probability of remission, especially if it is performed early after the symptoms appear.

Surgical Procedure

Thymectomy is performed in some children with severe generalized myasthenia gravis who fail to respond to other treatment, even if there is no thymoma. The best remission occurs in young children with thymic hyperplasia. Extended thymectomy (i.e., complete) is considered the surgical management of choice; however, this can now be accomplished via minimally invasive surgery. This is preferred for the myasthenic child because it significantly decreases postoperative problems with incisional pain.

Special Anesthesia Problems

1. Muscle weakness may lead to ventilatory failure.
2. Treatment with anticholinesterases increases the respiratory tract secretions.
3. Potential sudden deterioration in muscle power may be caused by:
   a. A myasthenic crisis or
   b. A cholinergic crisis induced by excessive dosage with anticholinesterase
4. Postoperative pain may limit ventilation. Regional analgesia for postoperative pain is ideal (e.g., epidural analgesia).
5. Chest physiotherapy postoperatively rapidly fatigues the child if it is too vigorous.
6. Extreme sensitivity to nondepolarizing relaxants may occur. Inhalational anesthesia has proved very successful.

Anesthesia Management

Preoperative

1. The child should be admitted to the hospital for a period of rest, and anticholinesterase drugs should be reduced or withdrawn.
2. Ensure that blood is available.
3. Do not give heavy premedication—avoid opioids.
4. In children with severe symptoms preoperative plasmapheresis may be useful.
5. Consult with pediatric neurology.

Perioperative

1. Induce anesthesia by inhalation of sevoflurane or halothane or with IV thiopental (5 to 6 mg/kg IV) or propofol (4 to 5 mg/kg).
2. Deepen anesthesia with N_2O and sevoflurane or halothane, or with TIVA (propofol and remifentanil)
3. Do not give any muscle relaxants; intubate the trachea when the child is adequately anesthetized and after applying topical analgesic to the larynx. For VATS surgery a double lumen tube or blocker is required (see previous discussion).
4. Control ventilation. Continue with TIVA or nitrous oxide/sevoflurane anesthesia. If a thoracotomy is performed, discontinue N_2O.
5. Ensure reliable intravenous infusion routes for possible transfusions.

6. At the completion of surgery, allow the child to recover and resume spontaneous respirations with the tracheal tube in place. Check the vital capacity; if this is adequate (more than 20 ml/kg), proceed cautiously with extubation.

Postoperative

1. Close observation and respiratory care in the PICU is essential.
2. Reduce or discontinue anticholinesterase therapy (to lessen the likelihood of a cholinergic crisis).
3. Edrophonium testing may be performed periodically as a guide to anticholinesterase therapy (i.e., administer a small dose of edrophonium to confirm that this produces an improvement in muscle power). If there is no improvement, an impending cholinergic crisis is likely.
4. Use caution with opioids—regional nerve block (e.g., continuous epidural) is preferable.
5. Plan physiotherapy carefully to avoid overtiring the child. (Time the physiotherapy to take advantage of the increased muscle power after each edrophonium test.)
6. If fatigue and/or serious retention of secretions occur, intubate the trachea and control ventilation.

Suggested Reading

White MC, Stoddart PA: Anesthesia for thymectomy in children with myasthenia gravis, Paediatr Anaesth 14(8):625–635, 2004.
Bagshaw O: A combination of total intravenous anesthesia and thoracic epidural for thymectomy in juvenile myasthenia gravis, Paediatr Anaesth 17(4):370–374, 2007.

Splenectomy

See Idiopathic Thrombocytopenic Purpura (page 575).

Pheochromocytoma

Pheochromocytoma is rare in children (fewer than 5% of all cases); when it appears, it is usually in the adrenal medulla and is bilateral in 20% of children. The principal symptoms are headache, nausea, and vomiting, with sustained or, less commonly, episodic hypertension. Abdominal pain may occur. If undiagnosed, this might prompt an unnecessary and dangerous exploratory operation in an unprepared child. The diagnosis is confirmed by the finding of increased catecholamines (or their metabolites) in urine (VMA). Sustained hypertension with vasoconstriction contracts the intravascular volume and increases hematocrit.

Associated Conditions

1. Neurofibromatosis
2. Thyroid tumor
3. Multiple endocrine adenomatoses (e.g., Sipple syndrome)

Special Anesthesia Problems

Note: Anesthesia is very dangerous in the unprepared child—extreme swings in BP may occur.

1. Management of the BP and volume status of the child can be difficult.
2. Major blood loss may occur from extensive surgery performed to locate and remove multiple tumors.
3. Avoid anesthetics that might increase the release of catecholamines (e.g., succinylcholine, pancuronium) or sensitize the heart to these substances (e.g., halothane). Pancuronium or droperidol may cause a hypertensive crisis. Drugs that release histamine (e.g., morphine, atracurium) should be avoided.
4. Good preoperative sedation and a smooth induction are essential to prevent release of catecholamines.

   N.B. Dangerous cardiac arrhythmias are extremely rare in children.

Anesthesia Management

General anesthesia may be required for special investigations to locate the tumor, and for its extirpation, and must be conducted with the same considerations.

Preoperative

1. The child should be treated with α-blocking drugs (e.g., phenoxybenzamine HCl, 0.25 to 1.0 mg/kg/day) for several days, until:
   a. BP is consistently normal or there are signs or symptoms of postural hypotension.
   b. Hematocrit has decreased (indicating expansion of intravascular volume).

It is not necessary to administer a β-blocker to children; ß-blockers are contraindicated when incomplete α-blockade is present (most of the time in children). (β-blockade without α-blockade may lead to cardiac failure.)

2. Ensure that adequate supplies of blood are available.
3. Check that drugs are at hand to treat any blood pressure disturbance or cardiac rhythm, including
   a. Phentolamine—to decrease BP (usually necessary)
   b. Isoproterenol—to increase heart rate
   c. Norepinephrine—to increase BP
4. Give adequate premedication (e.g., midazolam, 0.75 mg/kg PO) on the ward to prevent undue anxiety.

Perioperative

1. If the child appears apprehensive on arrival in the OR anteroom, give supplemental doses of midazolam intravenously (0.05 mg/kg) until the desired level of sedation is achieved before entering the OR.
2. Apply standard monitors.
3. Induce anesthesia with titrated doses of either propofol or thiopental.
4. Give rocuronium (0.6 to 1.0 mg/kg) or vecuronium (0.1 mg/kg) IV.
5. Ventilate with N_2O, O_2, and a clinically indicated dose of sevoflurane or isoflurane.
6. Give lidocaine 1.5 mg/kg IV and a dose of fentanyl and when the child is fully relaxed, intubate the trachea.
7. Maintain anesthesia with N_2O, O_2, and either isoflurane or sevoflurane with controlled ventilation.
8. Establish arterial and CVP access for monitoring. An epidural catheter may be useful to supplement intraoperative analgesia, postoperative pain control, and to improve hemodynamic stability. If so, be prepared to infuse intravenous fluids and/or initiate a Neo-Synephrine infusion as necessary as the block becomes established.
9. Infuse fentanyl 5 µg/kg when surgery commences and continue with an infusion of 2 µg/kg/hr.
10. When the tumor has been excised:
    a. Transfuse fluids rapidly to maintain arterial pressure. Large volumes may be required.
    b. Maintain CVP at 9 to 11 cm H_2O, and check the Hct periodically.
    c. If hypertension persists, suspect additional tumors.
11. When the tumor or tumors have been removed:
    a. Discontinue isoflurane.
    b. Continue anesthesia with N_2O, O_2, fentanyl, and muscle relaxant as indicated until the end of surgery.

Postoperative

1. Check blood glucose levels frequently. (Hypoglycemia may occur as a result of the fall in catecholamine level and a secondary rebound hyperinsulinism.)
2. Order maintenance intravenous fluids; these should contain dextrose.
3. Anticipate an increase in Hct as the effect of phenoxybenzamine wears off.
4. Maintain epidural analgesia or order analgesics as required.

Suggested Reading

Hack HA: The perioperative management of children with phaeochromocytoma, Paediatr Anaesth 10(5):463–476, 2000.

Ein SH, Pullerits J, Creighton R, et al: Pediatric pheochromocytoma. A 36-year review, Pediatr Surg Int 12(8):595–598, 1997.

Wilms Tumor (Nephroblastoma)

Wilms tumors constitute 50% of the retroperitoneal masses in children and cause 6% to 8% of deaths from cancer in children younger than 12 years. These tumors usually manifest as an abdominal mass; approximately 5% are bilateral. Abdominal pain and fever are common symptoms. Hypertension may develop, possibly as a result of ischemia of renal tissue adjacent to the tumor, but the BP may remain elevated after removal of the entire affected kidney.

Associated Conditions

1. Hemihypertrophy
2. Congenital absence of the iris (aniridia)

Special Anesthesia Problems

1. Massive blood loss may occur during surgery. Full hemodynamic monitoring should be instituted (arterial and CVP lines).
2. Surgical manipulations may kink the IVC and cause abrupt falls in cardiac output.
3. A thoracoabdominal approach may be required for large tumors.
4. The size of the tumor and previous whole-body radiation may impair pulmonary function.
5. Hypertension may be present (60% of cases) secondary to renin secretion. It may be severe in some children and may require preoperative and intraoperative therapy. Angiotensin-converting enzyme (ACE)-inhibiting drugs (e.g., captopril) have been suggested as most appro-

priate preoperatively. Vasodilating drugs such as sodium nitroprusside may be required during surgery.

6. Rarely, tumor may invade the IVC; in such cases intraoperative pulmonary tumor or thrombus embolism may occur.
7. A coagulopathy, acquired von Willebrand disease, may occur in association with Wilms tumor. This improves after resection of the tumor. Factor VIII concentrates may be required to reduce the bleeding time.
8. Anemia is commonly associated with nephroblastoma.
9. Large intraabdominal tumors are associated with delayed gastric emptying and regurgitation at induction of anesthesia.

Anesthesia Management

Preoperative

1. Check that an adequate supply of blood products is available.
2. Do not palpate the child's abdomen.
3. Consider the use of antacids and metoclopramide to reduce the risk of aspiration.
4. Anticipate a massive rapid blood loss. Be prepared.
5. Anticipate the need for vasopressors. Have them set up and in place ready for emergent use.
6. Anticipate possible severe hypocalcemia if rapid infusion of blood products (FFP or platelets) are needed.

Perioperative

1. Apply monitors and induce anesthesia. A RSI is preferred.
2. Start intravenous infusions in an upper limb or neck vein using a large-bore cannula.
3. Maintain anesthesia with isoflurane or sevoflurane, and a relaxant (rocuronium or vecuronium).
4. Insert an arterial line and consider a double lumen CVP to monitor volume status and provide a reliable route for vasopressors or vasodilators.
5. Beware of abrupt decreases in BP (due to surgical compression of the IVC). Notify the surgeon to desist immediately if this occurs.
6. If hypertension occurs (unusual), increase the inspired concentration of isoflurane.

   N.B. Significant blood losses may occur during wound closure: continue transfusion to match losses. (Do not relax as soon as the tumor is out!)

Postoperative

1. Hypertension may continue and may require therapy (e.g., hydralazine).
2. Blood loss into the wound may continue, requiring ongoing transfusions.

Suggested Reading

Whyte SD, Mark Ansermino J: Anesthetic considerations in the management of Wilms tumor, Paediatr Anaesth 16(5):504–513, 2006.

"Acute Abdomen"

In children, an "acute abdomen" most commonly represents acute appendicitis, intussusception, or perforated Meckel diverticulum.

Appendicitis

Appendicitis is the most common cause of acute abdomen in childhood. The concerns for the anesthesiologist are possible fluid and electrolyte disturbance (secondary to emesis) and the presence of sepsis and high fever. Adequate fluid resuscitation should be ensured before proceeding to general anesthesia.

Intussusception

Intussusception is the most common cause of obstruction between infancy and 5 years of age. A segment of bowel passes into more distal bowel and may become ischemic and gangrenous. Enlarged Peyer patches, caused by viral infection, may precipitate this lesion by providing the lead point. The diagnosis is confirmed by contrast enema, which may also serve to reduce the intussusception. If this fails, a second attempt at hydrostatic reduction under general anesthesia may be successful; inhalation anesthetics may facilitate the process by relaxing abdominal muscles, decreasing smooth muscle activity, and reducing splanchnic blood flow. Pneumatic pressure of air or oxygen has also been used to reduce an intussusception. In this case there is a risk of gas embolism, so N_2O should be omitted from the anesthesia technique. Laparotomy is indicated for peritonitis, failed reduction, and repeated episodes. It should be noted that occasionally significant and hidden blood loss may occur within the intussusception; some children will require transfusion.

Suggested Reading

Brenn BR, Katz A: General anaesthesia may improve the success rate of hydrostatic reductions of intussusception, Paediatr Anaesth 7(1):77–81, 1997.

Meckel Diverticulum

Meckel diverticulum is partial persistence of the omphalomesenteric duct, which is present in 2% of the population; it may provide a site for bleeding, perforation, or intestinal obstruction. Severe bleeding may occur from ectopic gastric mucosa within the diverticulum and may result in hypovolemic shock.

Special Anesthesia Problems

1. Full stomach: even if the child has been NPO for several hours (and even if the child has vomited), do not assume that the stomach is empty. Gastric secretions accumulate rapidly when intestinal ileus is present.
2. Fluid and electrolyte disturbances may occur secondary to vomiting.
3. The child may have a high temperature; this increases the metabolic rate for oxygen and compounds the risk should any interruption of ventilation occur. It also increases the maintenance fluid requirements by 10% to 12% per 1 °C increase in body temperature.

Anesthesia Management

Preoperative

1. Assess the child's general condition. Check the volume status, fluid intake, serum electrolytes, and urine output. Ensure that fluid replacement is sufficient to correct deficits and produce good urine output.
2. If the child's temperature is increased, avoid atropine or hyoscine.
3. Prepare and check all equipment for a rapid-sequence induction (Chapter 4) and have suitable assistance available.

Perioperative

1. Check that a reliable intravenous route is available.
2. Apply standard monitors.
3. Preoxygenate as tolerated
4. Perform a RSI; use an IV induction agent and muscle relaxant
5. Intubate the trachea as soon as the child has fasciculated and/or relaxed.
6. Maintain anesthesia with N_2O, isoflurane, or sevoflurane and a nondepolarizing muscle relaxant.
7. Children with high fever may benefit from intraoperative cooling, facilitated by the use of inhalational anesthetics and muscle relaxants.
8. At the end of surgery, stop all anesthetic agents and antagonize the relaxant.
9. When the child is fully awake, extubate the trachea with the child in the lateral decubitus position.

Postoperative

1. Order analgesics as required.
2. Monitor temperature postoperatively. Cool the child if fever persists.

Testicular Torsion

Testicular torsion requires immediate surgery. Therefore, in most cases, it is not possible to prepare the child. Always assume a full stomach is present.

Anesthesia Management

Preoperative

1. Prepare and check all equipment for a RSI (Chapter 4, page 98) and have suitable assistance available.

Perioperative and Postoperative

1. As for "Acute Abdomen" above.

Organ Transplantation

Transplantation of solid organs is now becoming common in children. Although transplantation (apart from kidneys) is limited to a few specialist centers, organ procurement may be performed in many hospitals. The anesthesiologist has a major role to play in the care of the donor to ensure that donated organs remain in optimal condition until harvesting.

Determination of Brain Death

Determination of brain death has been based on the following: the presence of deep coma, lack of brain-stem function, unresponsiveness to stimuli, together with a host of criteria (including EEG) that vary from jurisdiction to jurisdiction. Before brain death is declared, all local criteria for "brain death" in an infant or child must be satisfied.

Care of the Donor

When cerebral death occurs, a sequence of physiologic changes follow throughout the body that may compromise the survival of organs destined for transplantation. Hence, intensive measures to support these organs are indicated. The anesthesiologist will be involved in caring for the donor during organ retrieval. It is very useful to discuss management strategies with the surgical harvest teams as the goals of one (e.g., liver) may differ from that of another (e.g., heart).

After "brain death," the following occurs:

1. Hemodynamic instability: Widespread vasodilation occurs, and the child tends to become pink and hypotensive. This hypotension may be compounded by hypovolemia secondary to the use of diuretics for previous attempts at cerebral resuscitation. Myocardial function may also be depressed. As the brain stem fails or in the presence of raised intracranial pressure, hypertension may occur. In the gravest situations, wide swings from hypotension to hypertension occur.
2. Central diabetes insipidus leads to polyuria, dehydration, hyperosmolarity, and hypernatremia.
3. Arrhythmias, atrial or ventricular, are frequent owing to intracranial pressure changes, electrolyte disturbances, and myocardial injury.
4. Hypothermia is present owing to loss of central thermoregulation.
5. Coagulopathy occurs secondary to disseminated intravascular coagulation as a result of released substrates from a necrotic brain.

To counter these changes the following management regimen is suggested:

1. The circulating volume should be restored rapidly with large volumes of fluid (20 to 40 ml/kg). Overhydration should be avoided.
   a. Lactated Ringer's solution or normal saline. Use 5% dextrose in water if the Na concentration is greater than 150 mEq/L but avoid hyponatremia and hyperglycemia.
   b. Albumin 5%. Volume expansion to maintain the CVP greater than 8 cm H_2O and an adequate urine output.
   c. Packed red blood cells for Hct less than 30%. Warm all fluids to prevent hypothermia.
2. If hypotension persists despite adequate volume expansion, check electrolyte levels (Ca^{++}) and then commence vasopressors with:
   a. Dopamine 5 to 15 μg/kg/min first.
   b. Epinephrine up to 0.1 μg/kg/min.

Vasopressors should, if possible, be discontinued or reduced in infusion rate before organs are harvested to minimize the chance of ischemic injury. The use of dopamine in cardiac donors should be limited to that required to stabilize hemodynamics; excessive doses may deplete energy stores and damage the myocardium; doses greater than 20 μg/kg/min are contraindicated.

3. Renal function should be maintained by fluid loading:
   a. If urine output decreases to less than 2 ml/kg/hr, give furosemide 1 mg/kg.

b. For diabetes insipidus, give *either* 1-deamino-8-D-arginine vaso-pressin (DDAVP), 1 to 4 μg IV, *or* pitressin infusion, 0.01 to 0.02 units/kg/hr titrated to maintain the desired output.

c. Suitable electrolyte solutions should be administered to correct hypernatremia and hypokalemia.

4. Hepatic function should be preserved by maintaining oxygenation and perfusion.

5. Other measures:

  a. Measure esophageal and rectal temperature and maintain normothermia.

  b. Determine and correct acid-base and electrolyte status.

  c. Optimize ventilation (beware of pulmonary changes).

  d. Use careful aseptic technique. Prophylactic antibiotics may be used. Blood cultures are taken immediately before organs are harvested.

All of these measures should be continued throughout the surgical procedure of organ procurement.

Suggested Reading

Sarti A: Organ donation, Paediatr Anaesth 9(4):287–294, 1999.

Ali MJ: Essentials of organ donor problems and their management, Anesthesiol Clin North Am 12:655–671, 1994.

Otte JB, Squifflet JP, Carlier MC, et al: Organ procurement in children—surgical, anaesthetic and logistic aspects, Intens Care Med 15(Suppl 1):S67–S70, 1989.

Liver Transplantation

Major advances in the control of rejection and in surgical and anesthesia techniques have made liver transplantation an option for infants and children. A limitation is imposed by the lack of suitably sized donor organs, but transplantation of a portion of a living related donor organ or split liver cadaver donor have become possible alternatives. Common indications for pediatric liver transplantation include the following:

1. Biliary atresia

2. Metabolic disease (e.g., α_1-antitrypsin deficiency)

3. Liver tumors—The results are significantly better in infants and children older than 1 year of age who weigh more than 10 kg.

Special Anesthesia Problems

1. Major blood losses may occur requiring massive blood transfusion.

2. Intraoperative circulatory instability may result from preexisting myocardial disease, plus mechanical factors (surgical manipulation), electrolyte disturbances (K^+, Ca^{++}), acidosis, hepatic encephalopathy, and release of vasoactive and cardiotoxic factors on reperfusion.

3. Coagulation defects may preexist secondary to impaired preoperative hepatic function and are compounded by massive blood losses.

4. Metabolic derangements may occur including hypothermia, hypoglycemia (rare), hyperglycemia (more common), hypernatremia secondary to bicarbonate therapy, ionized hypocalcemia secondary to citrate, and hyperkalemia on reperfusion.

5. Pulmonary function may be impaired secondary to liver disease (hepatopulmonary syndrome), and severe hypoxemia may be present. However, this condition improves after successful transplantation. Restrictive disease may be present secondary to ascites.

6. Renal dysfunction may be present, as may hepatorenal syndrome, due to previous renal tubular damage.

7. Central nervous system dysfunction as a result of hepatic coma with increased ICP.

Anesthesia Management

Preoperative

1. Preoperative angiography to assess the vascular connections of the liver may require general anesthesia. Urgent admission at the time a donor organ becomes available is the norm.

2. Examine the child carefully to exclude the presence of acute disease that might influence anesthesia. Assess coagulation status and correct as possible.

3. Bowel preparation is performed.

4. Immunosuppressive therapy is initiated: high-dose steroid therapy and cyclosporin A administration.

5. Anticipate increased blood losses in children younger than 2½ years of age, in those who have had previous abdominal surgery and in those with increased prothrombin times, acute liver disease, bleeding varices, or encephalopathy. Be ready with a rapid infusion device.

6. Avoid intramuscular injections in children with coagulopathy. Midazolam (IV or PO) premedication is preferred.

7. Many children are at risk for pulmonary aspiration; possible recent feeding, delayed gastric emptying, and abdominal distention may be present.

8. Appropriate psychological support must be provided for the child and the family.

9. Anticipate the need for frequent (hourly) determination of glucose, electrolytes, acid-base, hematocrit and coagulation factors.

10. Prepare size appropriate infusions of dopamine and epinephrine.
11. Prepare infusions of fentanyl and muscle relaxant (pancuronium).
12. Prepare resuscitation drugs (dilute epinephrine, calcium chloride, calcium gluconate, bicarbonate).

Perioperative

First Stage:

The first stage includes mobilization of the diseased liver before its removal.

1. Apply basic monitors and induce anesthesia using a rapid-sequence induction. If a small intravenous infusion must be started for induction, insert the catheter in a lower extremity.
2. Continue anesthesia using air /O_2/isoflurane as tolerated, with fentanyl supplementation. N_2O is contraindicated because it may cause bowel distention and exacerbate an intraoperative air embolization. Control ventilation to produce normocapnia with positive end-expiratory pressure (PEEP) to prevent atelectasis.
3. Maintain neuromuscular block with pancuronium. All drugs, including fentanyl, pancuronium, dopamine, and magnesium sulfate, should infuse continuously via a central vein.
4. Insert at least three large-bore intravenous routes into the upper limbs and neck (20 gauge for infants, 14- or 16-gauge catheters for children; or 5 to 18 Fr double/triple lumen CVP line), and prepare rapid blood transfusion and warming devices. Insert an arterial line, preferably in the radial artery (the abdominal aorta may have to be clamped); and a urinary catheter. Place esophageal and rectal temperature probes. Remember that a multi-lumen CVP is not adequate for rapid blood administration because of the luminal resistance and that large bore IVs, rapid infusion catheters, or introducer sheaths are essential.
5. The child should be carefully positioned and padded. A forced air warmer should cover the legs and head.
6. Monitor blood gases, electrolytes, glucose, ionized calcium, Hct, platelet count, prothrombin time, and partial thromboplastin time at frequent intervals, performing as many tests as possible on equipment in the OR suite. Other studies of coagulation (e.g., thromboelastogram) may be helpful to guide replacement therapy.
7. During mobilization of the liver, major bleeding may occur (especially if postoperative Kasai), depending on the extent of intraabdominal adhesions from previous surgery. The intravascular volume should be replaced as necessary to maintain the CVP, BP, urine flow, and the Hct.

The surgeons generally will prefer that the CVP be kept in a lower range so as to minimize venous pressure.

8. Hypotension may occur as a result of manipulation of the liver on its pedicle and compromise of IVC flow, but it may also be a result of low ionized calcium levels. Mannitol (0.5 g/kg) may be administered before clamping to establish a brisk diuresis.

Second (Anhepatic) Stage:

1. When the IVC is clamped, venous return from the lower body becomes dependent on collateral anastomotic channels unless a venovenous bypass system is used. In this case, venous return is maintained but hazards of hypothermia, thromboembolism, and air embolism may be introduced. Venovenous bypass may, however, reduce blood loss and improve intraoperative splanchnic and renal blood flow, with associated reduced morbidity. Venovenous bypass is not usually used in infants weighing less than 10 to 15 kg because it is difficult to maintain flow in small cannulas and small infants seem to tolerate IVC clamping.

2. Hypoglycemia had been postulated as a problem of the anhepatic stage, but it is unusual because the dextrose content of infused blood products maintain normal to high blood levels. Monitor blood glucose levels frequently.

Third Stage:

1. When the donor liver is reperfused, the most worrisome physiologic changes may occur; severe hypotension, arrhythmias, heart block, and cardiac arrest. These arise from combined acute changes in acid-base and electrolyte levels and the effects of vasoactive and cardiotoxic factors released from reperfused, previously ischemic tissues.

2. To minimize these changes:
   a. Before reperfusion, the ionized calcium and bicarbonate (pH) levels should be increased.
   b. Volume expansion with crystalloid or colloid solutions to maintain a CVP greater than 10 mm Hg should be established. Further volumes should be immediately available for infusion.
   c. Rapid evaluation and correction of adverse electrolyte changes must be performed.
   d. Vasopressors should be prepared for instant infusion as required.

3. During the third stage, large blood losses may continue. Platelet transfusions are usually withheld until this stage to minimize the risk of vascular thrombosis in the transplanted liver.

4. The need to treat coagulopathy is based on both coagulation studies and observation of the surgical field; if oozing occurs, replacement therapy must be instituted.

5. Hypertension is common late in the operation and is often unresponsive to additional opioids and antihypertensive medication. It has been attributed to multiple factors: volume overload, impaired renal function, cyclosporine, and steroid therapy. Treatment with salt restriction, diuretics, and ACE inhibitors may be indicated.

6. There may be difficulty in closing the abdomen because of the size of the implanted liver and distention of the bowel. Ventilation may be compromised, and in extreme cases the use of a Silastic pouch to close the abdomen temporarily (as in children with omphalocele) may be required.

Postoperative

1. If surgery has been prolonged, the child is cold or unstable, he or she is returned to the ICU intubated, and maintained on IPPV for at least 12 hours. Pulmonary problems are common and require aggressive therapy. Some transplants may be completed within 6 hours, without blood and with normal homeostatic indices permitting extubation in the OR. A team discussion and decision as to the disposition of the child and airway management should occur.

2. In many cases, return to the OR is necessary to reexplore for continued bleeding, impaired liver perfusion, or biliary obstruction.

3. Renal function is often impaired, and hypertension may be a continuing problem. Acid-base and electrolyte disturbances must be anticipated and treated.

4. There is a high risk of infection, and careful aseptic precautions are essential.

5. Neurologic complications, manifesting as seizures, are common.

6. Acute rejection—evidenced by headache, fever, malaise, nausea, and abdominal pain—may occur in 7 to 14 days. Liver enzyme levels may rise and synthetic functions diminish. Modification of the immunosuppressive drug regimen is required. The use of living related donors may decrease the immunologic problems associated with liver transplantation.

Suggested Reading

Bennett J, Bromley P: Perioperative issues in pediatric liver transplantation, Intl Anesthesiol Clin 44(3):125–147, 2006.

COMMON MINOR SURGICAL PROCEDURES

N.B. Some children who require minor elective surgery have conditions that may complicate anesthesia and require special attention:

1. Anemia or an upper respiratory infection (see Chapter 6).
2. A history of prematurity and respiratory distress syndrome. These infants must not be considered absolutely normal even if they are now apparently healthy. See Chapter 6 for a discussion of these medical conditions.

Division of "Tongue-Tie"

If the frenulum is so short that the child has difficulty passing the tongue around the buccal sulcus, surgical division of the "tongue-tie" is probably advised. This is an outpatient procedure.

Special Anesthesia Problems

1. This is a very brief, minor procedure, but the surgeon must have good access to the oral cavity and a good airway must be ensured.
2. The surgeon may use one of several techniques to free the tongue: clamp the frenulum and then cut with scissors or cauterize the frenulum. Sutures may also be used.

Anesthesia Management

Preoperative

1. Premedication: sedative premedication (oral midazolam) if required.

Perioperative

1. Induce anesthesia by inhaled sevoflurane or halothane or IV propofol.
2. If the surgeon does not cauterize the frenulum, maintain deep anesthesia with 8% sevoflurane in N_2O and O_2 and hold the elbow of the circuit (facemask removed) over the mouth while the surgeon clamps the frenulum. Alternately, cut a RAE tube (distal end in the oropharynx) and insert at the angle of the mouth to insufflate gasses. (Both of these methods require ingenious attempts at scavenging.) Caution is advised with electrocautery and the potential for an airway fire; use an air/O_2 blend with the lowest FIO_2. Otherwise, a tracheal tube may be inserted. IV anesthesia is probably an ideal technique (it avoids the need to scavenge), administer intermittent propofol.

3. Suction the pharynx to remove blood. Apply lidocaine gel to the sublingual wound.
4. The child should be fully awake before extubation and transfer to the PACU.

Postoperative

1. Further analgesics are not usually required.

Inguinal Herniotomy

Inguinal hernia is the most common elective general surgical procedure in children. Because these hernias readily become incarcerated during the first year of life, their repair should not be unduly delayed in this age group. Once incarceration has occurred, conservative treatment is usually instituted. Virtually all of these hernias can be reduced, and then, after 24 to 48 hours, herniotomy can be performed.

If emergency surgery is to be performed as an outpatient procedure, select suitable anesthesia techniques.

The former preterm infant may benefit from spinal analgesia for herniotomy, especially if there is a history of residual pulmonary disease and as a means for reducing the potential for postanesthesia apnea (see Chapter 4, page 137).

Anesthesia Management

Preoperative

1. Assess the child's general condition carefully.
2. Infants at risk, with a history of prematurity, should be admitted for postoperative apnea monitoring (see Chapter 4, page 137).

Perioperative

The choice of anesthesia technique for hernia repair depends on the surgeon. There are pediatric surgeons who can perform a unilateral inguinal herniotomy in 10 minutes—there are also those who can stretch this procedure out to last well over an hour. For the faster surgeon, general inhalational anesthesia delivered by facemask or LMA, or spinal anesthesia is ideal; for more prolonged procedures, it is probably wise to use general anesthesia and intubate the trachea.

1. For general anesthesia, induce anesthesia by inhalation or with IV propofol or thiopental. Maintain anesthesia by mask with spontaneous ventilation and halothane or sevoflurane in N_2O/O_2.

2. For prolonged procedures, intubate the trachea after administration of a muscle relaxant, and maintain anesthesia with N_2O and sevoflurane or halothane and controlled ventilation.

3. Perform an ilioinguinal and iliohypogastric nerve block on the operative side (or sides) or a caudal block. Surgeons can perform these blocks during surgery while the nerves are exposed. Acetaminophen, 30 to 40 mg/kg PR is given before surgical incision, to prevent fever and augment postoperative analgesia. Opioids should generally be avoided because they increase the incidence of PONV.

Postoperative

1. Order additional analgesics as required.

Suggested Reading

Langer JC, Shandling B, Rosenberg M: Intraoperative bupivacaine during outpatient hernia repair in children: a randomized double blind trial, J Pediatr Surg 22:267–270, 1987.

Orchidopexy

Anesthesia management for orchidopexy is the same as for inguinal herniotomy.

A caudal block should be performed after induction of anesthesia, before the surgery commences, to provide for postoperative analgesia.

Circumcision

Indications for circumcision vary in different communities and from time to time. It remains a common (often outpatient) procedure in pediatric surgery.

Special Anesthesia Problems

1. Management of postoperative pain

Anesthesia Management

Preoperative

1. Assess the child's general condition carefully.

Perioperative

1. Induction and maintenance of anesthesia as for herniotomy. Facemask or LMA anesthesia is usually adequate.

2. Provide for analgesia postoperatively. Perform either or both of the following:
   a. Dorsal nerve block of the penis using 0.25% bupivacaine *without epinephrine;* maximal dose, 2 mg/kg.
   b. Apply lidocaine jelly to the wound.

Postoperative

1. If regional anesthesia is unsatisfactory, administer opioid analgesia (e.g., morphine 0.05 to 0.10 mg/kg), which can be repeated in the PACU until the child is comfortable.

Suggested Reading

Bacon AK: An alternative block for post-circumcision analgesia, Anaesth Intens Care 5:63, 1977.

Tree-Trakarn T, Pirayavaraporn S: Postoperative pain relief after circumcision: comparison among morphine, nerve block, and topical analgesia, Anesthesiology 62:519–522, 1985.

Heart surgery in children is performed almost exclusively for congenital heart disease (CHD). The incidence of CHD is approximately 6 per 1000 live births. The lesions listed in Table 14-1 account for more than 90% of all congenital heart defects. There are various classifications of CHD, but that given in the table is most useful for the anesthesiologist.

THE CHILD WITH CONGENITAL HEART DISEASE

Infants with CHD usually present early with respiratory distress and/or cyanosis and difficulty with feeding, or later with failure to thrive. Some malformations cause severe congestive cardiac failure during the neonatal period, evidenced by marked hepatomegaly. Cardiac failure results from the high pressures needed to compensate for obstruction to blood flow (valve stenosis or coarctation) or from high-volume flow through intracardiac or extracardiac shunts (i.e., ventricular septal defect [VSD] or patent ductus arteriosus [PDA]). Dyspnea may result from cardiac failure and/or changes in pulmonary blood flow.

The diagnosis of CHD in infants may be difficult; innocent murmurs are common, and serious lesions may be present with a deceptively soft

TABLE 14-1   Incidence of Congenital Heart Disease

Type of Lesion	Frequency (%)*
Lesions With Increased Pulmonary Blood Flow	
Ventricular septal defect (VSD)	16.6
Patent ductus arteriosus (PDA)	6.5
Endocardial cushion defect (AV canal)	5.3
Atrial septal defect (ASD)	3.1
Truncus arteriosus	1.5
Cyanotic Lesions	
Hypoplastic left ventricle	7.9
Tetralogy of Fallot	3.5
Transposition of great arteries	2.5
Tricuspid atresia	1.5
Obstructive Lesions	
Coarctation of the aorta	8.0
Pulmonary stenosis	3.5
Aortic stenosis	2.0

* Frequency of lesions symptomatic in the first year of life.
(From Fyler DC, Buckley LP, Hellenbrand WE et al: Report of the New England Regional Infant Cardiac Program. Pediatrics 65(Suppl):388, 1980, with permission.)

murmur (see page 460). The physiology of the neonatal cardiovascular system may obscure significant lesions; for example, increased PVR may limit left-to-right shunts, and a PDA may mask coarctation of the aorta. An ECHO is essential to make a definitive diagnosis and should be requested whenever CHD is suspected.

Older infants and children with CHD may have reduced exercise tolerance, chest pain, or syncope. Alternatively, a murmur may be discovered on routine medical examination. Children with CHD often experience repeated respiratory infections.

General Systemic Effects

Usually the child's height and weight are below average. Children with CHD, and especially those with cyanotic CHD, may also demonstrate some developmental delay. The underweight child with CHD, however, has a metabolic rate that is considerably greater than predicted from size or weight. Infants with cyanotic CHD are unable to increase their metabolic rate to meet the demands of physiologic stress (e.g., cooling) and hence tolerate such stress poorly.

Effects on the Respiratory System

CHD can have major effects on pulmonary function. Enlarged vessels or chambers of the heart may compress major airways.

Increased pulmonary blood flow results in small airway obstruction, decreased compliance, increased resistance, and ventilation-perfusion $\dot{V}/\dot{Q}$ imbalance. Excess pulmonary blood flow eventually results in irreversible pulmonary hypertension secondary to structural changes in the vessels; these include medial muscle hypertrophy and peripheral extension of the muscular layer into normally nonmuscular arterioles. These vascular changes may be prevented by pulmonary artery (PA) banding or more commonly by total repair during early life.

Children with decreased pulmonary blood flow have less efficient ventilation, requiring increased minute ventilation to eliminate carbon dioxide. The gradient between end-tidal and arterial carbon dioxide levels may be increased. The uptake of inhaled anesthetics into the blood is delayed; however, alveolar (and hence end-tidal) levels may rise rapidly. Cyanosis is associated with a reduced ventilatory response to hypoxemia.

Effects on the Heart

In addition to the special characteristics of the child's heart (see page 29), CHD may impose other changes:

1. Obstructive lesions impose a pressure load on the affected ventricle. This ventricle then hypertrophies (becomes less compliant and less able to increase stroke volume). The thickened ventricle is subject to myocardial ischemia and consequent arrhythmias.
2. Large shunts or valvular incompetence impose a volume load on the ventricle. This ventricle initially responds with an increased stroke volume but later dilates and fails. The dilated ventricle requires a high wall tension to effect pressure change within the chamber (Laplace's law); it therefore is vulnerable to myocardial depressants and cannot cope with additional loads.
3. Myocardial ischemia may result from reduced aortic diastolic pressures and rapid heart rates in some children (i.e., those with a PDA).

Effects on the Blood

Cyanosis induces compensatory changes in the blood: polycythemia and an increased blood volume. The increased hematocrit (Hct) may lead to thrombosis (especially cerebral) and abscess formation. Cyanotic CHD is also commonly accompanied by coagulopathy secondary to thrombocytopenia, impaired platelet function, and decreased vitamin K-dependent factors.

Effects on Hepatic and Renal Function

These functions are impaired in cyanotic CHD and especially in those children with CHF. Splanchnic blood flow is reduced. Clearance of drugs via the liver or kidneys is delayed (i.e., morphine clearance is reduced in many children with CHD).

GENERAL PRINCIPLES OF ANESTHESIA MANAGEMENT

1. Children with CHD and their parents are often very apprehensive and deserve careful and considerate attention. Older children and their families may have had to endure repeated surgery.
2. The techniques used must minimize demands on the cardiovascular system.
   a. Give adequate premedication to reduce anxiety, activity, and O_2 requirements.
   b. A rapid, smooth induction of anesthesia, with no crying or struggling, is very desirable.
   c. Give adequate doses of analgesics and general anesthetics perioperatively. Prevent tachycardia and/or hypertension. High-dose opioid anesthesia combined with good postoperative analgesia may favorably influence the neuroendocrine and metabolic responses to surgery and improve survival.
   d. Control ventilation but maintain normocarbia unless there is a specific indication to adjust the CO_2 tension. Avoid hypocarbia, which may:
      i. Reduce cardiac output.
      ii. Cause vasoconstriction and increase systemic resistance.
      iii. Decrease PVR and increase left-to-right shunts.
      iv. Shift the hemoglobin/oxygen (Hb/O_2) dissociation curve to the left and limit O_2 transfer.
      v. Decrease myocardial blood flow.
      vi. Decrease the serum K level, resulting in arrhythmias.
      vii. Decrease cerebral blood flow.

   Decide on an optimal level of ventilation for each child and maintain this level.

   e. Give adequate doses of muscle relaxants to prevent movement or ventilatory efforts, especially when the heart is open (danger of air emboli).

f. Maintain body temperature and prevent cold stress except when induced hypothermia is indicated.

g. When appropriate, consider left ventricular (LV) afterload reduction and/or measures to reduce PVR (see later discussion).

3. Optimal myocardial function and cardiac output must be maintained during surgery:

   a. Do not give agents that cause excessive myocardial depression.

   b. Adjust the fluid balance to maintain optimal cardiac filling pressures.

4. Prevent detrimental changes in cardiac shunts.

   a. Use anesthetic drugs that have minimal effects on SVR.

   b. Be aware of the possible effects of intermittent positive-pressure ventilation (IPPV) on shunts; avoid high intrathoracic pressures, but maintain the lung volume as necessary by the use of optimal positive end-expiratory pressure (PEEP). PVR is minimal at an optimal lung volume and increases at greater or lesser degrees of lung inflation.

   c. Drugs that produce a controllable degree of myocardial depression (e.g., halothane) may be useful when hyperdynamic ventricular muscle causes obstruction to blood flow and increased shunting (e.g., Tetralogy of Fallot).

   d. Children who depend on systemic-to-pulmonary shunts will desaturate if the systemic arterial pressure decreases.

   e. Anemia may increase left-to-right shunts. Conversely left-to-right shunting may be reduced by increasing Hct. Changes in blood viscosity have a greater effect on PVR than on SVR.

   f. Be prepared to use drugs or other methods to manipulate PVR or SVR.

5. Conditions that favor optimal myocardial perfusion must be maintained throughout surgery to prevent ischemic myocardial damage and subsequent impairment of cardiac function postoperatively.

   a. The duration of diastole and the diastolic pressure are important factors in maintaining perfusion of the myocardium, which is especially vulnerable if left-to-right shunting (causing low aortic root diastolic pressure) and ventricular hypertrophy are present. Inadequate anesthesia and analgesia produces tachycardia, which shortens diastole and therefore may impair myocardial perfusion. Replace blood and give adequate fluids to maintain the diastolic pressure.

   b. Maintain an optimal Hct to preserve oxygen transport to the myocardium. Significant anemia may compromise subendocardial blood flow.

   c. During CPB, it is preferable to maintain a regular rhythm until the aorta is cross-clamped and cardioplegia is induced; this preserves myocardial perfusion. If ventricular fibrillation occurs, greater perfusion pressures and an LV vent are needed to ensure adequate myocardial perfusion.

6. The cardiac workload must be minimized:
   a. Prevent hypertension and tachycardia during anesthesia by ensuring adequate analgesia and the use of vasodilators and/or β-adrenergic blocking drugs when appropriate.
   b. Avoid excessive doses of drugs that may produce hypertension (e.g., phenylephrine).
   c. Pulmonary hypertension must be controlled.

7. Heparin has a larger volume of distribution and a more rapid plasma clearance in infants than in adults. Therefore larger doses may be required initially, an activated clotting time (ACT) of 480 seconds or more is required before CPB, and the level of heparinization should be checked frequently (every 30 minutes). An ACT of 480 seconds is the commonly used threshold value to attain before and during CPB. However, some have questioned whether this is adequate to prevent thrombin formation in the hemodiluted, hypothermic infant, and suggest that a higher ACT is more appropriate (i.e., 600 seconds). Kaolin-activated ACT appears to produce more reproducible ACT results than Celite activated ACT. The determination of blood heparin levels* may provide a better means to monitor heparinization and is being performed in some units.

8. During CPB, the myocardium may be protected by:
   a. Cardioplegic solutions that are infused at a pressure of 100 to 150 mm Hg into the coronary circulation after aortic clamping. Controversy still exists concerning the most advantageous type of solution, and this may differ in infants and adults. Most solutions contain increased concentrations of potassium with added dextrose and pH buffers. The addition of free radical scavenger agents and calcium ion channel blockers has been suggested. The ideal cardioplegic solution:

      i. Produces immediate arrest and prevents energy depletion.
      ii. Provides substrate for anaerobic metabolism.
      iii. Buffers metabolic acidosis in the tissue.
      iv. Minimizes tissue edema by its osmolar effects.
      v. Stabilizes cell membranes.
      vi. Minimizes reperfusion injury.

---

* Hepcon, Medtronic, Minneapolis.

Blood cardioplegia is preferred by many institutions. Repeated doses of cardioplegic solution are normally given at 15- to 20-minute intervals.

  b. Hypothermia. Remember that the heart has a great tendency to rewarm because of surgical manipulation and heat from operating room lights. Therefore, during prolonged surgery, cold cardioplegic solutions should be repeatedly applied, and a pericardial cooling bath should be used.
  c. Pre-CPB systemic corticosteroids may help preserve myocardial tissue during periods of ischemic arrest, but this is controversial.
  d. An optimal reperfusate solution may be used after a period of ischemic arrest. This may flush out metabolites and prevent reperfusion injury. This solution should be warmed and alkaline and should contain a minimal concentration of ionized calcium and a slightly increased potassium concentration. In practice, a repeat dose of warmed cardioplegic solution is often given just before reperfusion.
9. After CPB, small infants and children may bleed excessively owing to dilutional thrombocytopenia and reduced concentrations of coagulation factors. This is primarily a result of the large pump-priming volume in relation to the child's blood volume. Be prepared to administer platelets and other factors as required. Fresh whole blood, if available, may be particularly advantageous in small infants. Make sure that infants do not cool after weaning from CPB; coagulopathy may result.

SPECIAL PROBLEMS

Large shunts may be present.

1. Right-to-left shunts result in:
  a. Reduced PaO_2. This is often only minimally improved by increasing the FiO_2.
  b. Delayed uptake of inhaled anesthetics into the blood.
  c. Extreme danger of systemic emboli from venous air embolism. Make certain all IV solutions are bubble free.
  d. Short arm-brain circulation time, with no pulmonary transit; therefore there is a danger of overdose with intravenous drugs.
  e. Less efficient ventilation and gas exchange; increased ventilation is necessary to maintain a normal $PaCO_2$, whether the child is awake or anesthetized.
  f. An increased arterial to $EtCO_2$ gradient; $EtCO_2$ levels underestimate arterial levels.

2. Left-to-right shunts result in:
   a. Pulmonary vascular overperfusion but good ventilatory efficiency and gas exchange initially.
   b. Later, pulmonary hypertension develops and progresses to irreversible increased PVR, which may limit the operability of associated cardiac lesions.
   c. Eventual CHF.
3. Obstructive lesions may result in:
   a. Fixed cardiac output, and therefore very limited ability to compensate for changes in metabolic demand or a decrease in SVR.
   b. Myocardial hypertrophy, with possible inadequacy of myocardial perfusion, especially to the subendocardium. Reduced ventricular compliance results in dependence on a high cardiac filling pressure.
   c. CHF.
   d. Sudden serious arrhythmias.
4. Heart failure is common in infants with CHD and is worsened by drugs that depress the myocardium (e.g., inhalational anesthetics).
5. Electrolyte disturbance
   a. Serum electrolyte (especially K^+) concentrations may be reduced, particularly after prolonged diuretic therapy. (Hypokalemia predisposes to cardiac arrhythmias, particularly with digitalis therapy and during hypothermia.)
   b. Neonates with CHD may have reduced blood Ca^{++} and glucose concentrations.
   c. Reduced serum magnesium concentrations may occur and predispose to arrhythmias.
6. Drugs essential for CHD therapy can cause problems:
   a. Digitalis: the therapeutic index is low, and toxicity is an ever-present hazard, especially in young children. Check a recent serum digitalis level (therapeutic range, 0.8 to 2 ng/ml). Hypothermia and hyperventilation increase the risk of digitalis toxicity because the serum K^+ concentration decreases.
   b. Diuretics: may deplete K^+, further increasing the risk of digitalis toxicity.
   c. β-Adrenergic blocking agents: they may impair cardiac contractility; however, this is not usually a problem with therapeutic doses. If being used in the treatment of cyanotic spells, these drugs should be continued until the day of surgery.
   d. Calcium channel-blocking agents: these are not commonly used in children. If used in infants, they may cause severe, persistent myocardial depression. The combination of β-blocking agents with calcium channel blockers is very dangerous and should be avoided.

7. Polycythemia. A high Hct (greater than 55% in cyanotic lesions) results in:
   a. Increased viscosity of the blood and therefore increased cardiac work
   b. Increased tendency to thrombosis
   c. Further increased risk of thrombosis if dehydration or venous stasis develops
   d. Coagulopathy
   e. Predisposition to cerebral abscess

   Despite the dangers of polycythemia, these children depend on a high Hct to ensure adequate O_2 transport. Hemodilution to normal Hct levels may be followed by severe cardiovascular collapse. Hemodilution before surgery, if indicated, must be very carefully controlled and the Hct not reduced below 40% to 45%.

8. Some infants with large left-to-right shunts are at extreme risk of pulmonary hypertensive crises during and after surgery (e.g., truncus arteriosus, arteriovenous [AV] canal). It is important to prevent such crises because they are difficult to reverse. The measures taken may include:
   a. Adequate anesthesia/analgesia during surgery, and minimal handling of the child postoperatively.
   b. Controlled hyperventilation ($PaCO_2$ = 25 to 30 mm Hg).
   c. Fentanyl infusion (e.g., 25 µg/kg loading dose plus 2 µg/kg/hr).
   d. Sodium nitroprusside (SNP) infusion 0.5 to 5 µg/kg/min.
   e. Inhalation of nitric oxide (NO). NO has specific pulmonary vasodilating properties and is a very useful drug to control PVR. It does require special equipment for its administration. It must be mixed in the inspired gases delivered to the child in a concentration of 20 to 80 ppm; this requires equipment to monitor its final concentration in the mixture. It cannot be premixed in oxygen containing mixtures of gases because nitrogen dioxide (NO_2) will be formed, which is damaging to the lungs. It should be mixed with the lowest FiO_2 that ensures adequate Hb saturation to minimize NO_2 formation. NO must not be suddenly withdrawn because severe rebound pulmonary hypertension may result. Large doses may result in the formation of methemoglobin.

9. Some infants depend on the patency of the ductus arteriosus as a route for shunting of blood until surgery can be performed (e.g., TGA with intact septum, interrupted aortic arch). Prostaglandin E_1 (PGE_1) is used to keep the ductus open in such infants. An infusion of 0.05 to 0.1 µg/kg/min should be continued until the appropriate surgical procedure is completed.

10. Associated malformations. Many children with CHD have additional defects (e.g., cleft palate, Down syndrome, subglottic stenosis) that may complicate anesthesia and require special considerations.

11. Induction of anesthesia. Different induction methods may be used, but if well conducted, all increase SaO_2, even in cyanotic children; therefore, the anesthesiologist may choose whichever seems best and most appropriate for a given child. In our practice, an intravenous induction using an opioid analgesic, a very small dose of barbiturate or propofol, and an intubating dose of a nondepolarizing relaxant are usually preferred; this allows for good ventilation, rapid airway control, and very stable conditions. Use of a topical local anesthetic cream and suitable sedation facilitate the ease of venous cannulation. Skillfully applied, the advantage of inserting venous access outweighs the potential for upsetting the child. Beware of using halothane or other myocardial depressant vapors in other than very small concentrations. Ketamine has been commonly used, but an intramuscular injection always upsets the child and leads to stress and crying.

12. Muscle relaxants. Nondepolarizing agents take a longer time to reach maximum effect in children with CHD; a more prolonged period of mask ventilation may be needed before intubation.

13. Temperature control. Temperature control may be especially poor in neonates with cyanotic CHD; body temperature decreases rapidly if they are exposed to a cool environment. Vasoconstriction in the cold child impairs efforts at insertion of intravenous lines and may result in metabolic acidosis. Keep the child warm.

14. Sepsis. This is a major threat to the success of cardiac surgery; great care must be taken to observe strict asepsis when invasive monitoring or infusion lines are being inserted. This is especially important in children undergoing transplantation.

15. Repeated surgery. Some children need repeated surgery, which imposes a severe psychological stress on them and their parents. A very considerate, careful approach by the anesthesiologist is essential.

ROUTINE PREOPERATIVE, PERIOPERATIVE, AND POSTOPERATIVE CARE

Preoperative Assessment and Preparation

Review all the medical records, obtain a history from the parents, and perform an independent physical examination, especially of the cardiovascular and respiratory systems, ears, nose, throat, teeth, and veins.

Look for evidence of associated disease or dysmorphic features that might complicate the anesthetic management. Look carefully for signs of cardiac failure: tachypnea, sweating, and hepatomegaly in infants. Carefully determine the respiratory status to exclude acute disease that might compromise the child perioperatively. If the child had a significant lower respiratory infection recently, elective surgery should be postponed for 2 to 3 weeks because of an increased susceptibility to pulmonary complications during this period.

Review the cardiology notes, ECHO, cardiac catheterization, and angiographic data to fully understand the current cardiac pathophysiology. Note salient abnormalities and findings on the anesthesia chart. Review previous anesthesia experience.

Many children with CHD take several medications regularly. β-blockers should be continued up to the day of surgery. With rare exceptions, digitalis and diuretics should be withheld on the day of operation. Calcium channel-blocking drugs are very infrequently used in children but, if they are used, they should be discontinued the day before surgery.

If the child requires O_2 therapy and/or maintenance of the sitting position during transit to the operating room (OR), order these specifically.

Plan in advance for postoperative pain management. In those whose tracheas may be extubated early, spinal or epidural opioids may be most useful. In most other cases, pain can be managed by an intravenous infusion of an opioid and/or PCA.

Blood Supplies

During any type of cardiac surgery, blood must be immediately available in the OR. In many centers, ordering blood is the responsibility of the surgical service. However, the day before surgery, the anesthesiologist should ensure that adequate supplies of blood and blood products will be available by operation time.

Some children have special requirements. For example:

1. For cyanotic children with an Hb greater than 16 g/dl, plasma should be available.
2. For all infants, check that the available blood is <3 days old and has been tested for cytomegalovirus. Washed cells should be ordered for small infants to prevent the danger of hyperkalemia. Radiated RBCs or leucocyte poor blood may be indicated for some children (immune deficient or transplant children).
3. For infants undergoing CPB, ensure that appropriate quantities of packed cells, FFP, and platelets (1 unit/5 kg) and cryoprecipitate

have been ordered. Alternatively, fresh whole blood is considered especially advantageous, and is reported to reduce bleeding after CPB, but may be difficult to obtain.

4. For all children likely to require prolonged CPB (longer than 1.5 hours), ensure that FFP and platelets have been ordered.

5. Where "relatively minor" surgery is planned for older children and those with an initially high Hct, hemodilution with a clear fluid prime in the pump oxygenator may avert the need for blood transfusion. At the end of CPB, modified ultrafiltration may be used to remove the fluid prime and restore the Hct. Alternatively, the contents of the pump circuit may be collected to be reinfused postoperatively. (Blood should be ordered to be available on a standby basis.)

Premedication

1. Children with CHD require adequate preoperative sedation to reduce excitement, anxiety, and crying (and thus reduce O_2 consumption). Order a hypnotic to be given the evening before surgery for anxious older children and preoperative sedation for all infants and children greater than 6 months of age.

2. In recent years, an oral regimen has come to be preferred:
   a. Midazolam 0.5 to 0.75 mg/kg PO (maximum 20 mg) is very effective; allow 10 to 30 minutes for the peak effect to be achieved. Alternately, oral ketamine (5 mg/kg) or a combination of midazolam (0.25 mg/kg) and ketamine (3 mg/kg) may be effective. (Children given this mixture should be constantly observed and SpO_2 monitored).
   b. Lorazepam 1 to 2 mg PO is effective for the adolescent patient. This premedication does not usually decrease SaO_2, even in cyanotic children. However, the child should be supervised as sedation occurs, and a pulse oximeter may be used as the child becomes settled.

   Topical local anesthetic cream should be applied to a predetermined site for intravenous cannulation, covered with an occlusive dressing, and allowed to remain in place until effective and then removed before induction.

3. For cyanotic children with a high Hct, ensure that oral fluids are regularly offered up to 2 hours before the operation to prevent dehydration. Alternatively, maintenance IV fluids should be administered during the preoperative fasting period.

Suggested Reading

Doshi RR, Qu JZ: Preoperative and postoperative anesthetic assessment for pediatric cardiac surgery patients, Int Anesth Clin 42(4):1–13, 2004.

ANESTHESIA MANAGEMENT

Routine Anesthesia Management

Preoperative

1. Check all anesthesia and monitoring equipment before the child enters the OR
2. Have the following available in case of emergency:
   a. Sodium bicarbonate, 8.4% solution 20 ml volume
   b. Atropine (0.4 mg/ml) diluted in 4 ml N saline (0.1 mg/ml solution).
   c. Calcium chloride, 10% solution: 10 ml volume
   d. Epinephrine, 1:10,000 preparation: 10 ml volume
   e. Phenylephrine, 0.1 mg/ml: 10 ml volume

Solutions of inotropic drugs should be prepared, loaded on appropriate infusion pumps with appropriate initial settings and primed. These should be made in a concentration that will permit their infusion at a therapeutic rate without adding an excessive fluid load and set up in such a manner that a carrier infusion of balanced salt solution assures timely delivery. In practice, for small infants and children, it is useful to use a dilution that will deliver the required dose when infused at 1 to 2 ml/hr (see Appendix 3).

3. Check that preoperative medication has been given as ordered and is effective.
4. On arrival in the OR, gently apply basic monitors: pulse oximeters (one probe to a finger, thumb, or ear and one probe to a toe), precordial stethoscope, BP cuff, and ECG electrodes. Record HR and rhythm and BP. Do not prolong this process, especially if the child is apprehensive, but proceed carefully and rapidly.

Perioperative

1. Administer O_2 by mask. Often the child will be happier if the mask is held slightly away from the face. Use a high flow.
2. Induce anesthesia, preferably intravenously, particularly in children with right-to-left shunts, which slow inhalation inductions. For most children, fentanyl 2 to 5 μg/kg followed by propofol (3 to 5 mg/kg) or thiopental (2 to 4 mg/kg) given slowly produces a smooth induction with minimal cardiovascular effects. In small infants, precede the fentanyl by a small dose of atropine (0.01 mg/kg) or an appropriate dose of pancuronium to prevent bradycardia. For the very unstable child,

omit thiopental but give incremental IV doses of fentanyl slowly up to a total of 30 μg/kg with midazolam up to 0.2 mg/kg for induction.

3. Drugs given intravenously should be administered in small doses, *slowly*. (If a right-to-left shunt is present, they act very rapidly; but if the circulation time is slow, their effect may be less rapid.) Be patient and wait for the desired effect. Beware of overdose.

4. For tracheal intubation: give an initial dose of nondepolarizing relaxant and ventilate the lungs until relaxation is adequate; pancuronium 0.1 mg/kg, rocuronium 1 mg/kg, or vecuronium 0.1 mg/kg produce good intubating conditions within 3 minutes (see also item 9 in this list).

   NB: Be aware of the possibility of subglottic stenosis in children with CHD, be prepared to use a smaller diameter tube.

5. Use a cuffed endotracheal tube to ensure ability to ventilate well. The tube should pass easily through the glottis and subglottic space; otherwise use a smaller diameter tube. Carefully position the tube and check bilateral ventilation. The cuff does not usually need to be inflated in infants to prevent leaks at normal ventilator pressures.

6. Maintain anesthesia with a suitable mixture of N_2O/O_2 or air/O_2 (It is rare to require >50% O_2. If a large right-to-left shunt is present, an increase in the FiO_2 has very little effect on the PaO_2.) It is probably advisable to avoid N_2O in the child with pulmonary hypertension, although the effect on PVR is small.

7. If myocardial function is good, for simple lesions, low concentrations of inhaled agents may be used. Otherwise, for all complex lesions, add opioids in adequate doses.

8. Control ventilation to produce desired carbon dioxide tension. Note that $EtCO_2$ is a satisfactory means to monitor $PaCO_2$ in acyanotic children but may underestimate the $PaCO_2$ in those with cyanotic CHD. Always compare the $EtCO_2$ against the $PaCO_2$; the $EtCO_2$ can then be used to follow trends.

9. The choice of muscle relaxant during maintenance of anesthesia should be influenced by the following:

   a. Rocuronium and vecuronium have very little effect on cardiovascular parameters, have an intermediate duration of action, and, if properly dosed, can readily be reversed for early extubation. They are probably the agents of choice for many infants and children.

   b. Pancuronium (to offset the bradycardic effects of high-dose fentanyl) combined with fentanyl is useful for the very unstable small infant with a complex lesion.

10. Insert a nasopharyngeal and rectal or bladder thermometer. An esophageal stethoscope cannot be inserted if a TEE probe will be used.

11. Insert adequate-bore intravenous routes, an arterial line, a double-lumen central venous line (see Chapter 4), and a urinary catheter. In older children who may be extubated early, it is preferred if possible to place the arterial line and the intravenous line in the same upper limb (usually the left). The other hand can then be used to operate a PCA pump.

12. Give maintenance fluids as outlined in Chapter 4. All fluid administration should be regulated by infusion pumps. If the child was polycythemic preoperatively, plasma may be preferable to blood as replacement fluid, especially if a systemic-pulmonary shunt is being performed. In these children, an Hct of at least 35% to 40% by the end of surgery is usually desirable. Use a fluid warmer for all infusions.

13. For those whose trachea may be extubated early after surgery, consider the use of epidural or spinal opioids (see Chapter 5).

Open Heart Surgery

1. Follow routine management (see previous discussion). Cerebral function monitoring may be useful during CPB if available, especially for complex lesions. Near infrared spectrometry and transcranial Doppler have been found to be most readily interpreted.

2. If a TEE probe is to be inserted, monitor ventilation, SaO_2, the $EtCO_2$ curve, and the BP very carefully. Passage of the probe may compromise ventilation, displace the tracheal tube, and/or compress the major vessels, especially in small infants; it may also trigger autonomic reflexes.

The TEE has proved most useful intraoperatively because the exact anatomy and pathophysiology can be defined and the adequacy of repair assessed immediately. Residual shunts can be detected and valve function, ventricular filling, and contractility assessed. The flow in conduits or shunts can also be assessed. TEE probes are available which can be inserted into very small infants.

3. Maintain anesthesia with:
   a. N_2O/O_2 in suitable proportions to ensure SaO_2 at an acceptable level. Use air/O_2 for children in whom N_2O is contraindicated. Very occasionally, it may be necessary to deliver an FiO_2 <0.21 to maintain pulmonary vasoconstriction and prevent overperfusion of the lungs (single ventricle physiology). In this instance, it is desirable to be able to mix nitrogen with the inspired gases and to monitor the oxygen content of the delivered gases.

    b. If tolerated, isoflurane 0.5% to 0.75% or sevoflurane 2%, depending on the lesion, may be given and supplemented with generous doses of fentanyl.

    c. Children with a history of CHF who may benefit from afterload reduction will probably do well with minimal isoflurane (e.g., VSD with left-to-right shunt). Children with dynamic ventricular outflow obstruction who may benefit from a degree of controlled myocardial depression usually do well with minimal (0.5%) halothane (e.g., tetralogy of Fallot, subaortic stenosis).

4. Give incremental doses of muscle relaxants as needed. Administer an additional generous bolus just before bypass to ensure complete immobility.

5. Give maintenance fluids, such as lactated Ringer's solution according to body weight to replace the calculated deficit during fasting (if any) and maintain urine output greater than 1 ml/kg/min. Additional "fluid loading" before CPB has not been shown to be advantageous. Avoid dextrose-containing fluids; hyperglycemia may increase neurologic injury in case of cerebral hypoxia/ischemia, but monitor blood glucose concentrations in small infants to detect hypoglycemia.

6. Blood loss from sponges, suction, drapes, and blood specimens (i.e., blood withdrawn for analysis) must be measured, and the volume replaced. It is seldom necessary to transfuse blood before CPB unless major blood loss occurs during opening of the chest or dissection around the heart (i.e., during repeat operations). In repeat operations, warmed lactated Ringer's solution should be ready for infusion at the time of sternotomy; blood should also be immediately available in the OR.

    a. Aim to maintain the Hct near the preoperative level and the intravascular volume at a level to maintain CVP.

    b. If the Hct was markedly increased preoperatively, replace initial losses with plasma, but refrain from hemodilution before CPB. Excess hemodilution may compromise oxygen delivery.

    c. During venous cannulation in small infants, a significant volume of blood may be lost into the cannulae. Ensure that this volume is replaced, usually by transfusion from the pump oxygenator circuit via the aortic cannula.

7. Children with cyanotic CHD may benefit from the administration of ε-aminocaproic acid (Amicar), an antifibrinolytic agent, to reduce bleeding. A loading dose of 75 to 100 mg/kg should be infused before skin incision. Alternatively, tranexamic acid, 50 to 100 mg/kg, may be administered.

8. In children having repeat procedures, administration of ε-aminocaproic acid or tranexamic acid may reduce blood loss.

9. During dissection around the heart, watch the BP closely; arrhythmias are common, although most are innocuous. If hypotension or arrhythmia persists, ask the surgeon to desist until the condition corrects itself. Continuing hypotension suggests hypovolemia; thus fluid should be infused so that the child can tolerate essential manipulations around the heart.

10. If N_2O is given, discontinue it before cannulation to prevent expanding any potential air embolism.

11. Before the heart is cannulated, give the initial dose of heparin.
    a. 400 units/kg for neonates
    b. 300 units/kg for older children.

Give this dose and recheck the ACT after 2 to 3 minutes; the ACT should be at least 480 seconds before initiation of CPB. Small infants may require more heparin and demonstrate more variation in dose requirements than older children.

N.B. *There is much discussion in the literature concerning heparin requirements in small infants and in children and whether the ACT is a reliable measure of the adequacy of heparinization during CPB. Current practice in most centers however continues to be as is outlined here. Some centers monitor blood heparin levels (See previous discussion).*

12. Once CPB is established, the pump flow should be increased to establish a satisfactory perfusion. Indicators of adequate perfusion are the cerebral function monitor, urine output, and the absence of metabolic acidosis on repeated acid-base studies. In children with cyanotic CHD, perfusion pressures may be low during early bypass because of the child's decreased vascular resistance (children with cyanotic CHD have larger vessels) and the use of a low-viscosity perfusate. Those with tetralogy of Fallot may also have extensive collateral flow into the lungs. High flows may be required initially, but the systemic pressure will increase progressively, especially as cooling progresses. The use of vasoconstrictors is not usually necessary but should be considered if hypotension persists. When the perfusion pressure is low, it is vital that the superior vena cava (SVC) pressure should also be at or near zero. Any increase in jugular venous pressure in these circumstances may have a serious effect on cerebral blood flow. Monitor CVP carefully to detect any compromise of SVC venous return because of obstruction of the cannulae.

13. During partial bypass, ventilate the lungs with 100% O_2. Never use N_2O because of the possibility of expanding an air embolism.

14. During total bypass:
  a. Keep the lungs inflated at a low pressure.
  b. Add 0.5% isoflurane to the oxygenator to continue anesthesia and improve perfusion during normothermic bypass, or give additional doses of fentanyl. Remember that fentanyl may bind to the plastic components of the CPB circuit, so blood levels decrease precipitously on bypass. Do not add inhalational agents to the oxygenator during hypothermic bypass; the increased tissue solubility of the agent at low body temperatures may result in residual cardiac depressant effects after rewarming and during weaning from CPB. Discontinue inhalational agents 15 minutes before the end of bypass.

15. Hypertension in the adequately anesthetized child may be treated by injection of phentolamine (0.2 mg/kg). During hypothermic CPB, children secrete catecholamines; phentolamine, by its α-adrenergic blocking action, improves perfusion and delays the development of metabolic acidosis.

16. During bypass (partial and total), repeat the ACT every 30 minutes and give additional doses of heparin as necessary to increase the ACT to more than 480 seconds.

17. Take blood samples for acid-base, electrolyte, and Hct determinations every 30 minutes and just before CPB is discontinued. Monitor glucose levels in small infants.

18. Before discontinuing CPB:
  a. Inflate the lungs, suction the trachea/bronchi, and check ventilation by observing the movement and full reexpansion of both lungs.
  b. Commence pacing if the heart rate is slow or if sinus rhythm is absent; infants and children need an atrial contraction to maintain a good cardiac output at this stage. Atrial pacing can be used for slow heart rates with normal conduction. AV sequential pacing is required if conduction is abnormal. If AV block is present, it is usually possible to sense the atrial contraction and use it to pace the ventricle (AV sequential pacing).
  c. If the cardiac action is impaired, inotropic agents should be commenced at a time well before weaning. A combination of dopamine 5 μg/kg/min, dobutamine 5 μg/kg/min, and milrinone 0.5 μg/kg/min is a common initial routine.
  d. If the myocardial contractility is very severely depressed, start an infusion of epinephrine 0.1 μg/kg/min.
  e. All neonates should have a calcium chloride infusion commenced at 5 mg/kg/hr. Alternatively any hypotension attendant upon the administration of blood or blood products in the intensive

care unit (ICU) must be immediately treated by injections of calcium chloride. In our unit we have preferred to use an infusion to prevent delays in administration.

19. For children with pulmonary hypertension, the following should be established before weaning:
    a. A PA line to monitor pressure.
    b. Hyperventilation with oxygen
    c. Correction of any preexisting metabolic acidosis
    d. In some children with mild increase of pulmonary artery pressure, it may be useful to commence an infusion of SNP at 0.5 to 2 μg/kg/min before weaning from bypass.
    e. Add nitric oxide to the inspired gases if necessary to control high PVR.

20. As CPB is discontinued:
    a. Administer calcium chloride (10 mg/kg) to improve cardiac action if necessary. (Calcium should never be given until the heart has resumed a steady regular rhythm).
    b. Request infusion of blood from the pump, and infuse cells until the CVP or left atrial pressure is adequate (8 to 12 mm Hg, depending on the cardiac lesion). The Hct on bypass is usually less, and it is advisable to infuse a mixture of cells to increase the Hct to 30% to 35% as CPB is discontinued. In small infants, fresh whole blood is preferred; otherwise, an appropriate mixture of packed red blood cells and recently thawed FFP may be infused to restore the Hct and administer coagulation factors. Older children, especially those having more minor procedures, may be weaned at a lower Hct, given a diuretic (furosemide), and have the pump contents reinfused over the ensuing period. In this way it may be possible to prevent the need for blood transfusion.

21. If the child remains hypotensive despite a good rate and rhythm:
    a. Adjust the dopamine infusion (5 to 10 μg/kg/min). Larger dopamine doses are often required in infants compared with older children and adults.
    b. Dobutamine 5 to 10 μg/kg/min may be added. This drug also increases inotropy, but it may also increase heart rate and decrease SVR in children.
    c. Calcium infusion may improve performance in some children, especially small infants. It is required in children with DiGeorge syndrome.
    d. If all else fails, an infusion of epinephrine 0.1 to 0.5 μg/kg/min may be indicated.

22. Modified ultrafiltration may be employed after CPB has been discontinued. The bypass circuit is modified to withdraw blood from the aortic cannula, pass it through an ultrafiltration unit, and return it to the right atrium. Ultrafiltration removes fluid and filters the blood. This removes excessive intravascular fluid and increases the child's Hct. In addition, it may remove some inflammatory substances released during CPB. It has been suggested that modified ultrafiltration may reduce bleeding and enhance postoperative cardiopulmonary function.

23. When the child's condition is stable and the cannulas have been removed, give protamine slowly, preferably via a peripheral intravenous route. Common practice is to give a dose of protamine (mg/kg) equal to that of the heparin (per 100 U/kg), which was administered before bypass. If hypotension occurs after protamine it usually can be reversed by calcium.

24. At 20 minutes after CPB, take blood samples for coagulation studies, electrolytes, and blood gases. Repeat ACT and give more protamine if indicated.

25. If bleeding persists, give platelets (1 unit/5 kg), FFP (20 ml/kg), and/or cryoprecipitate, according to coagulation indices.

N.B. Anticipate continued bleeding because of platelet dysfunction and other factor deficiencies:

    a. After a long pump run
    b. In children with cyanotic CHD
    c. In small infants, in whom the pump-priming volume is very large in relation to blood volume

All bleeding must be well controlled before the chest is closed.

26. After some complex intracardiac repairs, sternal closure may be delayed, and a plastic membrane sewn in place to cover the heart in the interim. This is appropriate when myocardial edema is present, as leaving the chest open prevents the constricting effects of the closed sternum on cardiopulmonary function and may increase BP and urine output while decreasing CVP. The sternum is closed when myocardial function is improved and it is judged that the child can tolerate this maneuver.

27. At the end of surgery, the decision must be made whether to extubate the trachea immediately or to continue with ventilatory support. The decision depends on the disease that was present and the intraoperative course.

28. The trend toward "fast-tracking" some children after cardiac surgery is now well-established; it may be combined with minimally invasive surgical approaches. After simple procedures (i.e., closure of ASD, resection of subaortic membrane), the trachea may be extubated in the OR and the child may be expected to have a very short stay in the ICU. In such cases:

  a. Employ an anesthesia technique that permits early brisk recovery; avoid large doses of opioids or ultra–long-acting relaxants.

  b. Plan for good postoperative analgesia; a single-shot caudal morphine injection is safe, effective, and easy (see Chapter 5).

  c. Ensure that excess pump priming fluid is removed by means of modified ultrafiltration after CPB is discontinued.

It may be more appropriate for some children to be transferred to the ICU for extubation on arrival or soon thereafter, depending on local circumstances.

29. Many children after CPB require postoperative ventilatory support.

  a. These include:

    i. Those with hypoxemia despite a high F_{IO_2}

    ii. Low cardiac output

    iii. Pulmonary hypertension

    iv. Diminished lung compliance

    v. Persistent arrhythmias

    vi. Hypothermia (<34 °C)

    vii. Continuing hemorrhage

  b. In such children:

    i. Plan for continuing IPPV and/or CPAP or pressure support ventilation. Controlled ventilation and CPAP are particularly beneficial during the immediate postoperative period; at this stage, the child predictably has a tendency toward reduced lung volumes and increased lung water (especially the infant). IPPV also permits excellent pain control by opioid infusion

    ii. *Do not antagonize the muscle relaxants.*

    iii. The choice of a nasal versus an oral tracheal tube for postoperative ventilation has varied from unit to unit. Children tolerate nasal tubes extremely well; they are less likely to kink and cannot be occluded by the teeth. They are also easier to secure at a specific depth. It has been suggested that nasal tubes might predispose to middle ear or sinus disease; this has not proved to be a major problem. The continued use of the oral tube removes the need to change the tube and proves quite satisfactory in some units.

N.B. If nasal intubation is chosen for the ICU, it is preferable to change the tube from an oral to nasal tube at the end of the procedure rather than pass a nasotracheal tube initially: this could cause a nosebleed perioperatively, especially when the child has been heparinized. During some surgeries, blood-stained secretions may accumulate in the tube. The change is then considered advisable to provide the child with a clean tube before transfer to the ICU. Ensure that the nasotracheal tube does not exert pressure on the margins of the nares or the nasal septum; necrosis, ulceration, and scarring can occur. The change to a nasotracheal tube should be made only if the child's condition is judged to be stable; otherwise, ventilation via the orotracheal tube is advised.

30. During transport to the ICU (all children):
   a. Attach a full bag of blood (or other appropriate fluid) to the IV line to ensure immediate replacement volume availability in case of sudden hemorrhage.
   b. Cover the child with warm blankets.
   c. Administer O_2 by mask or, if the trachea is still intubated, continue controlled ventilation with O_2. Make sure that the tank has an adequate supply of O_2 for the transfer to ICU.
   d. A battery-powered monitor should provide:
      i. Pulse oximetry
      ii. ECG
      iii. Intravascular pressures
      iv. $EtCO_2$ monitoring is desirable.
   e. Continue the infusions of inotropic drugs and/or vasodilators using battery-powered syringe pumps. If NO is used, this must be continued during transport and in the ICU. Beware of interruptions to the flow of any of these drugs during transport to the ICU.

Postoperative Management in the Intensive Care Unit

1. Auscultate the chest to ensure that ventilation is adequate when the ICU ventilator is used. Order a suitable FiO_2 concentration, and confirm ventilation and oxygenation by blood gas determination as soon as possible.
2. Ensure good analgesia; if regional analgesia has not been provided, order suitable opioids and sedative drugs:
   a. Morphine may be given intravenously as a continuous infusion (10 to 30 µg/kg/hr for children, 5 to 15 µg/kg/hr for infants) or less desirably, every 2 hours.
   b. Midazolam infusion 1 to 2 µg/kg/min or 0.1 mg/kg IV every 2 hours as needed.

3. Continue balanced salt solution for maintenance (with added KCL 2 mEq/kg/24 hr provided that urine output is 1 ml/kg/hr or more; otherwise withhold the KCL).

4. Check blood loss via the drainage tubes and instruct the nurses to replace this and further losses with reconstituted whole blood.

5. A chest radiograph should be obtained. Examine it carefully for pneumothorax, hemothorax, and atelectasis, and to ensure that the tip of the endotracheal tube is well above the carina. Check placement of all other indwelling lines; ensure that the tip of the CVP line is positioned at the level of the junction of the SVC and right atrium. (Cardiac perforation may complicate CVP line advanced to within the atrium.)

6. If bleeding persists order coagulation studies. Based on results, administer fresh frozen plasma or platelet concentrates as indicated.

Deep Hypothermia With Circulatory Arrest

Deep hypothermia with circulatory arrest is used for some neonates and infants undergoing cardiac surgery. It is particularly advantageous when surgery involves the aortic root.

Hypothermia is achieved by means of bloodstream cooling on CPB. The debate concerning the safety of profoundly hypothermic circulatory arrest versus continued perfusion is ongoing; many infants managed by DHCA and have shown little evidence of increased cerebral impairment as they grow to adulthood. However, many centers now prefer to limit the duration of DHCA and possibly to use antegrade cerebral perfusion (ACP) during aortic arch reconstruction procedures.

Anesthesia Management

Anesthesia management is as described previously, with the following modifications:

1. No dextrose-containing solutions should routinely be given because hyperglycemia may increase the risk of cerebral damage during total circulatory arrest. However, the blood glucose level should be monitored to detect and treat hypoglycemia should it occur. Large doses of fentanyl (more than 50 μg/kg) should be given and may limit the increase in blood glucose concentration that occurs as a metabolic response during hypothermic CPB.

2. Give methylprednisolone (Solu-Medrol) 15 to 25 mg/kg IV slowly, before cooling on CPB. Ensure that the child is given adequate doses

of relaxant drugs. (Once circulatory arrest has occurred, no additional drugs can be given.)

3. Phenytoin (Dilantin) 5 mg/kg may be added to the CPB prime solution as a neuroprotective agent.

4. After CPB is begun, ensure that the difference between the esophageal temperature and the temperature of the pump's output does not exceed 10 °C. Set cooling mattresses to 10 °C. Turn the room temperature down. Pack the head in ice bags.

5. The optimal management of blood gas tensions and acid-base balance during profound hypothermia has been the subject of much debate.
   a. The "alpha stat" approach measures blood gases at 37 °C whatever the child's body temperature (i.e., pH alkalotic when corrected for the actual body temperature) has been widely used in adults. Blood gas analysis shows a normal or low $PaCO_2$ during cooling.
   b. The "pH stat" approach corrects the blood gases for the child's body temperature and requires that CO_2 be added to the oxygenator gases during cooling. This has the advantages of increasing CBF and improving oxygen delivery and improves neurologic outcome in infants. It is now the recommended strategy for pediatric patients.

6. Administer phentolamine 0.2 mg/kg to improve tissue perfusion, ensure rapid even cooling, and minimize acidosis on rewarming.

7. When the esophageal temperature is 16 °C and the rectal temperature is <20 °C, CPB is discontinued, blood is drained to the oxygenator, and the venous cannulas are removed.

8. Record the duration of circulatory arrest. The duration of safe circulatory arrest at a given temperature is unknown, but it is generally preferred to limit it to 60 minutes at 15 °C to 18 °C core temperature.

9. Keep the lungs slightly inflated at 5 cm H_2O with an air/O_2 mixture.

10. When the repair is complete, the venous cannulas are replaced and the child is rewarmed until the esophageal temperature reaches 37 °C. The temperature of the blood from the pump should never exceed 39 °C, and the child's temperature should not exceed 37 °C.

11. Do not correct the metabolic acidosis often seen during rewarming. It will spontaneously correct as the child's metabolism resumes. Administration of sodium bicarbonate usually results in postoperative metabolic alkalosis.

12. It is suggested that the use of Hct levels of 30% during CPB cooling and rewarming may preserve neurologic functions better than with a reduced Hct.

Further Reading

Schlunt ML, Brauer SD: Anesthetic management for the pediatric patient undergoing deep hypothermic circulatory arrest, Semin Cardiothoracic Vasc Anesth 11(1):16–22, 2007.

Nelson DP, Andropoulos DB, Fraser CD Jr: Perioperative neuroprotective strategies, Semin Thorac Cardiovasc Surg (Pediatr Cardiac Surg Annual) 49–56, 2008.

PRINCIPLES OF POSTOPERATIVE CARE

Respiratory System

The status of the respiratory system after cardiac surgery in infants and children may be determined by the following factors:

1. Preexisting status
   a. Immaturity of respiratory system in young children (especially infants)
   b. Effects of the cardiac disease on the lungs
2. Effects of anesthesia, operation, and CPB on the respiratory system
   a. Decreased lung volume
   b. Increased lung water

Most children benefit from a period of controlled ventilation and/ or PEEP or CPAP. This assists in restoring the lung volume to normal and improves gas exchange. Levels of added O_2 and PEEP or CPAP can be reduced as the pulmonary status improves. Diuretic therapy may be indicated to reduce lung water. Special measures to control PVR may be required in children with pulmonary hypertension.

Cardiovascular System

After cardiac surgery, the cardiovascular status is determined by:

1. Preexisting status
   a. Immaturity of the heart and circulatory system in infants
   b. Effects of the cardiac disease on the cardiovascular system
2. Effects of anesthesia, surgery, and CPB, which are dictated by:
   a. Duration of anesthesia and surgery
   b. Duration of CPB
   c. Duration of induced cardiac arrest
   d. The success of myocardial protection techniques

After all but the most minor cardiac operations, a deterioration in cardiac function is to be expected. This deterioration progresses for the first few hours after the operation, probably associated with edema of the myocardium and other changes, which decreases the compliance of the ventricles and reduces contractility. Treatment at this time must be directed towards:

1. Ensuring optimal filling pressures. Because the compliance of the ventricles is reduced in infancy and reduced in all children after cardiac surgery, increased filling pressures (i.e., 8 to 12 mm Hg) may be required.
2. Producing an optimal cardiac rate and rhythm. This is most effectively achieved by the use of sequential pacing when necessary. Sinus rhythm (i.e., atrial contraction) significantly augments cardiac output.
3. Reducing afterload. The use of vasodilators in children with ventricular dysfunction increases cardiac output with little change in cardiac work or arterial BP. When vasodilators are used, the preload must be maintained by infusion of appropriate fluids; SNP infusion is commonly used to produce vasodilation (infusion rates start at 0.5 to 2 μg/kg/min and increase up to 5 μg/kg/min). Alternatively, milrinone may be used to provide afterload reduction. In some units phenoxybenzamine is administered to produce a long-lasting adrenergic blockade. Caution: some children do not tolerate LV afterload reduction well. For example, those with impaired RV function (e.g., after tetralogy repair).
4. Inotropic agents: If a low cardiac output persists despite these measures, resorting to an inotropic agent becomes necessary:
   a. Dopamine is infused at 5 to 10 μg/kg/min by infusion pump. In infants and children, dopamine has been shown effective in increasing cardiac output, *but*
      i. Larger doses are required than in adults.
      ii. The vasodilating effect is less than in adults. Hence the concurrent infusion of a vasodilator (SNP or milrinone) is usually warranted. The combined administration of dopamine and SNP may also be effective in reducing PVR in children with pulmonary hypertension, but it must often be given as soon as the child is weaned from bypass.
   b. Calcium is infused to maintain the serum Ca^{++} at a high-normal level (1 to 1.2 mmol/dl).
   c. If serious low output persists despite these measures, an epinephrine infusion 0.05 to 1 μg/kg/min may be needed.

Fluid and Electrolyte Therapy

1. Blood should be administered to maintain the hemoglobin level at near-normal levels (14 to 15 g/dl), especially when cardiac dysfunction is present.

2. Acid-base status should be monitored and acidosis corrected by sodium bicarbonate infusions.
3. Balanced salt solutions (i.e., lactated Ringer's solution) should be infused at rates sufficient to maintain urine output and CVP indices.
4. KCl 2 mEq/kg/day may be added, *provided* a urine output greater than 1 ml/kg/hr.
5. Hypomagnesemia may occur perioperatively, especially with aggressive diuretic therapy. Magnesium sulfate 1 meq/kg/day may be added to the intravenous fluid regimen if necessary.
6. If urine output decreases to less than 1 ml/kg/hr in the absence of hypotension, fluid orders should be reviewed to ensure an adequate intake, and a "fluid challenge" may be administered. If there is no result, a diuretic may be ordered (furosemide, 1 to 2 mg/kg IV).

Further Reading

Beke DM, Braudis NJ, Lincoln P: Management of the pediatric postoperative cardiac surgery patient, Crit Care Nurs Clin N Am 17(4):405–416, 2005.
Shime N: Contemporary trends in postoperative intensive care for pediatric cardiac surgery, J Cardiothor Vasc Anesth 18(2):218–227, 2004.

SPECIAL CONSIDERATIONS FOR ANESTHESIA IN NEONATES

Cardiac surgery in neonates should be performed only where the most expert, comprehensive medical and nursing care and all requisite facilities are available. The general principles of anesthesia in neonates are as follows:

1. Assess the child's condition carefully and ensure that the status is the best that can be achieved before surgery.
2. Ventilation may be indicated preoperatively, especially if heart failure or metabolic acidosis is severe. (Respiratory care is as important preoperatively as postoperatively.)
3. Metabolic acidosis must be corrected as far as possible by infusion of sodium bicarbonate together with efforts to improve the effective cardiac output.
4. CHF must be controlled as far as possible. The following therapy should be instituted:
   a. Optimal digitalization (check serum level)

    b. Diuretic therapy: furosemide infusion

    c. Place in a neutral thermal environment.

    d. Maintain slight head-up position.

    e. O_2 therapy to maintain PaO_2 at 70 to 90 mm Hg

    f. Correct any ongoing acidosis.

    g. In addition, if these measures fail:

        i. Intubation and controlled ventilation

        ii. Use of other inotropic agents (e.g., dopamine)

5. If the infant is severely hypoxic or in shock, correct the acid-base status, oxygenate, and administer methylprednisolone sodium succinate (25 mg/kg) with induction of anesthesia.

6. Control of body temperature is very important; avoid unintentional hypothermia.

7. If bradycardia occurs, assume it is caused by hypoxia until proved otherwise. Respond immediately:

    a. Discontinue anesthetics.

    b. Request removal of packs and retractors from the chest.

    c. Expand the lungs with 100% O_2.

8. If cardiac function deteriorates, suspect metabolic acidosis. Determine acid-base status and correct as necessary.

9. Ensure optimal postoperative care; all neonates require meticulous attention to respiratory care and constant, highest-quality nursing care, including

    a. Maintenance of body temperature at about 37 °C

    b. Avoidance of cold stress

10. Neonates should be nursed in a slight head-up position and moved frequently from side to side. Dressings and chest drains should be located to cause minimal restriction.

11. Controlled ventilation may be required for long periods. The infant with a soft chest wall is particularly vulnerable to decreases in lung volume and ventilatory muscle fatigue. PEEP or CPAP usually improves arterial oxygenation.

12. Atelectasis, particularly of the upper lobes, is a common complication. It is treated by aspiration of lung secretions and application of chest physiotherapy.

13. If the period of intensive care is prolonged, special attention must be paid to ensuring adequate nutrition.

14. Unexpected difficulty in weaning from ventilator support must raise the possibility of phrenic nerve damage during surgery.

15. The appearance of a pleural effusion in the early postoperative period suggests the possibility of thoracic duct injury.

SPECIAL CONSIDERATIONS FOR SPECIFIC OPERATIONS

Ligation of Patent Ductus Arteriosus

Patent ductus arteriosus is now usually treated by catheter occlusion (see Page 455)—general anesthesia is usually required to ensure absolute immobility—or by VATS (see Page 341)—exceptions may be made for the very large ductus in a small infant.

Older Infants and Children

1. PDA as the sole lesion in older infants and children usually presents few problems. The child is asymptomatic but ligation or catheter ablation is necessary to prevent potential later complications (i.e., pulmonary hypertension and cardiac failure, SBE, or aneurysm).
2. If VATS is planned, prepare for the possibility that thoracotomy may be necessary to manage bleeding. Always ensure that a reliable large bore IV route is available. Prophylactic antibiotics should be administered.
3. An arterial line is not considered essential. The BP must be monitored in the right arm; in the unlikely event of bleeding from the ductus, it may be necessary to clamp the left subclavian artery. Monitor SaO_2 in the right hand and a foot.
4. A single-dose of caudal morphine after induction provides for good postoperative analgesia when combined with intercostal nerve blocks by the surgeon. After VATS simple infiltration of the small incision sites provides good analgesia.
5. During the procedure, monitor:
   a. For bradycardia during dissection near the vagus nerve.
   b. For vital signs after ligation; normally the continuous murmur ceases and a soft systolic murmur remains. The BP (especially diastolic) may increase slightly at this time, but large changes are unusual.

   Major changes in BP might suggest that the wrong vessel has been ligated or occluded. If the aorta has accidentally been occluded, hypertension and loss of the oximeter signal from the foot will occur. If a PA has accidentally been ligated, the continuous murmur of the ductus will remain. If a bronchus has been ligated, airway pressures will increase and the murmur will persist unchanged.

   Intraoperative TEE may be used to monitor the closure.

6. Blood loss is usually minimal, seldom necessitating transfusion, but it may be sudden and massive if a major vessel is torn. Therefore check that blood is immediately available in the OR during the operation.

Postoperative Care

1. Routine postthoracotomy care should be applied. Good analgesia facilitates deep breathing exercises.
2. Rarely, the thoracic duct may be injured during PDA ligation. The resulting chylothorax may require drainage, and continued losses of chyle may impose a severe nutritional challenge.
3. Damage to the left recurrent laryngeal nerve in the region of the ductus is also a rare complication.

Preterm Infants

Persistence of the ductus arteriosus may occur in preterm infants, especially those weighing less than 1500 g. In addition to prematurity, respiratory distress syndrome, excessive fluid therapy, neonatal asphyxia, hypoxia, and acidosis predispose to this condition. PDA results in a large left-to-right shunt, with pulmonary vascular engorgement and CHF. Clinical signs include tachypnea, hepatomegaly, and "bounding pulses."

Diagnosis is confirmed by auscultation of the typical murmur, radiographic evidence of increased vascularity, and ECHO findings of a large left atrium:aorta ratio. PDA may prevent weaning from ventilatory support of infants with RDS.

Treatment for Patent Ductus Arteriosus

1. *Medical treatment.* Administration of indomethacin, a prostaglandin inhibitor, 0.1 to 0.4 mg/kg IV daily for several days may induce closure of the PDA. Indomethacin may also cause renal damage and suppress bone marrow. Therefore, it is contraindicated in children with renal failure or coagulopathy. Very small infants (those weighing less than 1000 g) do not respond as well with closure of the PDA after indomethacin as do larger, more mature infants.
2. *Surgical treatment (ligation).* This is necessary if indomethacin therapy fails or is contraindicated.

Special Anesthesia Problems

1. Observe all special precautions for the preterm infant.
2. Be prepared for sudden blood loss; the ductus is very thin and tears easily.
3. In some circumstances it may be preferable to operate on very small preterm infants in the neonatal ICU. This prevents transport problems but requires that the anesthesiologist adapt routines to safely administer adequate anesthesia and analgesia in the ICU setting. Check that the pulse oximeter and ECG function during electrocautery.

Preoperative

1. Assess the infant carefully. Anemia, if present, may predispose to CHF. In such circumstances, a transfusion of packed red blood cells may improve the cardiac status. The increased Hct improves myocardial oxygenation and may also reduce the extent of left-to-right shunting.
2. For those infants transferred to the OR, a heated transport incubator with a ventilator is required to maintain body temperature.
3. No premedication is required.

Perioperative

1. Ensure that the OR is heated and all warming devices are in position before transferring the infant to the OR table.
2. Attach monitors. Monitor SaO_2 in a preductal site (right hand) and in the foot; measure the BP in the right arm (see previous discussion).
3. Tracheal intubation:
   a. If the trachea is already intubated, ensure that the tube is firmly fixed, patent, and optimally positioned; otherwise, reintubate.
   b. If the trachea is not intubated, give atropine 0.02 mg/kg, fentanyl 10 µg/kg, and rocuronium 1 mg/kg or vecuronium 0.1 mg/kg. Ventilate with O_2 for 3 minutes and intubate.
4. Induce and maintain anesthesia with N_2O (in a concentration appropriate to ensure saturation) and isoflurane 0.5% to 1.0% or fentanyl 10 to 12 µg/kg.
5. Rocuronium (0.3 mg/kg) may be used to facilitate ventilation and prevent movement.
6. Establish a large intravenous line. Blood loss is usually minimal but can be catastrophic if a vessel is torn.
7. Give minimal intraoperative fluids. These infants are usually adequately hydrated preoperatively and do not have third-space losses.
8. Manual ventilation is often useful as the ductus is approached. Many of these infants have congested lungs and poor compliance. Watch for surgical retraction compromising cardiac output and oxygenation; if the infant becomes hypotensive or suddenly desaturates, ask the surgeons to remove the retractors.
9. Intercostal nerve blocks by the surgeons are encouraged.

Postoperative

1. Continued ventilation is necessary for most infants, with increased attention to respiratory care in view of possible postthoracotomy complications (e.g., atelectasis).

2. Improvement in respiratory status after ligation of PDA is dictated by the relative contributions of pulmonary vascular congestion and pulmonary disease (RDS or bronchopulmonary dysplasia) to the preoperative status.

Aortopulmonary Window

This anomaly presents a clinical picture much like that of PDA but is a result of failure of the aorta and PA to completely septate during development. The shunt is usually much larger than with PDA, and consequently most infants develop pulmonary vascular changes and CHF earlier. Repair on CPB is required, and pulmonary hypertensive crisis may be a problem postoperatively.

Division of Vascular Rings and Suspension of Anomalous Innominate Artery

Abnormalities of the great vessels may encircle or compress the trachea, bronchi, and esophagus. There may be a double aortic arch, a vascular ring that is completed by a PDA or ligamentum arteriosum, or an abnormal course of the subclavian artery. Severe compression by vascular rings leads to stridor and difficulty with feeding during early infancy.

The infant with a vascular ring often assumes a characteristic opisthotonic position. A chest radiograph with barium swallow is often diagnostic. Anomalous vessels may compress the bronchi and lead to gas trapping in an individual lobe of the lung, with compression of the adjacent lung by the resultant emphysematous lobe. Infants with vascular compression are prone to sudden cardiorespiratory arrest.

Children with repaired tracheoesophageal fistula are particularly prone to develop tracheal compression between the aorta and esophagus during feeding. The onset of symptoms of dyspnea and "dying spells" during feeding (i.e., parents report unresponsive infant, pale and apneic) is usually seen between 2 and 4 months of age. This condition is caused when an abnormally soft trachea becomes compressed against the aorta by a dilated esophagus. Aortopexy usually relieves symptoms, but in some children insertion of an external stent to reinforce the trachea may be necessary.

Special Anesthesia Problems

1. Respiratory failure may exist.
   a. Chronic or recurrent respiratory infection may have impaired pulmonary function.

b. Vascular compression may have resulted in emphysema of one or more lobes, compressing other lung tissue.

2. Airway compression may be at the level of the carina or main bronchi; if so, a normally situated endotracheal tube will not relieve the obstruction.

3. Endotracheal intubation may be required preoperatively to relieve serious symptoms. Air trapping in a lobe as a result of vascular compression can often be alleviated by the application of PEEP.

4. The use of an esophageal stethoscope in infants with vascular rings has been reported to cause acute airway obstruction.

5. VATS may be used for the procedure (see page 341). Be prepared for thoracotomy if problems arise.

Anesthesia Management

Preoperative

1. Order intensive respiratory care to achieve optimal pulmonary status. The infant should be allowed to remain in a position that permits optimal ventilation.

2. Bronchoscopy may be required to evaluate the site of airway compression and is useful for endobronchial suction.

Perioperative

1. For intubation, use a method that ensures a good airway past the obstructing lesion. If the obstruction is midtrachea, this is relatively simple. If the obstruction is low or at the carina, do one of the following:
   a. Pass a long endotracheal tube past the obstruction into a main bronchus. Add a side hole to the tube for the other bronchus if not already present. Or:
   b. Ventilate the lungs via a rigid bronchoscope (which can be placed accurately under direct vision and adjusted perioperatively if necessary).

2. Monitor the BP via an arterial line placed in the right radial artery. Operations on the great vessels can cause serious bleeding; establish a reliable, large-bore intravenous infusion route.

3. For aortopexy, a bronchoscope should be used to ensure that the compression is relieved. Compression of the trachea should always be assessed during spontaneous ventilation and coughing. If controlled ventilation is used, the trachea is held open and always appears widely patent.

4. If it is necessary to assess the airway during operation, use general anesthesia and spray the larynx with lidocaine before inserting the

bronchoscope. During the remainder of the operation, ventilation can be assisted or controlled. Do not give relaxants.

Postoperative

1. Order constant care with added humidified oxygen for at least the first 24 hours.
2. If residual obstruction persists, continue with tracheal intubation for 24 hours, then reassess.
3. Partial obstruction may be improved by placing a small bolster, 1 to 2 inches thick, below the shoulders.
4. Racemic epinephrine and/or dexamethasone may be required for postinstrumentation croup.

Suggested Reading

Kussman BD, Geva T, McGowan F: Cardiovascular causes of airway compression, Paediatr Anaesth 14(1):60–74, 2004.

Resection of Aortic Coarctation

Aortic coarctation (CoA) was classified according to its site in relation to the ductus arteriosus (i.e., preductal, juxtaductal, or postductal); it is now considered that all coarctations are juxtaductal. However, it is useful to recognize the two distinct presentations of CoA; in infancy with CHF or in later life with hypertension. The infantile type is usually accompanied by other anomalies (e.g., VSD, PDA) and manifests as cardiac failure in an infant < 6 months of age. In later life, CoA is usually diagnosed during investigation of hypertension in the upper limbs in preschoolers.

CoA is now usually treated by balloon angioplasty but surgical resection may be indicated for some children depending on local preferences. Controversy continues as to the optimal care, but there is some agreement that recoarctation is best treated by angioplasty and that long segment coarctation is best treated surgically. General anesthesia may be required for balloon angioplasty to ensure immobility (see Interventional Cardiology).

Coarctation of the aorta is now recognized as a life-long disease; later in life many children will have continuing problems with hypertension and its complications. This is thought to be because of alterations in the renin angiotensin system or baroreceptors, and is more likely in those with a long history of hypertension preoperatively.

Preductal (Infantile Type)

Special Problems

1. Most of these infants have severe cardiac failure and are being treated with digoxin and diuretics. Assisted ventilation is often required.
2. Severe associated cardiovascular anomalies are common.
3. Blood flow to the lower portion of the body depends on the ductus arteriosus. Prostaglandin (0.05 to 0.15 µg/kg/min) is infused to maintain patency until surgical repair is performed.
4. Hypoplasia of the arch of the aorta may be present and, if significant, may require repair with CPB (see later discussion).

Anesthesia Management

Preoperative

1. Blood gases should be determined and abnormalities corrected. Maintain prostaglandin infusion.
2. Ensure that supportive drugs are immediately available (i.e., epinephrine, dopamine).
3. Ensure that an adequate volume of blood is available in the OR and checked before incision.

Perioperative

1. Maintain normothermia.
2. While the aorta is clamped, do not allow the systolic pressure to exceed 100 mm Hg. In the (rare) event that a drug is necessary to reduce the BP, administer small concentrations of isoflurane and titrate this against the BP. A small dose of heparin (1 mg/kg) usually is given before clamping or balloon angioplasty. Check that the ACT has been prolonged to 250 seconds.
3. Be prepared to support the circulation when the aortic obstruction is removed; infusion of fluid and/or cardiotonic drugs may be required.
4. Prostaglandin may be discontinued once the ductus is ligated and the CoA relieved.
5. The decision to extubate the trachea at the end of the procedure depends on the conduct of the anesthetic/surgery.

Postoperative

The course is sometimes stormy. Therefore:

1. Transfer the child to the ICU with a tracheal tube in place.
2. Controlled ventilation is usually necessary for at least 48 to 72 hours.

Postductal (Adult Type)

Special Considerations for Surgical Repair

1. Clamping the aorta could compromise the blood supply to the spinal cord; hence the need to maintain an optimal BP in the distal aorta (~ 45 mm Hg).
2. While the aorta is clamped, severe proximal hypertension may occur and require treatment.
3. Hypertension can be troublesome postoperatively; this may be controlled by the use of short acting β-blockers during the perioperative period, but it may also require the use of SNP.
4. Although blood must be available for transfusion, few children require it. (Bleeding from chest wall collateral vessels is much less profuse than in adults.)
5. In the very rare event that severe proximal hypertension cannot be controlled after aortic clamping or if the distal pressure is very low, a temporary shunt must be placed to bypass the site of anastomosis, or left heart bypass must be used.

Anesthesia Management

Preoperative

1. Monitor BP and SaO_2 in the right arm. Place a second oximeter probe on a foot.
2. Establish reliable intravenous infusions at sites other than in the left arm.
3. Consider the use of an epidural catheter for administration of morphine and/or bupivacaine for postoperative pain management.

Perioperative

1. Maintain anesthesia with N_2O and isoflurane; use rocuronium or vecuronium for relaxation.
2. Place an arterial line into the right radial artery, and a central venous line; the latter may be used to infuse drugs as necessary to control hypertension.
3. During the period of aortic clamping, control the BP if necessary, by increasing the inspired concentration of isoflurane. The BP should not be allowed to exceed 140 mm Hg, but do not attempt to reduce the pressure if it remains below that level. Distal aortic pressure during clamp-off varies directly with the proximal pressure; distal pressure should be main-

tained at or above a mean of 45 mm Hg to ensure perfusion of the spinal cord.

4. The surgeon first removes the distal clamp and then (slowly) the proximal clamp. Monitor the BP continuously. If hypotension develops, infuse fluids; if this is unsuccessful, ask the surgeon to partly reapply the proximal clamp briefly. The BP may remain slightly reduced for a while, but usually it is back to above-normal levels by the end of the operation. Anticipate the need to treat postoperative hypertension by preparing:
   a. SNP 1 to 10 μg/kg/min to control hypertension
   b. Esmolol—a loading dose 500 μg/kg over 1 minute followed by an infusion of 100 to 250 μg/kg/min to control hypertension.

5. Blood loss is usually minimal and transfusion unnecessary.

6. In most cases, controlled ventilation is not required postoperatively and the child can be extubated at the end of the operation.

Postoperative

1. The child should be monitored continuously in the ICU, special attention being paid to signs of blood loss. Measure the chest drainage and observe the clinical indices.

2. Hypertension usually persists for several days postoperatively; if severe, it may necessitate therapy with SNP and/or esmolol (see previous discussion). Prevention of hypertension is essential to prevent arteritis (see later discussion).

3. Very rarely, the postoperative course is complicated by postcoarctectomy syndrome; intestinal ileus caused by mesenteric arteritis secondary to increased pulsatile flow in the mesenteric artery. In extreme cases, bowel resection may be required.

4. Other serious postoperative complications include recurrent laryngeal nerve palsy, phrenic nerve palsy, chylothorax, and paraplegia because of spinal cord ischemia during repair (very rare).

5. Recoarctation may occur in later years, particularly after repair in infancy. Repeat operation may be technically much more difficult and may involve major blood losses. Hence balloon angioplasty is now usually preferred.

Interrupted Aortic Arch

This lesion, which is frequently associated with VSD and DiGeorge syndrome, requires repair using CPB with profound hypothermic circulatory arrest. The patency of the ductus arteriosus must be maintained with a prostaglandin infusion until operation.

Palliative Surgery to Increase Pulmonary Blood Flow

The operations that may be used include the following:
1. Blalock-Taussig procedure (systemic artery anastomosed to the PA). A modified Blalock procedure using a synthetic graft between the aorta or innominate artery and the central portion of the PA is now the most commonly performed procedure.
2. The Potts operation (PA anastomosed to descending aorta) and the Waterston procedure (PA anastomosed to ascending aorta) are now rarely performed because they tend to become too large and may also cause unilateral pulmonary edema.

The operation is performed for infants and children with tetralogy of Fallot, tricuspid atresia, and other conditions in whom right-sided cardiac lesions result in decreased the pulmonary blood flow. They are usually performed during infancy to increase pulmonary blood flow and stimulate growth of the PAs; they may then be followed by total correction of the defect at an older age. The performance of total repair of CHD in infancy has resulted in much less use of these shunting procedures.

Special Anesthesia Problems

1. Many of these children are severely hypoxemic and polycythemic.
2. During surgery, the PA is partly occluded so that the anastomosis can be completed; this causes a further temporary decrease in pulmonary blood flow.
3. Children with polycythemia may have a coagulation defect, although this is rarely a problem.
4. In small infants, the narrow lumen of the new shunt is prone to thrombose. This may be prevented by using a small dose of heparin and appropriate fluid therapy.

Anesthesia Management

Preoperative

1. Ensure that the respiratory system is optimal, with no active infection or recent history of URTI.
2. If the child is taking digoxin, order the morning dose for the day of operation to be given at 6:00 AM. (Children having shunts to improve pulmonary blood flow frequently develop failure postoperatively; they need their morning digoxin!)

3. Order adequate sedation for older infants to prevent them from crying and becoming further desaturated.
4. If the child is taking β-blocking agents, they should be continued up to the evening before surgery.
5. Allow liberal fluids up to 3 hours before operation. Otherwise, order intravenous maintenance fluids during any prolonged preoperative fasting period for children with an Hb greater than 16 g/dl.

Perioperative

1. Follow routine management, as on page 407.
2. Induce anesthesia intravenously (most of these children have a right-to-left shunt); a small dose of propofol or thiopental followed by fentanyl and rocuronium is preferred.
3. An arterial line should be placed either in the radial artery—*in the rare event that the subclavian artery will be used, place the line in the opposite side*—or in the femoral artery.
4. Maintain anesthesia with sevoflurane, isoflurane, or halothane in at least 50% O_2.
   a. Halothane is useful for children with tetralogy because it tends to decrease the RV contractility and hence reduce obstruction to outflow.
   b. If desaturation occurs intraoperatively, it may be treated with esmolol (500 µg/kg IV slowly) and/or small doses of phenylephrine (1 to 10 µg /kg).
   c. If excessive hypotension occurs with halothane (rare), it will be necessary to substitute fentanyl.
5. Immediately before the PA is clamped, switch to 100% O_2, inflate the lungs well, and give a further dose of relaxant.
6. Once the clamps are in place and if oxygenation is stable, allow the surgeon to proceed with the anastomosis. (Once this is commenced, the PA will be open and the clamps cannot come off until the anastomosis is completed.)
7. Although the anastomosis is being performed: if there is a serious decline in BP or bradycardia occurs, infuse cardiotonic drugs (i.e., epinephrine 1 to 5 µg/kg, calcium chloride 10 mg/kg) until the anastomosis is completed and the clamps are removed.
8. A "modified" Blalock anastomosis is usually performed using a synthetic graft. In small infants, it is usual to give a small dose of heparin (100 units/kg) to prevent thrombosis of the shunt. A bolus of fluid after the clamps are released may enhance flow through the shunt.

9. Throughout the surgery, give 5% albumin as necessary to replace blood loss and decrease the Hct.

Postoperative

1. Auscultate the chest to document that a new murmur is present (this indicates that the shunt is functioning).
2. Extubate the trachea in the OR; this is preferred since spontaneous ventilation with reduced intrathoracic pressure may improve flow through the new shunt.
3. Review the digitalis dosage; the child may require a larger dose than previously (RV work is now increased, myocardial perfusion may be compromised by the lower diastolic pressure, and RV failure could ensue).
4. If the anastomosis is small and considered likely to be blocked by thrombosis, it is usual to order heparin in suitable dosage for several days postoperatively.

Palliative Surgery to Decrease Pulmonary Blood Flow

PA banding is performed to diminish blood flow to the lungs in infants who have a large left-to-right shunt, thereby improving systemic perfusion, decreasing pulmonary vascular congestion, and averting the development of fixed pulmonary hypertension. This is usually performed as an emergency procedure in the neonate.

Special Anesthesia Problems

Many of these infants have severe CHF.

Anesthesia Management

Preoperative

1. Follow routine management, as on page 407.
2. Check that the CHF is under control.
3. Apply all measures possible to improve the infants' general status before surgery (e.g., IPPV for several hours can be very beneficial).

Perioperative

1. Avoid myocardial depressants.
2. Monitor the infant closely as the band is applied. With an optimal band tightness:
   a. The systemic BP should increase, and the saturation may decrease slightly.

b. The distal PA pressure should decrease to approximately 30% to 50% of systemic pressure.

c. The EtCO$_2$ value may decrease very slightly. (A large decline indicates that the band is too tight.)

Postoperative

1. Controlled ventilation may be required for several days.

Specific Open Heart Procedures

The considerations discussed here are a supplement to all the other important general principles outlined previously.

Atrial Septal Defect (Secundum Type)

Atrial septal defect (ASD) may be associated with partial anomalous pulmonary venous drainage, in which case a baffle is required to redirect this flow to the left atrium. This may complicate and prolong the simple ASD closure procedure slightly. Simple small ASD is now commonly closed in the cardiac catheter laboratory using an 'Umbrella' device (see page 455). Large ASD requires surgical closure, though this may be performed using minimally invasive techniques (i.e., small incisions).

1. Plan to extubate the trachea at the end of surgery. A single dose of caudal morphine (33 µg/kg of Duramorph) given after induction before surgery provides for early postoperative analgesia and lasts up to 24 hours.

2. Closure of the ASD is performed either with cardioplegia or with induced ventricular fibrillation, so as to prevent the possibility that air may enter the LV and be pumped into the circulation. Ensure that the child is completely paralyzed during CPB to prevent the possibility that the child takes a breath while the atrium is open, which could draw air into the left side of the heart; give an additional dose of relaxant as the heart is being cannulated.

3. As the last suture is being tightened to close the defect, the surgeon may request sustained inflation of the lungs to promote flow of blood via the pulmonary veins into the left atrium to remove any residual air from the left side of the heart.

4. Bypass is short and post-CPB inotropic therapy is unlikely to be needed.

Total Anomalous Pulmonary Venous Drainage (TAPVD)

The pulmonary veins drain into the right atrium or its venous connections. There are three common types:

1. *Supracardiac (50% of cases):* Pulmonary veins drain into the left SVC.
2. *Cardiac (30% of cases):* Pulmonary veins drain into the coronary sinus or right atrium.
3. *Infracardiac (10% of cases):* Pulmonary veins drain into the inferior vena cava via a common trunk below the diaphragm.

TAPVD manifests in early neonatal life with severe cyanosis and acidosis. Obstruction of the pulmonary veins may be present and may cause pulmonary edema and cardiac failure. Survival depends on a right-to-left shunt, usually via an ASD or patent foramen ovale, which may need enlarging by balloon dilation. The presence of obstruction to the pulmonary veins exacerbates the symptoms.

Special Considerations

1. If the pulmonary veins are obstructed, pulmonary edema, pulmonary hypertension, and cardiac failure may be present.
2. Preoperative ventilation may be required to treat pulmonary edema and improve oxygenation.
3. The left atrium and LV may be small and the LV compliance reduced; aggressive inotropic therapy may be required after bypass.
4. The pulmonary vasculature may have a thick medial layer, and PVR may remain increased after repair.

Anesthesia Plan

1. Maintain controlled ventilation and PEEP; monitor acid-base status frequently.
2. High-dose opioid technique is preferred.
3. After repair, the LV may require generous inotropic support and afterload reduction to maintain cardiac output. High left atrial pressures should be avoided as these may lead to fluid overload.
4. Active measures to reduce PVR and prevent pulmonary hypertensive crisis must be instituted. The PA pressure should be monitored. Prepare to administer NO if it becomes necessary.

Cor Triatriatum

This lesion consists of a membrane within the left atrium that obstructs pulmonary venous return and requires surgical excision on CPB.

Ventricular Septal Defect

VSD is the most common single defect (20% of CHD cases). The position of the VSD is used to classify the disease and also may predict complications:

1. *Type I (supracristal, 5%):* under the annulus of the aorta; may affect the adjacent cusp and cause aortic valve incompetence; also associated with narrow aortic isthmus
2. *Type II (infracristal, most common, 80%):* in the membranous septum—often large with a big shunt
3. *Type III (AV canal type, 11%):* beneath the tricuspid valve
4. *Type IV (muscular 4%):* may be multiple ("Swiss cheese" defect)

The physiologic effects of the VSD depend on its size. If it is large (nonrestrictive), the left-to-right shunt is similarly large, resulting in early CHF and subsequent pulmonary vascular obstructive disease (PVOD). Small defects (restrictive) allow only a small shunt, which may be physiologically insignificant. Early operation is performed for large defects to prevent the onset of PVOD.

Special Considerations

1. Infants with severe CHF may benefit from intubation and ventilation preoperatively.
2. Infants with CHF cannot tolerate myocardial depressant drugs (e.g. halothane).
3. Postoperative conduction disturbances, which may be temporary (possibly due to edema around a suture), should be anticipated.
4. Pulmonary vascular crisis may occur in small infants postoperatively.

Anesthesia Plan

1. Avoid myocardial depressants; high-dose opioids are preferred. Titrate drugs slowly.
2. Bidirectional shunts are common; be careful to prevent air bubbles in IV lines.
3. Maintain PVR to prevent increasing left-to-right shunting; prevent hyperventilation. Minor reductions in SVR (perhaps minimal isoflurane) may be beneficial.
4. Be prepared to institute pacing if conduction is abnormal after repair.
5. In the case of large defects, postbypass therapy to reduce PVR and to prevent pulmonary vascular crisis may be required.

Atrioventricular Canal

AV canal is frequently associated with Down syndrome and may be complete (ASD, VSD, and cleft AV valve) or partial (ostium primum ASD plus cleft mitral valve). The most significant hemodynamic changes are a large left-to-right shunt, leading to pulmonary hypertension, and mitral incompetence. Early surgical repair in infancy is preferred.

Special Considerations

1. Down syndrome often present (see Chapter 6, page 196).
2. Pulmonary hypertension may be a problem postoperatively; prepare to measure PA pressure and institute therapy. Aggressive inotropic therapy may be required.
3. Disturbances of conduction are relatively common after repair and may persist; chronic pacemaker therapy may be required.
4. Mitral valve malfunction may occur in the early or late postoperative period, and reoperation to repair the valve may be required.

Tetralogy of Fallot

The clinical picture results from the large VSD in the presence of RV outflow obstruction, which together produce a large right-to-left shunt; the other features of tetralogy are overriding of the aorta and RV hypertrophy. RV obstruction may be infundibular (50%), valvular (10%), PA (10%), or combined (30%). Acute dynamic increases in infundibular obstruction may result in severe desaturation episodes ("tet" spells). Most children are now treated by complete repair in infancy, except those with small PAs, who are treated initially with a systemic-to-pulmonary shunt.

Special Considerations

1. Adequate preoperative sedation and sufficient anesthesia and analgesia to suppress any response to surgical stimulation are important to prevent "tet" spells. Avoid drugs that reduce SVR significantly (e.g., isoflurane); high-dose opioid technique is preferred. Titrate the drug carefully.
2. Halothane in low concentrations may be useful to depress the muscle of the RV infundibulum and prevent "tet" spells.
3. Otherwise, intraoperative "tet" spells should be treated with oxygen, fluid infusion, and esmolol 0.5 mg/kg slowly and/or phenylephrine 1 to 10 µg/kg IV.
4. After CPB, a high filling pressure may be required owing to the thickened, poorly compliant right ventricle. Rarely, conduction defects require AV pacing.
5. The use of LV afterload reduction may be poorly tolerated because the RV output is the limiting factor on overall cardiac output.

Transposition of the Great Arteries

The most common cause of cyanotic CHD in the neonate is transposition of the great arteries, whereby the aorta arises from the RV and the PA arises from the LV. The pulmonary and systemic circulations are thus separate and in parallel; survival depends on mixing via the patent foramen ovale (PFO), ASD, VSD, or PDA. Without treatment, 90% of infants with transposition of the great arteries die within 12 months. Current surgical treatment is to perform an arterial switch procedure; this must be performed in the neonatal period for infants with an intact septum but may be performed later in those with a large VSD.

Special Considerations

1. The neonate with an intact septum, dependent on mixing via the PFO and PDA, will become desperately hypoxic when the latter closes. Balloon atrial septostomy has been used to improve mixing, or, if the neonate is having early surgery, PGE_1 may be used to maintain the PDA.
2. The effective pulmonary or systemic blood flow is limited to that volume of blood that shunts between the circulations.

Anesthesia Plan

1. A technique that maintains myocardial function and cardiac output should be used; a high-dose opioid technique is preferred.
2. Moderate hyperventilation with a high FiO_2 may reduce PVR and thereby increase pulmonary blood flow, mixing, and arterial saturation.
3. PGE_1 infusion must be continued and may be useful after CPB for neonates at risk for pulmonary vascular crises.
4. Post-CPB measures to optimize blood flow in the reimplanted coronary arteries are required. An infusion of nitroglycerin (1 µg/kg/min) should be commenced before weaning from CPB. Maintain an optimal preload; the arterial BP should not be allowed to decrease!
5. Bleeding from multiple suture lines is to be expected. Order blood components to correct the coagulopathy that is common after CPB in neonates. Platelet suspensions, FFP, and cryoprecipitate are often required.

Aortic Stenosis

Critical aortic stenosis can cause severe CHF in the neonate. Older children with aortic stenosis may be asymptomatic, but they are at increasing risk for angina, syncope, and sudden death. Aortic stenosis may be subvalvular; valvular, usually with a bicuspid valve (80% of cases); or supravalvular (often associated with Williams syndrome [see Appendix 1]). Critical aortic stenosis is now usually treated by balloon dilation. On occasion an infant with a small aortic annulus or with associated cardiac lesions may require operation. The principles outlined below apply equally to those children who require anesthesia in the cardiac catheterization lab.

Special Considerations

1. Infants with critical aortic stenosis are hypotensive, poorly perfused, and acidotic, with respiratory distress and hepatomegaly. The disease often becomes apparent as the ductus arteriosus closes. The thickened LV is prone to ischemia and arrhythmias. Subendocardial fibroelastosis may also be present. These infants require aggressive resuscitation and early operation; even so, the mortality rate is high.
2. Older children with valvular aortic stenosis commonly have a bicuspid valve, and cardiac function is usually quite good despite a high gradient across the stenosed valve.

Anesthesia Plan—Infants

1. The infant will be receiving an infusion of prostaglandin to maintain the ductus arteriosus; this must be continued.
2. A high-dose opioid and pancuronium technique is preferred. (Pancuronium/fentanyl combination is particularly useful as the chronotropic effect of the relaxant is antagonized by the bradycardic effect of the opioid resulting in very stable conditions.)
3. Maintain body temperature carefully.
4. Serious arrhythmias, including ventricular fibrillation, may occur as the heart is manipulated, especially if any cooling has occurred. A very small dose of propranolol (10 µg/kg) may reduce this danger.

Anesthesia Plan—Older Children

1. The aim is to maintain the heart rate constant, prevent tachycardia or bradycardia, and prevent any major decline in SVR and aortic root pressure. Opioid plus rocuronium or vecuronium is usually satisfactory.
2. Halothane may be useful to reduce dynamic LV outflow tract obstruction in those with subvalvular aortic stenosis.
3. Children with supravalvular aortic stenosis and Williams syndrome may have airways that are difficult to intubate.
4. Postoperative hypertension is common after aortic valvotomy and SNP infusion may be required.

Hypoplastic Left Heart Syndrome (HLHS)

In HLHS, the LV and ascending aorta are hypoplastic and the LV is nonfunctional. Immediate survival depends on the pumping action of the RV and systemic flow via the PDA with retrograde flow in the aortic arch. Blood mixes in the right atrium (via an ASD or PFO), and pulmonary-to-systemic flow ratio depends on the size of the intraatrial communication, the PVR, and the SVR. Treatment of this condition is either by heart transplantation or by conversion to a univentricular series type of circulation by means of a staged repair:

1. *Stage 1:* Norwood procedure. Division of the PA, connection of the RV to a reconstructed aortic arch (neoaorta made from the PA and AO), atrial septectomy, and a modified Blalock-Taussig shunt. (Neoaorta to PA) A modification of the Stage 1 Norwood procedure is to place the shunt from RV to PA; this may improve myocardial perfusion.
2. *Stage 2:* Bidirectional Glenn (SVC-RPA) anastomosis or hemi-Fontan procedure (and take down of the B-T shunt). This procedure is designed to direct some of the blood flow directly to the lungs and so reduce the load on the RV.
3. *Stage 3:* Completion of the Fontan procedure, which connects the IVC to the PA by means of a lateral tunnel or Gortex conduit, and places the systemic and pulmonary circulations in series.

Special Considerations

1. Preoperative management is aimed at maintaining the ratio of pulmonary to systemic blood flow (Qp:Qs) close to 1. The ease with which this can be achieved depends first on the child's anatomy (i.e., the size of the interatrial communication).
   a. If it is large and unrestrictive, pulmonary blood flow is excessive and systemic hypoperfusion with metabolic acidosis occurs. These infants must be treated by tracheal intubation and controlled ventilation to increase the $PaCO_2$ and hence increase PVR. The FiO_2 must also be strictly limited, possibly less than 21% by the addition of nitrogen. It may not be possible to achieve the desired $PaCO_2$ and maintain SaO_2 if ventilation is simply reduced; it may then be necessary to add CO2 to the inspired gases. This management must be continued until CPB is instituted.
   b. Children with relative restriction (a high percentage) may achieve Qp:Qs near 1 when breathing room air. These infants must be managed to maintain the status quo (i.e., to prevent changes in ventilation or oxygenation.)
   c. Children with a very small or absent ASD have pulmonary hypoperfusion and are profoundly hypoxic at birth. These infants require immediate surgery to survive.
2. All infants require a continuous infusion of PGE_1 to maintain patency of the ductus arteriosus.
3. Some infants may require inotropic agents to increase cardiac output and systemic perfusion; these must be used with caution to prevent adverse changes in SVR.

Anesthesia Plan-Norwood Stage 1

1. Take great care to maintain F_{IO_2} and ventilation unchanged during transport to and from the OR. A transport ventilator is preferred. It is very easy to hyperventilate the lungs accidentally and cause a disastrous fall in PVR and systemic blood flow.
2. Care during the prebypass stage is similar for those undergoing either the Norwood procedure or transplantation. Carefully maintain the level of ventilation and oxygenation to balance the PVR:SVR ratio. The arterial saturation should be ±80%. In some cases it may be necessary to add N_2 to the inspired gases to achieve an F_{IO_2} less than 21%. CO_2 may be cautiously added if necessary to rapidly increase PVR.
3. High-dose opioid anesthesia is preferred, but fentanyl (50-75 µg/kg) must be titrated slowly, balancing surgical stimulation, to prevent hypotension. Pancuronium is the relaxant of choice.
4. Post-CPB after a Norwood procedure and measures to maintain the PVR and limit pulmonary blood flow may still be required, depending on the size of the shunt. Expect the saturation to be 70% to 80%. Inotropic therapy with standard doses of dopamine and dobutamine is usually adequate.
5. Rarely, if pulmonary blood flow is inadequate and the infant is severely hypoxic, measures to reduce PVR may be needed (i.e., NO). In some cases a larger shunt may be needed.

Tricuspid Atresia

Tricuspid atresia is a condition in which there is no communication between the right atrium and the RV, which is usually hypoplastic. Survival depends on the presence of an adequate atrial communication (PFO or ASD) and a systemic-to-pulmonary shunt (VSD or PDA). Palliation in the neonate is required, and the ASD may have to be enlarged by balloon septostomy. For those children with diminished pulmonary blood flow, a systemic-to-PA shunt (e.g., modified Blalock operation) is performed. Those with increased pulmonary blood flow, CHF, and systemic hypoperfusion need a PA band. Later in life, when PVR decreases, other procedures are possible. The Glenn procedure (SVC-PA anastomosis) was commonly used for these children but has now been superseded by the Fontan repair. The Fontan procedure and its modifications are now also used to treat other forms of CHD in which there is a single functional ventricle. After this operation, the right atrial pressure must serve to perfuse the lungs. A low PVR is obviously crucial.

Fontan Procedure

Special Considerations

1. After the operation, the total cardiac output is directed to the systemic circulation. The pulmonary circulation is driven by the pressure exerted by the venous return from the body. Hence a low PVR is vital. There is no shunting, so there is improved SaO_2 and there is also a reduced load on the ventricle.
2. For a successful operation, PVR less than 4 units/m^2 is desirable and PVR must not increase. However, in some children with mildly increased PVR, a Fontan operation is performed but a fenestration is left in the vena cava-to-PA baffle. This allows for some right-to-left shunting and relieves the right atrial pressure; cyanosis may occur, but ventricular filling and cardiac output are maintained.
3. Pleural and pericardial effusions are very common after the Fontan procedure and may require drainage for a prolonged period.
4. Plastic bronchitis leading to acute airway obstruction and requiring bronchoscopic removal of a membrane is described in post-Fontan children. The production of this membrane is considered to be because of the high venous pressures in these children.

Anesthesia Plan

1. Establish several reliable intravenous routes before the operation; postoperative edema may make later venous access difficult.
2. A reliable CVP line is essential for postoperative monitoring.
3. Before terminating bypass, ensure that sinus rhythm is present or institute sequential pacing. Sinus rhythm is essential. Commence an infusion of SNP to reduce PVR and SVR. Hyperventilate using a short inspiratory phase, minimal peak inspiratory pressure, and PEEP just adequate to maintain optimal lung volume.
4. After bypass, maintain the CVP at 14 to 16 mm Hg to maintain pulmonary blood flow. It is hoped that this will provide a left atrial pressure of 4 to 8 mm Hg. The gradient across the pulmonary bed should be less than 10 mm Hg.
5. Early return to spontaneous ventilation and extubation augment pulmonary blood flow.
6. Fluid retention with peripheral edema, pleural and pericardial effusions, and ascites is common. Protein-losing enteropathy may occur in some children.

Truncus Arteriosus

Truncus arteriosus occurs when the pulmonary artery fails to completely separate from the aorta resulting in a communication between the two vessels. Several types have been described:

1. *Type I:* PA arises from truncus and then divides
2. *Type II:* separate PAs arise from posterior truncus
3. *Type III:* separate PAs arise from sides of truncus
   The optimal time for repair is the first month of life.

Special Considerations

1. DiGeorge syndrome is present in 25% of cases (see Appendix 1). In such cases monitor the Ca^{++} level. Immune deficiency is present: use washed red blood cells.
2. Increased pulmonary blood flow predisposes to pulmonary vascular hypertensive crises.
3. Low aortic diastolic pressure may result in inadequate coronary flow and myocardial ischemia.
4. The truncal valve is semilunar and commonly is incompetent.

Anesthesia Plan

1. Children may require preoperative ventilation and inotropic support.
2. SVR and PVR should be maintained to support aortic diastolic pressure and coronary flow. Therefore, prevent hyperventilation, excess O_2, or vasodilating drugs.
3. High-dose opioid technique is preferred.
4. After CPB and postoperatively, institute measures to protect against pulmonary vascular crisis.

Suggested Reading

Textbook

Andropoulos D, Stayer SA, Russel IA: Anesthesia for congenital heart disease, Malden, Mass, 2005, Blackwell/Futura.

Anesthesia Management

Aronson LA, Spaeth JP: Frontiers in pediatric anesthesia: cardiac anesthesia, Int Anesth Clin 44(1):33–49, 2006.
Friesen RH, Williams GD: Anesthetic management of children with pulmonary arterial hypertension, Paediatr Anaesth 18(3):208–216, 2008.

Cardiopulmonary Bypass and Myocardial Protection

D'Errico C, Shayevitz JR, Martindale SJ: Age-related differences in heparin sensitivity and heparin-protamine interactions in cardiac surgery patients, J Cardiothorac Vasc Anaesth 10:451–457, 1996.

Jonas RA: Hypothermia, circulatory arrest, and the pediatric brain, J Cardiothorac Vasc Anesth 10:66–74, 1996.

Preisman S, Keidan I, Perel A, et al: Anesthesia for port-access cardiac surgery in a pediatric population, J Cardiothorac Vasc Anesth 19(5):626–629, 2005.

Transesophageal Echocardiography

Balmer C, Barron D, Wright JG, et al: Experience with intraoperative ultrasound in paediatric cardiac surgery, Cardiol Young 16(5):455–462, 2006.

Stevenson JG: Incidence of complications in pediatric transesophageal echocardiography: experience in 1650 cases, J Am Soc Echocardiogr 12: 527–532, 1999.

Neema PK, Manikandan S, Rathod RC: Endotracheal tube migration following transoesophageal echocardiography probe placement in a child, Euro J Anaesth 23(12):1060–1061, 2006.

HEART TRANSPLANTATION

The indications for heart transplantation in infants and children are:

1. Severe congenital malformations (e.g., HLHS) or failed previous surgical corrections of CHD not amenable to further surgery.
2. Cardiomyopathy - progressive with no chance of timely remission.
3. Myocardial tumors not amenable to resection (rare).

General Principles

1. The preoperative PVR is the most important determinant of the suitability of the infant or child for transplantation. Neonates have a high PVR, but a neonatal donor heart should be able to cope with this, and PVR may be expected to decrease over the first weeks of life. Otherwise, for older children, strategies must be used to reduce PVR or, failing this, heart-lung transplantation must be considered.
2. Other contraindications to transplantation include serious hepatic, renal, or central nervous system disease and chronic infections (i.e., hepatitis, cytomegalovirus, human immunodeficiency virus).
3. A stable family and social environment is most desirable to ensure the continued care that will be required after transplantation.

Care of the Donor

Care of the donor child during the organ harvesting is discussed in Chapter 13, page 387.

Anesthesia Management of the Recipient—Special Considerations

1. The basic management is similar to that for other open-heart procedures. However, the child may have been urgently admitted and may not have been fasted. Precautions for dealing with the full stomach may be necessary. If a rapid-sequence induction is planned, drugs and doses should be carefully worked out to prevent excessive cardiovascular effects. Ketamine or etomidate is useful for the child with minimal reserve.

2. Very strict attention to aseptic technique is required. All intravascular lines should be inserted with full sterile precautions (gown and gloves). The puncture site should be treated with antibiotic ointment and covered with a clear adhesive dressing.

3. Do not aspirate the stomach after induction if oral cyclosporin was recently given as a component of the antirejection therapy.

4. Most children have very poor cardiac function and a dilated heart; therefore take care to prevent inducing tachycardia, bradycardia, or any additional myocardial depression. A fentanyl-O_2 midazolam, pancuronium anesthetic is usually preferred. Continue solutions of inotropic agents and/or PGE_1. Some children may need additional inotropic support as surgery commences.

5. Children who have had previous cardiac surgery should be given tranexamic acid or Amicar to reduce postoperative bleeding.

6. Increased PVR should be managed to prevent any further pulmonary vasoconstriction.

7. Neonates with HLHS should be treated as for the Norwood procedure before CPB.

8. Infusions of dopamine and dobutamine, isoproterenol, and SNP should be primed for immediate use during weaning from bypass. An infusion of PGE_1 should be prepared for neonates.

9. On weaning from CPB, immediately give methylprednisolone (Solu-Medrol) 15 mg/kg and other antirejection drugs as indicated. Sinus tachycardia is often present at this stage, and the action of two atrial pacemakers may be observed (one from the remains of the child's native atrium and one from the implanted atrium). In the absence of sinus rhythm, AV pacing should be commenced. A slow sinus rhythm usually responds well to an isoproterenol infusion. Infuse other inotropic solutions (e.g., dopamine) as necessary to maintain good cardiac action (see later discussion).

10. Measures to minimize PVR should be continued.
11. Remember the special properties of the newly implanted but denervated heart:

  a. Cardiac drugs will exert *only their direct effects*; atropine will have no chronotropic effect; anticholinesterases will not affect heart rate. Epinephrine, isoproterenol, and norepinephrine will all cause an increase in heart rate. Dopamine and dobutamine are effective inotropic agents.

  b. Increased filling pressure will, through the Frank-Starling mechanism, result in increased stroke volume. A CVP of 10 to 12 mm Hg is usually optimal. Hypovolemia is poorly tolerated.

  c. There is no change in heart rate with the respiratory cycle or with a Valsalva maneuver.

  d. Arrhythmias are not common in children, but the response to those antiarrhythmic drugs that have both direct and indirect effects on the heart will be altered:

   i. Digoxin and procainamide normally exert a mixture of direct and indirect effects on the heart and will have a less predictable effect on the denervated heart.

   ii. The effects of lidocaine, phenytoin, β-adrenergic blocking drugs, and calcium channel-blocking drugs are direct and similar to those in the intact heart.

Suggested Reading

Williams GD, Ramamoorthy C: Anesthesia considerations for pediatric thoracic solid organ transplant, Anesth Clin N Am 23(4):709–731, 2005.
Schindler E, Muller M, Akinturk H, et al: Perioperative management in pediatric heart transplantation from 1988 to 2001: anesthetic experience in a single center, Pediatr Trans 8(3):237–242, 2004.

HEART-LUNG OR LUNG TRANSPLANTATION

Lung transplantation in children is usually performed with the aid of CPB; the considerations are similar to those for heart-lung transplantation.

Indications

1. The indications for heart-lung transplantation are
  a. Eisenmenger syndrome
  b. Other congenital defects with pulmonary vascular disease
  c. Complex CHD, inadequate pulmonary vessels not amenable to further repair

2. The indications for lung transplantation are
   a. Primary pulmonary hypertension
   b. Pulmonary fibrosis
   c. Cystic fibrosis

Care of the Donor

The general principles are outlined in Chapter 13. Selection of a donor for lung transplantation is more difficult:

1. Significant lung disease, infection, or damage from recent aspiration or pulmonary edema associated with resuscitative interventions and artificial ventilation must be excluded. It is suggested that a PaO_2 of 100 mm Hg or more with an FiO_2 of 0.4, and peak inflating pressures of 30 cm H_2O or less with a tidal volume of 15 ml/kg and PEEP of 5 cm H_2O, indicate acceptability for transplantation.
2. The lungs must be an appropriate size to fit the thorax of the recipient; if they are too large, atelectasis will result. Perfect match or slightly smaller donor lungs are accepted; otherwise, lobar transplantation or tailoring of the donor lung may be required.
3. Before harvesting the lungs, the donor should receive 30 mg/kg of methyl-prednisolone and an infusion of PGE_1 (25 ng/kg/min) increased until the systemic arterial pressure decreases by 10% to 20%. This produces maximal pulmonary vasodilation before infusion of the pulmoplegic solution.
4. Cardioplegia and pulmoplegia are induced, and the lungs are held inflated before tracheal clamping.
5. In selected cases, donor lung tissue may be obtained from living related donors (e.g., one lobe from each parent may be transplanted into a child).

Anesthesia Management of the Recipient for Lung Transplantation

Special Considerations

1. Older children with critical respiratory disease may be very apprehensive; consider the use of well-monitored preoperative sedation (e.g., midazolam or lorazepam intravenously with pulse oximetry in place and constant monitoring).
2. Before induction, verify administration of immunosuppressants and antibiotics as ordered.
3. Induction and maintenance of anesthesia should be planned as for CPB, bearing in mind the advanced respiratory disease.
4. Tracheal intubation: Use a cuffed tube and place the cuff just below the cords. For children with cystic fibrosis, suction the tube frequently during dissection of the native lungs.

5. Maintain meticulous aseptic technique for all procedures; remove all existing intravenous lines and replace them with new lines using strict asepsis. A pulmonary artery catheter should be inserted after induction.

6. Fluid therapy should be limited to basal rates.

7. Antifibrinolytic therapy (ε-aminocaproic acid or tranexamic acid) should be commenced after induction to decrease postoperative bleeding.

8. Plan for optimal postoperative pain management.

9. During bypass, be prepared to reintubate with a new sterile endotracheal tube, using appropriate aseptic technique. For children with pulmonary infections (e.g., those with cystic fibrosis), change the entire breathing circuit. In addition, once the native lungs are removed, the proximal trachea and bronchi should be lavaged with a solution of tobramycin.

10. Dopamine, dobutamine, and PGE_1 infusions should be available. For those with pulmonary infections, prepare a phenylephrine infusion (see later discussion). Nitric oxide should be available.

11. Immediately on weaning from CPB, administer methylprednisolone 15 mg/kg IV and furosemide 0.5 to 0.75 mg/kg. Give inotropic agents as required. Pulmonary function may be improved by albuterol inhalations and aggressive diuretic therapy.

12. Adjust the FiO_2 to maintain oxygen saturation at ±93% and to prevent hyperoxic damage to lungs. Hyperventilate slightly to maintain pulmonary flow using tidal volumes of 15 ml/kg. PEEP to 6 to 10 cm H_2O should be added to maintain optimal lung volume, minimize PVR, and prevent pulmonary edema.

13. Children with a history of severe lung infections (e.g., cystic fibrosis) may demonstrate signs of sepsis: low BP despite good cardiac action. In such cases, an infusion of phenylephrine may be required.

14. Persistent high PA pressures after transplantation should be treated by the addition of NO to the inhaled gases.

15. Extensive bleeding is to be expected, especially if the child has had a previous thoracotomy. Order appropriate supplies of replacement factors.

16. Postoperative problems may be related to damage to the phrenic, vagus, or recurrent laryngeal nerves.

Suggested Reading

Williams GD, Ramamoorthy C: Anesthesia considerations for pediatric thoracic solid organ transplant, Anesth Clin N Am 23(4):709–731, 2005.

CARDIOLOGIC PROCEDURES

Cardiac Catheterization

This is usually an elective procedure, and older children will benefit from preoperative teaching, a visit to the catheter laboratory, and familiarization with the procedures to be performed. Cardiac catheterization may be performed under general anesthesia or with a combination of sedation plus local or regional analgesia. The important prerequisites for gathering reliable catheterization data are as follows:

1. Hemodynamic parameters during sedation/anesthesia should be as close to awake values as possible.
2. The inspired O_2 concentration should remain constant throughout the procedure. Room air is preferred if safe for the child. Otherwise, a constant optimum inspired O_2 concentration should be selected.
3. Spontaneous ventilation is preferred when appropriate; controlled ventilation may change intracardiac shunts and modify intracardiac pressures.
4. The child should be maintained in an optimal physiologic state (normothermic, well hydrated, euglycemic, and so on).

Special Anesthesia Problems

1. The child may be seriously ill and in CHF.
2. The condition may further deteriorate during cardiac catheterization, especially if arrhythmias occur.
3. Contrast media used for angiograms may cause adverse effects.
4. Children with pulmonary hypertension are particularly prone to serious complications during cardiac catheterization and may require special consideration.
5. Cardiac perforation with tamponade is always a possibility.

Anesthesia Management

When the procedure is to be performed under sedation, the following technique has proved satisfactory:

1. Establish an intravenous route using local analgesia.
2. Apply monitors (ECG, pulse oximeter, BP cuff, temperature probe). If you have a Doppler probe positioned over an artery, it provides a very good means to monitor cardiac status moment by moment.
3. Maintain a thermoneutral environment, particularly in small infants (i.e., overhead warmer, forced air warming blanket).

4. Administer intravenous sedation. An infusion of propofol with or without small doses of midazolam has been found to be most useful. When combined with good local or regional analgesia, only very small doses of drugs are required to ensure sleep, and very stable cardiovascular parameters are maintained.

5. Small infants may be offered a "sucrose soother" and often settle with this alone.

6. Caudal analgesia may be useful for some children, especially if bilateral femoral catheterization is necessary or if large catheters are to be inserted (i.e., for balloon dilation).

7. Angiography requires that the child remain absolutely still; therefore augment the sedation if necessary. Contrast media are hyperosmolar (although new nonionic agents are less so); they can cause aggregation of erythrocytes and, rarely, anaphylaxis. The total dose administered should be carefully recorded, especially in small infants and recommended limits observed.

8. The procedure may be carried out in a darkened room.

9. When it is considered advisable to ventilate the lungs during the procedure, the same technique (propofol infusion) may be used with the addition of a suitable muscle relaxant (e.g., rocuronium) and tracheal intubation. Normocapnia should be maintained.

10. In some children, the response of the pulmonary circulation to hyperventilation, hyperoxia, or the inhalation of NO may be studied.

11. Postcatheterization care: The child should be carefully monitored until the effects of sedation resolve and smooth awakening occurs. It is necessary that the child lie quietly to prevent bleeding and bruising at the catheter site; additional mild sedation may be necessary to achieve this state. The catheterization site should be examined for bleeding, and the pulses distal to arterial cannulation should be evaluated regularly. The child should be discharged from the PACU when awake, with stable vital signs, and with no evidence of vascular complications.

Interventional Cardiology

Sedation and/or general anesthesia are now quite frequently required for complex interventional techniques. These include:

1. Balloon dilation of pulmonary or aortic valves, or recoarctation of the aorta

2. Occlusion of the ductus arteriosus

3. Closure of septal defects or other fistulas

Special Problems

1. The child may be critically ill.
2. Absolute immobility is essential during the critical stages.
3. An urgent call for open operation if complications occur is a real possibility. The heart may be perforated, vessels may be ruptured, or the occlusive device may become displaced. Complications are most likely during valve dilation procedures.
4. The procedure may be carried out in a darkened room.
5. A steady hemodynamic state is required for measurements to be made.
6. Simultaneous TEE may be required to monitor results.

Anesthesia Management

1. Prepare and monitor the child for an open procedure. A large-bore, reliable intravenous route should be established.
2. For some very simple procedures in older children, sedation with propofol with spontaneous ventilation and local analgesia may be suitable.
3. For more complex procedures (e.g., balloon dilation of a stenotic valve, "umbrella" closure of a septal defect), tracheal intubation with neuromuscular block and controlled ventilation is preferred. Anesthesia may be maintained with a propofol infusion.
4. Plans must be made for transfer to the OR should a complication occur. Supplies of blood for rapid transfusion should be immediately available.
5. During the procedure, the anesthesiologist must constantly monitor for signs of blood loss or cardiac tamponade.
   a. Cardiac perforation manifests with hypotension, and tachycardia with ectopic beats.
   b. Cardiac tamponade leads to hypotension, with reduced cardiac motion on fluoroscopy. Confirm by ECHO. Pericardiocentesis should be performed in either case. Continued bleeding from a cardiac perforation requires thoracotomy.
6. Children with pulmonary hypertension (PAH) require special considerations:
   a. During catheterization the response of the pulmonary vasculature to increased levels of oxygen and/or inhalation of NO may be assessed.
   b. Anesthesia management should be conducted to prevent precipitating increases in PVR.
      i. Excessive sedation leading to respiratory depression, increased $PaCO_2$, airway obstruction and hypoxemia must be prevented. Hypoventilation should be corrected early.

ii. An adequate level of anesthesia should be ensured during potentially painful stimuli or instrumentation of the airway. Tracheal intubation should be avoided if possible in those with severe PAH.

Suggested Reading

Bennett D, Marcus R, Stokes M: Incidents and complications during pediatric cardiac catheterization, Pediatr Anesth 15(12):1083–1088, 2005.

Taylor CJ, Derrick G, McEwan A, et al: Risk of cardiac catheterization under anaesthesia in children with pulmonary hypertension, Br J Anaesth 98(5):657–661, 2007.

ELECTROPHYSIOLOGIC STUDIES

Children may require anesthesia or sedation for electrophysiologic studies and radiofrequency catheter ablation of accessory conduction pathways in the treatment of dysrhythmias. These procedures are not painful, except during the moments of the actual radiofrequency ablation, but may be prolonged (consider inserting a urinary catheter), and absolute immobility is essential. Hence, general endotracheal anesthesia with controlled ventilation is recommended.

Isoproterenol may be infused during the procedure to elicit dysrhythmias to find accessory conduction pathways. If ablation of such pathways is the goal, defibrillation pads should be in place on the child's thorax before the procedure and antiarrhythmic drugs should be immediately at hand.

An important consideration is the possible effect of anesthesia or sedative drugs and anesthesia techniques on cardiac rhythm generation and conduction. Some anesthetics (e.g., halothane) have much greater effects than others (e.g., propofol). Deep sedation or anesthesia with propofol or balanced anesthesia with nitrous oxide and low dose isoflurane do not interfere with EP studies or the ability to trigger SVT or VT. Therefore these agents are acceptable during electrophysiologic studies.

Suggested Reading

Renwick J, Kerr C, McTaggart R, et al: Cardiac electrophysiology and conduction pathway ablation, Can J Anaesth 40(11):1053–1164, 1993.

CARDIOVERSION

Cardioversion is usually an emergency. The arrhythmia may be severe, markedly reducing cardiac output and producing shock.

Anesthesia Management

Preparation:

1. Give 100% O_2 by mask until cardioversion can be performed.
2. Ascertain whether the child has been fasting (see later discussion).
3. Prepare and check all equipment.
4. Apply monitors:
   a. Precordial stethoscope
   b. Pulse oximeter and BP cuff
   c. ECG
5. Establish reliable intravenous access.

During the conversion:

1. Continue 100% O_2 by mask.
2. When ready to cardiovert, premedicate with IV midazolam and induce anesthesia using a sleep dose of propofol (or ketamine if cardiac function is poor).
3. If the child has a full stomach:
   a. Continue 100% O_2.
   b. Give atropine 0.02 mg/kg IV.
   c. Inject propofol 2.5 to 3.5 mg/kg or ketamine 1-2 mg/kg or etomidate 0.2-0.3 mg/kg if a cardiomyopathy is present) and succinylcholine 1 to 2 mg/kg.
   d. Perform a RSI and secure the trachea.
4. As soon as anesthesia has been induced and good oxygenation achieved, countershock may be applied. Repeat propofol, ketamine or etomidate doses as needed.

Postprocedure

1. The period of recovery is short, but the child should be closely monitored (including ECG) for several hours afterward.
2. If the trachea was intubated, remove the endotracheal tube after the child is fully conscious.

ANESTHESIA FOR CARDIAC MRI

MRI studies now provide a very important tool for mapping the anatomy of the heart and this is very useful in CHD. Studies can be satisfactorily performed with sedation (e.g., propofol). However, general anesthesia with intubation may be required for MRI in unstable infants and small children and in some cases where the images are improved during apnea.

Special Anesthesia Problems

1. All considerations for sedation or anesthesia in the MRI unit must be observed (see page 525). For general endotracheal anesthesia, an MRI compatible ventilator must be available.
2. The specific considerations of the child's cardiac disease must be observed.
3. If tracheal intubation is required; children with potential difficult intubation should be intubated in the OR and then transferred to the MRI suite. All children should recover in a properly staffed and equipped PACU.

General Anesthetic Management

1. Monitors must all be applied and functioning before induction.
2. The technique chosen must depend on the physiologic status of the child; stable children may be induced by inhalation of sevoflurane or a titrated IV dose of propofol. Potentially unstable children may be managed by infusion of opioid analgesics (e.g., remifentanil) and small doses of midazolam.
3. Cisatracurium is preferred for neuromuscular blockade (brief duration of action).
4. The lungs are ventilated with a high FiO_2.
5. Oxygen saturation is carefully monitored during apnea periods.

Suggested Reading

Odegard KC, DiNardo JA, Tsa-Goodman B, et al: Anaesthesia considerations for cardiac MRI in infants and small children, Paediatr Anaesth 14(6):471–476, 2004.

ANESTHESIA FOR NONCARDIAC SURGERY IN INFANTS AND CHILDREN WITH CONGENITAL HEART DISEASE

CHD often occurs in association with other congenital defects, some of which may require surgery in the neonate or infant. Older children with CHD frequently require anesthesia for noncardiac procedures (e.g., dental surgery). Therefore, the anesthesiologist may be called on to provide care for children with CHD for other types of surgery. Some of these children have uncorrected cardiac lesions, others have undergone partial (palliation) procedures, and others have had complete repair of their defect. However, even after "complete repair" there may be important considerations, such as the need for prophylactic antibiotics (see page 462) the presence of a pacemaker for heart block, or other residual defects. After repair of complex lesions, the postrepair physiology (e.g., post Fontan repair) may demand special perioperative considerations. Remember that the appearance of an intraoperative arrhythmia may be a very important observation indicating the potential for a more serious sudden cardiac event and should be reported to the child's cardiologist.

Diagnosis of Congenital Heart Disease

The first problem may be to decide whether the child presented for anesthesia does indeed have CHD. Although some children with CHD may be diagnosed in utero, many still go unrecognized throughout the neonatal period. In neonates, the diagnosis of CHD can be quite difficult:

1. Heart murmurs are common in the perinatal period and may not be indicative of significant heart disease.
2. Serious cardiac lesions may be present in the absence of a loud murmur.
3. The transitional circulation of the neonate may obscure the diagnosis: high PVR limits left-to-right shunts, and the patency of the ductus arteriosus provides flow to the lower body (i.e., in children with coarctation).

Signs suggesting CHD in the neonate include murmurs, cyanosis, tachypnea, prominent precordial pulsations, bounding peripheral pulses, hepatomegaly, poor feeding, cyanotic spells, and large heart on radiography. The definitive diagnosis, however, is most likely to be confirmed by echocardiography. Therefore, all neonates with lesions that are commonly associated with CHD (i.e., tracheoesophageal fistula, diaphragmatic hernia, omphalocele) and those with the signs just listed should be screened with an ECHO.

Older children may be found to have a previously undetected and undiagnosed murmur when examined before anesthesia. The problem is to determine whether significant heart disease is present and whether it is necessary to refer the child to a cardiologist. First, it is important to determine whether the child has normal exercise tolerance. It is very unlikely that a child with unlimited activity has a lesion that will cause problems during anesthesia. On physical examination, the characteristics of the murmur should be analyzed:

1. *Innocent murmurs* are soft, systolic, and not radiated; they may vary with position, may disappear on exercise, are not characteristic of any lesion, and are heard in healthy children.
2. *Noninnocent murmurs* include all diastolic murmurs, all pansystolic and late systolic murmurs, all loud murmurs, all continuous murmurs (except venous hum), and all transmitted murmurs.

If a soft and presumably innocent murmur is heard in a healthy child, surgery usually is not delayed. If a murmur suggestive of a definite, previously undiagnosed cardiac lesion is heard, delay elective surgery and refer to a cardiologist. Emergency surgery must proceed, and the child should be managed with due regard for the cardiac disease; prophylactic antibiotics should be administered when indicated (see page 462) and appropriate monitoring established.

Anesthesia Management

Preoperative

1. Many of the potential problems during noncardiac surgery are similar to those associated with cardiac surgery, and the same considerations for each specific lesion apply. For any major surgery, the child should be monitored as for cardiac surgery.
2. The anesthesiologist must clearly understand the pathophysiology of the child's disease and carefully assess the current physical status. Read the introduction to this chapter (pages 399-402) to understand some of the physiologic alterations in children with CHD.
3. The child's current medication schedule must be reviewed and discussed with the parents. All cardiac medications should be continued up to the day of surgery. For those taking digoxin, a recent blood level should be available (therapeutic range, 0.8 to 2 ng/ml).
4. Care must be taken to avoid excessive fluid restriction, especially in children with cyanotic CHD. The parents should be instructed to encourage clear fluids up until 2 hours before the operation. If oral fluids cannot be taken, intravenous fluid therapy must be established.
5. Order appropriate preoperative sedation, but avoid producing respiratory depression. The child should be sedated but not depressed. Oral midazolam is ideal, but the child should be monitored with a pulse oximeter once sedation is achieved. Apply a topical analgesic cream to a likely intravenous site.
6. Ensure that equipment for cardiopulmonary resuscitation (including a defibrillator with paddles of suitable size) is available in the OR suite.
7. Check coagulation status in those children with cyanotic heart disease; coagulopathy is a common complication of polycythemia.
8. Anesthesia must be carefully planned to minimize the possibility of adversely affecting the cardiovascular status of the child.
   a. Use extreme care with potent inhalational agents or other cardiac depressants, especially in those with a history of or predisposition to CHF.
   b. Avoid causing major alterations in PVR or SVR.
      i. Carefully maintain ventilation and oxygenation.
      ii. Avoid vasodilating drugs (e.g., isoflurane >0.5 %)

TABLE 14-2   Antibiotic Routine for Patients with Cardiac Disease

Dental Procedures, Oropharyngeal Surgery, Instrumentation of the Respiratory Tract Including Nasotracheal Intubation
Standard oral regimen for children includes those having prosthetic heart valves and other high-risk factors *:
Amoxicillin 50 mg/kg PO 1 hr preoperatively to a maximum of 2 g
Regimen for children allergic to amoxicillin/penicillin:
Clindamycin 20 mg/kg PO 1 hr preoperatively
Alternative regimen for children unable to take oral medications:
Ampicillin 50 mg/kg IV or IM 30 min preoperatively
Regimen for children allergic to ampicillin/penicillin and unable to take oral medications:
Clindamycin 20 mg/kg IV 30 min preoperatively
Regimen for children with methicillin sodium–resistant staphylococcal infections:
Vancomycin 20 mg/kg (maximum, 1 g) IV given over 1 hr, starting 1 hr preoperatively
Gastrointestinal or Genitourinary Procedures or Instrumentation
Standard regimen for children at high risk:
Ampicillin 50 mg/kg (up to 2 g) plus gentamicin 1.5 mg/kg (up to 120 mg); IV/IM, 30 min preoperatively and repeat ampicillin 25 mg/kg IV/IM 6 hr later; or amoxicillin 25 mg/kg PO
Regimen for high-risk children allergic to ampicillin:
Vancomycin 20 mg/kg (maximum, 1 g) IV plus gentamicin 1.5 mg/kg (maximum 80 mg) IV 1 hr preoperatively
Alternative regimen for children at moderate risk:
Amoxicillin 50 mg/kg PO 1 hr preoperatively or ampicillin 50 mg/kg IV/IM 30 min preoperatively

* High-risk factors for subacute bacterial endocarditis include the presence of prosthetic valves or materials (e.g., Gore-Tex shunts), cyanotic lesions, and especially tetralogy of Fallot. (Wilson W, et al. see Suggested Reading)

iii. Be gentle during laryngoscopy and use a topical LA before intubation.

iv. Ensure adequate analgesia before surgery or anesthetic interventions.

v. Exercise extreme caution in children with pulmonary hypertension, anticipate their increased potential for complications and avoid precipitating a pulmonary hypertensive crisis (see page 407).

9. Ensure that suitable antibiotic prophylaxis is ordered when indicated (Table 14-2). Routine prophylactic antibiotic therapy is no longer recommended for the prevention of infective endocarditis in children undergoing gastrointestinal or GU surgery. However, check

with your gastroenterologist/pediatric surgeon and urologist for their recommendations. See page 315 for antibiotic prophylaxis regimens for children undergoing dental surgery.

10. Minimally invasive video assisted surgery is now used for many procedures and provides the same advantages of decreased postoperative pain and more rapid recovery for the cardiac patient. However, the special considerations for these procedures (see page 339) must be observed together with the requirements dictated by the cardiac lesion. Provided intraabdominal pressure is maintained at below 10 mm Hg most children will tolerate these procedures.

11. The child who has had a Fontan procedure demands special consideration. Most important requirements are to maintain preload constant, prevent myocardial depression, and to ensure that PVR remains optimal. Spontaneous ventilation is ideal but if IPPV is required, ventilator settings to minimize intrathoracic pressure should be selected (brief inspiratory times, limited peak inspiratory pressure, and minimal PEEP). Fluid therapy must be carefully monitored and managed to maintain preload.

Perioperative

1. Attach all monitors before inducing anesthesia.
2. Establish a reliable intravenous route, but be aware of the risk of paradoxic emboli. Be careful to remove all bubbles from intravenous lines, especially in children with right-to-left shunts, but remember that others also may have bidirectional shunts.
3. Give 100% O_2 by mask.
4. Induce anesthesia with titrated doses of intravenous thiopental or propofol. Otherwise, inhalation induction with sevoflurane may be acceptable in some children, but beware of producing unacceptable myocardial depression or allowing any airway obstruction with resultant hypoxemia induced pulmonary hypertension.
5. Intubate the trachea for all but the most minor procedure (e.g., myringotomy). Give a suitable relaxant, but remember that if the circulation time is prolonged, there will be a longer delay before muscle paralysis is complete.
6. Children with less severe disease tolerate low concentrations of inhalational agents well; for minor procedures, maintain anesthesia with N_2O and sevoflurane or isoflurane with spontaneous or assisted ventilation. Children with more severe disease and those with any history of CHF cannot tolerate the use of myocardial depressant potent volatile agents. These children should be managed with a high-dose

opioid, midazolam and relaxant (pancuronium or rocuronium) technique, with controlled ventilation.

7. Maintain an adequate inspired concentration of oxygen, and monitor the oxygen saturation carefully. Oximeters are less accurate at lower saturations; therefore err on the safe side.

8. For major noncardiac surgery, insert arterial and other lines and monitor the child as for cardiac surgery. Consider the effects of previous surgery (e.g., systemic-to-pulmonary shunts) in choosing the BP cuff location.

9. $EtCO_2$ may not correlate well and tends to underestimate $PaCO_2$ in those children with right-to-left shunts whose tracheas are intubated, but does, however, give valuable information about pulmonary blood flow. For example, a decrease in $EtCO_2$ in a child with tetralogy indicates a decrease in pulmonary blood flow and an impending cyanotic spell.

10. Replace blood and fluid deficits and losses accurately.

Postoperative

1. Continue to monitor the child (including ECG and oximeter) until the child has fully recovered from all effects of anesthesia. Transfer to the PICU or PACU as appropriate.

2. Give O_2 until recovery is complete. Those with cyanotic CHD have a reduced ventilatory response to hypoxemia.

3. Provide good pain control. Pain and restlessness increase oxygen demand.

4. Give maintenance fluids intravenously until oral intake is adequate, but avoid overhydrating.

Suggested Reading

Sumpelmann R, Osthaus WA: The pediatric cardiac patient presenting for noncardiac surgery, Curr Opin Anaesth 20(3):216–220, 2007.

Taylor KL, Holtby H, Macpherson B: Laparoscopic surgery in the pediatric patient post Fontan procedure, Paediatr Anaesth 16(5):591–595, 2006.

Litman RS: Anesthetic considerations for children with congenital heart disease undergoing noncardiac surgery, Anesth Clin N Am 15:93–103, 1997.

Wilson W, Taubert KA, Gewitz M, et al: Prevention of infective endocarditis: guidelines from the American Heart Association: a guideline from the American Heart Association Rheumatic Fever, Endocarditis, and Kawasaki Disease Committee, Council on Cardiovascular Disease in the Young, and the Council on Clinical Cardiology, Council on Cardiovascular Surgery and Anesthesia, and the Quality of Care and Outcomes Research Interdisciplinary Working Group, Circ 116(15):1736–1754, 2007.

Orthopedic Surgery 15

A considerable proportion of children who undergo elective orthopedic surgery have multiple congenital anomalies and/or neuromuscular disease (see Appendix 1). Underlying diseases, particularly those associated with muscle weakness, require special anesthesia care; even minor surgery may be fraught with major anesthesia complications.

GENERAL PRINCIPLES

1. Children with orthopedic deformities may require repeated surgery and spend much time in the hospital; sympathetic management is particularly important, and preoperative sedation should be chosen carefully.
2. Check the history carefully. Neuromuscular disease is particularly relevant. In general, muscle relaxants, particularly succinylcholine, should be avoided in children with myopathies (see Appendix 1). Drug selection is influenced by the underlying disease and the type of neuro-monitoring that will be used intraoperatively.
3. Major surgery of the vertebral column deserves special consideration; the operations are extensive and may involve massive blood loss. Be prepared for a major transfusion. Autotransfusion and acute normovolemic hemodilution may be appropriate in some cases. Amicar and tranexamic acid decrease blood loss in spine surgery.
4. Malignant hyperthermia, though very rare, is more common in children with orthopedic diseases. Maintain vigilance for the early signs of a reaction (see Chapter 6, page 197).

465

5. When a tourniquet is used, blood loss is negligible. In other cases, surgery involving bone may result in significant blood loss (e.g., innominate osteotomy). Therefore establish a reliable intravenous route and confirm that blood is available.

   a. When a tourniquet is inflated, there usually follows a progressive increase in the heart rate and blood pressure. The exact cause is unknown, but it has been attributed to sympathetic stimulation. If the anesthesiologist has been aggressively treating the tourniquet-induced hypertension by giving greater concentrations of inhaled agents, the blood pressure may decrease precipitously on tourniquet release. Therefore use caution with concentrations of potent inhalational agents and other drugs while the tourniquet is being used, and reduce the concentration in anticipation of tourniquet release.

   b. Hemodynamic and metabolic responses to tourniquet release in children are usually not clinically important. A transient decrease in arterial pH associated with an increase in base deficit and carbon dioxide tension ($PaCO_2$) does occur; this is most marked after long tourniquet times or with the use of double tourniquets. General recommendations include the following:

      i. Attempt to limit tourniquet times to less than 75 minutes.

      ii. Use controlled ventilation before and after tourniquet release to remove the respiratory component of the acidosis.

      iii. Do not release bilateral tourniquets simultaneously.

      iv. In children in whom metabolic or respiratory acidosis is not easily compensated for (i.e., those with renal disease or pulmonary disease), consider staged release of the tourniquets and close monitoring of SpO_2 and $EtCO_2$.

      v. Serious complications of tourniquet use in children are very rare; however, pulmonary embolism on release has been reported in an obese child. Consider subcutaneous heparin in such children and monitor cardiopulmonary function closely after release.

      vi. Ensure that the tourniquet is removed from the limb as soon as it is deflated. Residual pressure compromising perfusion of the limb has resulted in serious complications.

6. Orthopedic surgery is associated with high levels of postoperative pain. Plan for optimal management, using regional analgesia whenever possible. The introduction of continuous peripheral nerve blocks using disposable pumps has opened up new avenues for postoperative pain control after limb or trunk surgery.

7. Compartment syndrome may complicate orthopedic injuries, especially supracondylar fractures of the humerus, and forearm and tibial fractures.

There is a concern that effective analgesia may mask the presenting sign of this syndrome (i.e., increased pain). This is especially of concern when the limb cannot easily be examined (i.e., encased in a cast). Compartment syndrome is rare enough that many question withholding effective analgesia from the majority of children who will not develop this complication. There is a strong consensus that effective postoperative pain relief should be provided for every child. Means to monitor compartment pressure are now readily available; a compartment syndrome must be diagnosed either by direct means (frequent nurse examination) or by the increased need for analgesic medication.

8. Urinary retention may occur in children who have lower limb surgery and are treated with a regional block. This should be noted by postanesthesia care unit (PACU) staff and treated as necessary.

9. Children with cerebral palsy frequently present for orthopedic surgery. These children require special considerations (see Chapter 6).

10. Children with Duchenne muscular dystrophy may present for major scoliosis surgery and require careful assessment of their cardiorespiratory status and anticipation that the bleeding will be greater than usual (see later discussion and Appendix 1).

Suggested Reading

Tredwell SJ, Wilmink M, Inkpen K, et al: Pediatric tourniquets: analysis of cuff and limb interface, current practice, and guidelines for use, J Pediatr Orthop 21(5):671–676, 2001.

Sinicina I, Bise K, Hetterich R, et al: Tourniquet use in childhood: a harmless procedure? Paediatr Anaesth 17(2):167–170, 2007.

Dalens B: Some current controversies in paediatric regional anaesthesia, Curr Opin Anaesthesiol 19(3):301–308, 2006.

MISCELLANEOUS ORTHOPEDIC PROCEDURES AND ANESTHESIA CONSIDERATIONS

Hip Arthrogram

Hip arthrograms are performed in infants to assess the head of the femur and other aspects of the hip joint. As part of the procedure, a small amount of air may be injected into the joint to ensure that the tip of the needle is in the joint space before injecting contrast material; serious air embolism and cardiac arrest have occurred.

Recommendation: If a hip arthrogram is planned, determine whether air will be injected. Monitor the child very carefully during injection, omit nitrous oxide, and monitor for evidence of an air embolism.

Suggested Reading

Lamdan R, Sadun A, Shamir MY: Near-fatal air embolus during arthrography of the hip in a baby aged four months, J Bone Jt Surg (Br) 89(2):240–241, 2007.

Club Feet

Beware of the high incidence of myopathies in children having clubfeet. Examine the child and the medical history carefully for any indications of a myopathy. If positive, revise the anesthesia technique appropriately.

In some cases, regional analgesia techniques combined with intravenous sedation may be optimal for clubfoot surgery. Caudal epidural analgesia may augment intraoperative management and provide for postoperative pain management.

Suggested Reading

Zanette G, Robb N, Zadra N, et al: Undetected central core disease myopathy in an infant presenting for clubfoot surgery, Paediatr Anaesth 17(4):380–382, 2007.

Tobias JD, Mencio GA: Regional anesthesia for clubfoot surgery in children, Amer J Ther 5(4):273–277, 1998.

LIMB FRACTURES

Closed Limb Fractures

Injuries to upper limbs are common; many of these children are older; therefore regional analgesia can be used. If so:

1. Use a sufficient local analgesic drug to produce a profound block.
2. Perform the block well in advance of the scheduled surgery so that it has plenty of time to become well established.
3. If supplementary sedation is required, midazolam or ketamine is usually very satisfactory.

Fractures of the Forearm

1. Perform a block of the brachial plexus via the axillary route, see Chapter 5, page 164 for drugs and doses. Ultrasonography improves the success with brachial plexus blocks.
2. Intravenous blocks are not satisfactory for reduction of fractures. It is more difficult to apply an optimally tight cast to an exsanguinated limb.

Fractures of the Femur

1. A block of the femoral nerve with lidocaine or bupivacaine is easy to perform and relieves pain and muscle spasm as the traction apparatus is being applied.
2. A catheter may be introduced to the femoral sheath and a continuous femoral nerve block maintained with 0.5% bupivacaine (see continuous femoral block Chapter 5, page 166).

General Anesthesia

Every child with a recent fracture must be considered to have a full stomach and a rapid-sequence induction should be performed. Vomiting more frequently occurs during emergence from anesthesia; therefore, the child should be fully awake and in a lateral position before extubation.

Postoperative

1. Pain may be quite severe after routine orthopedic surgery, and should be controlled by either systemic analgesic drugs or regional analgesia or a combination of these:
   a. Regimens combining acetaminophen and a nonsteroidal anti-inflammatory drug (NSAID) are more effective than either drug alone. Acetaminophen (40 mg/kg PR or 15 mg/kg PO) with keto-profen (2 mg/kg IV) augmented by titrated doses of opioids as required is a suitable basic regimen. Pain should be assessed using standard objective measures (see Chapter 7).
   b. Patient-controlled analgesia (PCA) may be appropriate for many children (see Chapter 7).
   c. Regional analgesia provided by neuraxial or peripheral nerve block. When possible the latter should be chosen as this is less likely to cause complications. In children, it is customary to perform blocks and insert catheters under general anesthesia. Peripheral nerve blocks and catheter placement should be guided by ultrasonography when possible.
   d. Peripheral nerve blocks may be initiated in the operating room and continued through the PACU to the ward or even to home using a disposable elastomeric infusion pump. The decision to continue this at home will depend upon the home circumstances and the attitude and abilities of the parents. A postoperative infusion of ropivacaine 0.2% at a rate of 0.1 ml/kg/hr has been suggested for continuous peripheral nerve block.

Suggested Reading

Hiller A, Meretoja OA, Korpela R, et al: The analgesic efficacy of acetaminophen, ketoprofen, or their combination for pediatric surgical patients having soft tissue or orthopedic procedures, Anesth Analg 102(5):1365–1371, 2006.

Remerand F, Vuitton AS, Palud M, et al: Elastomeric pump reliability in postoperative regional anesthesia: a survey of 430 consecutive devices, Anesth Analg 107:2079–2084, 2008.

Ganesh A, Rose JB, Wells L, et al: Continuous peripheral nerve blockade for inpatient and outpatient postoperative analgesia in children, Anesth Analg 105(5):1234–1242, 2007.

KYPHOSCOLIOSIS

Kyphoscoliosis may be congenital (15% of cases), idiopathic (65%), or secondary to neuromuscular disease (20%). More than 80% of children with idiopathic scoliosis are female. Pulmonary function may be impaired, and some children with associated diseases (myopathies, cerebral palsy) may be severely disabled, wheelchair bound, and physiologically debilitated.

Pulmonary Function

Changes in pulmonary function are related to the underlying cause, the speed of development of the scoliosis, and the severity of the curvature. The cardiorespiratory effects of scoliosis are summarized in Figure 15-1.

The pulmonary abnormality is restrictive rather than obstructive; chest wall compliance is reduced. The vital capacity and the total lung capacity may be dramatically reduced, and the functional residual capacity somewhat less so. The residual volume tends to be maintained. The elastic resistance of the chest wall may be high, increasing the work of breathing. If left untreated, severe and prolonged lung compression impairs gas exchange, which becomes evident only in later stages of the disease.

The principal concern for young children with idiopathic scoliosis is the cosmetic effect of the spinal and pelvic or chest wall deformity, especially when the curvature increases during the years of rapid body growth. At this stage, respiratory symptoms are uncommon, but pulmonary function studies may reveal an abnormality. Although lung volumes can be normal, exercise tolerance may be reduced. In severe cases the mechanical effects of scoliosis on respiratory function are apparent even at rest.

Pulmonary function is relatively normal in most children who present for correction of idiopathic scoliosis with a curvature of less than 65%. Respiratory disability is more likely to occur in association with congenital scoliosis or curvature of paralytic etiology.

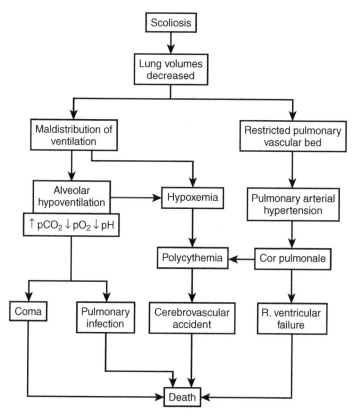

Figure 15-1. Pathophysiology of the cardiorespiratory effects of kypho-scoliosis. Progressive alveolar hypoventilation, leading to hypoxia, may be accompanied by pulmonary hypertension and right ventricular failure. *(Courtesy Henry Levison, MD, Former Director of Respiratory Physiology, The Hospital for Sick Children, Toronto.)*

The High-Risk Scoliotic Child

Scoliosis surgery may be recommended for severely incapacitated children for the purpose of facilitating their ongoing care and arresting the progression of cardiorespiratory compromise. There is a very high incidence of perioperative complications in this group of children and many require very aggressive and prolonged postoperative intensive care; however, the ultimate outcome is judged by many of these children and their caregivers to be worthwhile. It is very important that these children be optimally prepared for their surgery:

1. The nutritional status should be assessed and optimized using TPN or via a gastrostomy as may be appropriate to the individual.
2. The pulmonary system should be evaluated for reversible disease that might be improved by physiotherapy or antibiotic therapy. Those with neuromuscular disease and a preoperative FEV_1 less than 40% of predicted are likely to need postoperative ventilation.
3. The cardiac status should be evaluated by echocardiogram (i.e., myocardial contractility, RV function, etc.) and preoperative therapy initiated as indicated.
4. The pediatric intensive care unit (PICU) should be notified that the child will require admission and they should be familiar with his or her preoperative condition.

Surgical Procedures

1. Posterior spinal fusion may be performed using contoured metal rods to stabilize the spine postoperatively until bony fusion occurs. In some children with a flexible spine, the deformity is corrected solely by a posterior fusion. Adjustable rods may be placed in some young children to permit adjustments during growth.
2. In some, an anterior thoracoabdominal approach may be used to remove the intervertebral discs or a hemivertebra to correct a lateral curve. This may be an open procedure or an endoscopic procedure.
3. In others, the two procedures are combined: an anterior release followed by a posterior fusion. In this case, surgery is often prolonged, and associated with significant blood loss: a challenge for the anesthesiologist. Anterior release procedures may be carried out endoscopically, in which case the special considerations for endoscopic surgery apply (see Chapter 13, page 339).

Special Anesthesia Problems

1. Anesthesia management must take into account the following:
   a. The severity and cause of the curvature. The more severe the curve, the more pulmonary function is impaired, and greater the likelihood of postoperative pulmonary failure.

   If the scoliosis is secondary to neuromuscular disease:

   i. Pulmonary function impairment caused by the mechanical effects of the spinal curvature may be compounded by involvement of respiratory muscles in the disease process. Postoperative respiratory insufficiency is more likely.

    ii. Increased bleeding may be expected. This may be a result of altered vascular responses and platelet adhesion associated with myopathies (e.g., Duchenne muscular dystrophy).

    iii. Cardiomyopathy may occur in adolescents with Duchenne muscular dystrophy.

    iv. Selection of suitable drugs may be limited (i.e., avoid succinylcholine and inhalational anesthetics to prevent rhabdomyolysis if a myopathy is present. Titrate doses of nondepolarizing relaxants if required.

  b. The degree of respiratory and cardiovascular impairment:

    i. Surgery may be expected to stabilize the cardiorespiratory effects of the disease but may not improve these.

    ii. A further impairment of pulmonary function must be anticipated in the early postoperative phase and may require respiratory support.

  c. The type of corrective procedure proposed.

    i. Posterior fusion only

    ii. Anterior and posterior fusion combined

2. Preoperative assessment must include the following:

  a. Detailed history and examination for an indication of abilities, stamina, and the presence of any other significant medical conditions.

  b. Routine hematology studies, biochemistry, and cross matching for transfusion.

  c. Pulmonary function studies, including blood gas analysis. (These studies may not be possible in very young children due to lack of cooperation.)

  d. Echocardiogram to assess myocardial function for all children (particularly adolescents) with very severe curves or associated myopathy.

3. Be alert for signs of significant respiratory impairment (i.e., tachypnea at rest, severely reduced vital capacity, abnormal blood gas values, inability to cough effectively). Postoperatively, hypoventilation, secretion retention, and atelectasis are likely in response to pain, analgesic drugs, and immobilization that will further compound existing problems.

4. Severe impairment of respiratory function is not a contraindication to surgery, provided that resources are available for postoperative intensive respiratory care (including controlled ventilation, if necessary). Fixation of the spinal deformity is essential to prevent further deterioration of respiratory function (but usually does not result in significant improvement).

5. Children with a vital capacity less than 40% of normal may develop major respiratory complications postoperatively and likely require postoperative ventilation.

Corrective Surgery by the Posterior Approach

Special Anesthesia Problems

1. Because the child will be in the prone position, extra care should be taken to secure the tracheal tube and prevent it from becoming dislodged. If preoperative correction of the spinal curvature has been achieved with an exoskeletal apparatus, intubation will probably be difficult; fixation of the head and neck may render adequate direct laryngoscopy impossible, making a fiberoptic technique necessary.
2. Discuss with the family and the child the need for invasive lines, postoperative ventilation (if likely), the need for ICU, and the potential for an intraoperative wake-up test.
3. Blood loss may be severe (in excess of 50% of the estimated blood volume [EBV]). Most bleeding originates from the vertebral veins, which become engorged if there is any pressure on the anterior abdomen. Blood loss is also related to the extent of the surgery (length of spine to be fused) and to the surgeon's speed and expertise. Those with scoliosis secondary to a recognized neuromuscular disorder usually have a larger blood loss than those with idiopathic scoliosis. Alternatives to homologous transfusion should be considered:

   i. Autologous blood programs are very suitable for preoperative collections in these children.
   ii. Intraoperative acute normovolemic hemodilution may be used cautiously.

   (These procedures may be optimized by giving oral ferrous sulfate daily beginning 4 weeks before surgery and then administering twice-weekly intramuscular injections of erythropoietin commencing 2 weeks before surgery. The hematocrit (Hct) should not be allowed to exceed 55% preoperatively).

   iii. The cell saver may be used to salvage erythrocytes from suctioned blood. However, transfusion of large volumes of washed cells may lead to coagulopathy because of dilution of coagulation factors. Fresh-frozen plasma should also be administered if blood loss exceeds one blood volume.
4. Spinal cord function is usually monitored during surgery: the use of somatosensory evoked potentials (SSEPs) has been augmented by the addition

of motor evoked potentials (MEPs), stimulating the cord above the level of the surgery and recording the electromyogram from the limb.

Anesthetic techniques that permit the monitoring of evoked potentials limit inhalational agents to 0.5 MAC, although large doses of opioids may be given. Nitrous oxide decreases the amplitude of evoked potentials and is usually avoided. Propofol/opioid infusions are the mainstay for these anesthetics. Benzodiazepines may be used to induce amnesia. During the testing of MEPs, better results are obtained with minimal neuromuscular blockade (i.e., 2 to 4 twitches on a train of four); specifically, most electrophysiologists permit an intermediate-acting relaxant for tracheal intubation and then no further relaxant during surgery whereas others permit an infusion to maintain a limited degree of neuromuscular blockade. Because of the difficulty in assessing depth of anesthesia during TIVA, a depth of anesthesia monitor is often used.

Despite the use of multimodal neurophysiologic monitoring, a wake-up test may still be required (i.e., a surgical misadventure or failure of the monitoring system). Fortunately, the anesthesia technique that provides for neurophysiologic monitoring also allows for a rapid wake-up test should this be required.

Every child should be awake at the end of the operation, so that both sensory and motor function can be tested immediately. Any defects should be reported to the surgeon promptly.

5. Pulmonary function may be severely impaired. The anesthesiologist must check that the present state is optimal and exclude any superimposed acute respiratory disease.

6. Postoperative pain is considerable; intrathecal opioids administered intraoperatively have been effective for postoperative analgesia and may also facilitate intraoperative BP control and reduce blood loss. Otherwise epidural analgesia or PCA should be planned and these options discussed with the child and family.

7. Visual loss occurs rarely after spine surgery.

   a. The most common ocular injury is a corneal abrasion. Far less common is visual loss because of posterior ischemic optic neuropathy (PION) (occurring three times more frequently than anterior AION) or central retinal artery occlusion (CRAO) may rarely occur after spine surgery—especially when performed in the prone position.

   b. Age: occurs rarely in pediatric patients (<18 years).

   c. Factors associated with visual loss because of ION include preoperative anemia, prolonged surgery, intraoperative hypotension, low hematocrit, and major blood loss. CRAO results from direct facial-orbital compression.

d. A possible but unproven factor in the genesis of postspinal visual loss is excessive crystalloid fluid administration intraoperatively. This is known to increase intraocular pressure (IOP) and periorbital edema.

e. NB. Visual loss recovers in 44% of those with ION but in 0% of those with CRAO.

Procedures that reduce the risk of intraoperative visual loss:

1. Assess the child carefully and encourage staged procedures if the proposed operation may be excessively long (>6 hours) or associated with large blood losses (>45% estimated blood volume).
2. Position carefully:
   a. Avoid pressure on the eyes—check frequently during surgery and document this in the anesthesia record.
   b. Position the head in a neutral forward position (no neck flexion, extension, or rotation) so that it is level with or above the heart.
3. Monitor the hematocrit frequently and avoid markedly reduced levels intraoperatively.
4. Monitor central venous pressure and administer balanced crystalloid and colloid solutions to maintain an adequate blood volume.
5. Induced hypotension is an accepted practice for spine surgery but avoid excessively reduced levels from baseline (i.e., within 20% to 25% of baseline mean arterial pressure or a minimum systolic pressure of 80 to 90 mm Hg).

Check the child's vision immediately upon awakening and seek consultation if there are any defects.

Suggested Reading

Practice advisory for perioperative visual loss associated with spine surgery: a report by the American Society of Anesthesiologists Task Force on Perioperative Blindness, Anesthesiology 104:1319–1328, 2006.

Anesthesia Management

Preoperative

1. Premedication with oral midazolam is usually adequate if combined with reassurance and a full explanation of procedures to be performed. Lorazepam 1 to 2 mg PO 1 hour preop is very effective for adolescents.
2. Do not give respiratory depressant drugs to children whose respiratory function is impaired.

3. Ensure that all equipment and drugs are prepared in case of emergency.
4. Check that an adequate supply of blood and other fluid replacements is at hand.

Perioperative

1. If halo-loop traction is in place, check that instruments to release the connecting rods are at hand.
2. Tracheal intubation:
   a. In uncomplicated cases, induce anesthesia with propofol or thiopental followed by a low dose of an intermediate-acting relaxant (e.g., rocuronium 0.3 to 0.4 mg/kg) and intubate. If evoked potential monitoring is planned, allow the child to recover from the neuromuscular blockade then check the positioning and function of the stimulating electrodes over the posterior tibial nerve.
   b. If exoskeletal apparatus is present, direct laryngoscopy may not be possible.
      i. Avoid muscle relaxant drugs until tracheal intubation has been accomplished. Some older children may consent to and cooperate during "awake" fiberoptic intubation under sedation.
      ii. Select a suitable intubation technique (i.e., fiberoptic intubation awake or under general anesthesia).
3. Maintenance:
   There are several choices for maintenance: balanced anesthesia with inhaled anesthetic or propofol and opioid (i.e., total intravenous anesthesia [TIVA]). In both instances, an opioid infusion is generally required:
   a. Opioid infusions:
      i. Fentanyl-loading dose of 5 µg/kg; infusion at 3 µg/kg/hr
      ii. Morphine-loading dose of 100 µg/kg; infusion at 10 to 30 µg/kg/hr
      iii. Remifentanil infusion at 0.1 µg/kg/min and adjusted up or down to control blood pressure as needed.
   b. Limited concentrations of isoflurane (0.5% to 1%) or desflurane (3% to 5%) may control the BP as needed. This technique does not usually interfere with neurophysiologic monitoring. If MEPs are to be measured, neuromuscular block is generally permitted only for tracheal intubation.
   c. A TIVA protocol. This is a useful technique when multimodal neurophysiologic monitoring is to be performed. A propofol infusion is administered, though propofol decreases the amplitude of transcranial MEPs, these can still be acceptably monitored. Propofol is commonly administered with remifentanil as TIVA as follows:

Propofol 100 to 150 µg/kg/min with remifentanil 0.1 to 0.3 µg/kg/min.

The dose of propofol may be modified as surgery proceeds on the basis of BIS readings or other benchmarks of anesthetic depth. The remifentanil infusion may be adjusted according to hemodynamic parameters. It is also recommended that other sedative drugs may be administered during TIVA, including dexmedetomidine and midazolam, the latter to ensure amnesia.

    d. Nitrous oxide is usually avoided as it interferes significantly with neurophysiologic monitoring.

    e. Insert a nasogastric tube.

4. Position the child on a scoliosis operating frame that avoids any external pressure on the anterior abdominal wall (i.e., the Hall-Relton frame). Maintenance of the correct prone-suspended position is essential to ensure minimal blood loss. (If the child is malpositioned so that pressure on the abdomen causes vertebral venous engorgement, heavy blood loss is inevitable.) Ensure that there is no pressure on the eyes and that the considerations for the prevention of postoperative visual loss are observed (see previous discussion).

5. Monitor the following throughout:

    a. Ventilation-esophageal stethoscope, airway pressure, $EtCO_2$

    b. Circulation—ECG, pulse oximeter, arterial line, and central venous pressure (CVP)

    c. Temperature—rectal or esophageal probe

    d. Neuromuscular blockade—peripheral nerve stimulator

    e. Blood loss—gravimetric method and graduated suction bottles

    f. Urine output—indwelling catheter

    g. SSEPs and/or MEPs—before, during, and after correction

    h. Hematology and biochemistry—acid-base and blood gas status, Hct and coagulation status as indicated by the duration and severity of the procedure

    i. Head/neck position; no pressure on the eyes

6. Blood loss is minimized by:

    a. Proper posture (see item 5, previously) and muscle relaxation (if no MEPs)

    b. Deep infiltration of the wound site (by the surgeon) with a large volume of dilute epinephrine/saline solution (up to 500 ml of 1:500,000 solution may be used)

    c. Controlled ventilation, maintaining $PaCO_2$ at 30 to 35 mm Hg to avoid hypercarbia and vasodilation

    d. Surgical technique (firm packing and meticulous subperiosteal plane dissection)

e. Use of a propofol infusion to avoid high concentrations of anesthetic agents that cause vasodilation (e.g., isoflurane)

f. Hypotensive anesthesia—may be used, but the MAP should be kept within 20% to 25% of baseline. In the prone child, the spinal cord is above the heart and, if hypotension occurs, spinal cord ischemia may ensue, especially while it is manipulated or stretched, leading to paraplegia. Do not combine with hemodilution.

g. Acute normovolemic hemodilution (i.e., an alternative blood conservation method) is carried out as follows:

   i. A calculated volume of blood is withdrawn to reduce the Hct to 30%. Use the preoperative Hct and the EBV (in milliliters) to calculate the volume to be withdrawn:
   Volume withdrawn = (Hct − 30) × EBV/Hct

   ii. When the child is anesthetized and lines have been inserted, a weighed volume of blood is withdrawn via the arterial line into citrate-phosphate-dextrose bags for storage.

   iii. During blood withdrawal, a volume of warmed lactated Ringer's solution equal to three times the blood volume withdrawn is infused.

   iv. As surgery progresses, the blood that has been withdrawn is reinfused. This method results in loss of lower-Hct blood during surgery and conservation of the child's cells for reinfusion.

   v. Monitor the oxygen tension (PaO_2), pH, and plasma lactate levels to ensure an adequate tissue supply of oxygen.

h. Both Amicar and tranexamic acid have been recommended to decrease blood losses during extensive or repeat spine surgery. The selected drug should be initiated after induction of anesthesia but before skin incision and continuously infused until the completion of surgery.

7. If the neurophysiologic recordings show any changes or cannot be obtained for technical reasons, or if the surgeon requires confirmation of spinal cord integrity after application of the distraction and compression apparatus or other manipulation, a wake-up test may be necessary:

a. Discontinue inhaled anesthetics or TIVA infusions. Check the neuromuscular monitor for the extent of neuromuscular block (if present). Full antagonism is not advisable because it may lead to complications (see later discussion).

b. Decrease ventilation to return the $PaCO_2$ to normal levels. Flood the wound with saline to reduce the potential for air embolization. Ask the child to move the toes. (Voluntary dorsiflexion and plantarflexion of the feet confirms spinal cord integrity.) Reanesthetize the child using midazolam (0.1 mg/kg) and propofol (3 to 5 mg/kg) IV. Beware of allowing the child to awaken too much; excessive movements may result in dangerous loss of position on the frame, and attempts to breathe spontaneously against the ventilator. (This has been reported to result in air embolism).

Corrective Surgery by the Anterior Approach

For treatment of a curve in the lumbar region, the vertebral column is approached laterally on the convex side of the curvature. Thoracotomy is performed or using VATS; the diaphragm is divided at its peripheral attachments to provide access to the vertebrae.

N.B. This surgical trauma to the diaphragm and chest wall increases the risk of postoperative respiratory insufficiency.

Anesthesia management is the same as for the posterior approach— N_2O, controlled ventilation, muscle relaxation, and supplementary analgesia, with the following modifications:

1. Selective endobronchial intubation of the contralateral lung may be advantageous, permitting easier access to upper thoracic curvatures. (Serial blood gas measurements dictate the feasibility of continuing this technique throughout the procedure, but it is usually well tolerated.)

   The Arndt endobronchial blocker has proven useful for this procedure.

2. If bilateral ventilation is selected, ventilation of the exposed lung will be impeded by surgical packing and retractors. Periodically, expand the lung fully (to avoid prolonged atelectasis).

Spinal Osteotomy

Spinal osteotomy with wedge excision consists of local resection of deformed vertebrae. This procedure may result in excessive blood loss owing to the proximity of the vertebral and epidural venous plexuses. It may be difficult to control the hemorrhage.

Monitor blood loss by:

1. Gravimetric method (weigh sponges and measure suction losses)
2. Continuous CVP measurement and direct BP readings via an arterial line
3. Clinical observation (e.g., urine output)

If massive transfusion (>1 blood volume) is required:

1. Use packed cells in recently thawed FFP.
2. Warm all blood and intravenous fluids.
3. Monitor coagulation indices, especially platelets.
4. Order platelet concentrates (1 unit/5 kg) if the platelet count is less than 100,000/mm³. Administer platelets if < 50,000/mm³
5. Monitor the acid-base status and correct acidosis.
6. If citrate toxicity is suspected (hypotension despite volume replacement), administer calcium chloride (10 mg/kg) or calcium gluconate (30 mg/kg) intravenously (repeat as indicated).

Postoperative Care After Scoliosis Surgery

A. For the child with idiopathic scoliosis and good preoperative pulmonary function:
   1. The child should be awake and the trachea extubated before leaving the operating room.
      a. Check for movement of legs and feet.
      b. Check air entry throughout the lungs. (Pneumothorax is a possible complication of spinal surgery.)
   2. On arrival in the PACU:
      a. Give 40% O_2 by mask.
      b. Provide a detailed account of the intraoperative course to the PACU staff.
      c. Supplement analgesia as necessary (e.g., morphine infusion, patient-controlled analgesia). There is evidence that morphine requirements may be increased after a remifentanil-based TIVA protocol.
      d. Obtain plain radiographs of the chest and vertebral column. Check the lung fields, looking especially for pneumothorax.
      e. Obtain hemoglobin and Hct values; administer blood transfusion accordingly.
   3. The child must remain supine for at least 12 hours. Order physiotherapy; encourage breathing exercises.
   4. Ensure that the child is nursed in a warm environment. (Body temperature usually decreases 1 °C to 2 °C during surgery because of large wound exposure, air-conditioning, and so on.)
B. For the high-risk child with neuromuscular disease and impaired cardiopulmonary function.
   1. Transfer the child to the PICU intubated and ventilated. Anticipate that several days of IPPV may be required. X-ray chest on arrival; check endotracheal tube tip (ETT) position.

2. Provide a detailed account of the intraoperative course to the PICU staff.
3. Postoperative pulmonary insufficiency may result from:
   a. Underlying neuromuscular disease and residual neuromuscular blockade
   b. Acute conditions (e.g., pneumothorax, hemothorax, pleural effusion [check postop Chest x-ray])
   c. Retention of secretions and atelectasis (due to pain, analgesics, and/or immobilization)
   d. Perioperative aspiration of gastric contents
   e. Postoperative alteration in thoracic mechanics.
   f. Fat embolism syndrome (rare, but may be fatal).
4. Other medical complications may follow scoliosis surgery:
   a. Syndrome of inappropriate antidiuretic hormone secretion (SIADH)
   b. Abdominal conditions; pancreatitis; cholelithiasis; superior mesenteric artery syndrome; ileus; pneumothorax; hemothorax; chylothorax.

Continuing Pulmonary Management

1. IPPV may be required via the endotracheal tube for several days.
2. In some children, extubation may be possible with continuing assisted ventilation by means of noninvasive positive pressure ventilation.

Suggested Reading

Preoperative Assessment

Yuan N, Skaggs DL, Dorey F, et al: Preoperative predictors of prolonged postoperative mechanical ventilation in children following scoliosis repair, Ped Pulmonol 40(5):414–419, 2005.

Intraoperative Care

Anschel DJ, Aherne A, Soto RG, et al: Successful intraoperative spinal cord monitoring during scoliosis surgery using a total intravenous anesthetic regimen including dexmedetomidine, J Clin Neurophys 25(1):56–61, 2008.
Bird GT, Hall M, Nel L, et al: Effectiveness of Arndt endobronchial blockers in pediatric scoliosis surgery: a case series, Paediatr Anaesth 17(3):289–294, 2007.
Gibson PR: Anaesthesia for correction of scoliosis in children, Anaesth Intens Care 32(4):548–559, 2004.

Pelosi L, Lamb J, Grevitt M, et al: Combined monitoring of motor and somatosensory evoked potentials in orthopaedic spinal surgery, Clin Neurophys 113(7):1082–1091, 2002.

Schwartz DM, Auerbach JD, Dormans JP, et al: Neurophysiological detection of impending spinal cord injury during scoliosis surgery, J Bone Jt Surg Am 89(11):2440–2449, 2007.

Sethna NF, Zurakowski D, Brustowicz RM, et al: Tranexamic acid reduces intraoperative blood loss in pediatric patients undergoing scoliosis surgery, Anesthesiology 102(4):727–732, 2005.

Baig MN, Lubow M, Immesoette P, et al: Vision loss after spine surgery: review of the literature and recommendations, Neurosurg Focus 23(5):15, 2007.

Postoperative Care

Almenrader N, Patel D: Spinal fusion surgery in children with non-idiopathic scoliosis: is there a need for routine postoperative ventilation? Br J Anaesth 97(6):851–857, 2006.

Doherty MJ, Millner PA, Latham M, et al: Non-invasive ventilation in the treatment of ventilatory failure following corrective spinal surgery, Anaesthesia 56(3):235–238, 2001.

Shapiro G, Green DW, Fatica NS, et al: Medical complications in scoliosis surgery, Curr Opin Pediatr 13(1):36–41, 2001.

16 Urologic Investigation and Surgery

GENERAL PRINCIPLES

The anesthesia risk depends on the state of the child's renal function and any other disease process that may be present.

1. Most children who come for investigation or surgery of the lower urinary tract have good renal function.
2. Many of those who require renal biopsy have mild renal dysfunction (usually insufficient to influence anesthesia risk).
3. All children in renal failure are seriously ill and present multiple problems for the anesthesiologist.
4. Renal disease may be part of a syndrome and therefore requires consideration of all aspects of the condition (see Appendix 1).
5. Surgery of the genitalia may have significant psychological effects on small children; effective postoperative pain relief may minimize these effects.
6. Many urologic procedures are now performed endoscopically and the provisions for laparoscopy should be applied (see Chapter 13, page 339).

CHILDREN WITH GOOD RENAL FUNCTION

Anesthesia Management—Minor Procedures

Children almost always require general anesthesia for minor procedures, such as cystoscopy, retrograde pyelography, circumcision, or hypospadias repair. Healthy children undergoing brief investigative procedures or operations are almost all treated as outpatients.

Preoperative

1. Oral sedative premedication (midazolam) is useful for some children, especially those who require repeated surgery.

Perioperative

1. Induce anesthesia with inhalational or intravenous anesthetics.
2. Maintain anesthesia with N_2O, O_2, and sevoflurane or isoflurane by mask, laryngeal mask airway (LMA), or tracheal tube.
3. Provide regional analgesia for postoperative pain control whenever possible (see Chapter 5). If the block is performed before the surgery commences, less anesthetic drugs will be required during surgery and awakening will be rapid and pain-free.
   a. For circumcision: perform a penile block (see Chapter 5, page 161) using bupivacaine *without* epinephrine. Ropivacaine should not be used for this block because of its vasoconstrictor properties. EMLA cream may be applied to the incision to augment the block.
   b. For hypospadias repair, perform a caudal block (see Chapter 5, page 153).

Postoperative

1. Give supplementary analgesia as required; those children with a successful regional block will require few additional medications. Outpatients are usually discharged from the hospital 1 hour after recovery. Anticipate the need for additional analgesia at home as the block wears off. For optimal pain relief, instruct parents to administer a suitable analgesic (e.g., acetaminophen with codeine) *before* the pain occurs.

Anesthesia Management—Major Genitourinary

Surgical Procedures

Apply anesthesia management as for minor procedures (see previous discussion), plus the following:

1. Use general endotracheal anesthesia with muscle relaxants and controlled ventilation.
2. Be prepared for major hemorrhage: Insert a reliable large-bore intravenous line, measure blood losses carefully, and replace fluids as indicated.

3. Use regional analgesia when possible to provide postoperative pain relief. For example, for reimplantation of ureters, a single-shot caudal provides analgesia for the first few hours or an indwelling epidural catheter, provides analgesia for up to 3 days. Intercostal nerve blocks or, preferably, a lumbar epidural block provides good analgesia after renal surgery. Establish the block before surgery.
4. Children who have dilated ureters may develop hypertension postoperatively. This may require treatment.
5. For special considerations for Wilm's tumor, see Chapter 13.

CHILDREN WITH POOR RENAL FUNCTION OR RENAL FAILURE

These children may have many physiologic and psychological disturbances.

Special Anesthesia Problems

1. Anemia (usually normochromic, normocytic) may be present but with standard care under the supervision of a renal unit, this should not be severe, the objective of pretransplant care is to avoid significant anemia.

   Anemia in renal failure is caused by:

   a. Decreased erythropoietin production. If erythropoietin is reduced, the hemoglobin concentration (Hb) will not exceed 7 to 9 g/dl. Recombinant human erythropoietin therapy may not be effective if severe uremia is present
   b. Decreased erythrocyte survival and increased hemolysis
   c. Increased bruising and bleeding from increased capillary fragility
   d. Iron and/or folic acid deficiency
   e. Bone marrow depression due to increased blood urea nitrogen (BUN)

   The presence of anemia leads to compensatory changes; that is, increased cardiac output and increased red blood cell (RBC) 2,3-diphosphoglycerate (2,3-DPG), although the latter is minimal. The P_{50} values are similar to those of children with normal renal function.

   Treatment with erythropoietin and supplemental iron will increase the hemoglobin concentration to near 10 gm/dl, which is the target level. After successful renal transplantation, the Hb increases further.

   Blood transfusions, once contraindicated pre-transplant, are now recognized to improve post-transplantation graft survival.

2. Coagulopathy may be present, caused by:
   a. Increased capillary fragility
   b. Functional platelet defect (decreased adhesiveness), possibly due to increased guanidinosuccinic acid
   c. Thrombocytopenia due to bone marrow depression
   d. Drugs (e.g., heparin, acetylsalicylic acid)

Coagulopathy if present is usually of minor significance and does not usually represent a contraindication to epidural catheter placement.

3. Acid-base imbalance:
   a. Children produce even more acid than adults; when urinary ammonia production decreases, a metabolic acidosis predominates and plasma bicarbonate falls to 12 to 15 mEq/L. This is compensated to a variable degree by respiratory alkalosis.
   b. In long-standing stable renal failure, H^+ displaces Ca^{++} from bone and K^+ from intracellular fluid.

4. Fluid and electrolyte changes. Children undergoing dialysis (particularly hemodialysis) are likely to be slightly hypovolemic. The timing of the last dialysis is critical as hypovolemia may result in precipitous hypotension in response to inhalation agents or intravenous drugs. More information regarding the volume status may be obtained from the nephrology team (e.g., the number of liters of fluid that were removed during the most recent dialysis).
   a. "Sodium losers" are those children with polycystic kidneys or severe pyelonephritis (tubular damage is disproportionately greater than glomerular injury):
      i. Normotension or slight hypotension is present.
      ii. Edema is present uncommonly.
      iii. Hypokalemia is present in some.
      iv. Renal function is improved by increasing intake of sodium and water; sodium restriction may rapidly lead to severe hyponatremia.
   b. "Sodium retainers" are often children with glomerulonephritis; salt retention, hypertension, and edema predispose them to cardiac failure.
   c. Potassium shifts due to displacement of K^+ from the cells by H^+:
      i. High serum K^+ levels
      ii. Depressed excitability of muscles and nerves. This is particularly significant if the cardiac muscle is affected—further sudden rises in K^+ (e.g., with succinylcholine or increased acidosis) may precipitate cardiac arrest.

    d. Calcium shifts:

        i. If displacement of Ca^{++} by H^+ is prolonged, osteoporosis may develop.

    e. Anion changes:

        i. Plasma bicarbonate (HCO_3^-) is decreased.

        ii. Plasma (SO_4^-), (HPO_4^-) and (Cl^-) are increased.

5. Cardiovascular problems:

    a. Hypertension may result from abnormalities of extracellular fluid regulation, fluid overload, and derangement of the renin-angiotensin-aldosterone system:

        i. In many children (those with hypertension secondary to sodium and water retention), this can be controlled conservatively (i.e., by careful moderate salt restriction).

        ii. In some children, the BP can be titrated against sodium and water content during dialysis.

        iii. In others, drug therapy with diuretics and vasodilators is necessary.

        iv. In a few, even large doses of antihypertensive agents fail to control the hypertension (which is probably caused by overproduction of renin). Retinopathy and/or encephalopathy may develop, and bilateral nephrectomy may become necessary.

        v. Hypertensive crisis may occur, occasionally in the perioperative period. Diazoxide (5 mg/kg) has commonly been used for this indication, but a labetalol infusion is now the therapy of choice.

    b. Congestive heart failure may occur with advanced renal failure, as a result of hypertension, volume overload, anemia, electrolyte imbalance, and the effects of an arteriovenous (AV) fistula:

        i. Digitalis therapy is difficult to control.

        ii. Pericardial effusion and tamponade may occur.

    c. Fatty degeneration of the myocardium may occur secondary to chronic renal failure.

6. Pulmonary congestion:

    a. The alveolar-arterial partial oxygen pressure difference (A-aDO$_2$) may be large.

    b. Sodium and water retention, left ventricular failure, and hypoproteinemia contribute to the development of "uremic lung."

    c. Pleural effusions may develop.

7. Gastrointestinal disturbances:

    a. Anorexia, nausea, and vomiting (due to bacterial breakdown of urea to ammonia in the gastrointestinal tract) may aggravate the water, electrolyte, and acid-base imbalance. Gastric emptying may be delayed.

8. Multiple medications:
   a. Many of these children are receiving long-term steroid therapy with resultant osteodystrophy, Cushingoid state, and glycosuria. Continue steroid therapy perioperatively.
   b. Antihypertensive polypharmacy: potential cardiovascular instability under anesthesia must be anticipated. (Do not discontinue these drugs before surgery.)
   c. Digitalis and diuretic therapy may lead to K^+ depletion and thus to increased susceptibility to cardiac arrhythmias.
   d. Antibiotics (e.g., gentamicin) may prolong the effect of nondepolarizing muscle relaxants.
   e. Antimetabolites (e.g., azathioprine) that are highly protein-bound may increase the bioavailability of other protein-bound drugs by displacing them from the protein molecule.
9. Reduced immunity (risk of infection): it is vital to practice very careful asepsis.
10. Poor quality of life and potentially major psychological disturbances:
   a. Resulting from chronic debilitating disease
   b. Heightened by the uremic state and knowledge of a life-threatening condition

In summary, these children may have:

1. Reduced O_2 carrying capacity, which is dependent on a stressed cardiovascular system
2. Incipient or apparent cardiac failure:
   a. Left ventricular failure if hypertensive, hypervolemic, and anemic
   b. Right ventricular failure (late)
3. Greater risk of cardiac arrest (e.g., due to increased K^+ and acidosis)
4. Intolerance of inaccurate administration of blood, other fluids, and electrolytes
5. Cardiovascular instability due to long-term administration of antihypertensive drugs
6. Coagulopathy
7. Low resistance to infection
8. Very low tolerance to further discomfort, however minor (e.g., finger prick, movement from one bed to another)

Many of the problems of chronic renal failure may be significantly reduced when the child is on a renal dialysis program and under close medical supervision. However, some children are underweight, some are hypertensive, and other disease processes may be present. Every child should be very carefully assessed preoperatively.

N.B. Many children with impaired renal function are undergoing hemodialysis regularly and therefore have an AV shunt or fistula usually in the arm. Special care must be taken to ensure that this shunt is well protected and kept functioning throughout the perioperative period. The child must not be allowed to lie on that limb at any time, and it should not be used for blood pressure determinations. The function of the AV fistula should be monitored perioperatively (Doppler flowmeter).

Preoperative Assessment and Preparation

Pay careful attention to the following physical and psychological aspects:

1. Children in a dialysis program are usually dialyzed 12 to 18 hours before surgery. Check the postdialysis fluid and electrolyte status and body weight.
2. Plan ahead so that the child's discomfort is not increased and any necessary disturbances are minimized.
3. Psychological preparation and support are of special benefit to these children and are safer than depressant medication. Some sedation may help.
4. Check results of laboratory tests:
   a. Hemoglobin: blood transfusions may be given if deemed desirable and may help pretransplant. Packed RBCs are preferable. However, transfusion is of temporary benefit only.
   b. Serum potassium: values less than 5 mEq/L are acceptable, even in an emergency; levels greater than 6 mEq/L are unacceptable.
      i. If the serum K^+ level is increased, surgery is usually delayed until hemodialysis has been performed.
      ii. In an emergency, K^+ can be lowered rapidly by giving 0.5 g/kg glucose as a 10% solution with 1 unit of regular insulin added for each 5 g of glucose.
   c. Acid-base balance:
      i. A pH greater than 7.32 is acceptable. If necessary, administer sodium bicarbonate ($NaHCO_3^-$) for correction of acidosis, even if sodium (Na^+) levels are elevated.
      ii. Correction must be cautious and gradual. If the serum calcium (Ca^{++}) level is low, sudden correction may precipitate tetany or convulsions.

Anesthesia Management

1. Pay meticulous attention to details of asepsis.
2. For brief procedures (e.g., insertion of a peritoneal catheter) in a poor-risk child who is cooperative and emotionally stable, use local anesthesia (1% to 2% lidocaine without epinephrine; maximum, 3 mg/kg).
3. For all other cases and if in doubt, use general anesthesia.
4. Anesthesia drugs and renal failure:
   a. Children with renal failure vary in their response to opioids. Use these with caution. Morphine and meperidine may exert prolonged effects owing to a failure to excrete/dialyze active metabolites (M6G and normeperidine, respectively). In contrast, fentanyl, alfentanil, and sufentanil are relatively safe because their metabolites are inactive. Remifentanil may be the ideal intraoperative opioid for these children.
   b. Propofol and thiopental should be used cautiously in reduced doses; less protein binding results in an increased free active fraction. Ketamine and etomidate may result in less hypotension.
   c. Inhalational anesthetics are eliminated via the lungs and hence are most useful. Fluoride nephrotoxicity does not occur with the current ether anesthetics.
   d. Succinylcholine may be used as a single dose provided that the serum potassium (K^+) concentration is 5.5 mEq/L or less (serum K^+ increases 0.5 to 1 mEq/L after succinylcholine in children with renal failure; this produces no ECG changes because the hyperkalemia is chronic. If a peripheral neuropathy is present, however, succinylcholine may cause greater increases in serum K^+ and arrhythmias). Succinylcholine should only be used if a rapid sequence induction is deemed necessary and should be preceded by a small dose of a nondepolarizing relaxant.
   e. Muscle relaxants, nondepolarizing: *cis*-atracurium and vecuronium are drugs of choice. Rocuronium has a slower onset of action but a similar duration of action in children with and without renal failure. Pancuronium and gallamine are partially or completely excreted by the kidneys and should be avoided.
   f. Local anesthesia drugs have not been extensively studied in children with renal failure; they may be used in normal doses for "single-shot" techniques. Repeat doses or infusions might be dangerous if clearance of the drug is delayed.

Preoperative

1. Dose requirements for drugs in children with renal failure are more variable than in those with normal renal function; titrate doses carefully.

2. Do not discontinue antihypertensive drugs.
3. Premedicate when required (e.g., PO or IV midazolam).
4. Check all medications that have been given and note their last dose before surgery.
5. Check the location of a shunt or fistula. Avoid any pressure to this area, and monitor function (Doppler flowmeter).
6. Ensure that all supportive drugs are available in the operating room.
7. Ensure that adequate supplies of blood and other fluids are available (including washed cells if and when indicated).

Perioperative

1. Give 100% O_2 by mask.
2. Apply monitors:
   a. Precordial stethoscope
   b. ECG and pulse oximeter
   c. Automated blood pressure—*do not use a limb with a shunt or fistula*
3. Ensure that the limb with the shunt or fistula is easily accessible. Monitor function throughout the procedure.
4. Induce anesthesia with propofol (2 to 4 mg/kg), thiopental 2 to 3 mg/kg (more may be required) or if dehydrated, consider ketamine (1 to 2 mg/kg) or etomidate (0.3 mg/kg), followed by N_2O/O_2 and sevoflurane.
5. For intubation:
   a. Do not give succinylcholine unless the serum K^+ concentration is less than 5.5 mEq/L (see previous discussion)—and always pretreat with a nondepolarizing agent. Always limit succinylcholine to a single dose.
   b. Otherwise give cis-atracurium, rocuronium, or vecuronium for intubation.
6. Maintain anesthesia with N_2O/O_2 and isoflurane with a nondepolarizing muscle relaxant.
7. Control the ventilation in all procedures that last longer than 15 minutes. Use moderate hyperventilation to compensate for metabolic acidosis and to encourage K^+ movement back into the cells. In general, it is advised to control ventilation to maintain the arterial carbon dioxide pressure ($PaCO_2$) at the usual level for that particular child.
8. Administer fluids to ensure adequate blood volume for satisfactory BP, good peripheral perfusion, and function of an AV fistula or shunt.
   a. Give balanced salt solutions (but avoid all potassium-containing solutions [i.e., lactated Ringer's solution]) to replace the preoperative deficit and for perioperative maintenance.
   b. For small blood losses, replace with maintenance solution.

c. For significant blood losses, replace with washed RBCs and salt-poor albumin.
   i. Check Hb and hematocrit (Hct); keep Hct below 30%.
   ii. Avoid overtransfusion.
9. Antagonize muscle relaxants at the end of surgery.

Postoperative

1. Ensure good ventilation and oxygenation.
2. Carefully titrate opioid doses (repeated doses of morphine and its metabolites accumulate in renal failure; M6G cannot be removed by dialysis); monitor the effect and give supplements if necessary.
3. Ensure that the shunt or fistula is functioning; record this fact.
4. Check Hb, Hct, electrolytes, and blood gases.
5. Consult a nephrologist for continuing care.

RENAL TRANSPLANTATION

Transplantation offers the chance of a relatively normal life for the child with chronic renal failure. Organs for transplantation are in very limited supply. The anesthesiologist, by paying careful attention to the details of intraoperative management, can make a real difference in the probability that the graft will survive. An aggressive approach to attaining conditions that optimize graft survival should be taken.

Anesthesia Management

Preoperative

1. General management is the same as for children in renal failure.
2. Discuss with the nephrologist and urologist to ascertain the child's exact present status (state of hydration, electrolyte and acid-base status, renal function, cardiopulmonary state, coagulation issues).
3. If the child is not in optimal condition (e.g., volume overload), surgery should be postponed until after dialysis. The basic objective is to implant the kidney within 24 hours.
4. Review the immunosuppressive therapy plan for the child (i.e., drug dosage, timing). A typical plan includes administration of cyclosporin, methylprednisolone succinate (Solu-Medrol), and azathioprine; an antibiotic is also given.

Perioperative

1. General management is the same as for children in renal failure.
2. After induction of anesthesia:

   a. Insert a central venous line.
   b. Check its position with a pressure tracing and/or radiograph.
   c. Maintain the central venous pressure (CVP) at an acceptably high level to ensure diuresis (8 to 12 mm Hg). Normal saline is the preferred initial maintenance fluid (cf. lactated Ringer's solution, which contains K^+.)
   d. The objective is to adequately replace any existing deficit and ongoing losses. This may require infusions at four to five times normal maintenance rates (i.e., at 10 to 20 ml/kg/hr).

3. An arterial line may not be essential in uncomplicated cases. Leaving the radial artery untouched may be advantageous in case the child needs another shunt at some time in the future.
   a. If an external (Scribner) shunt is available, the arterial end may be used for monitoring and the venous end as an infusion route. (Use very careful aseptic technique.)
   b. If an arterial line is indicated, insert the catheter in the radial artery (in the arm opposite to the fistula), do not use a cannula larger than a 22 gauge, and arrange to have the catheter removed as soon as possible postoperatively to minimize damage to the artery.

4. Provided no significant coagulopathy is present, an epidural catheter may be inserted to augment surgical anesthesia, maintain hemodynamic stability, and ensure good postoperative analgesia.

5. Transfuse with packed RBCs to obtain an Hct value in the 35% to 40% range at the end of the operation. Children with chronic renal failure tend to lose third-space fluid extensively; greater Hct and colloid administration may limit this effect and improve graft perfusion.

6. During vascular anastomosis and before clamp release, give 1 mg/kg of furosemide and 1 g/kg of mannitol IV. Anticipate a decline in blood pressure as the clamps are removed, and prepare for fluid infusions. Some surgeons will request an RBC transfusion just before releasing the clamp.

7. Systolic blood pressure (100% to 120% of preoperative value) and a CVP greater than 14 mm Hg are preferred before the clamps are removed to initiate and maintain renal perfusion and function. Lighten anesthesia and use a dopamine infusion 5 µg/kg/min if necessary. A greater pressure at this time increases the perfusion of the graft and improves the chances for early good function and graft survival.

8. The solution used to preserve the kidney has a high potassium level; hyperkalemia and acidosis after release of the clamps has on rare

occasions resulted in cardiac arrest. This may be a greater danger in small children.

9. Placement of a large adult kidney in a small infant introduces some problems. The kidney should be well flushed by the surgeon before it is implanted. Blood must be rapidly infused as the clamps are released to fill the vascular space of the graft. The CVP should be increased to 15 to 20 mm Hg in anticipation of unclamping. The danger of hyperkalemia (due to preservative fluid) and acidosis (due to clamping of the aorta or iliac artery) is increased. Check acid-base status and give calcium chloride and sodium bicarbonate as necessary.

10. Maintain the CVP at a level that produces a good urine output (i.e., up to 15 to 18 mm Hg). If the CVP is adequate but urine flow is still low:
    a. Give furosemide 2 to 4 mg/kg IV.
    b. If necessary, add 20% mannitol 1 g/kg.

11. Anticipate the need to infuse large volumes of fluid (three to five times the normal) to compensate for third-space losses.

12. At the end of surgery, determine serum electrolytes:
    a. If urine output is adequate, serum K^+ should be within the normal range.
    b. If the serum K^+ is greater than 6 mEq/L and urine output is poor, continue to hyperventilate the lungs and plan to arrange for dialysis or therapy with glucose and insulin.

13. With such an aggressive approach to fluid management, pulmonary edema may threaten. In such cases, continue with controlled ventilation into the postoperative period.

Postoperative

1. General management is the same as for children in renal failure. Ensure good postoperative analgesia. Epidural analgesia is ideal.

2. The pulmonary status of all children should be monitored by pulse oximetry, blood gases, and periodic chest radiography. Small infants with large implanted kidneys may be at risk for pulmonary complications (especially atelectasis). This may be a combined result of the abdominal surgery, the mass of the implanted kidney, and aggressive fluid therapy. The need to "push fluids" to ensure diuresis may result in pulmonary edema; occasionally treatment may be required.

3. Renal function in the transplanted kidney is as follows:
    a. Glomerular function is initially normal but wanes during the first 48 hours as the kidney swells. Increased intravenous fluids are required to maintain diuresis at that time.

b. Some degree of tubular damage is always present. Diuresis and loss of sodium result, and replacement of sodium and water is required. Other electrolytes must be infused as indicated by serum studies.

c. Declining urine flow after 48 hours despite fluid loading is indicative of mechanical problems (vascular) or rejection of the transplant.

4. Hypoglycemia has been described as a late complication after renal transplantation in small children. This may have been associated with the use of β-blocking drugs.

Suggested Reading

Renal Transplantation

Coupe N, O'Brien M, Gibson P, et al: Anesthesia for pediatric renal transplantation with and without epidural analgesia—a review of 7 years experience, Paediatr Anaesth 15(3):220–228, 2005.

Uejima T: Anesthetic management of the pediatric patient undergoing solid organ transplantation, Anesth Clin N Am 22(4):809–826, 2004.

Anesthesia Drugs and Renal Disease

Driessen JJ, Robertson EN, Van Egmond J, et al: Time-course of action of rocuronium 0.3 mg.kg-1 in children with and without endstage renal failure, Paediatr Anaesth 12(6):507–510, 2002.

Geha DG, Blitt DC, Moon BJ: Prolonged neuromuscular blockade with pancuronium in the presence of acute renal failure: a case report, Anesth Analg 55:343, 1976.

Ghoneim MM, Pandya H: Plasma protein binding of thiopental in patients with impaired renal or hepatic function, Anesthesiol 42:545, 1975.

Hunter JM, Jones RS, Utting JE: Use of atracurium in patients with no renal function, Br J Anaesth 54:1251, 1982.

Koide M, Waud BE: Serum potassium concentrations after succinylcholine in patients with renal failure, Anesthesiology 36:142, 1972.

Miller RD, Way WL, Hamilton WK, et al: Succinylcholine-induced hyperkalemia in patients with renal failure? Anesthesiology 36:138, 1972.

Trauma, Including Acute Burns and Scalds

Children are commonly involved in accidents; trauma is the leading cause of death between 1 and 14 years of age. Even if the injury is relatively minor, some children require emergency anesthesia, the potential dangers of which may overshadow the injury.

Most children injured in accidents were previously healthy. Therefore considerations of past health are usually less important than in the adult. However, a complete medical history must be obtained as soon as possible. From the time of arrival in the emergency department, the anesthesiologist must be included in the treatment team. The anesthesiologist can contribute to immediate care while evaluating the child's condition for anesthesia and the need for further continuing care.

MAJOR TRAUMA

Diagnosis and treatment must proceed rapidly and simultaneously. Vigorous resuscitative measures must be continued without interruption during anesthesia. The common major problems for the anesthesiologist include:

1. To secure and maintain a safe, reliable airway and to optimize ventilation and oxygenation
2. To achieve adequate blood and fluid replacement
3. To optimize cerebral perfusion pressure in children with a head injury
4. To maintain body temperature

N.B. Injuries are often multiple. Although injuries may appear to be limited to a single anatomic site or body system, the possibility of serious injuries elsewhere must constantly be kept in mind. The fractured femur may be an obvious injury, but the as yet undiagnosed ruptured liver could be the greater threat to life.

Initial Urgent Procedures

1. Ensure a safe and protected airway, and optimize ventilation and oxygenation.
2. The cardiovascular status must be determined:
   a. If hypovolemia is present, it must be corrected.
   b. Effective cardiac output must be maintained or restored.
3. Blood is withdrawn without delay for type and cross-match. The blood bank should be advised immediately if a massive transfusion is likely to be necessary.

Establishing the Airway

Airway obstruction is common in head and facial injuries and can have a disastrous effect on the outcome.

1. All children with head injury should be given oxygen by mask immediately on admission.
2. For those with depressed consciousness, if simple positioning does not provide a clear airway or if the gag reflex is absent, intubate the trachea without delay.
3. Do not insert oropharyngeal airways in unconscious children. Resistance to ventilation is greater than with an endotracheal tube and they do not protect against aspiration of gastric contents.
4. Injury of the cervical spine must be suspected in all trauma; immobilize the neck using sandbags, a plaster shell, or a bean bag.* Avoid moving the neck. Note that a cervical spine injury may occur without any radiologic evidence (known as SCIWORA, **s**pinal **c**ord **i**njury **w**ithout **r**adiographic **a**bnormalities). Optimal airway management must be the first priority, but caution concerning cervical spine injury is required (see later discussion).
5. Be alert to the possibility of foreign bodies (i.e., teeth, bone fragments) in the mouth, pharynx, trachea, or bronchi, especially if there are facial injuries.

---

* Vac-Pac surgical positioning system, VenTech Healthcare Inc., Toronto.

6. "Awake" laryngoscopy and intubation can markedly increase intracranial pressure (ICP), which may be detrimental in the head-injured child. In children with suspected increased ICP, administer a general anesthetic with RSI: give IV lidocaine 1 to 2 mg/kg, propofol 2 to 3 mg/kg, or thiopentone 5 mg/kg; atropine 0.02 mg/kg; and succinylcholine 1 to 2 mg/kg before intubation. This regimen cannot, however, be safely followed if the child is hypovolemic; in such instances, ketamine (use cautiously with increased ICP), etomidate or midazolam (with IV lidocaine for the latter two) should be used for induction. All trauma patients must be assumed to have a full stomach, and an RSI should be used to secure the airway. Succinylcholine does not increase intragastric pressure in young children and therefore does not increase the risk of regurgitation. Succinylcholine does not increase ICP significantly and the advantages of rapidly securing a safe and clear airway and instituting controlled ventilation are more important. Beware of neck injury; stabilize the spine. (Remember: a cervical spine injury is a relative contraindication to cricoid pressure.)

7. Vomiting and aspiration commonly occur after an accident. Immediately after intubation, check air entry to all lung regions and suction via the endotracheal tube if necessary. Examine chest radiographs for tracheal tube position and evidence of pathology.

8. A gastric tube should be passed to decompress the stomach, especially in those with chest or abdominal injuries in whom acute gastric dilation is common. Even children with relatively minor injuries often swallow enough air to cause significant gastric distention; this interferes with ventilation and predisposes to vomiting and aspiration. Do not pass a tube through the nose in children who may have a basal skull fracture.

9. Be alert to the possibility of pneumothorax or hemothorax.

Intravenous Therapy

Large-bore intravenous lines must be established. These must be placed in the upper limbs or neck in children with injuries at the level of the thorax and below because flow through the inferior vena cava may be (or become) compromised. *All intravenous fluids should be warmed; hypothermia may rapidly develop in the injured child.*

Percutaneous cannulation of large veins, using at least 20-gauge catheters, is preferable. Alternatively, a cut-down or an intraosseous needle may be required. Internal jugular or subclavian lines may be inserted if no other venous access is available; beware of further worsening the cardiorespiratory status if a pneumothorax or hemothorax occurs.

A central venous catheter will be useful during the further management of the child, but it may be inserted after the initial acute fluid resuscitation (avoid IJ lines in head-injured children).

Clues to blood volume status are as follows:

1. Cardiovascular indices:
   a. Tachycardia suggests hypovolemia in children of all ages. A heart rate in excess of 140 beats/min in infants or 100 beats/min in older children is suggestive.
   b. In infants, the systolic blood pressure (BP) varies in parallel with the intravascular volume and is a very good guide to volume status.
   c. In older children, as in adults, hypovolemia stimulates early constriction of venous capacitance vessels. Therefore the systolic BP may remain near normal, despite a loss of up to 20% of the blood volume. The central venous pressure (CVP) may also be maintained initially. When such vasoconstriction can no longer compensate and maintain the venous return to the heart, rapid decompensation may occur. At this point the CVP decreases and becomes a more reliable guide to the adequacy of replacement of the blood volume. A 2 to 3 mm Hg decrease in CVP may represent as much as a 25% decrease of the circulating blood volume in a healthy, supine child.
2. General appearance: Pallor, mottling, sweating, and coolness of the skin, especially over the extremities, are signs of hypovolemia. The latter can be quantified by simultaneous measurement of skin and body core temperatures: a large difference indicates vasoconstriction, and lessening of the difference indicates improving skin perfusion as blood volume increases toward normal.
3. Confusion and irrational behavior are common signs of hypovolemia in children.
4. Urine output: The severely injured child should be catheterized and the urine output monitored. A urine flow of more than 1 ml/kg/hr indicates adequate renal perfusion and adequate volume replacement.
5. Biochemical studies: Metabolic acidosis (lactic acidosis) may result from impaired organ perfusion and is a confirmatory sign of a low circulating blood volume. This acidosis may be corrected by adequate volume replacement. Sodium bicarbonate administration is not recommended except for severe acidosis that may compromise cardiac action (i.e., pH <7.2 despite normocapnia or hypocapnia).

Selection of Fluids for Infusion. The types of fluid depend on (1) what is indicated and (2) what is available.

Frequently, initial fluid resuscitation includes balanced salt solutions rather than blood products. If at all possible, do not transfuse non–cross-matched universal donor blood. (A rapid cross-match can be performed in 20 minutes.) If blood loss is massive, and is in the chest cavity, consider autotransfusion.

A balanced salt solution (e.g., lactated Ringer's solution) can be used initially to expand the circulating blood volume, but if used to excess (more than 100 ml/kg), it may lead to pulmonary insufficiency and/or dilutional coagulopathy later. An initial rapid infusion of 20 ml/kg is appropriate for the hypotensive child and may be repeated. If the child has a head injury, then normal saline (isotonic) should be used for volume replacement to reduce the potential for cerebral edema.

Other plasma substitutes may be used (e.g., dextran 70, hetastarch). Note that dextrans may impair coagulation and interfere with cross-matching: do not exceed 7 ml/kg. Hetastarch does not impair coagulation, and may be used in volumes up to 25 ml/kg. (N.B. The starches have long resident times in the reticuloendothelial system in humans; limited data are available for their use in children.)

Dextrose-containing solutions should not be given (except, very rarely, to treat documented hypoglycemia); hyperglycemia may occur and may increase the severity of neurologic damage (blood glucose >200 mg/dl) should cerebral hypoxia/ischemia occur.

Expanding the blood volume with 5% albumin may be very effective in the immediate treatment of hypovolemic shock, but there is a concern that, if large quantities of albumin are infused, some may "leak" into the lungs and impair pulmonary function later.

Indications for Blood Transfusion. It is seldom possible to measure the volume of blood lost after trauma. Large amounts may be lost from the intravascular volume but remain within hematomas (e.g., after fracture of the femur) or body cavities. Volume replacement must therefore be judged on the basis of the clues listed previously. We recommend that sufficient fluid be replaced to correct clinical signs of hypovolemia and that blood be given in volumes sufficient to maintain hematocrit (Hct) at 30%.

The young child who is showing obvious signs of hypovolemia (pallor, sweating, hypotension) must be assumed to have lost at least 25% of the blood volume. Estimate the weight of the child [for children < 8 years old: $2 \times age (yr) + 9 = weight (kg)$ and for ≥ 9 year olds, $3 \times age (yr) = weight (kg)$] and assume the normal blood volume to be 70 ml/kg; 25% of this total is the initial volume to be replaced rapidly. The situation can then be reassessed. The need for continuous infusion to maintain the BP, or deterioration after an apparently stable period, indicates persistent bleeding.

Children who have lost large volumes of blood require transfusion with whole blood. The trend toward blood component therapy has made it difficult to obtain whole blood. Packed cells resuspended in plasma (preferably recently thawed FFP) may be substituted.

Massive Blood Transfusion. Loss of an amount of blood that would be negligible in an adult (500 ml) may constitute a major loss in a child. Indeed, massive blood transfusions may be required for severely injured children. For example, after thoracoabdominal injury, it may be necessary to replace more than 250% of the estimated blood volume.

Serious problems begin to develop after the rapid infusion of 200% of the estimated blood volume (i.e., transfusion of ~140 ml/kg). These problems include:

1. Hypothermia and accompanying cardiac arrhythmias. Warm all blood and fluids to 40 °C.
2. Coagulation problems
   a. Thrombocytopenia and impaired platelet function
      i. Check platelet count after each 50% blood volume replacement.
      ii. If the platelet count is less than $50,000/mm^3$, administer platelet concentrates (0.1 to 0.3 units/kg).
   b. Deficiency of coagulation factors
      i. Measure prothrombin time (PT) and partial thromboplastin time (PTT)
      ii. If these are prolonged, give recently thawed FFP (20 ml/kg). (Generally this occurs after loss of 1 to 1.5 blood volumes.)
   c. Disseminated intravascular coagulation (DIC).
      i. Likely if bleeding increases at all sites (i.e., old venipuncture sites).
      ii. Measure PT, PTT, clot lysis time, fibrinogen, and fibrin split product levels.
      iii. Prolonged PT and PTT, low fibrinogen level, and presence of fibrin split products suggest DIC.
      iv. If DIC is suspected, enlist the aid of a hematologist if possible. Treatment must include removal of the cause (i.e., correction of hypovolemic shock), replacement of coagulation factors, and possibly heparinization.
3. Acidosis
   a. Check acid-base status frequently.
   b. Correct metabolic acidosis with sodium bicarbonate.
4. Citrate toxicity (due to infusion of citrated blood or plasma)
   a. May cause more problems in infants and small children than in adults.
   b. Results in hypotension that persists despite adequate volume replacement. (**N.B. Remember that FFP and platelet suspensions**

contain more citrate per unit volume than whole blood and clinically important hypocalcemia will occur when infusions exceed 1 ml/kg/min FFP.)

   c. May be diagnosed by measuring the ionized Ca^{++} concentration or clinically by observing a prolonged rate-corrected Q-T interval on the ECG. But, in practice, if hypotension appears unresponsive to volume replacement, a therapeutic test using intravenous calcium chloride (10 mg/kg) is justified.

   d. Correct by administering 10% calcium chloride 10 to 30 mg/kg slowly under ECG control. Frequent small boluses (5 to 10 mg/kg calcium chloride or 15 to 30 mg/kg calcium gluconate) during rapid FFP infusions will prevent serious hypocalcemia.

5. Serum potassium disturbances: Monitor serum K^+ levels periodically. Contrary to expectation, hypokalemia may sometimes be found after massive transfusion. However, serious hyperkalemia may also occur, especially in the presence of a low cardiac output, transfusion of old cold blood and the use of a rapid infusion device. The cardiac manifestations of hyperkalemia (peaked T waves, ventricular irritability, ventricular tachycardia) may be treated acutely by slow administration of intravenous calcium chloride 10 to 30 mg/kg, sodium bicarbonate 1 to 2 mmol/kg, hyperventilation, administration of a β-agonist, and, if more severe, with glucose, insulin, and Kayexalate.

6. Posttraumatic pulmonary insufficiency. This is characterized by progressively decreasing pulmonary compliance, impaired gas exchange, and radiographic findings of diffuse infiltrates. The following factors may contribute:

   a. Excess use of balanced salt solutions and/or albumin

      i. Give diuretics (furosemide 1 mg/kg) if indicated.

   b. Microembolization of the pulmonary vessels by infused particulate matter (platelet or leukocyte clumps)

      i. Filter all blood given through an IV screen filter (140 μm) filter.

   c. Damage to alveolar-capillary membrane

      i. This results in low-pressure pulmonary edema.

      ii. Large doses of steroids may help to prevent this.

Autotransfusion. Autotransfusion can be life-saving for some trauma patients. Advantages are the ready availability of absolutely compatible warm red cells. In the extreme emergency, autotransfusion can be performed using only a large syringe and an in-line filter in the intravenous line. A collection of freshly shed uncontaminated blood in an accessible body cavity (e.g., the pleural cavity) is the main requirement. Do not use blood from the abdominal cavity if bowel injury is suspected.

Head Injury

Head injury is extremely common during childhood, and it is a cause of very significant mortality and morbidity, much of which might be reduced by early and efficient medical intervention. Children with head injury are less likely than adults to develop a mass lesion but are more likely to develop intracranial hypertension, secondary to diffuse hyperemia and edema. This secondary brain injury, which occurs after the primary trauma, must be minimized if recovery is to be optimized. Early aggressive treatment is essential to ensure cerebral oxygenation, control ICP and CPP, and minimize cerebral edema. The Glasgow coma scale is the most common means of initial assessment.

Glasgow Coma Scale and Pediatric Modifications

If consciousness is significantly depressed (GCS <8), airway obstruction is very common and seriously compromises the prognosis. The first priority of the anesthesiologist must be to ensure an absolutely clear airway, excellent oxygenation, and optimal ventilation. All children with head injury should receive oxygen. If there is any doubt about the child's ability to maintain the airway and ventilate:

1. Give oxygen and intubate the trachea without delay; use a cuffed oral tube. Suitable drugs should be given to obtund the cardiovascular responses to intubation (see previous discussion). Nasal tubes (and nasogastric tubes) are contraindicated in children with fractures of the base of the skull; perforation of the cribriform plate may occur. Beware of the possibility of cervical spine injury (see SCIWORA later discussion).

2. Apply controlled ventilation to produce normocapnia pending further evaluation of the child's injuries. Hyperventilation should be avoided because it may compromise cerebral perfusion. $PaCO_2$ should preferably be checked by arterial blood gas analysis as end-tidal CO_2 may be inaccurate.

3. Continue anesthesia as required, preferably with intravenous agents (e.g., propofol, opioids, and muscle relaxants). Inhalational agents should be limited to <1 MAC to prevent possible increases in ICP. MAP should be maintained to preserve CPP. Nitrous oxide may increase ICP. Avoid sufentanil, which increases ICP in head-injured patients.

4. Stabilize the hemodynamic state to ensure an optimal CPP. Glucose-free, isotonic fluids (normal saline) should be infused cautiously; excessive fluid therapy contributes to cerebral edema.

Glasgow Coma Scale and Pediatric Modifications

Standard	Score	Pediatric
Eye opening		
Spontaneous	4	Spontaneous
To speech	3	To speech
To pain	2	To pain
None	1	None
Verbal response		
Oriented	5	Coos, babbles (age appropriate)
Confused	4	Irritable, cries
Inappropriate words	3	Cries to pain
Incomprehensible sounds	2	Moans to pain
None	1	None
Motor response		
Follows commands	6	Spontaneous movement
Localizes to pain	5	Withdraws to touch
Withdraws to pain	4	Withdraws to pain
Abnormal flexion	3	Abnormal flexion
Extensor response	2	Extensor response
None	1	None

Utilize best score from each category for possible total score of 3–15.

The use of CT and MRI permits accurate anatomic mapping of traumatic lesions and removes the need for exploratory burr holes. CT or MRI is generally recommended for any child with GCS less than 13 or with vomiting. The characteristic appearance of diffuse cerebral damage on the scan can obviate the need for craniotomy and permit early specific monitoring and therapeutic measures, such as the following:

1. ICP monitoring—most commonly with the use of an extradural bolt connected to an external transducer. This is usually recommended for any child with a GCS less than 8. Once ICP monitoring is established, the CPP can be determined:

$$CPP = MAP - ICP.$$

Patients with a CPP between 40 and 70 mm Hg have a better prognosis than those with CPP < 40 mm Hg.

2. Initiate treatment to control ICP and CPP:
   a. Optimal positioning, 35° to 45° head up and face centrally forward. (No internal or external jugular lines in children with head injuries.)
   b. Diuretics—mannitol and/or furosemide

    c. Hypertonic saline infusions

    d. Barbiturates (thiopental 2 to 4 mg/kg), which may be more effective in controlling ICP in children than in adults and may also be useful to control seizures.

    e. Controlled ventilation, preferably adjusted on the basis of measurements of ICP, CPP, and $CMRO_2$. Excessive hyperventilation may be detrimental.

3. Maintenance of optimal CPP (>40 mm Hg), hemoglobin level, and arterial oxygenation: Glucose-free isotonic or hypertonic fluids should be used for volume expansion. Dopamine may be required to treat hypotension (but see caution in later discussion). Hyperglycemia should be avoided because it may exacerbate secondary brain injury. Fluid therapy must be guided by constant monitoring of physiologic and biochemical variables. Endocrine functions (especially pituitary/hypothalamic) may be disturbed after head injury, which may lead to;

    a. Diabetes insipidus, with a large urine volume and hypernatremia.

    b. Inappropriate secretion of antidiuretic hormone (SIADH) with oliguria and hyponatremia.

    c. Hyperglycemia is common after head injury, secondary to catecholamine release; the value of treating this is controversial. Hypoglycemia may develop later and should be corrected.

4. Control of seizure activity, as evident clinically or by EEG monitoring.

5. Control body temperature:

    a. To prevent hyperthermia, which commonly follows brain injury.

    b. Induced moderate (32.5 °C) hypothermia in children with severe traumatic brain injury does not improve neurologic outcome and may increase mortality.

    Caution: Head injuries do not normally cause shock. When anesthetizing or caring for the child with a head injury, be alert for evidence of other injuries. Do not ascribe signs of hypovolemic shock (i.e., tachycardia, hypotension) to the head injury. If such signs are present, search for bleeding from wounds in the scalp and/or other sites (intraabdominal, intrathoracic, or in the limbs). Be constantly aware that hemorrhage at another site may have been overlooked. Although anesthetizing a child for emergency neurosurgery, monitor the cardiovascular system closely and continue measurements (e.g., abdominal girth) to detect hemorrhage.

Suggested Reading

Hutchison JS, Ward RE, Lacroix J, et al: Hypothermia therapy after traumatic brain injury in children, NEJM 358(23):2447–2456, 2008.

Cervical Spine Injury

It was previously thought that cervical spine injury was rare in pediatric trauma patients. This was probably incorrect; it is now recognized that SCIWORA may occur. This means that many such injuries may have been overlooked in the past.

A pattern of high cervical spine injury occurs in children, often as a result of motor vehicle accidents. This is in contrast to the involvement of the lower cervical and upper thoracic spine in older patients. Severe high cervical spinal cord injury may result in apnea and cardiac arrest, and this possibility should be considered in children with absent vital signs.

The concern for the anesthesiologist is to achieve rapid, safe intubation of the injured child but to avoid causing injury to the spinal cord. Early relief of an obstructed airway and controlled hyperventilation are essential for optimal recovery from severe head injury. Current opinion suggests that some children may experience immediate damage to the spinal cord at the time of their accident; the outcome from such established injuries will not be altered by the technique of tracheal intubation chosen.

Techniques of intubation other than by direct vision are more difficult (and often more prolonged) in children, and it has been demonstrated that careful direct oral intubation can be performed without causing damage to the cord. Hence, it is recommended that careful direct laryngoscopy and intubation be performed in injured children. Unnecessary head and neck movement should be avoided by using manual in-line stabilization. Appropriate steps to prevent aspiration should be taken, although cricoid pressure is contraindicated in cervical spine injury.

Thoracoabdominal Injury

Blunt abdominal trauma is most commonly managed conservatively in children. Bleeding from the spleen or liver can be assessed by scanning techniques and usually resolves spontaneously; blood transfusion requirements are not increased beyond those for operation. Operation is necessary for penetrating wounds and if continued excessive bleeding causes hemodynamic instability. Occasionally, laparoscopy may be employed to assess intraabdominal injuries.

During initial assessment of the child with thoracoabdominal trauma, one must consider possible physiologic consequences of the injury and the additional effect of anesthesia on the child's condition. In those with intraabdominal injuries, the anesthesiologist's prime concerns are the amount of blood lost and the problem of securing a safe airway.

Special Anesthesia Problems

1. Major hemorrhage requiring massive blood transfusion (see Chapter 4)
2. The possibility of a full stomach (food or blood). Always use a cuffed tube in children with abdominal injuries.
3. Impaired cardiorespiratory function (in children with diaphragmatic or thoracic trauma); serious arrhythmias may follow blunt thoracic trauma.

Immediate Management

1. Prepare for transfusion:
   a. Insert a wide-bore cannula into an upper limb or neck vein, by cut-down if necessary.
   b. Send a blood sample for type and cross-match.
   c. Insert a central venous cannula via a second upper limb or neck vein (use the femoral vein if a head injury is present) for measurement of CVP and to provide an alternative route for transfusion if necessary.
2. Assess the extent of hypovolemic shock.
3. Infuse appropriate solutions with the use of a blood warmer.
4. Never infuse large volumes of cold fluids (or blood) via a central vein.

Anesthesia Management

During anesthesia, the anesthesiologist is responsible for continuing vigorous blood volume replacement and other resuscitative measures.

Preoperative

1. Before induction, make every effort to restore the blood volume to near-normal levels. (This may not be possible until the source of bleeding has been controlled surgically.)
2. Order adequate supplies of blood for transfusion and have them immediately available in the operating room (OR).
3. Premedication usually is not required.
4. If the patient is hypovolemic, give any necessary drugs in minimal doses, slowly, and only by the intravenous route.
5. Ensure availability of a rapid infusion device that will allow rapid administration of warmed blood and fluid.
6. Prepare appropriate vasopressors and administration pumps.
7. Prepare transducers for arterial and central venous access lines.
8. Consider a cerebral function monitor to provide trends for depth of anesthesia.

Perioperative

Induction:

1. Prepare and check all necessary equipment and drugs for RSI and tracheal intubation.
2. In the OR, re-examine the child to ascertain the exact current status.
3. Preoxygenate as tolerated.
4. Check intravenous lines.
5. Connect monitoring equipment.
6. Consider the possibility of persisting hypovolemia:
   a. If hypovolemia has been corrected, induce anesthesia intravenously with propofol (up to 3 mg/kg) or thiopental (up to 4 mg/kg), atropine (20 μg/kg), and succinylcholine 1 to 2 mg/kg or rocuronium 1.2 mg/kg if there is a contraindication to succinylcholine. Inject these agents directly into a wide-bore venous cannula (to avoid the delayed transit through intravenous lines).
   b. If the hypovolemia is present and anesthesia is urgently required, use ketamine 2 mg/kg IV or etomidate (0.3 mg/kg) instead of propofol.
7. Position the child supine and horizontally for intubation (to facilitate rapid insertion of a cuffed tube).
8. Do not inflate the lungs before laryngoscopy (ventilation may precipitate vomiting). Have an assistant apply cricoid pressure unless there is suspicion of cervical spine injury until an endotracheal tube is in place and the cuff inflated. If the spine has not been "cleared," cricoid pressure may be contraindicated.
9. Do not give any drugs (except atropine and midazolam) to moribund patients before intubating the trachea.

Maintenance

1. Give O_2, fentanyl, and a nondepolarizing neuromuscular blocking agent (vecuronium, rocuronium, or pancuronium). N_2O may cause distention of air-containing spaces (e.g., bowel, pneumothorax) and should be avoided. Low concentrations of inhalational agents or a propofol infusion may be appropriate. IV midazolam should be given to minimize the risk of awareness in trauma patients.
2. Control ventilation to produce a near-normal $PaCO_2$. If the hypovolemia is still uncorrected, avoid positive end-expiratory pressure and adjust the inspiratory:expiratory ratio to give a low mean intrathoracic pressure. Use a passive or heated humidifier.

3. Monitor ventilation, heart rate and rhythm, temperature, BP, CVP, pulse oximeter, end-tidal carbon dioxide, and urine output. A cerebral function monitor may provide useful trend information in older children.
4. Insert an arterial cannula for direct BP monitoring and for repeated blood sampling for serial determination of the acid-base status, blood gases, Hct, and coagulation studies.
5. Insert a double-lumen CVP line. This provides for monitoring and drug infusions.
6. Maintain body temperature carefully; use a forced air heater.
7. Be alert to the possibility of sudden hypotension as the abdomen is opened in the child who has intraabdominal bleeding requiring vigorous fluid resuscitation.

Postoperative

1. In the absence of chest injury or significant impairment of pulmonary function, remove the endotracheal tube after antagonizing the muscle relaxant and with the child awake, responding, and in a lateral position.
2. In the child with thoracic injuries or impaired pulmonary function, who remains unconscious—or whose condition is otherwise labile—continue ventilatory support and reevaluate later in the intensive care unit.
3. Plan for good postoperative pain relief.

Special Considerations

1. Overt or suspected hepatic injury: Drugs that are metabolized by the liver may have increased elimination half-lives. Cautious use of repeated doses of drugs that depend on liver for metabolism (barbiturates, opioids) is warranted to prevent overdose. Substitute those that are excreted relatively unchanged by the lungs or kidneys (i.e., isoflurane or desflurane, pancuronium or rocuronium).
2. Overt or suspected renal injury is usually treated conservatively unless the child is hemodynamically unstable. In this case, prepare for major volume replacement. Trauma patients with acute renal failure as a complication of prolonged hypovolemia and hypotension require special attention: Maintain a good mean arterial pressure, administer mannitol, avoid drugs that are excreted predominantly via the kidneys (e.g., pancuronium).
3. Ruptured diaphragm: Rupture of the diaphragm, as a consequence of blunt abdominal trauma, is more common in children than in adults and may be overlooked because respiratory distress is usually not severe. This condition requires thoracoabdominal repair.

    a. Insert a gastric tube to decompress the upper gastrointestinal tract.

    b. N_2O is contraindicated if the chest cavity contains a large volume of bowel.

4. Injury to chest wall and lungs:

    a. In young children, the ribs are relatively soft and less likely to fracture; however, the injury may separate the costochondral junctions, and this, in association with fractures of posterior ribs, may lead to "flail chest." If this results in hypoventilation, intubate the trachea and control the ventilation without delay.

    b. Trauma to the chest wall is usually accompanied by contusion of the underlying lung, even when there are no rib fractures. This results in shunting of blood through damaged lung tissue and the need for O_2 therapy and possibly positive-pressure ventilation to maintain arterial saturation levels.

Pneumothorax, hemothorax, or both may be present. If these are suspected, request insertion of a chest drain with a suitable valve or underwater seal before the child is anesthetized. Pneumothorax should be suspected in the child who is grunting and it may occur without rib fracture in children.

5. Overt or suspected tracheal or bronchial injury:

    a. If there is any evidence to suggest such injury, or if subcutaneous emphysema of the face, neck, or chest is present, bronchoscopy is required to define the extent of damage.

    b. Induce anesthesia with sevoflurane in O_2, or IV propofol (very smoothly and deeply, avoiding coughing and straining). Maintain spontaneous ventilation and avoid positive pressure, which may increase any air leak. Do not use N_2O. In the case of a penetrating wound, cover the wound with a sterile dressing.

    c. Give lidocaine 1.5 mg/kg IV, wait 3 minutes, then perform laryngoscopy and spray the larynx with lidocaine. The bronchoscope may then be inserted.

    d. During bronchoscopy, give sevoflurane in O_2 via the bronchoscope; alternately use a propofol infusion or a combination of the two techniques.

    e. If thoracotomy is required and damage is limited to one bronchus, intubate the uninjured main bronchus using a fiberoptic scope to guide correct placement (see Chapter 4, page 101) and use 100% oxygen.

    f. If a tracheal injury is present, tracheostomy may be required, although immediate surgical repair is sometimes possible. During such repair, the endotracheal tube may be passed almost to the carina. Check bilateral ventilation and allow spontaneous respiration.

6. Injury to the heart and pericardium is rare in children but may occur in association with severe thoracic trauma. Cardiac contusion may result in changes in ventricular function that are detectable by echocardiography and scanning techniques; the ECG usually is unchanged. The clinical significance of such changes is not yet fully understood.

7. Injuries to the great vessels are less common than in adults, owing to the greater elasticity and mobility of the mediastinal structures. However, rarely, a widened mediastinum indicates the need for immediate exploration.

   a. If cardiac tamponade develops secondary to hemopericardium, induction of anesthesia may be very hazardous because the fixed low cardiac output cannot compensate for any drug-induced alterations in systemic vascular resistance.

   b. In hypotensive patients with hemopericardium, the surgeon should drain the pericardium (under local analgesia) before inducing general anesthesia. If tamponade is less severe, induction with ketamine may be possible. (**N.B.** Until the pericardium is open, maintain spontaneous ventilation to augment venous return.)

Suggested Reading

General Considerations

Bricker SWR, McLuckie A, Nightingale DA: Gastric aspirates after trauma in children, Anaesthesia 44:721–724, 1989.

Dykes EH: Paediatric trauma, Br J Anaesth 83:130–138, 1999.

Myer CM 3rd: Trauma of the larynx and craniofacial structures: airway implications, Paediatr Anaesth 14(1):103–106, 2004.

Rasmussen GE, Fiscus MD, Tobias JD: Perioperative anesthetic management of pediatric trauma, Anesthesiol Clin North Am 17:251–262, 1999.

Head Injury

Einaudi S, Bondone C: The effects of head trauma on hypothalamic-pituitary function in children and adolescents, Curr Opin Pediatr 19(4):465–470, 2007.

Martin C, Falcone RA Jr: Pediatric traumatic brain injury: an update of research to understand and improve outcomes, Curr Opin Pediatr 20(3):294–299, 2008.

Moppett IK: Traumatic brain injury: assessment, resuscitation and early management, Br J Anaesth 99(1):18–31, 2007.

Thoracoabdominal Injuries

Eipe N, Choudhrie A: Tracheal rupture in a child with blunt chest injury, Paediatr Anaesth 17(3):273–277, 2007.

Graham J, Davidson AJ: Anaesthesia for major orthopaedic surgery in a child with an acute tracheobronchial injury, Anaesth Intens Care 34(1):88–92, 2006.

Tome R, Somri M, Teszler CB, et al: Delayed ventricular fibrillation following blunt chest trauma in a 4-year-old child, Paediatr Anaesth 16(4):484–486, 2006.

Acute Burns And Scalds

Children are often the victims of burns and scalds. Extensive burns have widespread systemic effects: massive fluid shifts occur, plasma protein is lost, and all the major organ systems are affected. The physiologic response to acute burns may be divided into early (days 1 through 3) and late (after day 3) (Table 17-1).

1. Early after a burn, direct injury to the upper airway and lungs may cause obstruction secondary to edema, bronchospasm, or sloughed tissue. Later, pulmonary function may be affected by infection (pneumonia) or pulmonary vascular changes.
2. The cardiovascular system is affected by changes in blood volume and also possibly by a circulating myocardial depressant factor. Early cardiac dysfunction is generally related to hypovolemia. However, a dilated cardiomyopathy may complicate an acute burn although this usually resolves. After day 3, a hypermetabolic state usually occurs. This necessitates a marked increase in cardiac output (two to three times baseline) to maintain oxygen delivery; this will persist until the child is fully grafted (see Table 17-1).
3. The kidneys are subject to direct damage from myoglobin and hemoglobin, and acute tubular damage may occur as a result of hypovolemia and hypoxia. After day 3, the marked increase in cardiac output leads to increased GFR, which in turn greatly reduces the half-life of many drugs excreted by the kidneys. In addition, hypertension will occur in approximately 50% of children with extensive burn injury. This is mediated by increased renin, endogenous catecholamines, atrial natriuretic factor, and aldosterone production. Some children will require β-blocker or calcium channel blocker therapy to control the hypertension.
4. The liver may be damaged as a result of hypotension, hypoxemia, inhaled toxins, or sepsis. After day 3, marked increases in hepatic blood flow will increase excretion of medications metabolized by the liver.
5. Anemia of burns (decreased erythropoietin production), thrombocytopenia, and a consumptive coagulopathy may occur. Later, a notable thrombocytosis and increased fibrinogen may occur; beware, a sudden decrease in platelet count often precedes developing sepsis.
6. Gastric distention, intestinal ileus, and bleeding secondary to stress ulcers may develop; appropriate antiacid production therapy is indicated.

The anesthesiologist will be involved in the early treatment, consisting of:

1. Airway management and fluid resuscitation

TABLE 17-1 Systemic Effects of Burn Injury

System	Early	Late
Cardiovascular	↓CO due to decreased circulating blood volume, myocardial depressant factor	↑CO due to sepsis ↑CO 2-3 times >baseline for months (hypermetabolism) Hypertension
Pulmonary	Upper airway obstruction due to edema Lower airway obstruction due to edema, bronchospasm, particulate matter ↓FRC ↓Pulmonary compliance ↓Chest wall compliance	Bronchopneumonia Tracheal stenosis ↓Chest wall compliance
Renal	↓GFR a) Secondary to ↓circulating blood volume b) Myoglobinuria c) Hemoglobinuria Tubular dysfunction	↑GFR 2° to ↑CO Tubular dysfunction
Hepatic	↓Function 2° to ↓circulating blood volume, hypoxia, hepatotoxins	Hepatitis ↑Function due to hypermetabolism, enzyme induction, ↑CO ↓Function due to sepsis, drug interactions
Hematopoietic	↓Platelets ↑Fibrin split products, consumptive coagulopathy, anemia	↑Platelets ↑Clotting factors

Neurologic	Encephalopathy
	Seizures
	↑ ICP
	Encephalopathy
	Seizures
	ICU psychosis
Skin	↑ Heat, fluid, electrolyte loss
	Contractures, scar formation, difficult intubation
Metabolic	↓ Ionized calcium
	↑ Oxygen consumption
	↑ Carbon dioxide production & gluconeogenesis
	↓ Ionized calcium
Pharmacokinetics	Altered volume of distribution
	Altered protein binding
	Altered pharmacokinetics
	Altered pharmacodynamics
	Tolerance to opioids, sedatives
	Enzyme induction, altered receptors
	Drug interaction

Early refers to the first 24 to 48 hours after injury. **Late** refers to days to weeks after injury. Legend: *CO*, cardiac output; *FRC*, functional residual capacity; *GFR*, glomerular filtration rate; *ICP*, intracranial pressure; *ICU*, intensive care unit. (With permission. Table 34-2 in A Practice of Anesthesia for Infants and Children. Cote, Lerman, Todres [eds], Philadelphia, 4th ed., 2009, Elsevier.)

2. Fasciotomy (electrical burns) and/or escharectomy (flame or scald burns) to improve adequacy of chest wall excursion or blood flow to extremities and digits.
3. Débridement and grafting

Special Anesthesia Problems

1. Airway and pulmonary involvement may lead to airway obstruction, severe intrapulmonary shunting, and respiratory failure; edema of the tissues surrounding the upper airway may occur very rapidly and make intubation extremely difficult (intubate the trachea as soon as possible). Airway burns must be suspected in all children involved in enclosed-space fires (house/automobile) (inhaled temperatures may reach 1000 °F) and whenever singeing of facial hair and/or eyebrows is present. These children may have macroglossia, macrouvula, epiglottitis, and croup simultaneously.

   Early intubation with a cuffed endotracheal tube is advised for airway burns. Heat injury is limited to the upper airway but inhalation of products of plastic combustion, such as NO_2 or SO_2, are carried far down into the tracheobronchial tree and combined with water to form sulfuric acid and nitric acid and a distal airway burn. Loss of ciliated epithelium and other respiratory protective mechanisms lead to early infection and airway obstruction. Bronchospasm is common. Acid aldehydes may cause pulmonary edema and inhaled cyanide may poison the cytochrome oxidase system. In addition, CO poisoning is the most common cause of impaired oxygen delivery in burns and necessitates therapy with 100% oxygen to reduce the elimination half-life of CO from 4 hours to 30 minutes.

2. Maintenance of fluid balance and renal function: several formulas may be used to calculate fluid regimens for the burned patient; these are based on the burn area (excluding erythema). The Parkland formula prescribes 4 ml/kg of lactated Ringer's solution for each 1% of burn area in addition to normal maintenance requirements. One half of this amount is given in the first 8 hours and the other half over the next 16 hours. Note that this formula will underestimate fluid requirements in children who weigh less than 10 kg; it should be further noted that the "rule of 9s" does not apply to toddlers and that burns of the head may account for 20% of the body surface area (it is easy to underestimate the severity of a burn). Many different resuscitation fluid regimens have been used and all are effective; the many variations are beyond the scope of this handbook. In practice, fluid therapy should frequently be adjusted as dictated by the child's clinical and biochemical status; urine output is an essential guide.

3. Acute gastric dilation: This commonly occurs and adds to the danger of regurgitation. The stomach should be decompressed, and special care should be taken during induction and emergence from anesthesia. Jejunal feeding tubes should not be removed.
4. Management of body temperature: Loss of normal skin severely impairs the patient's ability to conserve heat. Warm the operating room to maximal values (>90 °F or 32 °C); do not unwrap all of the dressings at one time.
5. In children with extensive burns:
   a. Monitoring may be difficult.
   b. Sites for intravenous infusions may be limited; subclavian and femoral lines are common.
6. Circumferential thoracic burns: These may lead to severely compromised ventilation requiring multiple escharotomies to restore chest wall compliance.
7. Danger of infection: Extreme care must be taken to observe strict asepsis with invasive procedures.

Anesthesia Management

Preoperative

1. If the fire occurred in a closed space or involved burning hydrocarbons, suspect respiratory tract burns.
   a. Look for burning around the face (e.g., singed eyebrows).
   b. Assess the airway very carefully. (Children with airway burns may have considerable swelling of the pharyngeal and laryngeal tissues making intubation difficult.)
   c. In the child with airway burns, early tracheal intubation with a cuffed tube should be performed before massive upper airway edema forms. This tube should be meticulously secured with cloth tracheostomy tape as adhesive tape will not adhere to burned tissue. Mark the appropriate distance of insertion with indelible ink so that misplacement does not occur with later dressing changes. Accidental extubation must be prevented as repeat intubation may be impossible.
2. Check the adequacy of fluid and blood replacement:
   a. The Hct should be greater than 25% to 30%; a low serum albumin concentration is usually corrected to greater than 2 g/dl.
   b. The bladder should be catheterized, and urine output should be at least 1 ml/kg/hr.
   c. FFP or platelets may be required to correct documented deficiency resulting in coagulopathy.

Beware of the use of excessive glucose-containing solutions for fluid resuscitation. Hyperosmolar, hyperglycemic nonketotic coma may occur in association with burns.

3. Ensure that the OR temperature is at least (>90 °F or 32 °C) and that heating blankets and lamps are ready for use. Humidify anesthetic gases. Warm blood and intravenous fluids.
4. Check whether the child has been given opioids. Analgesics and hypnotics should be given to prevent pain during transportation to the OR.

Perioperative

General endotracheal anesthesia may be required, but remember:

1. In acute burns, use caution with the dosing of thiopental or propofol if the child's volume status is uncertain; ketamine may be useful in such circumstances. Generally the child is induced in their hospital bed to prevent pain upon movement to the OR table.
2. Succinylcholine is contraindicated (after the first 24 hours) because it may cause cardiac arrest secondary to massive potassium release from muscle.
3. Resistance to nondepolarizing muscle relaxants is increased in proportion to the burn area. The drug must be titrated to achieve the desired effect. Monitor the neuromuscular blockade. Antagonism of very high doses is not a problem.
4. Potent inhalational agents may cause hypotension in those with extensive burns in the acute phase, but may be useful in controlling blood pressure during the hypertensive phase. Alternately, TIVA with propofol infusion and an opioid, or ketamine greatly simplify the anesthetic management of burned or scalded children.

For burn dressing changes, titrate either of the following:

a. Give atropine 0.02 mg/kg IV followed by ketamine 2 mg/kg IV.
b. Maintain anesthesia with ketamine 8 mg/kg IM or incremental doses of 2 mg/kg IV. Or:
c. A combination of propofol (1 mg/kg) and ketamine (1–2 mg/kg) IV.

For all children:

1. Carefully monitor the following:
a. Cardiac rate via an esophageal stethoscope and the ECG (peripheral or esophageal leads) plus pulse oximeter. The oximeter probe may be placed on the tongue or at the corner of the mouth if no other site is available.

b. BP—place a sterile BP cuff at any available site; for severe burns, insert an arterial line.

c. Temperature—esophageal and/or rectal.

d. Blood loss—it is often difficult to estimate loss. Replacement must then be dictated by cardiovascular parameters and urine output. Recall that blood loss is far greater with excision of eschar until bleeding is observed from viable tissue compared with full thickness eschar excision. Blood loss can be greatly reduced if the surgeon administers subcutaneous saline with dilute epinephrine into both the donor and excised areas. Beware of fluid overload when large quantities of tumescent solution are injected; this must be considered in overall fluid management as late pulmonary edema may occur as this fluid is absorbed into the vascular compartment.

e. CVP—consider necessity versus danger of introducing infection. (If BP can be measured, CVP measurement may be unnecessary.) With large burns, a CVP may be the only venous access; beware that the small lumen produces very significant resistance to blood flow and may be inadequate if rapid blood loss occurs. (Avoid rapidly transfusing cold blood through a central line.) Short-term cannulation of a femoral vessel with a single lumen catheter may be indicated just for the procedure and may be removed afterwards.

2. Replace blood losses carefully; large volumes may be required. Anticipate coagulation problems with massive transfusions.

3. Beware of hypocalcemia. Chronic low levels of ionized calcium have been described in burn patients. Plasma and platelet suspensions contain more citrate per unit volume than whole blood; give calcium chloride (5 to 10 mg/kg) or calcium gluconate (15 to 30 mg/kg) if unexpected hypotension occurs. If transfusion exceeds 1 ml/kg/min, anticipate hypocalcemia and administer calcium during these rapid infusions.

Postoperative

1. Order maintenance fluids:

a. Clear fluids to maintain urine output at more than 1 ml/kg/hr

b. Blood to maintain Hct at greater than 30%

c. Albumen may be indicated to maintain total serum protein at greater than 3 g/dl

d. Electrolyte supplements as indicated by serial determinations

2. Order analgesics as required. Burn patients require constant nursing supervision so that a generous dosage of analgesics can be safely administered. A long-term ketamine infusion combined with opioids has been found to be very effective in a child with very extensive burns.

Tolerance to opioids and sedatives rapidly develops. It is common for children with extensive burn injury to require up to 0.5 mg/kg/hr of morphine and 0.1 to 0.3 mg/kg/hr of midazolam just to sustain adequate analgesia with additional doses required intraoperatively.

3. Observe for evolving respiratory insufficiency. (This may occur during the first 24 hours, even if the chest appears clear initially.) Rhonchi and a decreasing level of arterial oxygenation are the usual first signs of trouble. Inhaled ß-adrenergic agents may be useful as may nebulized acetyl cysteine and heparin. In severe airway burns, beware of the possibility of sudden airway obstruction because of sloughed mucosa.

4. Ranitidine and antacids should be administered to protect against stress ulcer. Burn patients may require larger than usual doses to reduce acid secretion.

5. Children who have been intubated for a period in the intensive care unit are at increased risk for development of postextubation stridor, especially if there was no detectable leak around the tube before extubation. Such children require careful monitoring for 24 to 48 hours after extubation; treatment with racemic epinephrine, helium, and O_2, or even reintubation may be required.

Suggested Reading

Comprehensive Review

Sheridan RL: Comprehensive treatment of burns, Curr Prob Surg 38(9):657–756, 2001.

Anesthesia Management

Fuzaylov G, Fidkowski CW: Anesthetic considerations for major burn injury in pediatric patients, Pediatr Anesth 19:202–211, 2009.

Tosun Z, Esmaoglu A, Coruh A, et al: Propofol-ketamine vs propofol-fentanyl combinations for deep sedation and analgesia in pediatric patients undergoing burn dressing changes, Pediatr Anesth 18(1):43–47, 2008.

White MC, Karsli C: Long-term use of an intravenous ketamine infusion in a child with significant burns, Paediatr Anaesth 17(11):1102–1104, 2007.

Zabala LM, Parray T: Cardiac arrest because of unrecognized delayed dilated cardiomyopathy in a child with severe burn injury, Paediatr Anaesth 16(3):358–359, 2006.

Gunshot Wounds

Children frequently become victims of gunshot wounds, especially in the United States. The free access to weapons in the United States and the wide access that many children have to guns in the home contribute to this toll.

Anesthesiologists should be particularly aware of the tissue damage that is caused by modern high-velocity bullets. Tissue over an extensive area surrounding the path of the bullet is damaged or destroyed by the energy of the projectile. This is of particular importance when such wounds occur in the upper chest or neck region with the damage at the exit wound being far greater than the entrance wound. Tissue swelling can be expected to spread to involve a wide surrounding area, possibly jeopardizing the airway. The airway should be secured as early as possible, before distortion of the anatomy progresses further. If the child is relatively stable, ensure that adequate blood products are in the room and checked, otherwise O negative blood is necessary. Adequate venous access must be established in the upper extremities or central venous access before incision as tamponade of the intraabdominal or intrathoracic wound will be relieved upon surgical incision and rapid hypotension my ensue. Be prepared for rapid transfusion and the need for vasopressors.

MINOR TRAUMA

Children with minor trauma must be provided with anesthesia that is safe, as pleasant as possible, and suitable for a young patient who may be ready to go home in an hour or so. Usually there is no extreme urgency in these cases, permitting a considered approach to the selection of both the anesthetic and the optimal time for surgery. However, fractures with vascular compression may require immediate intervention.

Keep in mind the full stomach: gastric emptying may be considerably delayed after even minor injury. Some children starved for more than 8 hours after an accident still have a large volume of gastric contents. A safe period between oral intake, injury, and induction of anesthesia cannot be predicted. Hence, even if one can wait for a full normal fasting period, it is still advisable to use a regional technique or to induce general anesthesia using a rapid-sequence induction with cricoid pressure.

Although metoclopramide may help to speed gastric emptying, neither regional analgesia nor general anesthesia should be administered without fasting unless surgery is needed urgently. The need to convert an unsatisfactory regional anesthesia to general anesthesia arises more frequently in children than in adults.

18 Anesthesia in Remote Locations

REMOTE ANESTHESIA

There is an increased demand for pediatric anesthesiologists to travel outside the operating room to provide general anesthesia or monitored sedation for a variety of medical investigations or procedures in infants and children of all ages. The concept that treatment in a children's hospital should be a pain-and stress-free experience is now well accepted, and this has placed additional responsibilities on the anesthesia service.

Equipment for the Remote Location

Each area should be fully equipped for the anesthesia care of the child and for any resuscitation that might be required; much of this may be provided by means of a travel cart. Each area should be provided with:

1. Primary and backup oxygen supply (checked O_2 tank), and means to provide intermittent positive-pressure ventilation (IPPV).
2. Facilities for gas scavenging if any inhalation anesthetics are used.

3. Functioning suction apparatus.
4. Adequate lighting.
5. Electrical outlets (operating room standards).
6. Means of immediate communication to the operating room personnel.
7. Facilities and staff for the preparation and recovery of children according to published guidelines.*
8. Resuscitation cart and defibrillator (immediately available).

In addition, all drugs and equipment to manage the child during the procedure must be provided:

1. Monitoring for pulse oximetry, electrocardiography (ECG), end-tidal carbon dioxide, blood pressure, and body temperature.
2. Airway supplies; age and size appropriate facemasks, laryngoscope blades, endotracheal tubes, oropharyngeal airways, laryngeal mask airways, suction catheters, and breathing circuits.
3. Appropriate anesthesia equipment, infusion pumps, etc.
4. All necessary drugs for anesthesia and sedation, and, syringes, a variety of IV catheters, intravenous fluid and fluid administration sets.
5. Emergency resuscitation drugs.
6. Where indicated: equipment to maintain body temperature (e.g., forced air warmer for cardiac catheterization laboratory).

ADMINISTRATIVE PROCEDURE FOR REMOTE ANESTHESIA

For children anesthetized in remote locations, the following steps should be taken as in the OR setting:

1. A preanesthesia evaluation should be performed just before sedation.
2. Informed consent for anesthesia should be obtained or on file.
3. An anesthesia record should be completed.
4. The child should be recovered in an appropriately staffed and equipped recovery facility for children or go to the regular pediatric postanesthesia care unit (PACU).
5. A recovery record should be completed.
6. The child should be evaluated by the anesthesiologist when recovered and signed out of the unit (where appropriate this might be delegated using standard written criteria).

---

*Guidelines for non-operating room anesthetizing locations. American Society of Anesthesiologists, Park Ridge Il, 2003.

General Principles

1. The technique chosen should result in minimal (if any) postanesthesia sequelae.
   a. Use short-acting drugs that will not delay recovery and are not associated with postoperative nausea and vomiting. (Therefore, when possible, avoid opioids, barbiturates, and ketamine.) Propofol is ideal.
   b. Most children can be managed with an oxygen mask or nasal prongs, and a support to extend the neck. Occasionally an oral or nasopharyngeal airway may be required. The laryngeal mask airway (LMA) may be a useful alternative. Finally, if all of the above maneuvers still result in an obstructed airway, tracheal intubation may be required. In general, tracheal intubation is avoided in remote locations to minimize postextubation airway problems and to abbreviate the recovery time.
   c. When repeated anesthetics will be needed, a chronic intravenous line should be maintained: either a central line or a "Hep-Locked" peripheral line.
   d. Monitor every child as you would in the operating room.

Suggested Reading

Coté CJ, Wilson S: Guidelines for monitoring and management of pediatric patients during and after sedation for diagnostic and therapeutic procedures: an update, Pediatrics 118:2587–2602, 2006.

McFarlan CS, Anderson BJ, Short TG: The use of propofol infusions in paediatric anaesthesia: a practical guide, Paediatr Anaesth 9:209–216, 1999.

Roy WL: Anaesthetizing children in remote locations: necessary expeditions or anaesthetic misadventures, Can J Anaesth 43:764–768, 1996.

DIAGNOSTIC AND THERAPEUTIC MEDICAL PROCEDURES

Computed Tomography

1. CT scans require absolute immobility of the child throughout. However, modern CT scan times are exceedingly brief, most scans are complete (even when contrast is required) within 10 minutes. Hence many children can be managed without anesthesia and for the others, the anesthetic plan must be tailored accordingly. Small infants can be bundled and restrained during the procedure without sedation. Older children of normal intelligence can cooperate and do not require any form of sedation or anesthetic, they can be distracted and entertained for the short time necessary to complete a scan. It is sometimes necessary

to sedate infants and children less than 3 years, and cognitively challenged children. Very rarely a general anesthetic is required; usually for a child with significant comorbid disease or injury.

2. Intravenous sedation alone is suitable for many children:
   a. A propofol infusion is preferred.
   b. Intravenous pentobarbital is an alternative; an initial dose of 3 mg/kg of pentobarbital may be given. After 3 minutes, further doses of 1 mg/kg may be titrated up to a maximum of 7 mg/kg. (This is a regimen that may be used by specially trained nurses under supervision of the radiologist.)
   c. The child should be monitored with standard ASA monitors. All equipment required to establish an airway and ventilate the lungs should be immediately available.

3. If general anesthesia is required, use only plastic materials in the breathing circuit; metal components distort the image. Be aware that the metal spring in some LMA cuffs and tracheotomy tubes may also cause an artifact and need to be avoided or the spring needs to be taped away from the field.

4. Contrast media may be injected intravenously to enhance the images obtained; very rarely, reactions may occur (see later discussion); be aware to limit the dose in children with renal dysfunction.

Suggested Reading

Taghon TA, Bryan YF, Kurth CD: Pediatric radiology sedation and anesthesia, Intl Anesthesiol Clin 44(1):65–79, 2006.
Coté CJ: Strategies for preventing sedation accidents, Pediatr Ann 34:625–633, 2005.

Magnetic Resonance Imaging

Magnetic resonance imaging (MRI) scans are commonly used to secure accurate anatomic diagnoses, but they may also provide valuable information on the physiologic changes associated with disease. The MRI is increasingly being used to define vascular anatomy (Magnetic resonance angiography (MRA)) especially in children with congenital heart disease, and this requires special considerations (see later discussion). The basic component of the MRI system is a powerful superconducting magnet into which the child must be placed. This presents some problems:

1. The space is very confined, which frightens children, may cause claustrophobia, and also limits access to the child should an emergency occur.
2. There may be a high noise level within the magnet (approximately 95 decibels), and the unit may vibrate and scare the child. Because of

these considerations, deep sedation or general anesthesia is usually required for infants and children having MRI scans.

3. Ferrous metal objects are attracted to the magnet and become dangerous, life-threatening projectiles. Therefore all equipment including oxygen tanks, IV poles, etc., which are taken into the unit must be MRI compatible (nonferromagnetic).

4. It is essential that the child is screened for accompanied or implanted devices that might incorporate ferromagnetic material. These could be dangerously attracted to the magnet, their function could be affected by the magnetic field (e.g., cardiac pacemaker, transthoracic or transvenous pacing wires, vagal nerve stimulator) or they could seriously damage adjacent tissues (e.g., implanted prostheses, wires or vascular clips, cochlear implants, and metal foreign bodies).

N.B. For children with nonremovable ferromagnetic implanted material, an MRI is contraindicated.

5. The magnetic field may cause burns by inducing currents in wire leads (ECG or pulse oximeter cables) or temperature probes. These can produce heat and burn the child's skin. Prevent direct contact between the cables and the child's skin, avoid loops in the cables, and ensure that the cables are directed out of the center of the bore (not the sides) to minimize current induction. Most ECG cables today are carbon fiber lead electrodes. MRI compatible equipment and specifically, fiberoptic cables, are now available for ECG and pulse oximetry that precludes the risk of burns. Adolescents with tattoos may develop a burning sensation at the tattoo site if the dye contains ferromagnetic metals.

6. Implanted vagal nerve stimulators may contain wires that were coiled at the time of insertion so a screening x-ray may be indicated; the stimulator is generally shut off before entering the MR scanner. Cardiac pacemakers and implanted cardiac defibrillators are current not approved for use within any MRI scanner (although MRI compatible pacemakers have been patented).

7. The magnetic field may affect the performance of anesthesia delivery systems; syringe pumps may be unreliable, and vaporizers may become inaccurate (bimetallic strip is nonferromagnetic). Infusion pumps may be placed outside of the scanner room to avoid interference from the magnet. Extra long infusion tubing may be threaded through a conduit in the wall of the scanner room. Note that the long tubing may have significant resistance that could affect drug delivery by some infusion pumps; check proper function beforehand.

8. MRI is very motion sensitive; if the child moves at any stage, a whole scan sequence may need to be repeated.
9. The child may have a major life-threatening illness.
10. The child may have a difficult airway, in this case tracheal intubation should be performed in the operating room and the child transported to the MRI unit anesthetized, on a properly equipped gurney.
11. Resuscitation equipment *cannot* be brought into the MRI scan room should it be required. If resuscitation is required, the child must be rapidly moved from the MRI scan room to an adjacent room in which full resuscitation equipment is available.
12. Higher power magnets (3 Tesla) are now being installed and some equipment that was safe and reliable in the environment of a 1.5 Teslar shielded magnet may be unsafe and/or unreliable in a 3 Tesla unit. Currently units up to 8T are being studied. The shielding installed and the distance a piece of equipment is sited from the magnet are also vital safety concerns. The anesthesiologist should be very familiar with the safety concerns of the local unit.
13. Gadopentetate dimeglumine (gadolinium) is commonly used as a contrast agent to enhance the MRI image. This may cause minor side effects (dizziness, nausea), but may also very rarely cause anaphylaxis. If administered to children with renal impairment, it is poorly cleared and may result in very severe complications; nephrogenic systemic fibrosis (NSF) with multiorgan involvement. Hence the drug is contraindicated in children with renal impairment or immature renal function (infants under 2 years or those with <30 ml/min/1.73 m^2). (N.B. Radiology departments now have guidelines for gadolinium dose, weight, and BUN values, and these charts should be consulted.)

Suggested Reading

Kanal E, Barkovich AJ, Bell C, et al: ACR guidance document for safe MR practices: 2007, AJR 188:1447–1474, 2007.

Dempsey MF, Condon B: Thermal injuries associated with MRI, Clin Radiol 56:457–465, 2001.

Monitoring During MRI Scans

Monitoring during the scan is essential; a plastic precordial or esophageal stethoscope (without a thermistor probe) should be used, and MRI compatible equipment is essential:

1. Pulse oximetry may be used continuously, and various suitable machines are available. Caution must be taken that there are no loops in the cable leads to the child—otherwise currents may be induced and

the child may be burned. Fiberoptic sensors and cables that contain no magnetic or electrically conductive features should be used, eliminating the possibility of burns.

2. Blood pressure may be measured with most NIBP machines fitted with nylon connections.

3. The ECG may be monitored using nonferromagnetic fasteners, cables, and electrodes. The electrocardiogram waveform may be distorted in the MRI environment; all other monitored parameters are less affected. The heart rate may also be monitored from the pulse oximeter.

4. Temperature may be monitored using probes that have radiofrequency filters or nonferromagnetic skin temperature strips. Insulating the infant from the cool ambient magnet temperature is important; however, it is reported that children may increase their body temperature slightly during MRI scans (likely due to absorption of RF energy).

5. Complete MRI-compatible monitoring units are available, and preferably should include a remote slave monitor outside the MRI unit beside the viewing window. Each monitoring unit must be tested for compatibility with the local MRI magnet.

Management for Magnetic Resonance Imaging

Satisfactory immobilization of the child during the scanning process may be achieved by intravenous sedation/anesthesia or general anesthesia (with an LMA or endotracheal tube). IV sedation/anesthesia is most widely used for healthy children; general anesthesia is required for the critically ill child or neonate.

Intravenous Deep Sedation/Anesthesia

An intravenous propofol infusion has been demonstrated to be a safe and reliable method.

1. The child should fast as for general anesthesia.

2. Monitors are placed and sedation is initiated with the child in the supine position on the MRI table beginning with a bolus dose of propofol 2 to 3 mg/kg followed by an infusion of propofol at an initial rate of 250 μg/kg/min. The infusion pump should be MRI-compatible or placed outside the scan room. If IV access is unavailable, the child may undergo an inhalation induction to establish this route and then changed to total intravenous anesthesia (TIVA).

3. If the child moves, an additional bolus of 1 mg/kg of propofol is given. Alternately, the infusion rate of propofol may be increased. Cognitively challenged children and younger infants may require up to

400 µg/kg/min for the early period of anesthesia to achieve motionless conditions.

4. After 15 to 20 minutes, the infusion rate is reduced to 200 µg/kg/min, and after a further 15 to 20 minutes to a rate of 150 µg/kg/min.

5. A facemask or nasal prongs may be used to deliver oxygen during the scan. EtCO$_2$ should be monitored to assess adequacy of ventilation. CO$_2$ can be aspirated via an IV catheter that is inserted through the holes in the facemask with the tip positioned near the nares or mouth. Alternately, CO$_2$ can be aspirated from nasal prongs that are designed for administration of oxygen and sampling of expired gas simultaneously.

6. The airway is usually well maintained during propofol sedation, however:

   a. If airway obstruction occurs when placed on the scan table, reposition the head and place a small bolster under the shoulders and neck.

   b. If obstruction persists, insert an oral or nasopharyngeal airway or a laryngeal mask airway.

   c. If obstruction persists or ventilation/oxygenation is poor, the trachea may require intubation.

7. At the end of the scan, the infusion is discontinued; recovery in an appropriately staffed and equipped pediatric recovery area is usually complete within 20 to 30 minutes.

General Anesthesia

1. General anesthesia with an LMA or endotracheal intubation and controlled ventilation may be required for severely ill children, especially those with central nervous system disease or neonates and children with multiple injuries. All anesthetics can be delivered during MRI scans; the choice should suite the child's needs. **N.B.** There is no pain and no stimulation during MRI scans, so avoid an excessive depth of anesthesia.

2. Children with a possible difficult airway should be intubated in the operating room and transferred to the MRI suite when anesthetized. This will require a transport trolley with an oxygen supply, anesthesia circuit (usually a T-piece), and a battery powered transport monitor for ECG, SaO$_2$, and either invasive or noninvasive blood pressure monitoring. EtCO$_2$ monitoring during transport is desirable. Recall that all equipment to manage the child should unintended extubation occur should also accompany the child to the MRI suite.

Equipment

All equipment must be MRI compatible. Some MRI compatible equipment must remain outside the 5 gauss perimeter of the magnetic field.

Anesthesia machines with vaporizers built of nonferrous metals and with aluminum gas cylinders are available. Alternatively, the mixture of anesthetic gases can be delivered via a long fresh gas flow line (Mapleson system) or a long circle system circuit from outside the MRI suite (beware of kinking). For controlled ventilation, use either manual ventilation or an MRI compatible ventilator.

Standard vaporizers may deliver unpredictable concentrations if placed near the magnetic field; this has been attributed to the magnetic effects on the bimetallic strip, the temperature-compensation mechanism. When inhalational agents are used the expired anesthetic concentration must be measured to determine any possible effect on the vaporizer output.

Endotracheal intubation can be performed either inside or outside the MRI suite. Use nonferromagnetic laryngoscopes, blades, and batteries. Do not be misled; even plastic laryngoscopes may have batteries with ferromagnetic components.

If invasive arterial and/or central venous monitoring is planned, long, low-compliance extension tubing should be used to connect to transducers, which are placed at a distance from the magnet (recognizing that the waveforms may be altered).

Suggested Reading

Serafini G, Zadra N: Anaesthesia for MRI in the paediatric patient, Curr Opin Anaesthesiol 21(4):499–503, 2008.

Special Considerations for Cardiac MRI Imaging

Cardiac imaging in the MRI unit can very successfully demonstrate the exact anatomy of congenital heart diseases and has become a valuable diagnostic tool. To obtain consistent images, the scan must be successfully ECG "gated" to the cardiac cycle and obtained at a standard phase of ventilation.

Anesthesia for these children must recognize all the implications of their heart disease and must provide for periods of apnea at a standard lung volume (usually end-expiration). General endotracheal anesthesia with neuromuscular block is required. Comprehensive monitoring should be provided appropriate to their disease. Permissible periods of apnea should be applied by disconnection from the ventilator, and their duration limited by observation of the saturation monitor.

Suggested Reading

Odegard KC, DiNardo JA, Tsai-Goodman B, et al: Anaesthesia considerations for cardiac MRI in infants and small children, Paediatr Anaesth 14(6):471–476, 2004.

Other Radiologic Procedures

General anesthesia is often necessary for cerebral angiography in children because the procedure may be prolonged and uncomfortable and the child must remain immobile throughout.

Special Anesthesia Problems

1. Intracranial pressure (ICP) may be increased.
2. The radiologic examination may require special positioning and tilting of the child.
3. It may be difficult to maintain body temperature in infants.
4. Special attention must be paid to the total load of contrast material (milligrams/kilogram) particularly in infants with compromised renal function; low ionic contrast solutions are preferred. Reactions to contrast media may occur; this is now quite rare with the use of nonionic agents.
5. Children must recover rapidly so that their neurologic status can be checked.

Anesthesia Management

Preoperative

1. Assess the child's neurologic status and other underlying medical conditions carefully.
2. Check for a history of allergy, asthma, prior anesthetic experiences, or previous reactions to radiologic contrast media.
3. Avoid premedication if ICP is increased.

Perioperative

1. An intravenous induction is preferred. Give propofol or thiopental followed by relaxant.
2. For children with increased ICP, give lidocaine 1.5 mg/kg IV and a short-acting opioid (i.e., fentanyl 2 μg/kg) to attenuate the hypertensive response to laryngoscopy and intubation.
3. Insert an endotracheal tube. A nasal or armored tube should be used if the positioning or movement of the child might result in kinking of an oral tracheal tube.
4. Maintain anesthesia with sevoflurane or a propofol infusion (sevoflurane may provide more rapid awakening after a prolonged procedure).

Cerebral Arteriography

1. If a tumor or AVM is suspected, maintain anesthesia with N_2O, a low concentration of an inhalational agent and a muscle relaxant. Ventilation should be controlled to produce a carbon dioxide partial pressure (PetCO$_2$) of approximately 30 mm Hg (confirm by sampling from the arterial catheter). This degree of hypocapnia may improve radiographic definition by constricting the normal vessels while abnormal vessels remain dilated.

   N.B. If an AVM is suspected, preoperative management and induction of anesthesia should be as outlined on page 253.

2. Chart the total volume of contrast medium and flush fluid carefully, especially in small infants. Beware of fluid overload, especially in small infants with AVMs.
3. A transient bradycardia with hypotension may occur at the time of injection into the carotid artery owing to baroreceptor activity; atropine prevents this response.

Postprocedure Management

1. The child must be awake before transfer to PACU. After angiography, it is necessary to maintain pressure over the catheterization site to prevent hematoma formation; this is easier to achieve if the child is quiet and immobile.
2. Usually opioids are not needed; sedation with midazolam reduces restlessness.
3. Check arterial puncture sites frequently; if a limb artery was used, check the circulation to that extremity.

Additional Possible Complications

In addition to the complications that may develop during administration of any anesthetic, some special problems may occur during neuroradiologic procedures.

1. Hypothermia due to difficulty in keeping blankets and heating lamps in place during frequent changes in the child's position and the cold temperature of the angiography suite.
2. Acute increase in ICP, leading to coning of the brain stem, usually occurring with bradycardia. In this event:
   a. Hyperventilate the lungs.
   b. Request that a ventricular tap be performed as soon as possible.

c. Give an osmotic diuretic (mannitol 0.5 to 1 g/kg) or furosemide 0.5-1 mg/kg) and full doses of atropine to counter bradycardia.
3. Allergic reaction to contrast media (hives, bronchospasm, hypotension). Nonionic contrast media containing iodine are most commonly used (i.e., iopamidol [Isovue]). Such agents have much less tendency to trigger adverse reactions. However, such a possibility must always be anticipated, especially in the child with a history of allergy or asthma.
4. Stroke may occur if the embolizing glue or coil plugs a blood vessel for which it was not intended.

Reactions to Contrast Media

1. Although very rare in children, the anesthesiologist must be prepared for this possibility.
2. Minor allergic reactions (i.e., skin rashes) may be treated with diphenhydramine, 1 mg/kg IM or IV.
3. Major anaphylactic shock (very rare) must be treated aggressively (see page 205).
    a. Ventilation with oxygen; cardiopulmonary resuscitation as required.
    b. Epinephrine 10 µg/kg IV, followed by an epinephrine infusion 0.05 to 0.2 µg/kg/min.
    c. Hydrocortisone 10 mg/kg by IV injection.
    d. Intravenous fluids as necessary to maintain the blood pressure.
    e. H1 blocker (diphenhydramine 1 to 2 mg/kg IV) and H2 blocker (ranitidine 1.5 mg/kg IV) may be useful (no data in children).
4. Contrast media may cause sickling in children with sickle cell disease.

Suggested Reading

Castagnini HE, van Eijs F, Salevsky FC, et al: Sevoflurane for interventional neuroradiology procedures is associated with more rapid early recovery than propofol, CJA 51(5):486–491, 2004.

RADIATION THERAPY

Infants and small children usually require general anesthesia or deep sedation to render them immobile for the period of radiotherapy. Treatments may have to be repeated daily or twice daily for many days. Therefore a technique should be used that minimally interferes with the child's lifestyle and nutrition and causes the least emotional upset; intravenous sedation with propofol has been demonstrated to be very effective.

These children usually will have a central venous access device inserted to facilitate their care for the duration of their therapy. This can be used to administer the drugs, but:

1. Be meticulous with aseptic precautions to prevent catheter infection.
2. Carefully flush the catheter clear of propofol after the treatment. Residual propofol in the catheter might predispose to infection or to unexpected apnea when flushed later in PACU, on the ward, or at home.
3. Flush the system with an appropriate heparin solution so as to preserve device function and avoid clotting.

Alternatively, an intravenous catheter should be painlessly introduced (using a topical anesthetic cream) at the first treatment and maintained by the use of a splint and "Hep-lock" connection for use during subsequent sessions.

If the child is positioned and prepared with the parent in attendance, the treatment can sometimes be completed with a single bolus dose of propofol. Alternatively, an infusion should be used.

For radiotherapy to the head region, an immobilization frame that applies suction to the hard palate is commonly used. Surprisingly, this frame maintains the airway extremely well without the need for further interventions. Child specific fiberglass masks crafted during preradiation therapy planning CT scan sessions that lock into position are also used for this purpose.

Expired CO_2 is monitored by inserting an IV catheter into the oxygen mask and locating the tip near the nose or mouth for optimal sampling. SaO_2 and NIBP monitoring are routine. All parameters can be monitored by closed-circuit television when the patient care team leaves the radiation suite during treatments. Recovery is very rapid after short procedures using propofol, and the child's appetite soon returns. The child must be recovered in an appropriately staffed and equipped pediatric recovery facility.

INVASIVE MEDICAL PROCEDURES (ONCOLOGY)

Children who need lumbar puncture, bone marrow aspiration, or other painful procedures should be provided with optimal sedation and analgesia. This is particularly important for the child with a malignant disease who requires repeated sessions; an optimal management plan should be instituted at the outset of treatment. Apart from the use of well-selected sedative and analgesic drugs, there are some other important considerations:

1. The child and the parents must be well-prepared for the procedure and know exactly what to expect. Psychological preparation and behavioral training may be of value for the child.
2. The planned procedure should be performed in comfortable, pleasant surroundings. The parents should be encouraged to accompany the child. The area should be provided with oxygen, suction, and emergency equipment to deal with potential complications; this equipment can be discreetly covered but should be immediately available.
3. A suitable recovery area should be provided, and the parents should be allowed to remain with the child during awakening.

Suggested Routine

1. Fasting guidelines as for general anesthesia should be used.
2. The child's current health status should be fully assessed and informed consent for the procedure should be obtained or on file.
3. If the child does not have an established intravenous route (e.g., Hickman line), prepare to establish one by placing topical local anesthetic cream over a suitable vein as soon as the child arrives at the clinic. If the Hickman line is accessed be meticulous with asepsis.
4. If the child is anxious, premedicate with oral midazolam.
5. Hypnosis for the procedure may be provided by intravenous propofol, supplemented, if necessary, by small doses of fentanyl or alfentanil. Frequently, if local analgesics are properly administered, propofol alone is adequate. It is preferable to avoid opioids as they increase the risk of post-procedure nausea and vomiting. Small doses of ketamine (0.25 to 1 mg/kg) may be added to the propofol prescription to provide additional analgesia. This will not increase vomiting but may delay recovery slightly.
6. During the procedure, standard monitoring should be followed.
7. Age and size appropriate equipment to establish an airway and ventilate the lungs should be immediately available.
8. Monitor ventilation carefully; when propofol is being used, the child may be positioned in the lateral decubitus position, or even prone on bolsters; usually a clear airway is maintained without the need for tracheal intubation. Minor degrees of airway compromise usually can be corrected by repositioning the head or by insertion of an oropharyngeal airway, which is well tolerated during deep propofol sedation/anesthesia.

Gastrointestinal Endoscopy

Infants and children may require anesthesia during diagnostic upper or lower endoscopy and for therapeutic procedures such as injection of esophageal varices and percutaneous endoscopic gastrostomy.

Gastroduodenoscopy

There are two alternative methods for upper endoscopy and therapeutic procedures; use of a tracheal tube or no tube. Many of these children have a history of gastroesophageal reflux, and in these cases appropriate measures to ensure preoperative fasting, decrease gastric acidity, and rapidly secure the airway are usually taken. If the trachea is to be intubated, then the larynx may be sprayed with lidocaine to reduce coughing and bucking. The maintenance may include propofol with or without remifentanil infusions, titrating the doses to the child's requirements or sevoflurane. Alternatively, as these procedures are almost always performed in the lateral decubitus position (which facilitates the drainage of any fluids out of the mouth rather than into the larynx), with an endoscope in the esophagus/stomach (that can evacuate liquid in the stomach easily), many accept an unprotected airway in children. In such cases, after an inhalational induction and placement of an IV anesthesia is maintained with either intermittent propofol (1 to 1.5 mg/kg) or a continuous infusion of propofol with or without remifentanil. This method should only be used in those children free of the danger of regurgitation, vomiting, or major bleeding. In all children, care should be taken to prevent nerve compression in the lateral decubitus position. The endoscopist should be reminded to empty all air from the esophagus and stomach after the procedure.

In infants (<10 kg), the trachea must be intubated during EGDs because the pediatric gastric scope compresses the trachealis muscle and obstructs the upper airway. Similarly, if injection of varices is planned in any age child, the trachea should be secured with a tracheal tube and a large-bore intravenous line should be in place. The stomach should be aspirated at the end of the procedure in all cases before the endoscope is removed, and the child should be awake before tracheal extubation. If a child is to undergo insertion of a gastrointestinal camera (PillCam), then intubation may be the safest method of airway management since this device is quite large and could accidentally be deployed obstructing the airway.

Colonoscopy

Colonoscopy may follow the EGD or be a separate procedure. If it follows the EGD, anesthesia may be continued as per the EGD or administer 70% N_2O by facemask (or LMA) recognizing that one or possibly two doses of propofol may be required when passing the colonoscope by the splenic or hepatic flexure. If it is a separate procedure, general anesthesia is required although tracheal intubation is usually unnecessary. The child is positioned either supine or in the left lateral decubitus position and care must be directed at preventing nerve compression. The extent of abdominal distention caused by insufflation of air into the bowel should be monitored. The endoscopist should be encouraged to remove all air possible before terminating the procedure.

Percutaneous Endoscopic Gastrostomy (PEG)

Insertion of a PEG requires the same considerations as above with the addition that the skin area at the proposed gastrostomy site should be infiltrated with a local anesthetic. Endotracheal intubation is preferred to guarantee the airway while the rather large gastrostomy tube bulb is pulled through the esophagus.

Suggested Reading

Hussein SA: Anesthesia for pediatric endoscopies, Int Anesthesiol Clin 44(1): 81–93, 2006.

Anesthesia Implications of Syndromes and Unusual Disorders*

This Appendix contains brief descriptions of many common syndromes and their associated anesthetic considerations for safe pediatric anesthesia practice. Also described are some quite rare syndromes that have important anesthesia considerations. Many of these share features that make precise identification difficult, and the reader should consider all the information given in the description. *Whenever possible, the referenced literature should be consulted before anesthesia* is undertaken. A brief list of several excellent resources that are up-to-date follow this introduction. In some rare syndromes, the only references are in foreign language journals; we have listed these when an English abstract was appended. Very occasionally, the reference refers to the disease in adults; we still include it when no published pediatric literature was available and where we thought that the adult information provided might be useful. Space limits a complete literature review for each condition but we have attempted to list the most important and recent publications or case reports.

There are now more than 10,000 medical syndromes recorded, so it is inevitable that this list is incomplete. Genetic studies have identified many new syndromes and increased our knowledge of old ones. Although the number of syndromes has increased and existing syndromes have become better understood, anesthesiologists may still encounter unreported difficulties and complications. When in doubt as to the identity and implications of a syndrome, the anesthesiologist should make preparations that take into account all possible associated disorders.

There are a number of recurring problems associated with these syndromes that influence the choice of an anesthetic technique, predominantly difficult airway management and the management of cardiac conditions. The reader is encouraged to refer to the chapters that provide

---

*Adapted from Jones EP, Pelton DA: Can Anaesth Soc J 23:207, 1976 and extensively augmented and revised.

general advice on management of the difficult airway and congenital heart disease, which may be adapted to the particular syndrome presented and in accordance with the practice and experience of the anesthesiologist. Those conditions that include impaired renal function demand special care when administering radiologic contrast media. Classic descriptions of the clinical problems of a syndrome may allow the reader to decide when newer drugs and techniques can be used safely in individual cases.

Suggested Reading

Bissonnette B, Luginbuehl I, Marciniak B, et al. (eds.): Syndromes: rapid recognition and perioperative implications. McGraw-Hill Medical Publishing Division, New York, 2006.

Baum VC, O'Flaherty JE (eds.): Anesthesia for genetic, metabolic, & dysmorphic syndromes of childhood, 2nd ed. Lippincott, Williams & Wilkins, Philadelphia, 2007.

Fleisher LA (ed.): Anesthesia and uncommon diseases, 5th ed. Elsevier-Saunders, Philadelphia, 2005.

Kliegman RM (ed.): Nelson textbook of pediatrics, 18th ed. Elsevier-Saunders, Philadelphia, 2007, Online at: www.nelsonpediatrics.com.

Name	Description	Anesthesia Implications
Achondroplasia	Most common form of dwarfism. Defective fibroblastic growth factor (FGFR3) at chromosome 4. Defective bone formation with decreased rate of endochondreal ossification leads to shorter tubular bones. Foramen magnum or spinal stenosis may occur. Sleep apnea may be related to brain stem compression. May need suboccipital craniectomy, laminectomy, or cerebrospinal fluid (CSF) shunts.	Intubation may be difficult but usually is not. Tracheal tube size and depth of insertion are best judged by weight (not age)—most require a smaller tube than indicated by their age. Caution with neck movements—avoid excessive extension. IV access is difficult due to excess lax skin. High incidence of complications when operated on in the sitting position.
Krishnan BS, Eipe N, Korula G: Anaesthetic management of a patient with achondroplasia. Paediatr Anaesth 13(6):547–549, 2003.		
Acrocephalopolysyndactyly	See Carpenter syndrome, Saethre-Chotzen syndrome.	
Acrocephalosyndactyly	See Apert syndrome.	
Adrenogenital syndrome	Inability to synthesize hydrocortisone; virilization of females. All need perioperative steroid supplementation, even if not salt-losing.	Preoperatively check electrolytes, ensure that supplementary corticosteroids are ordered even if anesthesia is unaccompanied by surgery (i.e., for MRI or other investigation).
Abel M, von Petrykowski W: Perioperative substitution therapy in congenital adrenogenital syndrome with salt loss. [German-English abstract]. Anaesthesist 33(8):374–376, 1984.		
Adrenoleukodystrophy	See Leukodystrophy.	
Aicardi syndrome	Absent corpus callosum, chorioretinopathy and infantile spasms. Marked myotonia and drowsiness. Repeated aspiration pneumonia.	Caution with muscle relaxants. No other special recommendations.
Mayhew J: Anesthesia in a child with Aicardi syndrome. Paediatr Anaesth 17(12):1223, 2007.		

Table continues on the following page.

Name	Description	Anesthesia Implications
Alagille syndrome	Disorder of the bile ducts with cholestasis. May have cardiac (97%), musculoskeletal (inc. vertebral), ocular, facial, and neurologic abnormalities. Variable presentation of an autosomal dominant inherited condition. Severe cases necessitate liver transplantation.	Bilirubin, coagulation profile, and vitamin K level should be checked preoperatively. Hepatosplenomegaly encourages regurgitation; a rapid-sequence induction may be necessary to prevent aspiration. Caution with drugs handled by the liver. Avoid drugs that decrease hepatic blood flow (HBF); isoflurane has least effect on HBF. Maintain intravascular volume to preserve HBF. Epidural anesthesia may be preferred over opioids but check clotting state, and vertebral anatomy (check x-rays). Caution with transport and positioning; osteoporosis may be present (vitamin D deficiency)
	Choudry DK, Rehman MA, Schwartz RE, et al: The Alagille's syndrome and its anaesthetic considerations. Paediatr Anaesth 8:79, 1998. Subramaniam K, Myers LB: Combined general and epidural anesthesia for a child with alagille syndrome: a case report. Paediatr Anaesth 14(9):787–791, 2004.	
Albers-Schönberg disease (marble bone disease; osteopetrosis)	Disorder of osteoclasts and bone overgrowth. Infantile malignant form presents at less than 1 yr of age with failure to thrive and seizures because of hypocalcemia. Lethargy, macrocephaly, frontal bossing, obligate mouth breathing (overgrowth nasopharyngeal bone) are common. Hydrocephalus may occur. Brittle bones, pathologic fractures. Anemia from marrow sclerosis; hepatosplenomegaly.	Check anemia and Ca++ level preoperatively. Care in moving, positioning, and use of restraints. Nasal airway unreliable; may obstruct when anesthetized; prepare airways and laryngeal mask airway (LMA). N.B. Limited mobility of joints.
	Armstrong DG, Newfield JT, Gillespie R: Orthopedic management of osteopetrosis: results of a survey and review of the literature. J Ped Ortho 19(1):122–132, 1999.	
Albright-Butler syndrome	Renal tubular acidosis, hypokalemia, osteomalacia, rickets, renal calculi. Treated with alkali Rx and K+ supplementation.	Check and correct electrolytes to normal values. Renal impairment; caution with renally excreted drugs and fluid therapy.
	Unwin RJ, Capasso G: The renal tubular acidoses. J Royal Soc Med 94(5):221–225, 2001.	

Albright hereditary osteodystrophy (pseudohypoparathyroidism)	Ectopic bone formation, mental retardation. Hypocalcemia: possible ECG conduction defects, neuromuscular problems, convulsions. May present for cataract surgery.	Preoperatively check ECG and electrolytes. Prevent hyperventilation and respiratory alkalosis (exacerbates hypocalcemia). Monitor ECG carefully for increasing Q-T interval or conduction defects. Extreme caution with muscle relaxants.

Sunder RA, Singh M: Pseudohypoparathyroidism: a series of three cases and an unusual presentation of ocular tetany. Anaesthesia 61(4):394-398, 2006.

Aldrich syndrome	See Wiskott-Aldrich syndrome.	
Alexander disease	See leukodystrophy.	
Alport syndrome	Nephritis and nerve deafness; renal pathology variable. Renal failure in second to third decade. May present for renal transplantation.	Use caution with drugs excreted by kidneys, Check ECG as A-V conduction defects may occur.

Ferrari F, Nascimento P Jr, Vianna PT: Complete atrioventricular block during renal transplantation in a patient with Alport's syndrome: case report. Sao Paulo Med J, Revista Paulista de Medicina. 119(5):184-186, 2001.

Alström syndrome	Obesity, blindness by 7 years, hearing loss, diabetes after puberty, hepatic dysfunction, and glomerulo-sclerosis. Decreased liver function and renal impairment.	Check liver function. Diabetes and obesity require special consideration. Use caution with drugs excreted by kidneys.

Awazu M, Tanaka T, Sato S et al: Hepatic dysfunction in two sibs with Alstrom syndrome: case report and review of the literature. Am J Med Gen 69(1):13-16, 1997.

Amaurotic familial idiocy	See Gangliosidosis GM2 (Tay-Sachs disease).	
Amyotonia congenital (infantile muscular atrophy)		
Anterior horn cell degeneration	Sensitive to thiopental and propofol (due to reduced muscle mass) and respiratory depressants. Avoid muscle relaxants where possible: unpredictable response to non-depolarizing relaxants.	

Table continues on the following page.

543

Name	Description	Anesthesia Implications
Amyotrophic lateral sclerosis	Degeneration of motor neurons. Progressive muscular weakness and respiratory failure. Prone to aspiration pneumonia.	Check baseline ventilatory status (spirometry). Do not use succinylcholine: possible K^+ release and cardiac arrest. Use minimal doses of thiopental, propofol, and relaxants (cisatracurium preferred and monitor neuromuscular block.). Avoid respiratory depressants. Consider regional analgesia.
	Moser B, Lirk P, Lechner M et al: General anaesthesia in a patient with motor neuron disease. Euro J Anaesthesiol 21(11):921–923, 2004.	
Analbuminemia	Extremely low level of serum albumin (4–100 mg/dl).	Very sensitive to drugs that bind to protein (i.e., propofol, thiopental, pancuronium).
	Koot BGP, Houwen R, Pot DJ et al: Congenital analbuminemia biochemical and clinical implications. A case report and literature review. Eur J Pediatr 163:664-670, 2004.	
Analphalipoproteinemia	See Tangier disease.	
Andersen disease (glycogen storage disease type IV)	Deficiency of glucosyl transferase (brancher enzyme). Early severe hepatic cirrhosis; liver failure; splenomegaly; hemorrhagic tendency.	Check coagulation factors; treat excessive bleeding with fresh-frozen plasma. Possibility of hypoglycemia under anesthesia; infuse dextrose perioperatively.
Andersen syndrome	Periodic paralysis, long Q-T interval, dysmorphic features; severe midfacial hypoplasia → relative mandibular prognathism; abnormal structure and angle of mandible (triangular facies), kyphoscoliosis.	Possible airway problems; mask ventilation and intubation may be difficult. Assess respiratory status. Observe cautions for long Q-T syndrome. Avoid succinylcholine.
	Young DA: Anesthesia for the child with Andersen's syndrome. Paediatr Anaesth 15(11):1019–1020, 2005.	
Angelman syndrome	Mental retardation, craniofacial anomalies, drooling, ataxia, seizures, paroxysmal laughter, muscle atrophy. Genetic defect in maternal 15q chromosome in 75% of cases affecting $GABA_{A\beta}$ subunit receptors may alter response to anesthetic drugs. Vagal hypertonia.	Usually uncooperative. Continue anticonvulsants. Caution with IV hypnotics ($GABA_{A\beta}$) and muscle relaxants (myopathy). Normal response to inhaled agents and opioids. Possible difficult airway. Prophylactic anticholinergic to limit vagal overactivity.
	Ramanathan KR, Muthuswamy D, Jenkins BJ: Anaesthesia for Angelman syndrome. Anaesthesia 63(6):659–661, 2008. Gardner JC, Turner CS, Ririe DG: Vagal hypertonia and anesthesia in Angelman syndrome. Paediatr Anaesth 18(4):348-349, 2008.	

| **Angioedema** (hereditary angioneurotic edema) | Episodic brawny edema of extremities, face, trunk, airway abdominal viscera, lasts 4 hr to 1 wk. Mutation on chromosome 11 responsible. Onset in childhood differentiates this from idiopathic form. Etiology: (1) Deficiency of C1 esterase inhibitor, reduced to 20% normal levels or (2) normal levels of dysfunctional type of C1 esterase inhibitor. Accumulation of vasoactive substances → increased vascular permeability → edema. Usually painless; may have prodromal focal tingling or "tightness." Often induced by trauma or vibration. May have bouts of abdominal pain, diarrhea; hemoconcentration leading to hypotension, shock, pharyngeal edema (usually develops slowly). Most deaths from laryngeal edema; mortality rate up to 33%. Treatment with antifibrinolytic and hormonal agents. | Check complement assay, Hct, fluid status, treatment history, previous drug reactions. Note voice change or dysphasia. Prophylaxis (i.e., for dental manipulation): EACA and/or fresh-frozen plasma for 1–3 days, preoperatively. Continue EACA IV perioperatively and postoperatively. Danazol (androgen) is useful. Acute attack: epinephrine, steroids, antihistamine (in case diagnosis is a true anaphylaxis), fresh-frozen plasma or purified C1 inhibitor. If pharyngeal edema develops: tracheal intubation (leave in place for 24–72 hr); if this is not possible, perform tracheotomy. Regional anesthesia when possible. Otherwise, extreme care when instrumenting airway. Preoperatively and postoperatively: monitor vital signs. |

Wall RT, Frank M, Hahn M: A review of 25 patients with hereditary angioedema requiring surgery. Anesthesiology 71(2):309–311, 1989.

| **Angio-osteohypertrophy** | See Klippel-Trénaunay-Weber syndrome. |
| **Anhidrotic ectodermal dysplasia** | See Christ-Siemens-Touraine syndrome. |

Table continues on the following page.

Name	Description	Anesthesia Implications
Antley-Bixler syndrome	Recessive condition with bony and cartilaginous abnormalities: craniosynostosis, midface hypoplasia, choanal atresia, and joint contractures. May have cardiac, gastrointestinal, and renal abnormalities. Respiratory obstruction may require early intervention (including tracheostomy). Need major cranial surgery in neonates to relieve craniosynostosis.	Potential respiratory problems and difficult intubation. Care with positioning. Extremity deformities may preclude easy vascular access.
	Boswell D, Mayhew J: Anesthesia for an infant with Antley-Bixler syndrome. Paediatr Anaesth 17(5):497–498, 2007.	
Apert syndrome (acrocephalosyndactyly)	Mental retardation. Hypoplastic maxilla and exophthalmos. Craniosynostosis, possibly with increased ICP; fused cervical vertebrae. Trachea may be narrow with fused rings ("Bamboo trachea") CHD may be present.	Mask anesthesia may be difficult; orotracheal intubation is almost always easy. Nasotracheal intubation may be difficult because of narrowed nasal passages. ICP may be increased. High incidence of respiratory complications— caution if history of recent URI.
	Elwood T, Sarathy PV, Geiduschek JM et al: Respiratory complications during anaesthesia in Apert syndrome. Paediatr Anaesth 11(6):701–703, 2001.	
Arachnodactyly	See Marfan syndrome.	
Arima syndrome	Malformation of the brain stem with congenital amaurosis and psychomotor retardation. Renal dysfunction or failure because of polycystic kidneys. May also have hepatic failure.	Preoperatively check serum electrolytes if chronic renal failure present. Caution with renally excreted drugs. Hyperkalemia during surgery can produce ECG changes necessitating treatment.
	Koizuka S, Nishikawa K-I, Nemoto H et al: Intraoperative QRS-interval changes caused by hyperkalaemia in an infant with Arima syndrome. Paediatr Anaesth 8:425, 1998.	

Arthrogryposis multiplex	Multiple congenital contractures, stiffness of joints; CHD in about 10% of cases. Intraoperative hyperthermia may occur but without classic biochemical or genetic markers for MH.	Minimal thiopental/propofol required—muscles replaced by fat. Sensitivity to nondepolarizing muscle relaxants. Difficult intubation and airway problem because of limitation of temporomandibular movement. Tachycardia and increase in body temperature often observed for unclear reasons. (Not prone to MH). Monitor body temperature and be prepared for cooling measures.

Kanaya N, Nakayama M, Nakae Y et al: Hyperthermia during sevoflurane anaesthesia in arthrogryposis multiplex congenita with central nervous system dysfunction. Paediatr Anaesth 6(5):428–429, 1996.

Asplenia syndrome	Absent spleen; malposition of abdominal organs. Very complex cardiovascular anomalies (i.e., single ventricle); cyanosis and heart failure in many cases. Increased susceptibility to overwhelming infection.	Assess cardiovascular status including preoperative echocardiogram; SBE prophylaxis if indicated; use sterile technique, reverse isolation. Do not use cardiodepressants; ketamine, midazolam, and fentanyl recommended.

Uchida K, Ando T, Okuda C et al: Anesthetic management of an infant with a single ventricle (asplenia syndrome) for non-cardiac surgery. [Japanese] English abstract - Masui - Jap J Anesth 41(11):1793–1797, 1992.

Ataxia telangiectasia	Cerebellar ataxia, skin and conjunctival telangiectasia; decreased serum IgA or IgE. Defective immunity → recurrent pulmonary and sinus infections; bronchiectasis. Severe anemia may be present. RES malignancy in about 10% of cases.	Check Hb and Hct levels and pulmonary function if indicated. Treat anemia. Use antibiotic prophylaxis if indicated. Use sterile technique (reverse isolation).

Peterson RDA, Good RA: Ataxia-telangiectasia. Birth Defects 4:370, 1968.

Table continues on the following page.

Name	Description	Anesthesia Implications
Bardet-Biedl syndrome Bauman ML, Hogan GR: Laurence-Moon-Biedl syndrome. Am J Dis Child 126:119, 1973.	Mental retardation, pigmentary retinopathy, polydactyly, obesity, hypogenitalism, diabetes, and hypertension. (Spastic paraplegia, typical in Laurence-Moon syndrome, is absent.) May have renal abnormalities and congenital heart defects.	Assess cardiac status (echocardiogram), renal (BUN/creatinine), endocrine, and fluid status. SBE prophylaxis if indicated. Use contrast material with caution.
Bartter syndrome Kannan S, Delph Y, and Moseley HSL: Anaesthetic management of a child with Bartter's syndrome. Can J Anaesth 42:808, 1995.	Hypokalemic, hypochloremic metabolic alkalosis. Normotensive but hypovolemic. Chloride reabsorption defect with urinary potassium loss. Juxtaglomerular cell hyperplasia, hyperaldosteronism, prostaglandin overproduction and activation of the rennin angiotensin aldosterone system.	Check acid-base status: electrolyte abnormalities difficult to correct. Hemodynamic instability; invasive monitoring is recommended. Careful attention to electrolytes and volume status. Regional anesthesia is suitable.
Beare-Stevenson syndrome Upmeyer S, Bothwell M, Tobias JD: Perioperative care of a patient with Beare-Stevenson syndrome. Paediatr Anaesth 15(12):1131–1136, 2005.	Craniosynostosis with clover-leaf skull, hydrocephalus, proptosis, choanal atresia, cleft palate, cutis gyratum, and abnormal genitalia. Associated cervical spine and foramen magnum abnormalities.	Airway maintenance and intubation may be very difficult. IV access may be complicated by skin changes. Caution with neck movement. Protect the eyes by lubricating and closing (with tape) or protecting (with eye shield). Monitor ventilation postoperatively.
Becker syndrome	See Duchenne muscular dystrophy.	
Beckwith syndrome (Beckwith-Wiedemann syndrome, infantile gigantism)	Rare disease caused by genetic defect with variable inheritance patterns. Birth weight greater than 4000 g, macroglossia, and exophthalmos. Omphalocele,	Airway problems and difficult intubation because of large tongue. Trachea may be large for age - use a cuffed tube. Monitor blood glucose carefully and treat

	visceromegaly, hyperviscosity syndrome, umbilical hernias and hypoglycemia are common (See Neonatal hypoglycemia) Cleft palate may be associated, and if this is repaired tongue reduction should be performed or severe airway obstruction may occur.	hypoglycemia by slow infusion of dextrose (bolus dose may cause rebound hypoglycemia). Nasopharyngeal airway useful for postoperative airway obstruction. May require phlebotomy to reduce high hematocrit.

Suan C, Ojeda R, Garcia-Perla JL et al: Anaesthesia and the Beckwith-Wiedemann syndrome. Paediatr Anaesth 6:231, 1996.
Kimura Y, Kamada Y, Kimura S et al: Anesthetic management of two cases of Beckwith-Wiedemann syndrome. J Anesth 22(1):93–95, 2008.

Behçet syndrome	Gross ulceration of mouth (usually first sign; may extend to esophagus) and genital area; uveitis, iritis, conjunctivitis, skin lesions, nonerosive arthritis. May have vasculitis, myocardial, and CNS involvement; risk of sepsis at sites of skin punctures, etc.	Preoperative echocardiogram and ECG to rule out cardiac involvement. Use sterile technique. May have history of steroid therapy; nutritional status may be very poor. Tracheal intubation may be very difficult because of scarring in pharynx.

Turner ME: Anaesthetic difficulties associated with Behçet's syndrome. Br J Anaesth 44:100, 1972.

Binder syndrome	Maxillonasal dysplasia; if severe, may be corrected surgically.	Advancement of maxilla and wiring of maxilla and mandible may cause airway problems perioperatively and postoperatively.

Henderson D, Jackson IT: Naso-maxillary hypoplasia-the Fort II osteotomy. Br J Oral Surg 11:77, 1973.

Blackfan-Diamond syndrome	Congenital idiopathic RBC aplasia. Liver and spleen enlarged: hypersplenism, thrombocytopenia. Treatment with steroids and repeated transfusions; hemochromatosis may develop. Bone marrow transplant may be successful. Increased incidence of malignancy (leukemia).	Coagulation studies preoperatively; treat anemia and have platelets available. Give additional steroids. Considerations of hemachromatosis.

Table continues on the following page.

Name	Description	Anesthesia Implications
Bland-White-Garland syndrome	Coronary artery malformation with left coronary arising from the pulmonary trunk. Myocardial ischemia leading to acute heart failure. Lethal if not corrected early.	Preoperative echocardiogram. Anesthesia as for coronary artery disease. Left ventricular dysfunction may require aggressive therapy to wean from CPB.
	Kleinschmidt S, Grueness V, Molter G: The Bland-White-Garland syndrome: clinical picture and anaesthesiological management. Paediatr Anaesth 6:65, 1996.	
Bowen syndrome	See cerebrohepatorenal syndrome.	
Brachmann-de Lange syndrome	Mental retardation with craniofacial, cardiac and GI malformations, hirsutism and strabismus. Gastroesophageal reflux and aspiration leads to frequent pulmonary infections.	Preoperative echocardiogram, check pulmonary status, anticipate difficult airway and intubation. SBE prophylaxis if indicated.
	Fernandez-Garcia R, Perez Mencia T, Gutierrez-Jodra A et al: Anesthetic management with laryngeal mask in a child with Brachmann-de Lange syndrome. Paediatr Anaesth 16(6):698-700, 2006.	
Branchio-Oto-Renal syndrome (BOR) (Melnick-Fraser syndrome)	Branchial cysts or fistulae, hearing loss, pre-auricular pits, external ear malformations, renal abnormalities.	Monitor heart rate carefully. Episodic bradycardia requiring atropine or epinephrine treatment may occur during sevoflurane administration. Paediatr Anaesth 17(1):80–83, 2007.
	Taylor MH, Wilton NC: Bradycardia with sevoflurane in siblings with Branchio-oto-renal syndrome. Paediatr Anaesth 17(1):80–83, 2007.	
Brugada syndrome	Rare in Occidentals but more common in SE Asia. Results from Na$^+$ channel defect in the myocardium. ST segment elevation in precordial leads and incomplete RBB with anatomically normal heart. Prone to V tach & VF.	Avoid parasympathetic stimulation (Give anticholinergic, caution with reversal agents), caution with drugs that affect Na$^+$ channels (Local analgesics). Thiopental/propofol and inhaled agents probably OK. Maintain normothermia. Apply defibrillator pads intra-op. Monitor ECG postoperatively.
	Baty L, Hollister J, Tobias JD: Perioperative management of a 7-year-old child with Brugada syndrome. J Intens Care Med 23(3):210–214, 2008.	
Canavan disease	See leukodystrophy.	

Cantrell pentalogy	Defect in the recti muscles of the abdominal wall above the umbilicus, agenesis of sternum and diaphragm, pericardial defect and cardiac malformations: cardiac septal and valvular defects present. Prone to develop severe respiratory distress.	Preoperative echocardiogram, monitor for arrhythmias. Caudal epidural anesthesia during general anesthesia for noncardiac surgery has been employed successfully.

Laloyaux P, Veyckemans F, Van Dyck M: Anaesthetic management of a prematurely born infant with Cantrell's pentalogy. Paediatr Anaesth 8:163, 1998.

Capillary angioma with thrombocytopenic purpura syndrome	See Kasabach-Merritt syndrome.

Carcinoid tumors	Carcinoid tumors (secrete vasoactive peptides) are more common in adults but may occur in children, often in the appendix but also at other sites (i.e., testis, bronchus, GI tract). Usually the diagnosis is made at histology. Carcinoid syndrome (flushing, hypotension, etc.) is very rare in children but may occur especially with malignant carcinoid tumors.	Slow stress-free induction and maintenance of anesthesia. Avoid drugs that stimulate the sympathetic system (i.e., ketamine) or release histamine (morphine, atracurium, meperidine). H_1 and H_2 blockers and ondansetron may be useful to prevent a crisis.

Vaughan DJ, Brunner MD: Anesthesia for patients with carcinoid syndrome. Int Anesth Clin 35(4):129–142, 1997.

Cardioauditory syndrome	See Jervell-Lange-Nielsen syndrome.

Carpenter syndrome (acrocephalopolysyndactyly)	Obesity, mental retardation, oxycephaly, peculiar facies, syndactyly, deformed extremities, CHD, hypogenitalism.	Preoperative echocardiogram, SBE prophylaxis if indicated. Hypoplastic mandible may make intubation difficult.

Davies DW, Munro IR: The anesthetic management and intraoperative care of patients undergoing major facial osteotomies. Plast Reconstr Surg 55:50, 1975.

Table continues on the following page.

Name	Description	Anesthesia Implications
Central core disease	Muscular dystrophy; hypotonia without muscle wasting. Increased risk of malignant hyperthermia.	Preoperatively, assess respiratory status carefully. Sensitive to thiopental, propofol, and respiratory depressants: use muscle relaxants with caution (postoperative ventilation may be required). Do not use succinylcholine. Do not give drugs that might trigger malignant hyperthermia (See page 197).
	Eng GD, Epstein BS, Engel WK et al: Malignant hyperthermia and central-core disease in a child with congenital dislocating hips. Arch Neurol 35:189, 1978.	
Cerebrohepatorenal syndrome (Bowen syndrome, Zellweger syndrome)	Neonatal jaundice, hepatomegaly, polycystic kidneys, muscular hypotonia, coagulopathy, and mental retardation. CHD may be present. Hypotonia and gastroesophageal reflux predisposes to recurrent pneumonia.	Assess pulmonary status carefully. Treat hypoprothrombinemia, fresh-frozen plasma may decrease surgical bleeding. Drug metabolism is impaired; use small doses, extreme care with muscle relaxants and other drugs excreted by kidneys.
	Platis CM, Kachko L, Peled E et al: Anesthesia for the child with Zellweger syndrome: a case report. Paediatr Anaesth 16(3):361–262, 2006.	
Catch 22 syndrome	See DiGeorge syndrome.	
Charcot-Marie-Tooth syndrome (peroneal muscular atrophy)	Hereditary polyneuropathy. Muscle weakness in legs and arms. Cardiac involvement: arrhythmias, conduction defects, cardiomyopathy. MH has been described in two patients with CMT syndrome; however, a relationship is not established and is very doubtful.	Responses to nondepolarizing muscle relaxants are usually normal.[54] MH triggering agents have been used in many patients without problems.
	Antognini JF: Anaesthesia for Charcot-Marie-Tooth disease: a review of 86 cases. Can J Anaesth 39(4):398–400, 1992.	
CHARGE association	An association of Coloboma, congenital Heart disease, choanal Atresia, Renal abnormalities, Genital hypoplasia, and Ear defects.	Difficult airway and intubation, possible impaired renal function. Difficulty with tracheal intubation increases with age.
	Stack CG, Wyse RK: Incidence and management of airway problems in the CHARGE association. Anaesthesia 46:582, 1991.	

Chédiak-Higashi syndrome	Disorder of neutrophil function, histiocyte infiltration of multiple organs. Partial albinism, immunodeficiency, pancytopenia, hepatosplenomegaly, recurrent bacterial infections. Neurologic disorders and mental retardation. Steroid therapy and cytotoxic drugs may be given to induce remission.	Use sterile technique (reverse isolation). Use disposable equipment. Repeated pulmonary infections may have impaired pulmonary function. Aggressive therapy to prevent postoperative complications is required. Give supplemental steroids. Thrombocytopenia may require platelet transfusions.
	Ulsoy H, Erciyes N, Ovali E et al: Anesthesia in Che'diak-Higashi syndrome—case report. Mid East J Anesth 13(1):101–105, 1995.	
Cherubism	Fibrous dysplasia of mandibles and maxillas with intraoral masses may cause respiratory distress.	Tracheal intubation may be extremely difficult; if there is acute respiratory distress, tracheotomy may be required. Profuse bleeding may occur during surgery of the disease mass.
	Monclus E, Garces A, Artes D et al: Oral to nasal tube exchange under fibroscopic view: a new technique for nasal intubation in a predicted difficult airway. Paediatr Anaesth 18(7):663–666, 2008.	
Chotzen syndrome	Craniosynostosis; associated renal anomalies.	Airway and tracheal intubation may be difficult. Renal excretion of drugs may be impaired.
	Easely D, Mayhew JF: Anesthesia in a child with Saethre-Chotzen syndrome. Paediatr Anaesth 18(1):81, 2008.	
Christ-Siemens-Touraine syndrome (anhidrotic ectodermal dysplasia)	Absence of sweating and tearing. Heat intolerance due to inability to control temperature by sweating. Poor mucus formation → persistent respiratory infections.	Hypoplastic mandible may make tracheal intubation difficult; monitor body temperature carefully and be prepared to institute cooling. Humidify inspired gases. Tape eyes closed. Use chest physiotherapy preoperatively and postoperatively.
	Hotta M, Koitabashi T, Umemura N et al: Anesthetic management of a patient with hypohidrotic ectodermal dysplasia. [Japanese] English abstract. Masui - Jap J Anesth 49(4):414–416, 2000.	

Table continues on the following page.

Name	Description	Anesthesia Implications
Chronic granulomatous disease	Inherited disorder of leukocyte function: recurrent infections with nonpathogenic organisms (Bacteria or fungi) and disordered inflammation. Poor pulmonary function. Multiple organ system involvement. Hepatomegaly in 95% of cases, advanced liver disease leads to portal hypertension. Thrombocytopenia may be present. GI lesions predispose to regurgitation and aspiration. Bone marrow transplant may be effective therapy.	Assess respiratory status carefully. Check coagulation. Use sterile technique (reverse isolation). Consider rapid sequence induction. Caution with drugs metabolized in the liver.
Wall RT, Buzzanell CA, Epstein TA et al: Anesthetic considerations in patients with chronic granulomatous disease. J ClinAnesth 2(5):306-311, 1990.		
Chubby puffer syndrome See also sleep apnea syndromes.	Obesity, upper airway obstruction, daytime somnolence, and respiratory distress when sleeping. May be hyperactive and aggressive. Blood gases may show hypoxemia and hypercapnia. Cor pulmonale may develop. May present for tonsillectomy.	Avoid preoperative sedation. Monitor carefully postoperatively for airway obstruction (Nasal CPAP may help). Extreme caution with opioids; sensitivity has been demonstrated. Titrate one third to one half the normal dose of opioid. Low dose ketamine may be useful for analgesia. Those with severe airway obstruction may require tracheostomy. Postoperative monitoring is essential. Do not send home the same day of surgery unless observed for 6 or more hours.
Stool SE, Eavey RD, Stein NL et al: The chubby puffer syndrome: upper airway obstruction and obesity, with intermittent somnolence and cardiorespiratory embarrassment. Clin Pediatr 16:43, 1977.		
CINCA syndrome	Chronic infantile neurologic cutaneous articular syndrome. Genetic autoinflammatory syndrome characterized by repeated attacks of fever and skin and joint inflammation starting in infancy.	Concern that stress of anesthesia and surgery may exacerbate inflammatory state. TIVA with propofol and remifentanil recommended on this basis. Caution with relaxant drugs. Potential difficult tracheal intubation.

Progressive mental retardation and muscle wasting may occur. Facial dysmorphia may be associated.

Hohne C, Burkhardt U: Anesthesia in an infant with a CINCA syndrome. Paediatr Anaesth 18(6):575–577, 2008.

Cockayne syndrome	Dysmorphic dwarfism, mental retardation, and premature senescence; patients present in early childhood. Prominent maxillae, large teeth, and sunken eyes. Ataxia, peripheral neuropathy, and flexion contractures. Associated hypertension, arteriosclerosis, and renal disease. Survival beyond second decade is unusual.	Difficult tracheal intubation; use of the LMA before fiberoptic intubation may be required. Subglottic stenosis; require a small-diameter tube (weight vs. age appropriate). May be difficult to position. Considerations of associated cardiovascular and renal disease. A preoperative ECG for evidence of myocardial ischemia/infarction may be indicated.
Raghavendran S, Brown KA, Buu N: Perioperative management of patients with Cockayne syndrome—recognition of accelerated aging with growth arrest. Paediatr Anaesth 18(4):360–361, 2008.		
Collagen diseases (dermatomyositis; polyarteritis nodosa; rheumatoid arthritis; systemic lupus erythematosus)	Systemic connective tissue diseases with variable systemic involvement. Osteoporosis, fatty infiltration of muscle, anemia, pulmonary infiltration with fibrosis. Renal involvement common. Frequently receiving steroid therapy.	Temporomandibular or cricoarytenoid arthritis may cause airway and intubation difficulties. Risk of fat embolism after osteotomy, fracture, or minor trauma. Supplement steroid therapy.
Smith BL: Anaesthesia for patients with juvenile chronic arthritis (Still's disease) Anaesthesia 53(3):314, 1998.		

Table continues on the following page.

Name	Description	Anesthesia Implications
Congenital heart block	Comprises less than 1% of congenital heart disease, may be associated with other CHD lesions. Defect of conduction between atrioventricular node and bundle of His, or within bundle of His. Supraventricular arrhythmias may occur, and up to 20% progress to congestive heart failure and Stokes-Adams attacks. Heart rates less than 55 are poorly tolerated by infants and the response to chronotropic drugs is usually minimal.	Preoperative consultation with the cardiology team is highly recommended. Because of possibility of intraoperative arrhythmia or increased atrioventricular block, preoperative insertion of a temporary transvenous pacemaker is usually recommended, this may be achieved via the umbilical vein in the neonate. Alternatively, transcutaneous pacing via pads may be considered. Transesophageal pacing is often not effective in infants. Sevoflurane may be useful for anesthesia as it tends to increase heart rate.
	Kussman BD, Madril DR, Thiagarajan RR et al: Anesthetic management of the neonate with congenital complete heart block: a 16-year review. Paediatr Anaesth 15(12):1059–1066, 2005.	
Congenital Insensitivity to Pain and Anhidrosis (CIPA)	Rare autosomal recessive disorder due to deficient nerve growth factor. Insensitivity to pain and temperature, lack of sweating, and possible mental retardation. Hyperpyrexia may occur.	Anesthesia is required for surgical procedures to block tactile hyperesthesia and unpleasant sensations. The use of the BIS monitor may prevent excessive doses. Careful monitoring of body temperature and maintenance of normothermia required. Avoidance of anticholinergics not essential. Paediatr Anaesth 16(4):466–470, 2006.
	Brandes IF, Stuth EA: Use of BIS monitor in a child with congenital insensitivity to pain with anhidrosis. Paediatr Anaesth 16(4):466–470, 2006.	
Conradi syndrome (chondrodysplasia epiphysealis punctata; chondrodysplasia calcificans congenita; koala bear syndrome)	Chondrodystrophy with contractures, saddle nose, macroencephaly or microcephaly, mental retardation, dwarfing, congenital cataracts. CHD and renal anomalies in some other cases.	
	Tasker WG, Mastri AR, Gold AP: Chondrodystrophia calcificans congenita (dysplasia epiphysealis punctata): recognition of the clinical picture. Am J Dis Child 119:122, 1970.	

Cori disease	See von Gierke disease.
Cornelia de Lange syndrome	Short stature, microcephaly, mental retardation, hirsute. Short or dysmorphic extremities, hypoplastic nipples, rib and sternal defect. Low hairline, thin lips, and downturned ("cod") mouth. Cry is low-pitched growl. CHD in 30%. Pulmonary aspiration is common, susceptible to infections (immune system defect).	Care with asepsis. Intubation may be difficult, and airway obstruction develops easily.

Tsusaki B, Mayhew JF: Anaesthetic implications of Cornelia de Lange syndrome. Paediatr Anaesth 8(2):181, 1998.

Costello syndrome	Mental retardation and delayed growth, coarse facies, redundant skin (neck, palms, soles) and papillomata (oral, nasal, anal). Cardiac involvement is common. CHD in 30%, hypertrophic cardiomyopathy in 20%. Endocrine problems include hypopituitarism, hypothyroid and hypoadrenal states. Hypoglycemia may occur. Potential airway problems include short neck, choanal atresia, macroglossia, and laryngeal papillomata.	Check endocrine status. Caution with airway; monitor postoperative ventilation carefully. Monitor blood glucose during long procedures.

Katcher K, Bothwell M, Tobias JD: Anaesthetic implications of Costello syndrome. Paediatr Anaesth 13(3): 257–262, 2003.

Cretinism (congenital hypothyroidism)	Goiter; hypothyroidism secondary to defective synthesis of thyroid hormone. Large tongue. Respiratory center very sensitive to depression; CO_2 retention common. Hypoglycemia, hyponatremia, hypotension, low cardiac output. Early treatment with levothyroxine is essential to prevent mental changes.	Correct hypothyroidism and anemia preoperatively if possible. Intravenous triiodothyronine may be useful. Airway problems due to large tongue. Monitor body temperature; use forced hot air warming blankets. Do not use myocardial depressants. Transfuse carefully; overtransfusion is poorly tolerated because of decreased myocardial contractility.

Mason KP, Koka BV, Eldredge EA et al: Perioperative considerations in a hypothyroid infant with hepatic haemangioma. Paediatr Anaesth 11(2):228–232, 2001.

Table continues on the following page.

Name	Description	Anesthesia Implications
Cri du chat syndrome	Chromosome 5p abnormality causing mental retardation, abnormal catlike cry, microcephaly, round face, hypertelorism. In some, ears abnormal, micrognathia, epiglottis and larynx small. CHD may be present.	Airway problems: stridor, laryngomalacia. Tracheal intubation may be difficult; small size tube may be required. Risk of postextubation croup.

Brislin RP, Stayer SA, Schwartz RE: Anaesthetic considerations for the patient with cri du chat syndrome. Paediatr Anaesth 5(2):139–141, 1995.

Name	Description	Anesthesia Implications
Crouzon syndrome	Craniosynostosis, hypertelorism, parrot beak nose, hypoplastic maxilla, and exophthalmos because of chromosomal bony defect causing premature closure of cranial sutures and intracranial hypertension.	Eye protection important. Mask ventilation difficult, requires jaw thrust ± oral airway. Tracheal intubation usually quite easy. Postoperative airway obstruction is common; elective tracheostomy may be indicated. Beware of additional airway problems related to external fixation devices postsurgery for maxillary distraction; may limit access to the mouth, lead to trismus.

Payne JF, Cranston AJ: Postoperative airway problems in a child with Crouzon's syndrome. Paediatr Anaesth 5:331, 1995.

Name	Description	Anesthesia Implications
Cutis laxa	Elastic fiber degeneration: pendulous skin, frequent hernias. Recurrent pulmonary infections, emphysema and cor pulmonale, arterial fragility.	Assess pulmonary status carefully. Use sterile technique. Difficulty maintaining IV line due to poor tissues. Excess soft tissues around larynx may cause upper airway obstruction.

Wooley MM, Morgan S, Hays DM: Heritable disorders of connective tissue: surgical and anesthetic problems. J Pediatr Surg 2:325, 1967.

Name	Description	Anesthesia Implications
Dandy-Walker syndrome	See hydrocephalus (page 246).	

Deletion 9p syndrome	Partial deletion of short arm of chromosome 9 is associated with mental retardation, trigonocephaly, dysmorphic facies, small mouth, cleft palate, choanal stenosis, cardiac and renal disease. Gastroesophageal reflux and aspiration leading to repeated pulmonary infections.	Difficult airway and intubation; smaller diameter endotracheal tube may be required. Use short-acting drugs for rapid recovery of airway reflexes.
Cakmakkaya OS, Bakan M, Altintas F et al: Anesthetic management in a child with deletion 9p syndrome. Paediatr Anaesth 17(1):88-89, 2007.		
Dermatomyositis	See collagen disease.	
Yotsui-Tsuchimochi H, Higa K, Matsunaga M et al: Anesthetic management of a child with chromosome 22q11 deletion syndrome. Paediatr Anaesth 16(4): 454-7, 2006.		
Passariello M, Perkins R: Unexpected postoperative tachycardia in a patient with 22q11 deletion syndrome after multiple dental extractions. Paediatr Anaesth 15(12):1145-1146, 2005.		
DiGeorge syndrome (Catch 22 syndrome, deletion 22q syndrome, third and fourth brachial arch/pharyngeal pouch syndrome)	Aortic arch abnormalities. Thymus and parathyroids absent, hypoparathyroidism, low serum Ca resulting in tetany and stridor. Often associated with chromosome 22 defect. Immune deficiency: susceptibility to fungal and viral infections; recurrent chest infections. Treated by thymic transplants.	Use sterile technique (reverse isolation). Donor blood must be previously irradiated (30 Gy) to prevent graft-versus-host reaction. Check calcium levels-Ca^{++} infusion may be required. Caution with epinephrine containing local analgesics, prolonged tachycardia has been reported.
Yotsui-Tsuchimochi H, Higa K, Matsunaga M et al: Anesthetic management of a child with chromosome 22q11 deletion syndrome. Paediatr Anaesth 16(4): 454-7, 2006.		
Passariello M, Perkins R: Unexpected postoperative tachycardia in a patient with 22q11 deletion syndrome after multiple dental extractions. Paediatr Anaesth 15(12):1145-1146, 2005.		
Donohue syndrome	See leprechaunism.	
Down syndrome (See page 196).		

Table continues on the following page.

Name	Description	Anesthesia Implications
Duchenne muscular dystrophy	Progressive pseudohypertrophy of muscles with cardiomyopathy in most cases. Predominantly occurs in males; a milder form, Becker syndrome, also occurs in females. Genetic cause: X-linked recessive mutation in dystrophin gene at chromosome 21. May be subclinical until 2–6 yr and many die before 20 yr of age.	Assess cardiac status particularly in adolescents (preoperative echocardiogram). Succinylcholine contraindicated (may cause hyperkalemic cardiac arrest). DMD may be undiagnosed in infancy, leading to recommendation to avoid succinylcholine in boys less than 6 yr of age. Inhalational agents may cause rhabdomyolysis; TIVA is preferred by some. Respiratory depression occurs easily: titrate drug dosage carefully to limit cardiorespiratory depression. Give nondepolarizing muscle relaxants carefully and monitor block. Use local analgesia whenever possible. IPPV support postoperatively.

Yemen TA, McClain C. Muscular dystrophy, anesthesia and the safety of inhalational agents revisited; again. [Editorial] Paediatr Anaesth 16(2):105–108, 2006. Sethna NF, Rockoff MA, Wonhen HM et al: Anesthesia related complications in children with Duchenne muscular dystrophy. Anesthesiology 68:462, 1988.

Name	Description	Anesthesia Implications
Dutch-Kentucky syndrome	See Trismus-pseudocamptodactyly.	
EEC syndrome (ectrodactyly, ectodermal dysplasia, and cleft lip and palate)	Congenital anomaly complex. Lobster claw deformity, dysplasia of all ectodermal elements (including central nervous system), with disordered temperature control (hypohidrosis plus central defect). Decreased tearing, conjunctivitis, blepharitis. Cleft lip and palate, respiratory tract infections, genitourinary anomalies, malnutrition, and anemia. Mental retardation in 8%.	Assess nutrition and anemia. Preoperative chest physiotherapy advised; avoid anticholinergics (i.e., atropine [effect on sweating]). Extreme care with skin required; position and pad carefully. Protect eyes. Tracheal intubation may be difficult with cleft palate. Be prepared to maintain normothermia using heating/cooling blankets, etc.

Mizushima A, Satoyoshi M: Anaesthetic problems in a child with ectrodactyly, ectodermal dysplasia and cleft lip palate: the EEC syndrome. Anaesthesia 47:137, 1992.

Edwards syndrome (trisomy 18[E])	Mental retardation and dysmorphic changes, micrognathia in 80%, hypotonia. CHD in 95%, renal malformations in 50%–80%. Most die in infancy.	Airway and tracheal intubation may be difficult; succinylcholine may cause muscle rigidity. Use caution with drugs excreted by kidney.
Courreges P, Nieuviarts R, Lecoutre D: Anaesthetic management for Edward's syndrome. Paediatr Anaesth 13(3):267–269, 2003.		
Ehlers-Danlos syndrome (cutis hyperelastica)	Collagen abnormality: hyperelasticity and fragile tissues; dissecting aneurysm of aorta, fragility of other blood vessels; ECG conduction abnormalities. Bleeding diathesis; hernias. May have heart, lung, and gastrointestinal malformations.	Difficult to maintain IV line and prevent complications of IV infusions. Poor tissues and clotting defect may lead to increased surgical bleeding. Spontaneous pneumothorax may occur. Monitor for ECG conduction abnormalities. Caution with neck movement. Neuraxial anesthesia relatively contraindicated (risk of bleeding).
Lane D: Anaesthetic implications of vascular type Ehlers-Danlos syndrome. Anaesth Intens Care 34(4):501–505, 2006.		
Eisenmenger syndrome	Association of high pulmonary vascular resistance (pulmonary hypertension), and an intracardiac or extracardiac R-L shunt. Dyspnea, fatigue, cyanosis, finger clubbing, and cardiac failure. Often associated with Down syndrome.	Assess severity of R-L cardiac shunt; shunt may increase with hypoxia, hypercarbia, or acidosis. Inhalation induction with halothane has been effective. Alternately, a slow intravenous induction may be performed as rapid effect from IV agents may occur. Avoid drugs or airway events that may increase PVR (i.e., N_2O, hypercarbia, hypoxemia, acidosis) or decrease SVR (i.e., high dose thiopental or propofol, SNP) significantly. Caution with IPPV to maintain lung volume but minimize intrathoracic pressure. Care with fluid therapy, hypovolemia is not well-tolerated, overtransfusion may lead to R ventricular failure. Polycythemia increases viscosity but caution required if hemodiluting as it decreases oxygen carrying capacity.

Table continues on the following page.

Name	Description	Anesthesia Implications
		Despite all the potential problems, many children tolerate a well-conducted anesthetic. Epidural anesthesia has been used successfully. Can J Anaesth 42:904, 1995.

Lyons B, Motherway C, Casey W et al: The anaesthetic management of the child with Eisenmenger's syndrome. Can J Anaesth 42:904, 1995.

Name	Description	Anesthesia Implications
Elfin facies syndrome	See Williams syndrome.	
Ellis-van Creveld syndrome (chondroectodermal/ mesoectodermal dysplasia)	Ectodermal defects causing skeletal dwarfism, cardiac anomalies (50%), chest wall defects, and poor lung function. Short limbs, polydactyly, and hypoplastic nails. May have abnormal maxillae, cleft palate, cleft lip, hepatosplenomegaly. Patients often die in infancy.	Tracheal intubation can be routine, but airway problems may make intubation difficult; assess carefully and be prepared.

Wu CL, Litman RS: Anaesthetic management for a child with the Ellis-van Creveld syndrome: a case report. Paediatr Anaesth 4:335, 1994.

Name	Description	Anesthesia Implications
Eosinophilic granuloma	See Histiocytosis X.	
Epidermolysis bullosa (Herlitz syndrome)	Skin cleavage at dermal-epidermal junction, resulting in erosions and blisters from minor trauma to skin or mucous membrane. The disease occurs in several forms: Simplex: Dominant, maps to chromosome 17. Relatively mild with rapid healing and little scarring. Lethalis: Recessive, maps to chromosome 12. Junctional epidermolysis bullosa. Severe, presents at birth, leads to extensive scarring and death (often from sepsis) usually before 2 yr of age.	Antibiotic prophylaxis perioperatively to prevent secondary infections. Check history of steroid therapy. Use sterile technique (reverse isolation). Airway difficulty: oral lesions, adhesion of tongue, intraoral scarring; avoid tracheal intubation and/or instrumentation of the airway if possible as bullas may develop; otherwise, lubricate tube and laryngoscope generously. Prevent trauma to skin or mucous membranes, especially from friction or shearing movements. Use very generous lubricated padding. Use insufflation or a well

	Dystrophic: Recessive, maps to chromosome 12. Very rare but severe; lesions heal slowly with extensive scarring. Strictures may form and involve the pharynx, larynx, and esophagus. Digital fusion occurs ("mitten hand"). Nutritional deprivation leads to growth retardation and anemia. Infections are common.	padded and lubricated mask for inhalation anesthesia or use propofol or ketamine. Care with a tourniquet. Do not tape eyelids shut (skin may slough); use optical ointment. Avoid adhesive tapes (patients/parents often know which, if any, tapes can be tolerated); an oximeter probe may be held in place with a lubricated gauze bandage. ECG pads should be coated with surgical lubricant and placed under the child. Regional analgesia may be appropriate for limb surgery.

Herod J, Denyer J, Goldman A et al: Epidermolysis bullosa in children: pathophysiology, anaesthesia and pain management. Paediatr Anaesth 12(5):388–397, 2002.
Cakmakkaya OS, Altindas F, Kaya G: Anesthesia in children with epidermolysis bullosa. Plastic Reconstruct Surg 122(1):34e-35e, 2008.

Erythema multiforme	See Stevens-Johnson syndrome.	
Eulenburg periodic paralysis	See paramyotonia congenita.	
Escobar syndrome (Multiple pterygium syndrome)	Autosomal recessive progressive disease; multiple joint contractures, facial and genital anomalies, severe kyphoscoliosis. Normal intellect.	Difficult airway and intubation—difficulties increase with age. IV access may be limited. Caution with padding and positioning. Epidural analgesia may be appropriate despite deformity.

Kuzma PJ, Calkins MD, Kline MD et al. The anesthetic management of patients with multiple pterygium syndrome. Anesth Analg 83:430–432, 1996.
Kachko L, Platis CM, Konen O et al: Lumbar epidural anesthesia for the child with Escobar syndrome. Paediatr Anaesth 16(6):700–702, 2006.

Fabry disease (angiokeratoma corporis diffusum)	X-linked lipid storage disorder. Lipid deposition in blood vessels causes periodic very severe pain and fever crises. Corneal opacities. Dark telangiectasia, particularly around genitals and buttocks; hypertension, myocardial ischemia, renal failure. Hypertension and myocardial ischemia.	Preoperative echocardiogram for myocardial function; ECG for myocardial ischemia; BUN and creatinine for renal function; caution with drugs excreted by the kidneys if renal dysfunction is present.

Wise D, Wallace HJ, Jellinek EH: Angiokeratoma corporis diffusum. Queensland J Med 31:177, 1962.

Table continues on the following page.

Name	Description	Anesthesia Implications
Familial dysautonomia	See Riley-Day syndrome.	
Familial osteodysplasia	See Andersen syndrome.	
Familial periodic paralysis	Periodic muscle weakness secondary to serum K⁺ disturbance (hypokalemia or hyperkalemia). Muscle weakness in the hypokalemic variety is caused by massive uptake of K⁺ into muscles and thus decreased serum K⁺.	Monitor serum K⁺, glucose, and the ECG; maintain normokalemia and normoglycemia. Avoid muscle relaxants; maintain body temperature. Avoid excessive glucose solutions. TIVA with propofol and remifentanil has been successful in adult patients.
O'Neill GN: Inherited disorders of the neuromuscular junction. Int Anesthesiol Clin 44(2):91-106, 2006.		
Fanconi syndrome (anemia with renal tubular acidosis)	Usually secondary to cystinosis. Proximal tubular defect: impaired renal function; acidosis, K loss, dehydration. Older children may have thyroid and pancreatic dysfunction secondary to cystine deposition. May present for renal transplant in second decade.	Treat electrolyte and acid-base abnormalities: Caution with drugs excreted by kidneys. Cisatracurium is the preferred muscle relaxant. Be aware of possibility of other metabolic or endocrine defects.
Ray TL, Tobias JD: Perioperative care of the patient with nephropathic cystinosis. Paediatr Anaesth 14(10):878-885, 2004.		
Farber disease (lipogranulomatosis)	Sphingomyelin deposition: widespread visceral lipogranulomas, especially in CNS. General systemic involvement leading to cardiac, renal failure.	Preoperatively assess cardiac and renal status. Deposits in oral cavity, pharynx, and larynx; possible difficult intubation.
Asada A, Tatekawa S, Terai T et al: The anesthetic implications of a patient with Farber's lipogranulomatosis. Anesthesiology 80:206, 1994.		

Favism (glucose-6-phosphate dehydrogenase (G6PD) deficiency)	Diathesis for spontaneous/induced (drugs, fava beans, infection) hemolytic anemia.	Do not give drugs that cause hemolysis (i.e., acetylsalicylic acid, phenacetin, sulfonamides, quinidine, methylene blue). Midazolam, sevoflurane, nitrous oxide, and rocuronium are all acceptable drugs. Anemia: transfuse if necessary.

Wada R, Hino H, Ando Y: Case of laparoscopic cholecystectomy in a patient with glucose-6-dehydrogenase deficiency. [English abstract.] Masui - Japanese J Anesth 57(2):200–202, 2008.

Fetal alcohol syndrome	Abnormalities of the infant due to maternal heavy alcohol consumption: growth retardation, intellectual impairment, craniofacial abnormalities (microcephaly, microphthalmia, hypoplastic upper lip, flat maxilla), cardiac defects (especially ventricular septal defect), renal abnormalities, and inguinal hernia.	May have difficulty with intubation. Evaluate for cardiac and renal diseases.

Clarren SK, Smith DW: The fetal alcohol syndrome. N Engl J Med 298:1063, 1978.
Finucaine BT: Difficult intubation associated with the fetal alcohol syndrome. Can Anaesth Soc J 27:574, 1980.

Fibrodysplasia ossificans progressiva	See myositis ossificans.
Focal dermal hypoplasia (Goltz syndrome)	Multifarious features, including multiple papillomas of mucous membranes, skin.	Airway may contain papillomas resulting in difficulties with ventilation.
Forbes disease (glycogen storage disease type III)	See von Gierke disease.

Holzman RS. Airway involvement and anesthetic management in Goltz's syndrome. J Clin Anesth 3(5):422–425, 1991.

Table continues on the following page.

Name	Description	Anesthesia Implications
Freeman-Sheldon syndrome (whistling face syndrome)	Progressive congenital myopathy and dysplasia with autosomal or X-linked recessive inheritance. Increased tone and fibrosis of facial muscles. Hypertelorism, microstomia, and micrognathia. Leads to flexion contracture of limbs. Strabismus and inguinal hernia common. Later, kyphoscoliosis causes restrictive lung disease.	Very difficult intubation primarily due to microstomia and micrognathia: tight facial muscles will not relax with neuromuscular blockade, and muscle rigidity may follow halothane or succinylcholine. Venous access difficult due to limb flexion contractures. Pulmonary function may be impaired (late). Insertion of an LMA (if microstomia is not severe) facilitates fiberoptic bronchoscopy and intubation. Regional analgesia may be useful for surgery and/or postoperative pain.

Madi-Jebara S, El-Hajj C, Jawish D et al: Anesthetic management of a patient with Freeman-Sheldon syndrome: case report. J Clin Anesth 19(6):460–462, 2007.

Name	Description	Anesthesia Implications
Friedreich ataxia	Progressive degeneration of cerebellum, lateral and posterior column of spinal cord; scoliosis; myocardial degeneration and fibrosis, leading to failure and serious arrhythmias. Glucose intolerance; 10% are diabetic.	Assess metabolic state carefully. Care with cardiac depressant drugs; monitor ECG carefully. TIVA with propofol and remifentanil has been recommended. BIS responses appear normal. Response to relaxants uncertain; avoid if possible. Otherwise cisatracurium with block monitor suggested.

Pancaro C, Renz D: Anesthetic management in Friedreich's ataxia. Paediatr Anaesth 15(5):433–434, 2005.

Name	Description	Anesthesia Implications
Gangliosidoses GM1, type 1 GM1, type 2 GM2 (Tay-Sachs disease: Sandhoff disease)	Invariably fatal. Supportive measures only treatment. Acute onset in infancy: Rapid neurologic decline, severe bone abnormalities; pulmonary infiltration common. Death by 2 yr of age. Onset in early childhood: Few somatic changes. Death from cardiopulmonary causes by 10 yr of age.	Progressive neurologic loss leads to respiratory complications; assess cardiopulmonary status carefully.

	Onset in infancy: Progressive psychomotor deterioration; blindness, seizures. Predominantly in Ashkenazi Jewish heritage. Death by 5 yr (by 2 yr in most cases). Rare juvenile variants: same features; longer survival.	
Gardner syndrome	Familial polyposis of colon; bone tumors, sebaceous cysts, fibromas.	No specific anesthesia problems described.
Gaucher disease	Cerebroside accumulation in CNS, liver, spleen, etc. Serum acid phosphatase increased. Pulmonary disease from aspiration (pseudobulbar palsy); hepatosplenomegaly. Hypersplenism may cause platelet deficiency. If obvious neurologic signs: usually fatal in infancy (neuronopathic type 2 and 3). If nonneuronopathic (type 1), course is more chronic with bone pain, fractures, etc.	Assess pulmonary status carefully; beware of aspiration. Tracheal intubation usually routine but may be difficult if trismus, neck, or airway infiltration. Surgical bleeding may be a major problem; treat coagulation disorders and correct anemia.
Ioscovich A, Briskin A, Abrahamov A et al: Uncomplicated outcome after anesthesia for pediatric patients with Gaucher disease. Can J Anaesth 52(8):845-847, 2005.		
Glanzmann disease (thromboasthenia)	Abnormal platelet function, leading to mild thrombocytopenic purpura; abnormality of high-energy phosphate mechanisms. Considerable bleeding risk with any surgical procedure.	No specific therapy for bleeding; platelet transfusions disappointing. Therapy with recombinant activated factor VII plus antithrombolytic agents may be helpful. May have history of steroid therapy.
Gunaydin B, Ozkose Z, Pezek S: Recombinant activated factor VII and epsilon aminocaproic acid treatment of a patient with Glanzmann's thrombasthenia for nasal polipectomy. J Anesth 21(1):106-107, 2007.		
Glucose-6-phosphate dehydrogenase (G6PD) deficiency	See favism.	

Table continues on the following page.

Name	Description	Anesthesia Implications
Glycogen storage disease		
Type I	See von Gierke disease.	
Type II	See Pompe disease.	
Type III (Cori disease; Forbes disease)	See von Gierke disease.	
Type IV	See Andersen disease.	
Type V	See McArdle disease.	
Type VI (Hers disease)	See muscle phosphofructokinase deficiency.	
Type VII	See hepatic phosphorylase kinase deficiency.	
Type VIII		
Goldenhar syndrome (oculoauriculovertebral syndrome; hemifacial microstomia)	Unilateral mandibular hypoplasia; CHD in 20%. Embryonic malformation due to chromosome 22 trisomy. Vertebral abnormalities may limit neck extension.	Airway problems; may be extremely difficult to hold a mask in place and maintain an airway once anesthesia induced. Tracheal intubation may be very difficult (bilateral) or very easy (unilateral or left-sided lesion). If right TMJ and mandible are involved or bilateral disease, increased difficulty for intubation. Have an LMA ready plus all difficult airway supplies. TIVA with propofol and remifentanil may facilitate rapid emergence. Extubate trachea awake. Problems of associated cardiac disease.

Altintas F, Cakmakkaya OS: General anesthesia for a child with Goldenhar syndrome. Pediatr Anesth 15(6):529-530, 2005.
Nargozian C, Ririe DG, Bennun RD et al: Hemifacial microstomia: anatomical prediction of difficult intubation. Pediatr Anesth 9:393-398, 1999.

Goltz syndrome	See focal dermal hypoplasia and Gorlin-Goltz syndrome.	

Gonadal dysgenesis	See Turner syndrome.
Gorham syndrome (disappearing bone disease)	Massive osteolysis and lymphangiomatosis. Pathologic fractures and bony deformities with neurologic and respiratory complications. Severe kyphoscoliosis may be present. Problems relate to bony involvement: cervical spine subluxation, thoracic deformity leading to respiratory failure. Pleural effusions or chylothorax may be present. Normal intellect.	Tracheal intubation may be difficult. Cervical spine precautions indicated. Caution with protein bound drugs if chylothorax has caused hypoproteinemia. Avoid succinylcholine to prevent fasciculations that break bones. Caution with transport and positioning. Postoperative ventilation may be required.

Szabo C, Habre W: Gorham syndrome: anaesthetic management. Anaesthesia 55(2):157–159, 2000.

Gorlin-Chaudhry-Moss syndrome	Craniofacial dysostosis, patent ductus arteriosus, hypertrichosis, hypoplasia of labia majora, dental and eye anomalies. Normal intelligence.	Asymmetry of head—difficult airway.

Ortalli G, Tiberio I, Mammana G: Gorlin-Goltz syndrome. Observation of a case. [Italian] English abstract. Minerva Anesthesiol 57(4):161-163, 1991.

Gorlin-Goltz syndrome (basal cell nevus syndrome)	Multiple nevoid basal cell carcinomas, hypertelorism, mandibular prognathism, multiple jaw cysts and fibrosarcomas, kyphoscoliosis, incomplete segmentation of cervical and thoracic vertebrae; congenital hydrocephalus, mental retardation, etc.	Extreme care in positioning and intubating; cervical spine movement may be limited. Increased ICP may be unrecognized.

Grönblad-Strandberg syndrome (pseudoxanthoma elasticum)	Degeneration of elastic tissue in skin, eye, and cardiovascular system; rupture of arteries, especially in gastrointestinal tract; hypertension; arterial calcification; occlusion of cerebral and coronary arteries.	Assess cardiovascular status; ECG and echocardiogram. Manage as for coronary artery disease. Difficult to maintain IV cannula in situ. Prevent tachycardia or hypertension (rupture of aneurysms). Prevent arterial line (vessel damage). Avoid NG tube (bleeding).

Krechel SL, Ramirez-Inawat RC, Fabian LW: Anesthetic considerations in pseudoxanthoma elasticum. Anesth Analg 60(5):344-347, 1981.

Table continues on the following page.

Name	Description	Anesthesia Implications
Guillain-Barré syndrome (acute [idiopathic] polyneuritis)	Acute polyneuropathy; progressive peripheral neuritis; usually involving cranial nerves; bulbar palsy with hypoventilation and hypotension. May follow an infection or surgery. Early treatment by plasma exchange and immunotherapy is highly desirable to limit the disease. Some require tracheotomy and ventilatory support.	Do not use succinylcholine for at least 3 months after onset of polyneuritis and until lower motor neuron deficit resolves (⇑ K⁺ release). May have serious hemodynamic instability. Disease may first present in the postoperative period with weakness and loss of tendon reflexes, etc.
	Jones GD, Wilmshurst JM, Sykes K et al: Guillain-Barre syndrome: delayed diagnosis following anaesthesia. Paediatr Anaesth 9(6):539–542, 1999.	
Hallervorden-Spatz disease	Autosomal recessive disorder of basal ganglia: leading to dementia, dystonia, and chorea. Torticollis, scoliosis, and trismus develop. Episodes of airway obstruction and desaturation may occur during posturing. Stereotactic thalamotomy may improve the neurologic state considerably.	Assess pulmonary status carefully. Inhalation induction of anesthesia leads to relaxation of abnormal posturing and trismus and facilitates intubation. Avoid succinylcholine (⇑ K⁺ release may intensify rigidity) or rapid-sequence induction (in case of difficult intubation). Reaction to usual anesthetics is normal.
	Keegan MT, Flick RP, Matsumoto JY et al: Anesthetic management for two-stage computer-assisted, stereotactic thalamotomy in a child with Hallervorden-Spatz Disease. J Neurosurg Anesthesiol 12(2):107–111, 2000.	
Hand-Schüller-Christian syndrome	See Histiocytosis X.	
Harlequin syndrome	Skin color changes with demarcation line bisecting the body. Hemifacial sweating and flushing due to unilateral sympathectomy.	No contraindications to routine anesthesia. Hemifacial flushing may develop during neck surgery due to interference with sympathetic ganglia.
	Kil HK, Kim WO, Cho JE et al: Transient postoperative harlequin syndrome combined with Horner's syndrome in a pediatric patient after neck mass excision. Paediatr Anaesth 17(6):597–68l, 2007.	
Hecht-Beals syndrome	Mental retardation, arachnodactyly, kyphoscoliosis, and multiple congenital joint contractures.	Difficult airway due to limited mouth opening—not obvious preoperatively.
	Nagata O, Tateoka A, Shiro R et al: Anaesthetic management of two paediatric patients with Hecht-Beals syndrome. Paediatr Anaesth 9(5):444–447, 1999.	

Hemangioma with thrombocytopenia	See Kasabach-Merritt syndrome.	
Johnson GD, Rosales JK: The haemolytic uraemic syndrome and anesthesia. Can J Anaesth 34:196, 1987.		
Hemolytic uremic syndrome	Usually occurs in 1- to 2-year-olds; prodromal (usually gastrointestinal) infection followed by sudden onset of renal failure, hemolytic anemia, and thrombocytopenia. All systems may be involved: Cardiovascular system: severe hypertension, myocarditis, and congestive cardiac failure; respiratory-pulmonary insufficiency. Central nervous system: depression progressing to drowsiness, seizures, and coma. Hepatosplenomegaly with hepatic dysfunction, seizures, and coma. Coagulopathy: thrombocytopenia, decreased platelet function, prolonged prothrombin time and bleeding time. Treatment is by blood transfusion, renal dialysis, and symptomatic therapy for other disorders.	Comprehensive respiratory assessment required. Correct electrolyte, acid-base, and coagulation abnormalities. May have full stomach (gastrointestinal dysfunction) requiring RSI. Isoflurane and cisatracurium are agents of choice. Intensive continuous monitoring of biochemistry needed intraoperatively and postoperatively.
Johnson GD, Rosales JK: The haemolytic uraemic syndrome and anesthesia. Can J Anaesth 34:196, 1987.		
Hepatic phosphorylase kinase deficiency (glycogen storage disease type VIII)	Hepatomegaly; increased liver glycogen concentration. Minor growth retardation and delayed motor development. Mild to moderate hypoglycemia may occur. Many children are asymptomatic and lead normal lives on a diet. Occasionally this is more severe with hypoglycemia and acidosis. Very rarely a form of this disease may cause severe neonatal hypoglycemia.	Assess metabolic status and history carefully. No specific anesthesia complications reported. Monitor glucose levels (and acid/base if indicated) perioperatively.
Tuchman M, Brown BI, Burke BA et al: Clinical and laboratory observations in a child with hepatic phosphorylase kinase deficiency. Metab Clin Exp 35(7):627-633, 1986.		

Table continues on the following page.

571

Name	Description	Anesthesia Implications
Herlitz syndrome	See epidermolysis bullosa.	
Hermansky-Pudlak syndrome	Albinism: bleeding diathesis due to platelet abnormality.	Monitor coagulation. May require platelet transfusion during surgery.
Haddadin AS, Ayoub CM, Sevarino FB et al: Evaluation of hemostasis by the Clot Signature Analyzer: a potentially valuable device for the anesthesiologist. J Clin Monit Comp 15(2):125–129, 1999.		
Hers disease	See von Gierke disease.	
Histiocytosis X (eosinophilic granuloma: Hand-Schüller-Christian disease, Letterer-Siwe disease)	Lesions in bones and viscera (larynx, lungs, liver, and spleen). Clinical course similar to acute leukemia. Hypersplenism, pancytopenia, anemia, purpura, hemorrhage; hepatic involvement. Pulmonary-diffuse hilar infiltration: respiratory failure, cor pulmonale. Gingival inflammation and necrosis, with loss of teeth. Diabetes insipidus if sella turcica involved. Many die in first year of life.	Correct anemia and coagulation defects. Assess cardiorespiratory status carefully. Check electrolytes and fluid balance. May have history of steroid therapy. Laryngeal fibrosis; intubation may be difficult. Beware of loose teeth.
Broscheit J, Eichelbroenner O, Greim C et al: Anesthetic management of a patient with histiocytosis X and pulmonary complications during Caesarean section. Euro J Anaesth 21(11):919–921, 2004.		
Holt-Oram syndrome (heart-hand syndrome)	Upper limb abnormalities; CHD in 80% (usually ASD) but arrhythmias may occur with normal cardiac anatomy; possibility of sudden death from arrhythmia, pulmonary embolus, coronary occlusion.	Preoperatively assess for cardiac disease (ECG and echocardiogram as indicated). Upper limb venous system may be abnormal. No other anesthesia problem.
Shono S, Higa K, Kumano K: Dan K: Holt-Oram syndrome. Br J Anaesth 80(6):856–857, 1998.		

Homocystinuria	Thromboembolic phenomena due to intimal thickening; ectopia lentis, osteoporosis, kyphoscoliosis. Hypoglycemia may occur. Angiography may precipitate thrombosis, especially cerebral.	Give fluids to maintain urine output plus dextran 40 to reduce viscosity and platelet adhesiveness and increase peripheral perfusion. Pneumatic stockings to prevent venous stasis. Infuse dextrose and monitor glucose level. Avoid nitrous oxide (impairs conversion of homocysteine to methionine and increases level).

Lowe S, Johnson DA, Tobias JD: Anesthetic implications of the child with homocystinuria. J Clinical Anesth. 6(2):142–144, 1994.
Koblin DD: Homocystinuria and administration of nitrous oxide. J Clinical Anesth 7(2):176, 1995.

Hunter syndrome (mucopolysaccharidosis type II)	Similar, but less severe than Hurler syndrome (See page 574). See also mucopolysaccharidoses.	As for Hurler syndrome. Difficult intubation due to large tongue. Attempts to secure airway using the LMA have not always been successful. Delayed recovery from anesthesia and postobstructive pulmonary edema reported.

Busoni P, Fognani G: Failure of the laryngeal mask to secure the airway in a patient with Hunter's syndrome (mucopolysaccharidosis type II). Paediatr Anaesth 9:153, 1999.

Kreidstein A, Boorin MR, Crespi P et al: Delayed awakening from general anaesthesia in a patient with Hunter syndrome. Can J Anaesth 41:423, 1994.

Hurler syndrome (mucopolysaccharidosis type I H; formerly classed as type I)	Mental retardation, gargoyle facies, deafness, stiff joints, dwarfing, pectus excavatum, kyphoscoliosis. Abnormal tracheobronchial cartilages; severe coronary artery disease at early age, valvar and myocardial involvement. Hepatosplenomegaly.	Preoperatively evaluate cardiac status, echocardiogram, and ECG. Antibiotic prophylaxis and chest physiotherapy preoperatively. Give atropine preoperatively to dry airway. Upper airway obstruction due to profuse lymphoid tissue infiltration. Caution with neck movement;

Table continues on the following page.

Name	Description	Anesthesia Implications
	Most die from respiratory and cardiac failure before 10 yr of age; sudden death common after 7 yr of age. See mucopolysaccharidoses.	hypoplasia of the odontoid, atlantoaxial subluxation may occur. Difficult intubation, especially in older children, due to micrognathia, short neck, and limited movement of temporomandibular joint. LMA may not relieve obstruction. Propofol, sevoflurane, cisatracurium are agents of choice. Epidural analgesia may fail (due to lymphoid deposition).

Belani KG, Krivit W, Carpenter BL et al: Children with mucopolysaccharidosis: perioperative care, morbidity, mortality, and new findings. J Ped Surg 28(3): 403–8, 1993.

Walker RW, Colovic V, Robinson DN et al: Postobstructive pulmonary oedema during anaesthesia in children with mucopolysaccharidoses. Paediatr Anaesth 13(5):441–447, 2003.

Name	Description	Anesthesia Implications
Hurler-Scheie compound syndrome (type I HS)	See Scheie syndrome.	
Hutchinson-Gilford syndrome	See Progeria.	
Hyalinosis, cutaneous-mucosal	See Urbach-Wiethe disease.	
Hyperexplexia	See stiff baby syndrome.	
Hyperpyrexia/ hyperthermia, malignant	See page 197.	

I-cell disease (mucolipidoses)	Mental retardation, Hurler-type bone changes, severe joint limitation, chronic pulmonary disease; cardiac involvement, valvar insufficiency common. Atlantoaxial subluxation. Death in early childhood common but some survive 1 or 2 decades.	Preoperatively assess cardiac status: echocardiogram and ECG. Tracheal intubation and airway maintenance difficulty, limited jaw movement, stiffness of neck and rib cage. Caution with neck movement. No specific anesthesia recommendations. May be difficult to wean from ventilatory support.
	Gonzalez Gonzalez G, Jimenez Lopez I: Anesthetic management of a boy with sialidosis. [Spanish, English abstract] Revista Espanola de Anestesiologia y Reanimacion 53(4):253–256, 2006.	
Idiopathic thrombocytopenic purpura	Autoimmune disease in which an antiplatelet factor is present, resulting in destruction of platelets in the spleen with thrombocytopenia and the potential for bleeding. May be acute or chronic; severe gastrointestinal and intracranial bleeding is rare in children, most recover in a few weeks. Chronic ITP is more likely in children over 10 yr of age. Treatment with high dose steroids and γ-globulin is effective in raising the platelet count (i.e., for a surgical procedure). Splenectomy is very rarely recommended in children.	May have history of steroid therapy. Platelet counts may be very low, but platelet transfusions are ineffective. Do not give NSAIDs. Avoid intramuscular injections. (If splenectomy is performed, do not give platelets until the spleen is out.)
	British Committee for Standards in Haematology General Haematology Task Force. Guidelines for the investigation and management of idiopathic thrombocytopenic purpura in adults, children and in pregnancy. Br J Haematol 120(4):574–596, 2003.	
Ivemark syndrome	See asplenia syndrome.	

Table continues on the following page.

Name	Description	Anesthesia Implications
Jervell and Lange-Nielsen syndrome (Romano-Ward syndrome, congenital long QT syndrome)	Congenital deafness and cardiac conduction defects: arrhythmias and syncopal attacks (may be misdiagnosed as epilepsy). ECG shows large T waves, prolonged Q-T interval. Sudden death may occur. Serious arrhythmias (ventricular fibrillation) under anesthesia. Acquired long QT syndrome may be a result of drug therapy.	Assess cardiac status carefully; consult with the child's cardiologist. General anesthesia may precipitate arrhythmias; pretreat with β-blockers to decrease risk. Avoid atropine, sevoflurane, and halothane. Propofol may improve rhythm disturbances. TIVA with propofol and remifentanil (or other opioid) may be the optimal technique. Left stellate ganglion block is recommended to decrease the Q-T interval. Ventricular fibrillation may respond to lidocaine and defibrillation. Watch for hypoglycemia as a complication of β-blockade.

Curry TB, Gaver R, White RD: Acquired long QT syndrome and elective anesthesia in children. Paediatr Anaesth 16(4):471–478, 2006.
Saussine M, Massad I, Raczka F et al: Torsade de pointes during sevoflurane anesthesia in a child with congenital long QT syndrome. Paediatr Anaesth 16(1):63–65, 2006.
Yanagida H, Kemi C, Suwa K: The effects of stellate ganglion block on the idiopathic prolongation of the Q-T interval with cardiac arrhythmia (The Romano-Ward syndrome) Anesth Analg 55:782–787, 1976.

Name	Description	Anesthesia Implications
Juvenile hyaline fibromatosis	Autorecessive disease; multiple subcutaneous nodules, flexion contractures of large and small joints, radiolucent bone destruction (especially femur and humerus), hypertrophic gingiva. Systemic manifestations may involve pleura, lung, renal, and digestive system. Entrapment of nerves and vessels may occur. Intelligence normal.	Check preoperatively for evidence of other organ involvement. Difficult intubation due to gingival hyperplasia and limited motion at neck and temporomandibular joints. Careful positioning and padding required.

Norman B, Soni N, Madden N: Anaesthesia and juvenile hyaline fibromatosis. Br J Anaesth 76(1):163–166, 1996.

Jeune syndrome (asphyxiating thoracic dystrophy)	Severe thoracic malformation leading to neonatal asphyxia. Associated pulmonary hypoplasia. Milder forms may present in older children. Cystic renal changes, progressing to renal failure.	Avoid high pressure ventilation (hypoplastic lungs). Surgery to enlarge thorax may necessitate prolonged periods of assisted ventilation. Care with drugs excreted by kidneys.

Borland LM. Anesthesia for children with Jeune's syndrome (asphyxiating thoracic dystrophy). Anesthesiology 66(1):86–88, 1987.

Joubert syndrome (Mohr syndrome variant, familial cerebellar vermis agenesis)	Rare autosomal recessive disorder. Cerebellar vermis dysplasia or agenesis and brain stem cysts. Hypotonia, ataxia, jerky eye movements, and tongue protrusion. Mental retardation. Abnormal respiration: alternating tachypnea and apneic spells. May be lethal in early childhood.	Life-threatening respiratory problems perioperatively. Very sensitive to anesthetic agents and opioids. Inhalational induction, controlled ventilation, and local or regional analgesia advised. Apnea monitoring postoperatively; caffeine may be useful.

Habre W, Sims C, D'Souza M: Anaesthetic management of children with Joubert syndrome. Paediatr Anaesth 7(3):251–253, 1997.

Kabuki syndrome	Mental retardation and craniofacial anomalies; 50% have CHD and 25% have renal disease. Muscular hypotonia may be present but muscle biopsies are normal. Scoliosis develops in many.	May have difficult airway but no other specific anesthesia problems reported.

Johnson G, Mayhew JF: Anesthesia for a child with Kabuki syndrome. Paediatr Anaesth 17(9):900–901, 2007.

Kartagener syndrome	Dextrocardia, situs inversus. Immotile cilia, deficient mucociliary clearance; sinusitis, bronchiectasis. Defective immunity.	Order physiotherapy preoperatively. Use careful aseptic technique (reverse isolation). Assess respiratory status carefully. Affected lung lobes may need to be carefully isolated for lobectomy.

Sahajananda H, Sanjay OP, Thomas J et al: General anaesthesia for lobectomy in an 8-year-old child with Kartagener's syndrome. Paediatr Anaesth 13(8):714–717, 2003.

Table continues on the following page.

Name	Description	Anesthesia Implications
Kasabach-Merritt syndrome	Hemangioma suddenly increases in size; thrombocytopenia, hypofibrinogenemia → purpura, bleeding, anemia, increased fibrinolytic activity. Treated by radiotherapy (surgery may precipitate disseminated intravascular coagulation). Recovery follows destruction of tumor.	If any surgery planned prepare for major blood losses! Correct anemia, hypovolemia, and coagulation defects. Fresh whole blood, FFP, and platelet transfusions required. Steroids may help.
	Kawahara M, Takeshita T, Akita S: Anesthetic management of a patient with Kasabach-Merritt syndrome. Anesth Prog 34(1):17–19, 1987.	
Kawasaki syndrome (mucocutaneous lymph node syndrome)	Acute febrile exanthematous disease secondary to vasculitis with cardiac involvement (pancarditis, valvular dysfunction, arrhythmias, and coronary artery vasculitis). Seen in infants and young children, endemic in Japan. Signs include fever, conjunctivitis, oral erythema, strawberry tongue, red hands and feet. Cardiac involvement in 20% of cases: ranges from asymptomatic ECG changes to severe congestive failure and massive myocardial infarction. Salicylates are used in treatment and may reduce coronary lesions. Biliary tract or bowel symptoms may require laparotomy. Hepatic involvement in 10% of patients. Consult with cardiology for cardiac status.	Avoid myocardial depressants and anesthetize as for a patient with coronary artery disease. Monitor for cardiac ischemic changes (V_5 and lead II). Be prepared with vasoactive and antiarrhythmic drugs. Sympathetic nerve blocks may improve ischemic limb circulation. Sevoflurane anesthesia has been used satisfactorily. Salicylates may increase surgical bleeding.
	Morrison JE, Anderson M, Chan KC et al: A 15-year review of children with Kawasaki's syndrome having general anesthesia or deep sedation. Paediatr Anaesth 15(12):1053–1058, 2005.	
Kenny-Caffey syndrome	Normal intellect. Dwarfism, macrocephaly, thoracic skeletal abnormalities, anemia, hypocalcemia, and can have mandibular hypoplasia.	Intubation may be difficult. Use of the LMA is an option for securing the airway. Monitor ionized calcium levels perioperatively.
	Janke EL, Fletcher JE, Lewis IH: Anaesthetic management of the Kenny-Caffey syndrome using the laryngeal mask. Paediatr Anaesth 6(3):235–238, 1996.	

Ketonuria, branched-chain	See maple syrup urine disease.
Klinefelter syndrome (gonosomal aneuploidy with tubular dysgenesis)	Confined to males. Sex chromosome defect (47 XXY). Tall, reduced intelligence, behavior problems, hypogonadism, vertebral collapse due to osteoporosis. May have diabetes mellitus. Androgen replacement therapy is applied at puberty.	No anesthesia problem reported, except as related to diabetes. Position very carefully to prevent spinal cord damage (osteoporosis).

Wattendorf DJ, Muenke M: Klinefelter syndrome. Amer Fam Phys 72(11):2259–2262, 2005.

Klippel-Feil syndrome	Congenital fusion of two or more cervical vertebrae, causing neck rigidity. Occipital encephalomyelocele may be associated in the neonate. Arnold-Chiari malformation and/or scoliosis may be associated. Rib defects, cardiac and renal disease occasionally related.	Assess for other significant conditions. Intubation may be very difficult because of immobile neck: should be done awake if possible; otherwise inhalation induction without muscle relaxant. Have an LMA available. Do not extubate until fully awake.

Cakmakkaya OS, Kaya G, Altintas F et al: Anesthetic management of a child with Arnold-Chiari malformation and Klippel-Feil syndrome. Paediatr Anaesth 16(3):355–356, 2006.

Klippel-Trénaunay-Weber syndrome (angio-osteohypertrophy)	Hemangiomas with hypertrophy of adjacent bone; thrombocytopenia. AV fistulas and anemia lead to high cardiac output, with possible cardiac failure; thrombocytopenia in association with visceral hemangiomas. Macrocephaly, scoliosis, and pectus excavatum. Severe bleeding may occur from hemangiomas.	Check cardiac status carefully, correct bleeding disorders. Assess airway carefully.

Ezri T, Szmuk P, Panksy A et al: Anaesthetic management for Klippel-Trenaunay-Weber syndrome. Paediatr Anaesth 6(1):81–82, 1996.

Krabbe disease (globoid cell leukodystrophy)	See leukodystrophy.

Table continues on the following page.

Name	Description	Anesthesia Implications
Larsen syndrome	Multiple congenital dislocations: knees, elbows, hips. Characteristic facies, hydrocephalus, cleft palate, flat face, upturned nose. Connective tissue defect of cartilage of ribs, epiglottis, arytenoids, and tracheomalacia. Cervical spine abnormal, kyphoscoliosis, chronic respiratory problems, and CHD.	Check for cardiac defects and respiratory status. Intubation may be difficult and subglottic stenosis may be present. Caution with neck; cervical spine instability. Possible increased ICP.
Malik P, Choudhry DK: Larsen syndrome and its anaesthetic considerations. Paediatr Anaesth 12(7):632–636, 2002.		
Laurence-Moon-Biedl syndrome	Mental retardation, pigmentary retinopathy, hypogenitalism, and spastic paraplegia. (Polydactyly and obesity, typical in Bardet-Biedl syndrome, are absent.) May have renal abnormalities and CHD.	Appropriate investigations are indicated in children with renal or CHD.
Banman ML, Hogan GR: Laurence-Moon-Biedl syndrome. Am J Dis Child 126:119, 1973.		
Leigh disease (subacute necrotizing encephalomyelopathy)	A genetic neurologic and metabolic disease. May occur in infancy or childhood. Infants develop hypotonia, somnolence, optic atrophy, deafness, and pyramidal tract signs. Altered respiratory patterns may occur and may lead to sudden infant death syndrome. Impaired intracellular metabolism secondary to mitochondrial involvement. Older children have acute neurologic deterioration and respiratory failure. General anesthesia may be followed by respiratory failure and death.	Preoperatively, assess pulmonary status carefully and treat acute infections. Ensure adequate hydration, give dextrose infusion, and monitor glucose levels. Use normal saline and avoid lactated Ringer's solution. Treat acidosis. Monitor ventilation carefully in the perioperative period. Propofol may be useful for many procedures.
Gozal D, Goldin E, Shafran-Tikva S et al: Leigh syndrome: anesthetic management in complicated endoscopic procedures. Paediatr Anaesth 16(1):38–42, 2006.		

LEOPARD syndrome	A cardio-cutaneous syndrome; multiple large freckles; hypertelorism, eyelid ptosis, deafness. CHD, progressive hypertrophic cardiomyopathy (pulmonary stenosis in 95%); ECG anomalies include aberrant conduction; serious arrhythmias may occur. Growth retardation common; pectus carinatum, kyphosis, etc., in some. Genitourinary anomalies (hypospadias cryptorchidism, ovarian hypoplasia, etc.).	Preoperatively assess cardiorespiratory function. Intubation may be difficult. Problems of associated cardiac disease; monitor ECG.
	Torres J, Russo P, Tobias JD et al: Anaesthetic implications of LEOPARD syndrome. Paediatr Anaesth 14(4):352-356, 2004.	
Leprechaunism (Donohue syndrome)	A severe insulin resistance disease; many organ systems involved. Elfin face. Failure to thrive, endocrine disorders, severe mental retardation. Hypoglycemia due to hyperinsulinism from hyperplastic islets of Langerhans; renal tubular defects → impaired renal function. Lungs may be dysmorphic. Most die before 1 yr of age.	Assess for multiple organ disease. Check metabolic status; monitor blood glucose. Intubation may be difficult. Use drugs excreted by kidneys with caution.
	Kallo A, Lakatos I, Szijarto L: Leprechaunism (Donohue's syndrome). J Pediatr 66:372, 1965.	
Lesch-Nyhan syndrome	Disorder of purine metabolism, occurs in males. Mental and growth retardation, malnutrition, choreoathetosis. Very aggressive with compulsive self-destructive behavior. Hyperuricemia leads to renal calculi; RBC damage, hypertension, and coronary artery disease. Renal failure by age 20 yr.	Use drugs excreted by the kidney with caution. Beware of regurgitation, give metoclopramide. Diazepam for behavior management. Midazolam, propofol, thiopental, isoflurane, and cisatracurium (Hoffman degradation independent of renal dysfunction) are recommended. Caution with catecholamines.
	Larson LO, Wilkins RG: Anesthesia and the Lesch-Nyhan syndrome. Anesthesiology 63(2):197-199, 1985.	
Letterer-Siwe disease	See Histiocytosis X.	

Table continues on the following page.

Name	Description	Anesthesia Implications
Leukodystrophy (Alexander disease, Canavan disease, Krabbe disease, Pelizaeus-Merzbacher disease, adrenoleukodystrophy, metachromatic leukodystrophy)	Inherited disorder of myelin formation. Progressive degenerative disease with spasticity; gait disturbance, poor motor development, seizures, extrapyramidal movements, and choreoathetosis. Disordered swallowing and gastroesophageal reflux lead to aspiration pneumonia. Malnutrition and anemia.	Assess pulmonary status and anticonvulsant medications. Copious oral secretion, use an antisialogogue. Danger of pulmonary aspiration. Position and pad carefully. Avoid succinylcholine (theoretical risk of hyperkalemia). Phenytoin therapy results in increased requirements for vecuronium and fentanyl. Maintain body temperature carefully. Extubate awake, monitor carefully postoperatively. (N.B. Adrenal dysfunction in adrenoleukodystrophy; give steroids. Lumbar epidural analgesia may be appropriate for postoperative pain.) Paediatr Anaesth 13(8):733–734, 2003.
	Hernandez-Palazon J. Anaesthetic management in children with metachromatic leukodystrophy. Paediatr Anaesth 13(8):733–734, 2003.	
Lipoatrophy with diabetes (Seip syndrome)	Generalized loss of all body fat, fibrotic liver leading to failure, portal hypertension; splenomegaly, nephropathy, diabetes. May have renal failure. Hypersplenism may lead to anemia and thrombocytopenia.	Check coagulation and renal function preoperatively. Considerations for diabetes. Caution with drugs metabolized by liver and those excreted by the kidneys.
	Oral EA. Lipoatrophic diabetes and other related syndromes. Rev Endocr Metab Disord 4(1):61–77, 2003.	
Lipogranulomatosis	See Farber disease.	
Long QT syndrome	See Jervell and Lange-Nielsen syndrome (Romano-Ward syndrome).	
Lowe syndrome (oculocerebrorenal syndrome)	Affects males. Cataract, glaucoma, mental retardation; hypotonia, renal acidosis, proteinuria, osteoporosis, and rickets.	Check electrolyte and acid-base balance, correct acidosis and hypokalemia, and low serum Ca^{++} (treated with vitamin D and Ca^{++}). Use reduced doses of nondepolarizing muscle relaxants; use a block monitor. Caution with opioids. Avoid hyperventilation or excess glucose infusion (decreases serum K^+). Caution with drugs excreted by kidneys.

Lupus erythematosus disseminatus	See collagen diseases.
Maffucci syndrome	Enchondromatosis and hemangiomas with malignant change. Pathologic fractures, gastrointestinal bleeding from hemangiomas, orthostatic hypotension.	Transport and position carefully. May show orthostatic hypotension and be sensitive to vasodilator drugs. Caution with intubation (airway hemangiomata).
Chan SK, Ng SK, Cho AM et al: Anaesthetic implications of Maffucci's syndrome. Anaesth Intens Care 26(5):586–589, 1998.		
Malignant hyperpyrexia/ hyperthermia	See page 197.	
Mandibulofacial dysostosis	See Treacher Collins syndrome.	
Mannosidosis Type I (severe), Type II (milder)	Primary metabolic deficiency of α-mannosidases A and B → lysosomal accumulation of mannose-rich substrates. Abnormal neutrophil immunologic function. Hepatosplenomegaly, severe recurrent infections, and early death. Hearing loss, mental retardation, Hurler-like skeletal changes, gargoylelike facies, clumsy motor function, weak connective tissues.	Be alert for hepatic dysfunction, and for hypoventilation perioperatively and postoperatively.
Desnick RJ, Sharp HL, Grabowski GA et al: Mannosidosis: clinical morphologic, immunologic, and biochemical studies. Pediatr Res 10:985, 1976.		
Maple syrup urine disease (MSUD; branched-chain ketonuria)	Inability to metabolize leucine, isoleucine, and valine and accumulation of branched chain amino acids and keto acids leads to severe neurologic damage and respiratory disturbances. Episodes of hypoglycemia. Treated by diet only from birth. Acute, life-threatening episodes may require peritoneal dialysis or exchange transfusion.	Check acid-base balance, plasma amino acids preoperatively. Check serum glucose before, during, and after operation. Start glucose infusion (at least 10–15 mg/kg/min) preoperatively and continue until diet is reestablished. Prevent overhydration. Propofol infusion has been suggested.
Kahraman S, Ercan M, Akkus O et al: Anaesthetic management in maple syrup urine disease. Anaesthesia 51(6):575–578, 1996.		

Table continues on the following page.

Name	Description	Anesthesia Implications
Marfan syndrome (arachnodactyly)	Tall, thin predominantly male patients with long fingers, long face, and high arched palate. Mutant gene at chromosome 15 for fibrillin causes connective tissue disorder leading to joint instability and dislocation (including cervical spine), dislocation of lens, kyphoscoliosis, hernia, pectus excavatum, lung cysts. High incidence (~4%) of spontaneous pneumothorax. Aortic root dilation may lead to aortic incompetence or aneurysm; pulmonary artery or mitral valve may be diseased.	Preoperative cardiac assessment usually indicated. Intubation may be difficult. Laryngoscopy should be gentle to prevent cervical spine or temporomandibular joint damage. Tracheomalacia leading to difficult ventilation has been described. Position carefully to prevent dislocations. Avoid myocardial depressants, but do not allow the patient to become hypertensive (danger of aortic dissection). Beware of pneumothorax with controlled ventilation.
Keane MG, Pyeritz RE: Medical management of Marfan syndrome. Circ 117(21):2802–2813, 2008. Oh AY, Kim YH, Kim BK et al: Unexpected tracheomalacia in Marfan syndrome during general anesthesia for correction of scoliosis. Anesth Analg 95(2): 331–332, 2002.		
Maroteaux-Lamy syndrome (mucopolysaccharidosis type VI)	Normal intellect. Kyphoscoliosis with poor lung reserve; chronic respiratory infections; hypersplenism, anemia, thrombocytopenia. Myocardial involvement; heart failure by 20 yr of age.	See mucopolysaccharidoses. Preoperatively assess cardiac status, chest x-ray, and platelet count. Care with cardiac depressant drugs. Spinal cord compression may occur. May require ventilation postoperatively.
Linstedt U, Maier C, Joehnk H et al: Threatening spinal cord compression during anesthesia in a child with mucopolysaccharidosis VI. Anesthesiology 80:227, 1994.		
Marshall-Smith syndrome	Skeletal dysplasia and dysmorphic facial features. Hypotonia and failure to thrive. Possible atlantoaxial instability. Respiratory tract anomalies lead to complications.	Flexion/extension lateral neck films to rule out atlantoaxial instability. Airway problems and difficult intubation. Association with laryngomalacia and tracheomalacia described as a cause of failure to ventilate. Require oropharyngeal or nasopharyngeal tube during induction and recovery. Cautious use of muscle relaxants if hypotonia present.
Dernedde G, Pendeville P, Veyckemans F et al: Anaesthetic management of a child with Marshall-Smith syndrome. Can J Anaesth 45(7):660–663, 1998.		

Mastocytosis syndrome (urticaria pigmentosa)	Abnormal aggregates of histamine- and heparin-containing mast cells; skin lesion is a brownish-red maculopapular rash mainly on trunk. Mast cell degranulation with systemic histamine and heparin release may occur with trauma, temperature changes, alcohol, and drugs (including salicylates, opioids, curare, gallamine, papaverine, polymyxin, and atropine). Often with a history of gastroesophageal reflux. Minor surgical procedures have lead to generalized anaphylaxis and death, but most are uneventful.	Avoid stimuli and drugs known to cause mast cell degranulation. Prophylactic treatment with antihistamines (i.e., diphenhydramine, ranitidine) and steroids has been recommended. Inhalation anesthetics may be safely used. Propofol, rocuronium, succinylcholine, fentanyl, remifentanil, and/or meperidine (Demerol) may safely be used. Caution with NSAIDs. Bleeding secondary to heparin release may require protamine therapy.

Carter MC, Uzzaman A, Scott LM et al: Pediatric mastocytosis: routine anesthetic management for a complex disease. Anesth Analg 107(2):422-427, 2008.
Borgeat A, Ruetsch YA: Anesthesia in a patient with malignant systemic mastocytosis using a total intravenous anesthetic technique. Anesth Analg 86(2): 442–444, 1998.

McArdle myopathy (glycogen storage disease type V)	Muscle phosphorylase deficiency; serum lactate not increased by exercise. Initially, increased fatigability; progresses to muscle cramps and weakness (all skeletal muscles affected), myoglobinuria may lead to renal failure. Myocardium may be involved; ECG abnormalities have been reported. Patients may test positive for MH with the in vitro contracture test but no reports of clinical MH have been reported.	Preoperative echocardiogram and ECG. Do not use tourniquets; maintain infusion of dextrose during surgery; do not use succinylcholine. Care with cardiac depressant drugs; monitor ECG.

Bollig G, Mohr S, Raeder J: McArdle's disease and anaesthesia: case reports. Review of potential problems and association with malignant hyperthermia. Acta Anaesth Scand 49(8):1077–1083, 2005.

Meckel syndrome (dysencephalia splanchnocystica)	Microcephaly, micrognathia, and cleft epiglottis, CHD, renal dysplasia, polydactyly. Most die in infancy.	Preoperatively assess cardiac status. Airway and intubation may be difficult. Care with drugs excreted by kidneys.

Salonen R, Paavola P: Meckel syndrome. J Med Gen 35(6):497-501, 1998.

Table continues on the following page.

Name	Description	Anesthesia Implications
Medium chain acyl-CoA dehydrogenase deficiency (MCAD)	A disorder of fatty acid metabolism secondary to deficiency of mitochondrial enzyme. Hypoglycemia and seizures or coma may result. Treated with carnitine.	Avoid prolonged fasting, give IV dextrose infusion and check blood glucose perioperatively. Avoid propofol due to its high fat content. Avoid lactated Ringer's solution, use normal saline.
Justiz AC, Mayhew JF: Anesthesia in a child with medium-chain acyl-CoA dehydrogenase deficiency. Paediatr Anaesth 16(12):1293–1294, 2006.		
Median cleft face syndrome	Various degrees of cleft face; lipomas and dermoids over frontal bone. Other intracerebral deformities are often present. Choanal atresia may be present.	Assess for associated defects. Cleft nose, lip, and palate may cause intubation difficulties. Caution with instrumentation; nasal encephaloceles may be present.
Bomelburg T, Lenz W, Eusterbrock T: Median cleft face syndrome in association with hydrocephalus, agenesis of the corpus callosum, holoprosencephaly and choanal atresia. Euro J Ped 146(3):301–302, 1987.		
Menkes syndrome (kinky hair disease)	X-linked disorder of copper metabolism. Onset in first months of life; retarded growth and development, seizures, progressive cerebral degeneration. Gastroesophageal reflux commonly leads to pneumonia. Death from seizures or pneumonia in a few years.	Assess anticonvulsant therapy (check blood levels) and optimize; continue therapy through perioperative period. Risk of acid aspiration. Prone to hypothermia. Avoid succinylcholine (neurologic disease). Phenytoin increases vecuronium requirements. Possibly use pancuronium. Postoperative ventilation may be required.
Tobias JD: Anaesthetic considerations in the child with Menkes' syndrome. Can J Anaesth 39(7):712–715, 1992.		
Methylmalonyl-coenzyme A mutase deficiency	Autosomal recessive defect of protein metabolism. Protein metabolism leads to high plasma methylmalonic acid levels, producing lethargy, vomiting, dehydration, acidosis, ketonemia, and hyperammonemia. Treated by limiting protein intake, plus supplemental bicarbonate and cobalamin. Anesthesia and surgery may increase protein metabolism and lead to acidemia.	Avoid excessive fasting or accumulation of blood in gastrointestinal tract. Maintain intravascular volume. Monitor blood gases, electrolytes, and ammonia level. Avoid nitrous oxide. (May exacerbate metabolic defect).
Sharar SR, Haberkern CM, Jack R et al: Anesthetic management of a child with methylmalonyl-coenzyme A mutase deficiency. Anesth Analg 73(4):499–501, 1991.		

Moebius syndrome (congenital oculofacial paralysis)	Congenital paralyses of sixth and seventh cranial nerves results in inability to smile. Limb deformities, micrognathia. Feeding difficulties and aspiration may cause chronic pulmonary problems.	Assess respiratory status carefully. Intubation may be difficult (but not usually). May be sensitive to opioids, central apnea may occur. Monitor ventilation carefully postoperatively.

Ames WA, Shichor TM, Speakman M et al: Anesthetic management of children with Moebius sequence. Can J Anaesth 52(8):837–844, 2005.

Morquio syndrome (mucopolysaccharidosis type IV)	Normal intellect. Severe dwarfing; aortic incompetence; kyphoscoliosis with poor lung function (cardiorespiratory symptoms and pulmonary hypertension by second decade). Unstable atlantoaxial joint leading to spinal cord compression; deafness. Inguinal hernia common. See mucopolysaccharidoses.	Preoperative cardiac investigation as indicated. Care with cardiac depressant drugs. Assess respiratory status. Assess atlantoaxial stability preoperatively. Care with positioning and avoid excessive neck manipulation; may require fiberoptic intubation. Regional analgesia may be appropriate for some patients. Monitor ventilation carefully postoperatively.

Morgan KA, Rehman MA, Schwartz RE: Morquio's syndrome and its anaesthetic considerations. Paediatr Anaesth 12(7):641–644, 2002.
Tobias JD: Anesthetic care for the child with Morquio syndrome: general versus regional anesthesia. J Clin Anesth 11(3):242–246, 1999.

Mucopolysaccharidosis type VII (β-glucuronidase deficiency)	Severe mental retardation. Skeletal anomalies similar to type IV.	Same as type IV: preparation and anesthetic.

Moschcowitz disease (thrombotic thrombocytopenic purpura)	Hemolytic anemia and thrombocytopenia, arteriolar and capillary disease, neurologic damage, renal disease. Treatment: plasmapheresis and steroids; splenectomy for resistant cases. Assess for history of steroid therapy.	Check platelet count and hemoglobin. Assess BUN/creatinine. Possible steroid supplement. Avoid IM injections. Smooth induction and intubation (prevent hypertension as might cause CNS bleed). Nasotracheal intubation contraindicated (due to risk of bleeding). Care with drugs excreted by kidneys. Platelet transfusions or fresh blood should be avoided (may exacerbate disease); transfuse with PRBC and FFP.

Pivalizza EG: Anesthetic management of a patient with thrombotic thrombocytopenic purpura. Anesth Analg 79(6):1203–1205, 1994.

Table continues on the following page.

Name	Description	Anesthesia Implications
Moyamoya disease	Severe carotid artery stenosis with a fine network of vessels around the basal ganglia. Cerebral ischemia leads to paroxysmal hemiplegia. Treatment is by surgical revascularization using scalp vessels.	Hypocapnia leads to severe cerebral ischemia: prevent hyperventilation, maintain normocapnia. Isoflurane may be useful as a cerebral vasodilator, propofol may provide cerebral protection. Prevent hypothermia. Maintain cerebral perfusion pressure.

Soriano SG, Sethna NF, Scott RM: Anesthetic management of children with moya moya disease. Anesth Analg 77:1066, 1993.
Baykan N, Ozgen S, Ustalar ZS et al: Moyamoya disease and anesthesia. Paediatr Anaesth 15(12):1111–1115, 2005.

Mucopolysaccharidoses Type I H, I HS, II, VII Type III Type I S, IV, VI	Affects bones and intellect. Affects intellect only. Affects bones only. See previous classifications: I H: Hurler syndrome. I S: Scheie syndrome; formerly classified as type V. HS: Hurler-Scheie compound (See Scheie syndrome). II: Hunter syndrome. III: Sanfilippo syndrome. IV: Morquio syndrome. V: Formerly Scheie syndrome. VI: Maroteaux-Lamy syndrome. VII: β-Glucuronidase deficiency (See Morquio syndrome).	All may be difficult to intubate. LMA may not relieve obstruction. Spinal cord compression may occur because of thickening of dura and odontoid hypoplasia; preoperative MRI of spinal cord suggested. Preoperative echocardiogram and ECG warranted to assess severity of cardiac dysfunction. All are subject to postobstructive pulmonary edema.

Walker RW, Darowski M, Morris P et al: Anaesthesia and mucopolysaccharidoses. A review of airway problems in children. Anaesthesia 49(12):1078–1084, 1994.
Walker RW, Colovic V, Robinson DN et al: Postobstructive pulmonary oedema during anaesthesia in children with mucopolysaccharidoses. Paediatr Anaesth 13(5):441–447, 2003.

Multiple endocrine adenomatoses Type I Type II	See Wermer syndrome. See Sipple syndrome.	

Muscle, eye, brain disease (MEB)	Muscle dystrophy, eye disease (glaucoma, strabismus, nystagmus), and mental retardation. Severe muscle weakness, secretion retention, bedridden.	Caution with all muscle relaxants. Succinylcholine results in very high CK levels and should be avoided.

Karhunen U: Serum creatine kinase levels after succinylcholine in children with "muscle, eye and brain disease." Can J Anaesth 35:90, 1988.

Muscle phosphofructo-kinase deficiency (glycogen storage disease type VII) (Tarui disease)	Neither glycogen nor glucose can be used as metabolic fuels. Reduced RBC life span (13–16 days).	Monitor glucose levels. Infuse dextrose. No specific anesthesia complications have been reported.

Toscano A, Musumeci O: Tarui disease and distal glycogenoses: clinical and genetic update. Acta Myologica 26(2):105–107, 2007.

Myasthenia congenita	Similar to myasthenia gravis in older children. See page 378.	Do not use respiratory depressants or muscle relaxants: Ventilatory support may be required postoperatively. Possibility of cholinergic crisis with anticholinesterase therapy.

White MC, Stoddart PA: Anesthesia for thymectomy in children with myasthenia gravis. Paediatr Anaesth 14(8):625–635, 2004.

Myositis ossificans (fibrodysplasia ossificans progressiva)	Bony infiltration of tendons, fascia, aponeuroses, and muscle. Thoracic involvement greatly reduces thoracic compliance: progressive respiratory failure. Risk of any further minor trauma causing progression of disease	Check respiratory function, history of steroid therapy. Airway and intubation problems if neck rigid and mouth fixed. Forced manipulation of jaw may cause local progression of disease; very gentle fiberoptic intubation indicated. Avoid IM injections. Careful padding and prevent all trauma to joints and tissues. Specific recommendations at www.IFOPA.org

Tumolo M, Moscatelli A, Silvestri G: Anaesthetic management of a child with fibrodysplasia ossificans progressiva. Br J Anaesth 97(5):701–703, 2006.

Table continues on the following page.

Name	Description	Anesthesia Implications
Myotonia congenita (Thomsen disease)	Decreased ability to relax muscles after contraction; diffuse hypertrophy of muscle (similar to myotonia dystrophica but more benign and nonprogressive). Paradoxical response to nondepolarizing muscle relaxants possible (generalized muscle spasms); avoid succinylcholine (possible hyperkalemia). If muscle relaxants needed use short-intermediate acting agents.	Use short-intermediate acting nondepolarizing muscle relaxants with caution; avoid succinylcholine; avoid inhalation anesthetics; TIVA technique recommended; use opioids with caution. Postoperative respiratory complications common due to poor cough. Regional nerve blocks for analgesia recommended.
Russell SH, Hirsch NP: Anaesthesia and myotonia. Br Anaesth 72(2):210–216, 1994.		
Myotonia dystrophica (myotonic dystrophy, Steinert disease)	Weakness and myotonia; eyelid ptosis, cataracts, frontal baldness; cardiac conduction defects and arrhythmias, possible cardiomyopathy. Reduced pulmonary function, very sensitive to respiratory depressants. Esophageal motility disorder; dysphagia and tendency to GERD and aspiration. Endocrine abnormalities (hypothyroidism, diabetes) may be present in older patients. May present in the neonate with weakness and hypotonia.	Assess cardiac function: preoperative echocardiogram and ECG. Assess respiratory function. Do not use succinylcholine (which causes myotonia in 50%). Cautious use of inhalational agents as may cause myocardial depression. Monitor ECG continuously. Nondepolarizing relaxant drugs may produce poor relaxation and may interact with patients medication (i.e., phenytoin). Caution with reversal; neostigmine may induce myotonia; halothane may cause shivering and myotonia postoperatively. Extremely sensitive to respiratory depressants—use regional analgesia. Anticipate postoperative pulmonary complications; ventilatory support may be necessary.
White RJ, Bass SP: Myotonic dystrophy and paediatric anaesthesia. Paediatr Anaesth 13(2):94–102, 2003.		

Syndrome	Features	Anesthetic Implications
Nager syndrome	Micrognathia, fishlike face, cleft palate (similar to Treacher Collins), limb deformities. Tetralogy of Fallot may be associated. Cervical spine anomalies.	Assess cardiac function preoperatively; SBE prophylaxis if indicated. Very difficult intubation. Mouth opening can be very limited and intubation only possible by a fiberoptic technique. Upper airway obstruction may necessitate tracheostomy in the neonate. Postoperative ventilatory obstruction may occur; monitor carefully.

Groeper K, Johnson JO, Braddock SR et al: Anaesthetic implications of Nager syndrome. Paediatr Anaesth 12(4):365–368, 2002.

Syndrome	Features	Anesthetic Implications
Nail-patella syndrome (arthro-osteoonychodysplasia)	Dysplasia of nails and absent or hypoplastic patellas. Fragile teeth. May have "iliac horns" abnormality of elbows, nephropathy, increased mucopolysaccharide excretion. Vasomotor instability. Distal sensory changes.	Caution with intubation (fragile teeth). Monitor heart rate and BP. Care with drugs excreted by kidneys. Position and pad carefully (abnormal muscle insertions).

Hennessey TA, Backman SB, Meterissian SH et al: Nail-Patella syndrome: a case report and anesthetic implications. Can J Anaesth 54(10):835–839, 2007.

Syndrome	Features	Anesthetic Implications
Nemaline rod myopathy	Congenital myopathy, may be related to central core disease. Commonly present as neonates with hypotonia, weak cry, and poor feeding. Dysmorphic features, micrognathia, slender face, high arched palate. Motor development delayed, muscle weakness of trunk and limbs plus respiratory and pharyngeal; leads to respiratory failure, aspiration pneumonia. Congenital heart disease may be associated.	Preoperatively assess airway and cardiac and pulmonary status carefully. Preoperative physiotherapy and antibiotics for infection if indicated, intubation may be difficult. Brisk vagal responses noted; prescribe atropine. Possible central sensitivity to depressant drugs. Avoid succinylcholine (abnormal response); response to pancuronium is reported to be normal. Postoperative ventilation may be required. Link to central core disease suggests possibility of MH but not yet reported in nemaline myopathy. Regional analgesia may be appropriate. TIVA technique may be the best alternative.

Cunliffe M, Burrows FA: Anaesthetic implications of nemaline rod myopathy. Can Anaesth Soc J 32(5):543–547, 1985.
Shenkman Z, Sheffer O, Erez I et al: Spinal anesthesia for gastrostomy in an infant with nemaline myopathy. Anesth Analg 91(4):858–859, 2000.

Table continues on the following page.

Name	Description	Anesthesia Implications
Neonatal hypoglycemia, symptomatic	Symptomatic hypoglycemia in infants: (1) small for gestational age, (2) of diabetic mothers, (3) premature. If untreated: convulsions, lethargy, and mental retardation; no ketosis. Rarely, insulinoma or pancreatic hypertrophy requiring subtotal pancreatectomy. See also Beckwith syndrome.	Start IV glucose infusion (5–10 mg/kg/min; no bolus) preoperatively and monitor blood glucose until condition stable postoperatively. (Boluses would precipitate rebound hyperglycemia.) The child may be receiving steroids, diazoxide, and glucagon. (N.B. Normal full-term neonates may occasionally be found to have asymptomatic "hypoglycemia" <40 mg/dl).
Cole MD, Peevy K: Hypoglycemia in normal neonates appropriate for gestational age. J Perinatol 14(2):118–120, 1994. McGowan JE: Neonatal hypoglycemia. Ped Rev 20:e6-e15, 1999.		
Nevoid basal cell carcinoma syndrome	See Gorlin-Goltz syndrome.	
Niemann-Pick disease (See also Wolman disease) Types A, C, D (onset in infancy) Type B	Hepatosplenomegaly and accumulation of sphingomyelin and other lipids throughout body. Bone marrow, liver, and spleen involvement lead to anemia and thrombocytopenia. Diffuse foam cell infiltration of lungs leads to pulmonary insufficiency, pneumonia. Mental retardation. Epilepsy, ataxia. Death usually by third year (type A) to 15th year (type C). Normal intellect. Pulmonary disease (foam cells in alveoli). Not fatal.	Check coagulation studies and cardiorespiratory function. Anticipate difficulty with ventilation (pulmonary restrictive disease and ascites) and possible requirement for postoperatively ventilatory support. Caution with drugs metabolized in the liver.
Bujok LS, Bujok G, Knapik P: Niemann-Pick disease: a rare problem in anaesthesiological practice. Paediar Anaesth 12(9):806–808, 2002.		
Noack syndrome	Craniosynostosis and digital anomalies; obesity.	Intubation may be difficult because of skull deformity.

Noonan syndrome	Short stature, web neck, hypertelorism, mild mental retardation. Similar to Turner syndrome. Cardiac anomalies: usually pulmonary stenosis, hypertrophic cardiomyopathy. Micrognathia, hydronephrosis, platelet dysfunction.	Preoperative evaluation of CHD. Check coagulation. Possible difficult intubation. Check BUN/creatinine; care with drugs excreted by kidneys.

Nakagawa M, Kinouchi K, Matsunami K et al: Anesthetic management of a child with Noonan syndrome and hypertrophic obstructive cardiomyopathy. [Japanese English abstract] Masui - Jap J Anesth 55(1):92–95, 2006.

Oculoauriculovertebral syndrome	See Goldenhar syndrome.
Oculocerebrorenal syndrome	See Lowe syndrome.
Oculodento-osseous dysplasia (ODOD)	Microphthalmia and microcornea, small nose with anteverted nostrils, cleft palate, dental enamel dysplasia, plus a generalized defect of bony modeling; mandibular dysplasia, thick ribs, abnormal long bones.	Airway difficulties due to nasal, oral, and mandibular defects. Brittle teeth. Difficult intubation.

Colreavy F, Colbert S, Dunphy J: Oculodento-osseous dysplasia: a review of anaesthetic problems. Paediatr Anaesth 4:179, 1994.

Oculofacial paralysis, congenital	See Moebius syndrome.
Ollier syndrome	See also Maffucci syndrome (enchondromatosis with cavernous hemangioma). Multiple chondromas within bones, usually unilateral; pathologic fractures	Position carefully. Hemangioma considerations as for Maffucci syndrome.

Table continues on the following page.

Name	Description	Anesthesia Implications
Opitz-Frias syndrome (G syndrome, hypospadias, dysphagia syndrome)	X-linked or autosomal dominant, affects males more than females. Craniofacial and genital abnormalities (bifid scrotum). Dysphagia and recurrent aspiration, achalasia, hiatal hernia. Hypertelorism, micrognathia, and a high arched palate. Laryngeal malformations (including laryngotracheal cleft and subglottic stenosis) and pulmonary hypoplasia.	Difficult airway, small larynx (prepare small endotracheal tubes). Danger of regurgitation; empty stomach before induction.
	Bolsin SN, Gillbe C: Opitz-Frias syndrome. A case with potentially hazardous anaesthetic implications. Anaesth 40(12):1189–1193, 1985.	
Oral-facial-digital syndrome (Mohr syndrome)	Cleft lip and palate, lobed tongue, hypoplastic mandible and maxilla, digital anomalies; hydrocephalus, polycystic kidneys. Possible tracheolaryngomalacia. Corpus callosum anomaly (may result in delayed recovery from anesthesia).	Assess respiratory status. Airway problems and intubation may be difficult; assess BUN/creatinine; possible renal impairment; caution with drugs excreted by the kidneys.
	Gercek A, Dagcinar A, Ozek MM: Anesthetic management of a newborn with Mohr (oro-facial-digital type II) syndrome. Paediatr Anaesth 17(6):603–604, 2007.	
Osler-Weber-Rendu syndrome (hemorrhagic telangiectasia)	Multiple capillary and venous dilation, most commonly of skin and nasal mucosa, but any organ may be affected. High incidence of pulmonary and hepatic AV fistula.	Anemia; internal hemorrhage may occur perioperatively. Blood loss difficult to control. Difficult to maintain IV due to fragile vessels. Check pulmonary status. Positive pressure ventilation may decrease oxygenation in patients with pulmonary AV malformation.
	Sharma D, Pandia MP, Bithal PK: Anaesthetic management of Osler-Weber-Rendu syndrome with coexisting congenital methaemoglobinaemia. Acta Anaesth Scand 49(9):1391–1394, 2005.	

Osteogenesis imperfecta (fragilitas ossium)	I. Congenita—Usually stillbirth or rapidly fatal. II. Tarda—Pathologic fractures, blue sclera, deafness. Osteoporosis → kyphoscoliosis → lung pathology. Fragility of vessels results in subcutaneous hemorrhage. Dentine deficiency results in carious, fragile teeth.	Use extreme care in positioning (to prevent breaking bones) and intubating. Teeth are easily broken. Difficulty in maintaining IV due to fragile vessels. Intraoperative hyperthermia (not MH) has been described in patients receiving inhaled anesthetics; temperature remains unchanged or may decrease during TIVA. Paediatr Anaesth 14(6):524–525, 2004.
Karabiyik L, Capan Z: Osteogenesis imperfecta: different anaesthetic approaches to two paediatric cases. Paediatr Anaesth 14(6):524–525, 2004.		
Osteopetrosis	See Albers-Schönberg disease.	
Paramyotonia congenita (Eulenburg periodic paralysis)	Myotonia on exposure to cold; paroxysmal weakness; serum K^+ may be high or low	Check serum K^+ level. Unpredictable response to non-depolarizing muscle relaxants; avoid succinylcholine. (See also myotonic dystrophy).
Ay B, Gercek A, Dogan VI et al: Pyloromyotomy in a patient with paramyotonia congenita. Anesth Analg 98(1):68–69, 2004.		
Patau syndrome (trisomy 13 syndrome)	Mental retardation, microcephaly, micrognathia, cleft lip or palate. May have cardiac anomalies (usually ventricular septal defect and/or dextrocardia). Patients die in infancy.	Preoperative echocardiogram and EKG, SBE prophylazis if indicated. Possible difficult intubation.
Pollard RC, Beasley JM: Anaesthesia for patients with trisomy 13 (Patau's syndrome). Paediatr Anaesth 6:151, 1996.		
Pelizaeus-Merzbacher disease	See leukodystrophy.	
Pendred syndrome	Deafness and goiter; incomplete block of thyroxine production. May be euthyroid or hypothyroid.	Preoperatively ensure that patient is euthyroid; otherwise as for cretinism.
Fraser GR, Morgans ME, Trotter WR: The syndrome of sporadic goitre and congenital deafness. Queensland J Med 29:279, 1960.		
Periodic paralysis	See familial periodic paralysis and paramyotonia congenita.	

Table continues on the following page.

Name	Description	Anesthesia Implications
PHACE syndrome	Posterior fossa brain malformations, hemangiomas, arterial anomalies, coarctation of the aorta, eye defects. May be associated with bilateral agenesis of the carotid arteries, cerebral perfusion via the vertebral arteries. Airway hemangioma may be present. Renal artery stenosis may cause hypertension.	Assess cardiac status preoperatively. Risk of cerebral ischemia, CVA. Review vascular anatomy carefully. Monitor cerebral function. Hypertension may need therapy.
	Javault A, Metton O, Raisky O et al: Anesthesia management in a child with PHACE syndrome and agenesis of bilateral internal carotid arteries. Paediatr Anaesth 17(10):c989–993, 2007.	
Phenylketonuria	Phenylalanine hydroxylase deficiency. Vomiting, CNS irritability, mental retardation, hypertonia, convulsions. Phenylalanine-deficient diet must be maintained; may present with megaloblastic anemia if poorly controlled.	Induction and maintenance by inhalation technique. Control ventilation. Give dextrose infusion and monitor glucose levels perioperatively (tendency to hypoglycemia). Ensure adequate phenylalanine and hemoglobin concentration (no megaloblastic anemia) preoperatively; otherwise, avoid nitrous oxide. Sensitive to opioids and other CNS depressants; monitor body temperature carefully. If patient has epilepsy, continue drugs.
	Dal D, Celiker V: Anesthetic management of a strabismus patient with phenylketonuria. Paediatr Anaesth 14(8):701–702, 2004.	
Pierre Robin syndrome	Cleft palate, micrognathia, glossoptosis due to first branchial arch embryologic defect. CHD may be present. Neonates: upper airway obstruction may occur and can lead to cor pulmonale. Maintain airway by nursing prone on a frame: may require tongue suture, intubation, or tracheostomy.	Micrognathia and airway improve with growth. Assess for cardiac defect preoperatively. Intubation may be extremely difficult. Fiberoptic intubation techniques should be anticipated; topical airway analgesia with nebulized lidocaine will facilitate awake insertion of an LMA, used to induce anesthesia, and as a conduit for intubation. The child should be fully awake before extubation.
	Asai T, Nagata A, Shingu K: Awake tracheal intubation through the laryngeal mask in neonates with upper airway obstruction. Paediatr Anaesth 18(1):77–80, 2008.	

Plott syndrome	Vocal cord paralysis, psychomotor retardation, and sixth nerve palsy. Stridor at rest, respiratory distress, and cyanotic or choking spells.	Anticipate airway obstruction and potential for aspiration perioperatively.
Poland syndrome	Absent pectoral muscles with chest deformity. Ipsilateral syndactyly or microdactyly. May have CHD, renal and gastrointestinal anomalies. Extreme form: Moebius syndrome has facial paralysis. Lung herniation on crying: paradoxical movement of chest wall on inspiration.	Assess preoperatively for cardiac and renal disease. Controlled ventilation is recommended due to the chest deformity.

Sethuraman R, Kannan S, Bala I et al: Anaesthesia in Poland syndrome. Can J Anaesth 45(3):277–279, 1998.

Polyarteritis nodosa	See collagen disease.	
Polycystic kidneys	Associated cysts in liver, pancreas, spleen, lungs, bladder, thyroid in one third; cerebral aneurysm in 15%.	Preoperatively, assess renal function. Lung cysts may lead to pneumothorax; prevent high peak inflation pressures. Prevent hypertension (possible associated cerebral aneurysm).
Polyneuritis, acute	See Guillain-Barré syndrome.	
Pompe disease (glycogen storage disease type II)	Deposits of glycogen in muscles, severe hypotonicity; large tongue; massive cardiomegaly. Death from cardiorespiratory failure before 2 yr of age. Recently replacement therapy with recombinant human α-glucosidase enzyme (rhGAA) has proven effective in extending the life span.	Preoperatively assess cardiac function: echocardiogram and EKG, SBE prophylaxis if indicated. Extreme care required: use respiratory or cardiac depressants or muscle relaxants with caution; etomidate and ketamine are recommended agents. Large tongue may cause airway problem. Maintain intravascular volume. Monitor ECG for rhythm and ST segment changes; serious arrhythmias may occur. TIVA is recommended. Paediatri Anaesth

Ing RJ, Cook DR, Bengur RA et al: Anaesthetic management of infants with glycogen storage disease type II: a physiological approach. Paediatri Anaesth 14(6):514–519, 2004.

Table continues on the following page.

Name	Description	Anesthesia Implications
Porphyrias	Paralysis, psychiatric disorder, autonomic imbalance—hypertension, tachycardia; abdominal pain precipitated by drugs, stress, infection, etc. High incidence of diabetes.	Avoid prolonged fasting and dehydration. Do not give barbiturates (including thiopental) and certain other IV agents (i.e., etomidate, some sedatives and, niketh-amide, hydantoin, derivatives, sulfonamides, antipyretics, or hypoglycemic agents). See Jensen et al (ref below) for drug concerns in porphyria. The following have been used safely: atropine, glyco-pyrrolate, propofol (brief exposure), succinylcholine, N_2O, sevoflurane, vecuronium, atracurium, cisatracurium, fentanyl, morphine, epinephrine, neostigmine, chloral hydrate, chlorpromazine, and bupivacaine.

Jensen NF, Fiddler DS, Striepe V: Anesthetic considerations in porphyrias. Anesth Analg 80:591–599, 1995.
Sheppard L, Dorman T: Anesthesia in a child with homozygous porphobilinogen deaminase deficiency: a severe form of acute intermittent porphyria. Paediatr Anaesth15(5):426–428, 2005.

Name	Description	Anesthesia Implications
Prader-Labhart-Willi syndrome	Sporadic mutation. Cytogenetic deletion at chromosome inherited from father (same genetic defect in Angelman syndrome is inherited from mother). Hypothalamic type "Pickwickian syndrome." Neonate: hypotonia, poor feeding, reflexes absent. Second phase: hyperactive, uncontrollable polyphagia, thermoregulation disturbed, mental retardation. Extreme obesity leading to cardiorespiratory failure.	Danger of hypoglycemia developing: monitor blood glucose carefully and infuse IV glucose solution before, during, and after anesthesia. Obesity makes venous cannulation difficult. Low-grade pyrexia may occur during scoliosis, strabismus, or hernia surgery. No relationship to MH. Hypothermia may also occur. Sleep apnea common: assisted or controlled ventilation may be necessary during and after operation, or apnea monitoring postoperatively. Beware of postoperative airway obstruction; nasal CPAP may improve airway. Regional analgesia may be appropriate in some patients for intraoperative management and/or postoperative pain.

Dearlove OR, Dobson A, Super M: Anaesthesia and Prader-Willi syndrome. Paediatr Anaesth 8(3):267–271, 1998.

Progeria (Hutchinson-Gilford syndrome)	Premature aging starts at 6 mo to 3 yr; cardiac disease-ischemia, hypertension, cardiomegaly. Diabetes may be present. Death from coronary artery disease may occur before 10 yr of age.	Carefully assess cardiac status preoperatively particularly evidence of coronary artery disease and myocardial ischemia. Intubation may be difficult because of small mouth and receding mandible. Anesthesia as for adults with coronary artery disease and myocardial ischemia.

Capell BC, Collins FS, Nabel EG: Mechanisms of cardiovascular disease in accelerated aging syndromes. Circ Res 101(1):13–26, 2007.
Liessmann CD: Anaesthesia in a child with Hutchinson-Gilford progeria. Paediatr Anaesth 11(5):611–614, 2001.

Proteus syndrome	A highly variable disease with progressive overgrowth of connective tissues, bone, skin lesions (nevi), and abnormal distribution of fat. Cystic lung lesions. Scoliosis is common. The neck may be elongated and twisted because of vertebral deformities. Vascular malformations may be present and pulmonary emboli without venous thrombosis have been reported.	Check preoperative chest x-ray for cystic lesion. If present, avoid N_2O and high peak inflation pressures; possible pneumothorax. Caution with airway—intubation may be very difficult. Postoperative airway obstruction may occur—monitor ventilation carefully.

Cekmen N, Kordan AZ, Tuncer B et al: Anesthesia for proteus syndrome. Paediatr Anaesth 14(8):689–692, 2004.

Prune-belly syndrome	Agenesis of abdominal musculature with renal anomalies. Poor cough; risk of postoperative atelectasis, respiratory infections, and respiratory failure.	Preoperatively assess renal function. Treat as for a full stomach: intubate and control ventilation. (But intubation may be difficult in some, so assess carefully). Use muscle relaxants and drugs excreted by kidneys with caution. Thoracic epidural useful for postoperative analgesia and may prevent respiratory compromise.

Baris S, Karakaya D, Ustun E et al: Complicated airway management in a child with prune-belly syndrome. Paediatr Anaesth 11:501–504, 2001.
Henderson AM, Vallis CJ, Sumner E: Anaesthesia in the prune-belly syndrome. A review of 36 cases. Anaesth 42(1):54–60, 1987.

Pseudohypoparathyroidism	See Albright osteodystrophy.

Name	Description	Anesthesia Implications
Pseudoxanthoma elasticum	See Grönblad-Strandberg syndrome.	
Pyle disease (metaphyseal dysplasia)	Craniofacial abnormalities; enlarged mandible; cranial nerve paralyses.	Assess airway carefully; possible difficult intubation.
Rett syndrome	Disabling neurologic disorder affecting only females. Underweight, mental retardation, autism, seizures, scoliosis, abnormal pain sensation, vasomotor instability, cardiac arrhythmias (long QT syndrome), marked irregular respiration: hyperventilation alternating with apneic spells.	Preoperative ECG. Assess pulmonary function carefully. Severe risk of respiratory complications. Often present for spinal surgery for scoliosis. SSEPs can be monitored but MEPs may be contraindicated if history of seizures. Postoperatively, apnea monitoring or ventilatory support needed. Insensitive or hypersensitive to pain. May be sensitive to respiratory depressant drugs. Benzodiazepines to control seizures. Cautions as for long QT syndrome; prevent tachycardia.
Dearlove OR, Walker RW: Anaesthesia for Rett syndrome. Paediatr Anaesth 6(2):155–158, 1996.		
Reye syndrome	Severe metabolic encephalopathy and fatty degeneration of viscera (especially liver): hyperaminoacidemia; increased prothrombin time, blood ammonia, serum transaminases. Suspected cofactor is ingestion of ASA (aspirin) during prodromal illness. Most reliable diagnosis is by liver biopsy. If untreated, increased ICP is usually fatal.	Anesthetize for investigation of and decompression of increased ICP. Patient may be receiving steroids and controlled hypothermia. Avoid drugs metabolized by liver. Control ventilation and continue hypothermia and all supportive measures.
Rheumatoid arthritis	See collagen diseases.	

Rieger syndrome	Hypodontia, malformations of anterior chamber of eye, myotonic dystrophy. May have other developmental abnormalities including maxillary hypoplasia.	Possible difficult airway. Avoid succinylcholine; use nondepolarizing muscle relaxants with caution (unpredictable response). Anesthetic requirements dictated by muscle disease: See also amyotonia congenita, myotonia congenita, myotonia dystrophica.

Asai T, Matsumoto H, Shingu K: Difficult airway management in a baby with Axenfeld-Rieger syndrome. Paediatr Anaesth 8(5):444, 1998.

Riley-Day syndrome (familial dysautonomia)	Recessive disorder of autonomic ganglia and sensory neurones found in Ashkenazi Jews. Deficiency of dopamine-β-hydroxylase: autonomic dysfunction and decreased sensation, paroxysmal hypertension, and orthostatic hypotension. Emotional lability, absent lacrimation, abnormal sweating, poor sucking and swallowing. Recurrent aspiration pneumonia and chronic lung disease. Dysautonomic crisis (vomiting, profuse sweating, heart rate and hemodynamic instability) can occur in response to stress.	Avoid prolonged fasting. Premedication with midazolam and H_2-receptor antagonist. Parental presence may help. Atropine can be given. Require IV hydration; replace fluid losses carefully to maintain volume status (monitor CVP if extensive blood loss is anticipated). Sensitive to anesthetic agents: titrate inhalational agents to effect; can use barbiturates, propofol, etomidate, opioids, and relaxants. Respiratory center unresponsive to CO_2; use opioids with caution, may require postoperative ventilation. Risk of aspiration, postoperatively and at induction. Diazepam often controls an autonomic crisis, ranitidine for gastric acidity, and clonidine may be useful to manage postoperative hypertension. Epidural anesthesia was thought to be contraindicated but has been used uneventfully in a few cases with increased cardiovascular stability and superior analgesia reported. Caution with eyes, lubricate and cover.

Ngai J, Kreynin I, Kim JT et al: Anesthesia management of familial dysautonomia. Paediatr Anaesth 16(6):611-620, 2006.

Robin Pierre syndrome	See Pierre Robin syndrome.

Table continues on the following page.

Name	Description	Anesthesia Implications
Robinow syndrome (fetal face syndrome)	Limb-shortening, facial (midface hypoplasia), and spinal deformities, CHD, renal disease, and hypoplastic genitalia. May be associated with Crigler-Najjer liver disease. (Both diseases a result of consanguinity.)	Preoperatively, assess cardiac, renal, and liver (if Crigler-Najjer suspected) function. If Crigler-Najjer is present, evaluate coagulation status. Caution with airway recommended, but usually not difficult.
Lirk P, Rieder J, Schuerholz A et al: Anaesthetic implications of Robinow syndrome. Paediatr Anaesth 13(8):725–727, 2003.		
Romano-Ward syndrome	See Jervell and Lange-Nielsen syndrome.	
Rubinstein-Taybi syndrome	Broad thumb and great toes, mental retardation, microcephaly. May have CHD (usually pulmonary stenosis), frequent chest infections, repeated aspiration leading to pneumonia and chronic lung disease. Estimated frequency: 1 of every 500 institutionalized mentally retarded persons.	Preoperative assessment for cardiac and pulmonary diseases. Anticipate difficult intubation. Caution with respiratory depressants. Beware of postoperative ventilatory depression or apnea.
Altintas F, Cakmakkaya S: Anesthetic management of a child with Rubinstein-Taybi syndrome. Paediatr Anaesth 14(7):610–611, 2004.		
Russell-Silver syndrome	See Silver-Russell dwarfism.	
Sandhoff disease	See gangliosidosis GM2.	
Saethre-Chotzen syndrome	Acrocephalosyndactyly III premature closure of cranial sutures with syndactyly hands and feet. Hypoplastic maxilla, hypertelorism, malformed ears may be present. Intelligence usually normal.	Caution with airway. No other special considerations.
Easely D, Mayhew JF: Anesthesia in a child with Saethre-Chotzen syndrome. Paediatr Anaesth 18(1):81, 2008.		

Sanfilippo syndrome (mucopolysaccharidosis type III)	CNS malfunction in childhood progresses to mental retardation and dementia. Emotional disturbance and agitation. No hepatosplenomegaly, cardiac problems, or major bone problems.	See mucopolysaccharidoses. No other specific anesthesia problems described.
Sanjad-Sakati syndrome (SSS)	Congenital hypoparathyroidism, hypocalcemia, hyperphosphatemia, seizures, dwarfism, mental retardation, and dysmorphic features. Recurrent pulmonary infections. Confined to children of Arab descent.	Assess respiratory status carefully and check electrolytes and ionized calcium preoperatively. Airway and intubation may be difficult. Use short-acting drugs. Monitor postoperative respiratory status.
Platis CM, Wasersprung D, Kachko L et al: Anesthesia management for the child with Sanjad-Sakati syndrome. Paediatr Anaesth 16(11):1189–1192, 2006.		
Scheie syndrome (mucopolysaccharidosis type IS, formerly classified as type V)	Normal or almost normal intellect. Corneal clouding, hernias; joint stiffness, especially of hands and feet; aortic insufficiency. Sleep apnea may occur.	Preoperatively evaluate cardiac status. See mucopolysaccharidoses. Monitor carefully for apnea. Position with care.
Perks WH, Cooper RA, Bradbury S et al. Sleep apnea in Scheie syndrome. Thorax 35, 85, 1980.		
Schwartz-Jampel syndrome	Dwarfism, microstomia, myotonia limiting joint movement, bowing of long bones, thermoregulatory disorder. Usually normal intellect (some degree of mental retardation in 25%).	Difficult intubation. Larynx may be anterior. Awake LMA-assisted fiberoptic intubation has been recommended. Succinylcholine contraindicated; possible abnormal response to nondepolarizing relaxants, avoid inhalation agents. (See also myotonia and paramyotonia.)
Ray S, Rubin AP: Anaesthesia in a child with Schwartz-Jampel syndrome. Anaesthesia 49(7):600–602, 1994.		

Table continues on the following page.

Name	Description	Anesthesia Implications
Scleroderma	Diffuse cutaneous stiffening. May have hemifacial atrophy. Plastic surgery required for contracture and constrictions. May have cardiac fibrosis or cor pulmonale (rare in children—but common cause of death). Esophageal dilation leads to GERD. Children have less multiple organ involvement than adults—more arthritis and myositis. Raynaud phenomena may rarely be present. Therapy may include steroids, methotrexate, Ca^{++} channel blockers.	Preoperatively assess cardiac function. Check history of steroid therapy and other drug history. Scarring of face and mouth—possible difficult airway and intubation. Chest restriction—poor compliance. Diffuse pulmonary fibrosis—hypoxia. Veins may be invisible, impalpable, difficult to enter. Prevent hypothermia.

Zulian F: Systemic sclerosis and localized scleroderma in childhood. Rheum Dis Clin N Am 34(1):239–255, 2008. Roberts JG, Sabar R, Gianoli JA et al: Progressive systemic sclerosis: clinical manifestations and anesthetic considerations. J Clin Anesth 14(6):474–477, 2002.

Name	Description	Anesthesia Implications
Sebaceous nevi syndrome, linear	Linear nevi from forehead to nose; hydrocephalus, mental retardation; may have coarctation and/or hypoplasia of aorta.	Assess cardiac status as indicated. May have increased ICP.
Seckel syndrome	Autosomal recessive disorder, mental retardation, dwarfism, microcephaly ("Birdlike" facies), prominent maxilla, micrognathia, pointed nose.	Check airway carefully; prepare for difficult mask ventilation, intubation, and venous access.

Gurkan Y, Hosten T, Dayioglu H et al. Anesthesia for Seckel syndrome. Pediatr Anesth 16:359–360, 2006.

Name	Description	Anesthesia Implications
Seip syndrome	See lipoatrophy with diabetes.	
Shy-Drager syndrome	Orthostatic hypotension; diffuse degeneration of central and autonomic nervous systems; lability of pulse and blood pressure possibly because of defective baroreceptor response; decreased sweating; hypersensitivity to catecholamines and angiotensin.	Caution with potent inhalation anesthetics; accurate fluid replacement important; treat hypotension with IV fluids and phenylephrine; vasopressin may be the best agent to treat refractory hypotension. Use muscle relaxants with caution.

Hutchinson RC, Sugden JC: Anaesthesia for Shy-Drager syndrome. Anaesthesia 39(12):1229–1231, 1984. Vallejo R, DeSouza G, Lee J: Shy-Drager syndrome and severe unexplained intraoperative hypotension responsive to vasopressin. Anesth Analg 95:50–52, 2002.

Silver-Russell dwarfism	Short stature, skeletal asymmetry, micrognathia. Low birth weight. Café au lait spots, endocrine abnormalities, hypogonadism. Wilms tumor in 10%.	Check endocrine status (esp adrenal). Possible difficult mask ventilation and intubation. Monitor blood glucose level. Prone to hypothermia. Caution with relaxants; monitor block. (See page 383 for Wilms tumor.)
	Dinner M, Goldin EZ, Ward R et al: Russell-Silver syndrome: anesthetic implications. Anesth Analg 78(6):1197–1199, 1994.	
Sipple syndrome (multiple endocrine adenomatosis (MEN2) type 2)	Three forms: MEN 2A, Familial medullary thyroid carcinoma and MEN 2B. Pheochromocytoma more common in 2A and 2B (bilateral in 75% of cases), medullary thyroid carcinoma, parathyroid adenoma (common in MEN 2A), multiple endocrine neoplasia. MEN 2B also presents with mucocutaneous neuromas and muscular hypotonia.	See pheochromocytoma. See page 380. Problem of multiple endocrine disorders. For MEN 2B, evaluate for presence of muscular hypotonia before considering muscle relaxants.
Sleep apnea syndromes	See also Chubby puffer syndrome. Disorders of breathing during sleep, including the following: (1) Central sleep apnea due to CNS immaturity (sudden infant death syndrome), trauma, infections, or neoplasms, and primary central alveolar hypoventilation (Ondine curse). Apnea occurs without evidence of respiratory muscle activity. (2) Obstructive sleep apnea due to obesity, adenotonsillar hypertrophy, Pierre Robin syndrome, or any other condition causing chronic airway obstruction. Apnea occurs because of obstruction and is accompanied by increased respiratory muscle activity. Response to CO_2 is decreased. Ventilatory depression with opiates	Review sleep study if done with attention to severity of nocturnal desaturation (Nadir <90 = caution). Assess airway carefully. Avoid preoperative sedation. Intubate and ventilate during anesthesia. Beware of acute obstruction during induction of anesthesia. Intubation may be difficult. Caution with opioids during and after anesthesia. Awaken patient completely before transfer to postanesthesia care unit (PACU). Monitor closely for apnea postoperatively. (See Chapter 10 for sleep apnea strategy during anesthesia).

Table continues on the following page.

Name	Description	Anesthesia Implications
	is markedly increased and opiate requirements for analgesia decreased. (3) Mixed forms. Medical history may include daytime somnolence, loud snoring, restless sleep, insomnia, fatigue. Children may be hyperactive and aggressive.	

Bandla P, Brooks LJ, Trimarchi T et al: Obstructive sleep apnea syndrome in children. Anesth Clinics N Am 23(3):535–549, 2005.

Name	Description	Anesthesia Implications
Smith-Lemli-Opitz syndrome	Inborn error of cholesterol synthesis. Microcephaly, mental retardation, genital and skeletal anomalies (including micrognathia), thymic hypoplasia, hypotonia; may have increased susceptibility to infection.	Use sterile technique. Airway and intubation problems. Use muscle relaxants with caution. Muscle rigidity with inhalational anesthetics has been described, but this disease is not associated with MH and has not been associated with rhabdomyolysis. Consider TIVA. Anesthesiology

Quezado ZM, Veihmeyer J, Schwartz L et al: Anesthesia and airway management of pediatric patients with Smith-Lemli-Opitz syndrome. Anesthesiology 97(4):1015–1019, 2002.

Name	Description	Anesthesia Implications
Sotos syndrome (cerebral gigantism)	Macrocephaly, dilated cerebral ventricles but normal ICP. Developmental delay. Hypotonia. Accelerated growth during childhood. Prone to hernias. Cardiac and GU abnormalities in a few patients. Reduced immune response.	Preoperative echocardiogram and EKG, SBE prophylazis if indicated. Care with asepsis. Intubation reported to be easy. Care with padding and positioning head. Hyperthermia during anesthesia is reported (not MH); monitor temperature and institute cooling as indicated.

Adhami EJ, Cancio-Babu CV: Anaesthesia in a child with Sotos syndrome. Paediatr Anaesth 13(9):835–840, 2003.

Name	Description	Anesthesia Implications
Stevens-Johnson syndrome (erythema multiforme)	Urticarial lesions; erosions of mouth, eyes, genitalia. Possible hypersensitivity to exogenous agents (drugs, infections, etc.). If pleural blebs are present, pneumothorax may occur. Dehydration and malnutrition are common. May have myocarditis,	Preoperatively, assess cardiac status, fluid status, and pulmonary function. Check for recent steroid therapy. Use sterile technique (reverse isolation). Oral lesions—avoid intubation and insertion of esophageal stethoscope, gentle pharyngeal suctioning. Use soft

		pericarditis. Medical care is similar to that of children with a burn injury; some may be on high-dose steroid therapy.	face mask with Vaseline gauze on skin. If intubation is required, secure tracheal tube with tracheostomy tape that is well padded; do not use adhesive tape. Monitoring is difficult (because of skin lesions) but essential; cover ECG pads with surgical lubricant and place beneath the patient. Warm the operating room to approximately 35-37 °C; danger of severe hypothermia. Monitor closely; serious arrhythmias and ventricular fibrillation may occur. IV infusion essential but avoid cutdowns if possible (possibility of infection). Ketamine is probably the best anesthetic agent.

Smith GB, Shribman AJ: Anaesthesia and severe skin disease. Anaesthesia 39(5):443-455, 1984.

Stickler syndrome	Autosomal dominant disorder with midface hypoplasia, retromicrognathia, cleft palate, and "Moon-face" appearance. Progressive myopia and retinal degeneration.	Anesthesia problems similar to Pierre Robin patients. Airway maintenance and intubation may be very difficult.

Kucukyavuz Z, Ozkaynak O, Tuzuner AM et al: Difficulties in anesthetic management of patients with micrognathia: report of a patient with Stickler syndrome. Oral Surg Oral Med Oral Pathol Oral Radiol Endodont 102(6):e33-e36, 2006.

Stiff baby syndrome (hyperekplexia, "startle disease")	Rare, genetic syndrome. Severe muscle rigidity appears at birth and persists for several years. Exaggerated startle response is present. Life-threatening spasms may be terminated by flexing the head and legs toward the trunk. Choking, vomiting, and difficulty swallowing may occur. EMG shows continuous muscle activity.	Use caution with muscle relaxants; monitor effects carefully. (Sevoflurane may cause fade on TOF monitor.) May be resistant to succinylcholine but have normal response to nondepolarizing muscle relaxants. Effect of neostigmine is normal. Opioids increase rigidity. Propofol may be appropriate. Monitor for perioperative apnea.

Garg R, Ramachandran R, Sharma P: Anaesthetic implications of hyperekplexia—'startle disease'. Anaesth Intens Care 36(2):254-256, 2008.

Table continues on the following page.

Name	Description	Anesthesia Implications
Still disease (juvenile rheumatoid arthritis)	See collagen diseases.	
Sturge-Weber syndrome	Cavernous angioma over trigeminal nerve distribution, usually unilateral. Developmental mesodermal capillary defect. Glaucoma. Intracranial calcification, convulsions, mental retardation. Possible laryngeal and tracheal involvement.	Often have port wine stains treated. Care with instrumentation of larynx in case of undiagnosed angioma. Care to prevent hypertension or raised intracular pressure during intubation or extubation. Often treated with repeat laser therapy. No other specific anesthetic problems.
Batra RK, Gulaya V, Madan R et al: Anaesthesia and the Sturge-Weber syndrome. Can J Anaesth 41(2):133–136, 1994.		
Supravalvar aortic stenosis with idiopathic infantile hypercalcemia	See Williams syndrome.	
Tangier disease (analphalipoproteinemia)	Low plasma high density lipoproteins; accumulation of cholesterol esters in large orange tonsils, spleen, and lymph nodes. Anemia and thrombocytopenia. Peripheral neuropathy and abnormal EMG; premature coronary disease (lipid deposits found in coronary arteries of a 6 year old).	Preoperatively assess cardiac/coronary arteries; Hb and platelet counts. Use caution with cardiac depressants and muscle relaxants. Monitor for cardiac ischemia. (No reports of ischemic heart disease in children.)
Mentis SW: Tangier disease. Anesth Analg 83(2):427–429, 1996.		
Tay-Sachs disease	See gangliosidosis GM2.	
Thomsen disease	See myotonia congenita.	
Telangiectasis, hemorrhagic	See Osler-Rendu-Weber syndrome.	
Thalassemia major (Cooley anemia)	Hereditary disease—may affect any race, but most common in Mediterranean and Southeast Asia.	Preoperatively assess cardiac function. Hemosiderosis may affect heart and hepatic function. Anemia may be

	Slow rate of Hb synthesis—high percentage of HbF is present. Low Hb levels require repeated transfusion leading to hemosiderosis.	severe. Facial deformity—overgrowth of maxilla may cause difficult intubation. Anesthesia considerations for the anemic patient (see page 180). Heterozygous form (thalassemia minor) poses no special anesthesia problems.
Thromboasthenia	See Glanzmann disease.	
Thrombocytopenia with absent radius	Episodic thrombocytopenia precipitated by stress, infection, surgery, etc. Platelets increase to normal by adulthood. CHD in 30% of cases.	Preoperatively assess cardiac function if CHD present. Platelet transfusion for surgery or bleeding. Avoid elective surgery in first year (35%–40% mortality from intracranial hemorrhage).

Hall JG, Levin J, Kuhn JP et al: Thrombocytopenia with absent radius. Medicine (Baltimore) 48:411, 1969.

Thrombocytopenia with eczema and repeated infections	See Wiskott-Aldrich syndrome.	
Thrombotic thrombocytopenic purpura	See Moschcowitz disease.	
Tourette syndrome	Complex neuropsychiatric disorder with onset in childhood. Attention deficit disorder progresses to spasmodic repetitious movements that may become powerful muscle jerks. Patient also may exhibit coprolalia (profane speech) and echolalia (repetitions). Treated with haloperidol, clonidine, or pimozide.	Establish rapport with patient and family. Continue medications. Sedate preoperatively. No specific anesthesia regimen is indicated, except that pimozide may cause prolonged Q-T interval syndrome (see page 47).

Morrison JE Jr, Lockhart CH: Tourette syndrome: anesthetic implications. Anesth Analg 65(2):200–202, 1986.

Table continues on the following page.

Name	Description	Anesthesia Implications
Treacher-Collins syndrome (mandibulofacial dysostosis)	Micrognathia, aplastic zygoma, microstomia, choanal atresia, coloboma of eyelids. Patients often have cleft palate and cardiac anomalies. Very like Pierre Robin syndrome.	Preoperatively assess cardiac function and airway. Possible very difficult mask airway and difficult tracheal intubation. LMA can be useful in facilitating fiberoptic intubation. Some children require tracheotomy.

Inada T, Fujise K, Tachibana K et al: Ororacheal intubation through the laryngeal mask airway in paediatric patients with Treacher-Collins syndrome. Paediatr Anaesth 5:129, 1995.
Nargozian CN: The airway in patients with craniofacial abnormalities. Pediatr Anesth 14:53–59, 2004.

Name	Description	Anesthesia Implications
Trismus-pseudocampto-dactyly (Dutch-Kentucky syndrome)	Autosomal dominant condition. Decreased mouth opening due to enlarged coronoid process of the mandible and/or abnormal ligaments plus flexion deformity of the fingers when wrist is extended. Short stature and foot deformities may occur. May present for surgery to mandible.	Extremely difficult intubation. May require blind nasal or fiberoptic technique.

Browder FH, Lew D, Shahbazian TS: Anesthetic management of a patient with Dutch-Kentucky syndrome. Anesthesiology 65(2):218–219, 1986.
Vaghadia H, Blackstock D: Anaesthetic implications for the trismus pseudocampodactyly (Dutch-Kentucky or Hecht Beals) syndrome. Can J Anesth 35:80–85, 1988.

Name	Description	Anesthesia Implications
Trisomies Trisomy 13 Trisomy 18[E] Trisomy 21	See Patau syndrome. See Edwards syndrome. See Down syndrome.	

Tuberous sclerosis	Neurocutaneous condition with hamartoma growth in body. Multisystem disease: sebaceous adenoma of skin, epilepsy, mental retardation, intracranial calcification, seizures. May have tumors in brain, lungs, and kidneys; pyelonephritis and renal failure may occur. Cardiac rhabdomyomas are benign but may occur in up to 90% of neonates. These tumors tend to remain the same in size (as the heart grows less important) or resolve spontaneously.	Preoperatively assess renal and cardiac function indicated; cardiac tumors tend to resolve spontaneously but may cause right outflow tract obstruction, particularly in infants. Care with drugs excreted by kidney. Possible cardiac arrhythmia and rupture of lung cysts. Anesthetic management depends on preoperative examination and limitations of organ functions found. Maintain normothermia and normocarbia to prevent seizures. Check anticonvulsant levels postoperatively.

Diaz JH: Perioperative management of children with congenital phakomatoses. Pediatr Anesth. 10:121–128, 2000.

Turner syndrome (gonadal dysgenesis)	XO females. Short stature, infantile genitalia, webbed neck; possible micrognathia. CHD coarctation, dissecting aneurysm of aorta or PS. Hypothyroidism in some cases. Renal anomalies in more than 50% of cases.	Preoperatively assess cardiac and renal function. Intubation may be difficult. Care with drugs excreted by kidneys.

Loscalzo ML: Turner syndrome. Ped Rev 29(7):219–227, 2008.
Mashour GA, Sunder N, Acquadro MA: Anesthetic management of Turner syndrome: a systematic approach. J Clin Anesth 17(2):128–130, 2005.

Umbilical hernia in infancy	Be alert to possibility of Beckwith syndrome.	

Urbach-Wiethe disease (cutaneous mucosal hyalinosis)	Hoarseness or aphonia (hyaline deposits in larynx and pharynx) and skin eruption. Tongue may be thickened. Mucous membranes thickened, dry, and friable. Intracranial calcification and epilepsy may develop.	Avoid anticholinergics (excessive drying). Gentle laryngoscopy and intubation to prevent mucosal trauma. Vocal cords may be thickened. Airway and intubation may be difficult; requiring fiberoptic intubation. If epilepsy is diagnosed, halothane, isoflurane, and TIVA are the preferred anesthetics.

Kelly JE, Simpson MT, Jonathan D et al: Lipoid proteinosis: Urbach-Wiethe disease. Br J Anaesth 63(5):609–611, 1989.

Table continues on the following page.

Name	Description	Anesthesia Implications
VATER association (VACTERL association)	A nonrandom association of defects: V-vertebral anomalies (congenital scoliosis); A-anal atresia; T-tracheoesophageal fistula; E-esophageal atresia; R-renal anomalies; (C-cardiac disease and L-limb defects also in VACTERL).	Examine neonates with any of these features carefully for other congenital lesions. Preoperatively assess cardiac and renal function. Anesthesia management dictated by considerations of individual lesions.
Bleicher MA, Melmed AP, Bogaerts XV et al: VATER association and unrecognized bronchopulmonary foregut malformation complicating anesthesia. Mt Sinai J Med 50(5):435–438, 1983.		
Velocardiofacial syndrome	A phenotypic variant of the 22q deletion syndrome. Speech difficulties due to velopharyngeal anomalies, learning disability (mild), CHD (especially VSD), and characteristic facies: large nose with broad nasal bridge, vertically long face, narrow palpebral fissures, and retruded mandible.	Preoperatively assess cardiac function if indicated. Airway and intubation may be difficult. May present for pharyngoplasty. Obstructive sleep apnea may occur after pharyngoplasty and may cause death. Postoperative monitoring for apnea is recommended.
von Gierke disease Type I (glycogen storage disease)	Mental retardation, hepatomegaly, renal hyperplasia, stomatitis, lactic acidosis, leucopenia, and bleeding diathesis. Fasting causes hypoglycemia and convulsions. Severe biochemical disturbances; unresponsive to epinephrine and glucagon. May also have Fanconi syndrome (see Fanconi syndrome).	Continuous IV glucose infusion preoperatively and perioperatively. Monitor blood sugar and acid-base balance. Caution with propofol —report of postoperatively pancreatitis in a patient with this disease. Type III (Cori disease; Forbes disease) Similar to but milder than type I. Type VI (Hers disease) Similar to but milder than type I.
Shenkman Z, Golub Y, Mereyk S et al: Anaesthetic management of a patient with glycogen storage disease type 1b. Can J Anaesth 43:467–470, 1996. Bustamante SE, Appachi E: Acute pancreatitis after anesthesia with propofol in a child with glycogen storage disease type IA. Paediatr Anaesth 16:680–683, 2006.		

von Hippel-Lindau syndrome	Retinal angiomas and cerebellar hemangioblastomas; pheochromocytoma in some; may have pulmonary, pancreatic, hepatic, adrenal, renal cysts. Paroxysmal hypertension due to cerebellar tumor or pheochromocytoma.	Preoperatively assess renal and hepatic function and investigate for pheochromocytoma (urinary vanillylmandelic acid). Hypertensive crises may occur.

Gurunathan U, Korula G: Unsuspected pheochromocytoma: von Hippel-Lindau disease. J Neurosurg Anesthesiol 16:26-28, 2004.

von Recklinghausen disease (neurofibromatosis)	Café au lait spots (>5): tumors in all parts of the CNS and peripheral tumors associated with nerve trunks. Tumors may occur in the larynx or trachea and right ventricular outflow tract); Kyphoscoliosis in 50%; neck may be unstable. May have fibrosing alveolitis "honey comb (cystic) lung" predisposing to pulmonary problems. Renal artery dysplasia (hypertension) common. Pheochromocytoma in 1% (All these patients should be investigated—urinary vanillylmandelic acid).	Check pulmonary, renal, and cardiac function as indicated. Intubation could be complicated by tumor. Caution with neck. Test response to neuromuscular drugs: effects of depolarizing and nondepolarizing muscle relaxants may be prolonged. If kidneys are involved, care with drugs excreted by kidneys.

Delgado JM, de la Matta Martin M: Anaesthetic implications of von Recklinghausen's neurofibromatosis. Paediatr Anaesth 12:374, 2002.

von Willebrand disease (pseudohemophilia)	Prolonged bleeding time (decreased von Willebrand factor and associated decreased factor VIII activity leading to defective platelet adhesiveness) and capillary abnormality. History of bruising and bleeding (menorrhagia, epistaxis, etc.). Several types of the disease exist and determine the response	Do not use salicylates (effect on platelets, possible gastrointestinal bleeding). Monitor factor VIII and bleeding time, maintain factor VIII at > 50% activity.

Table continues on the following page.

Name	Description	Anesthesia Implications
	to therapy. IV desmopressin acetate (DDAVP) is effective therapy for type 1 and some type 2 patients, but may exacerbate others. (Consult your hematologist.) Type 2 and type 3 patients require factor VIII concentrates. Bleeding may be controlled by transfusions of fresh blood or fresh-frozen plasma and/or cryoprecipitate. Antifibrinolytics may help.	
	Lee JW: Von Willebrand disease, hemophilia A and B, and other factor deficiencies. Int Anesth Clin 42:59–76, 2004.	
Weaver syndrome	Skeletal overgrowth leading to craniofacial and digital abnormalities. Relative micrognathia, short neck, and anterior larynx lead to difficult intubation.	Caution with airway and intubation. Difficulties may be less in older children.
	Crawford MW, Rohan D: The upper airway in Weaver syndrome. Paediatr Anaesth 15:893–6, 2005.	
Weber-Christian disease (chronic nonsuppurative panniculitis)	Necrosis of fat in any situation, including the following: Retroperitoneal tissue: may cause acute or chronic adrenal insufficiency. Pericardium: leads to restrictive pericarditis. Meninges: causes convulsions.	Preoperatively assess cardiac and renal function. Prevent trauma to fat by heat, cold, or pressure. Maintain blood volume; use cardiac depressant drugs and drugs excreted by the kidneys with caution.
	Spivak JL, Lindo S, Coleman M: Weber-Christian disease complicated by consumption coagulopathy and microangiopathic hemolytic anemia. Johns Hopkins Med J 126:344, 1970.	
Welander distal myopathy (late distal hereditary myopathy)	Initially involves distal muscles. Onset after third decade of life. Prognosis for life good, for ambulation poor. See also Werdnig-Hoffman disease.	May require spinal fusion. Use extreme care with propofol, thiopental, and muscle relaxants; use respiratory depressant drugs with caution.

Werdnig-Hoffman disease (infantile muscular atrophy)	Onset in infancy; more severe than Welander muscular atrophy. Feeding difficulties; aspiration of stomach contents. Chronic respiratory problems. Most patients die before puberty.	Minimal anesthesia required. Succinylcholine is contraindicated (due to hyperkalemia). Use muscle relaxants or respiratory depressant drugs with caution. Ventilatory support may be required, and weaning may be difficult.
Werner syndrome (multiple endocrine adenomatosis (MEN1) type 1)	Hyperparathyroidism, tumors of pituitary and pancreatic islet cells (hypoglycemia), gastric ulcer. Carcinoid tumors of bronchial tree are common. Renal failure due to stones. Preoperatively assess for renal and pituitary dysfunction: presence of carcinoid tumor. Preoperative consult with endocrinologist for specific management issues. Administer glucose at maintenance rates and monitor perioperative glucose values.	Control blood glucose carefully. See also carcinoid tumors (p. 551).
Capell BC, Collins FS, Nabel EG: Mechanisms of cardiovascular disease in accelerated aging syndromes. Circ Res 101:13–26, 2007.		
Werner syndrome	Premature aging; diabetes in 50%, mental retardation in 50%, early cataracts, osteomyelitis-like bone lesions, cardiac infarction and failure.	Preoperatively assess for evidence of myocardial ischemia and dysfunction, and diabetes.
Valkenburg AJ, de Leeuw TG, Machotta A et al: Extremely low preanesthetic BIS values in two children with West syndrome and lissencephaly. Pediatr Anaesth 18:446–448, 2008.		
West syndrome	Infantile spasms, hypsarrhythmia on EEG, and psychomotor impairment. Seizures, neurologic deficits, lissencephaly, and severe mental deficiency. Long-term treatment with anticonvulsants required.	Very low BIS values noted in "awake" patient with paradoxical changes during anesthesia induction. BIS monitor may be unreliable to monitor anesthesia depth. Parents may be helpful in determining when their child is "awake."

Table continues on the following page.

Name	Description	Anesthesia Implications
Williams syndrome (elfin facies syndrome)	Cardiac anomalies: usually supravalvular aortic stenosis, peripheral pulmonary artery obstruction, and mental retardation (IQ 40–80), elfin facies. Fixed cardiac output and myocardial ischemia leading to dyspnea and angina. Very high anesthetic risk and difficult to resuscitate. Sudden death may occur. Hypercalcemia, require low calcium diet, steroids, and cardiac corrective surgery. Hypothyroidism and renal abnormalities may be present.	Preoperatively assess cardiac and renal function, and calcium. Check steroid history. Monitor calcium levels perioperatively. Mask ventilation and intubation may be difficult. High incidence of cardiac arrest during induction of anesthesia. A careful smooth slow inhalation induction with modest doses of inhalation agent may be used, but an intravenous induction with an opioid based anesthetic is recommended. Avoid cardiac depressants and drugs causing tachycardia. Transesophageal echocardiography may aid anesthetic management. Also check website: www.williams-syndrome.org
Medley J, Russo P, Tobias JD: Perioperative care of the patient with Williams syndrome. Pediatr Anaesth 15:243–247, 2005.		
Wilson disease (hepatolenticular degeneration)	Decreased ceruloplasmin; copper deposits, especially in liver and CNS motor nuclei. Renal tubular acidosis; hepatic failure due to fibrosis.	Muscle relaxants: succinylcholine prolonged apnea rare despite pseudocholinesterase reduction. Nondepolarizing relaxants unpredictable due to globulin binding; titrate drugs and monitor block. Vecuronium predominantly hepatic degraded, caution use. Sevoflurane for induction; isoflurane and desflurane slightly preferred for maintenance. Care with drugs excreted by kidneys.
Green DW, Ashley EM: The choice of inhalation anaesthetic for major abdominal surgery in children with liver disease. Paediatr Anaesth 12:665–673, 2002.		
Wilson-Mikity syndrome	Prematurity (<1500 g birth weight); severe chronic lung disease leading to generalized fibrosis with cystic areas, repeated chest infection, aspiration,	Check respiratory and cardiac status preoperatively. May have a history of steroid therapy. Monitor carefully postoperatively for apnea.

	right ventricular failure. Steroids may be given to try to prevent pulmonary fibrosis. Pathogenesis unknown; possibly due to O_2 toxicity or barotrauma.
	Stasic AF: Perioperative implications of common respiratory problems. Sem Pediatr Surg 13:174–180, 2004.
Wiskott-Aldrich syndrome	Decreased production of platelets; hypersusceptibility to severe herpes simplex infections (disordered immune mechanism), eczema, asthma. May have RES malignancies. Most die before 10 yr of age, many from generalized herpes or opportunistic infection.	Antibiotic prophylaxis may be indicated preoperatively. Transfusions of blood and platelets may be required; bone marrow transplantation has been used. All blood products must be irradiated to prevent graft-versus-host reaction. Use sterile technique (reverse isolation).
	Notarangelo LD, Miao CH, Ochs HD: Wiskott-Aldrich syndrome. Curr Opin Hemat 15:30–36, 2008.	
Wolf-Parkinson-White (WPW) syndrome	Anomalous conduction path between atria and ventricles. ECG: Short P-R interval; prolonged QRS with phasic variation in 40%. Prone to paroxysmal supraventricular tachycardia (SVT). May have other cardiac defects. Infants, especially preterm, are very prone to SVT. May be associated with CHD. Prone to arrhythmias. Paroxysmal SVT on induction of anesthesia has been reported; treat with countershock.	Preoperatively review cardiac status with cardiologist. Avoid atropine, halothane, or pancuronium. Thiopental, isoflurane, and vecuronium are suitable agents; also rocuronium, sevoflurane, and opioids. Avoid use of neostigmine. During electrophysiologic studies, propofol may be anesthetic of choice having little effect on abnormal conduction pathways.
	Perez ER, Bartolome FB, Carretero PS et al: Electrophysiological effects of sevoflurane in comparison with propofol in children with Wolff-Parkinson-White syndrome. [Spanish] Revista Espanola de Anestesiologia y Reanimacion. 55(1):26–31, 2008.	
Wolman disease (familial xanthomatosis)	Failure to thrive because of xanthomatous visceral changes: adrenal calcification. Resembles Niemann-Pick disease, with hepatosplenomegaly, hypersplenism, and foam cell infiltration (of all tissues, including myocardium.) Death usually by 6 mo of age.	Treatment entirely supportive.
Zellweger syndrome	See cerebrohepatorenal syndrome.	

Cardiopulmonary Resuscitation, Including Neonatal Resuscitation

Cardiopulmonary resuscitation (CPR) is concerned with the restoration of pulmonary and cardiovascular function, and the prevention of neurologic damage. Initially, it consists of artificial ventilation and artificial circulation by whatever means are immediately available. This is termed *basic life support*. Its object is to prevent clinical death from progressing to biologic death before other remedial measures (i.e., *advanced life support*) can be instituted.

As in adults, heroic resuscitative efforts may not be indicated in children with lethal terminal disease. This is a decision that should be made in advance and clearly documented and communicated.

The overall success rate for pediatric CPR is possibly worse than for adults, especially if success is defined as long-term survival without neurologic deficit. A possible reason is that the majority of cardiac arrests in children result from hypoxemia. In such children, it must be assumed that by the time the heart has suffered hypoxia enough to stop it, the brain has also suffered hypoxia enough to severely damage it. This being so, every effort must be directed at detecting and treating any respiratory compromise before it leads to serious hypoxemia.

PREVENTION OF CARDIAC ARREST

Awareness of precipitating factors is essential in preventing cardiac arrest in children.

Common causes include:

1. Failure of ventilation:
   a. Due to central depression, airway obstruction, or primary pulmonary disorders
   b. Secondary to regurgitation and pulmonary aspiration. As a result of neurologic and neuromuscular disorders (i.e., residual neuromuscular block)
2. Hypovolemia.
3. Toxicity (drugs, poisons, toxins).
4. Primary cardiac disorders. (These account for only a small percentage of cardiac arrests on the general wards of a pediatric hospital.)

Prevention requires:

1. Recognition of potential causes
2. Constant surveillance
3. Early recognition of respiratory failure

Special Hazards for Children

Anesthesiologists should constantly be aware of factors that may be insignificant in the adult but may rapidly be life-threatening in infants and children.

1. The upper airway may become obstructed by:
   a. Laryngospasm (common); due to small amounts of mucus or blood or inadequate or unwisely planned anesthesia (see Chapter 4, page 92).
   b. Hypertrophied adenoidal tissue and/or enlarged tonsils, which may completely block the airway.
   c. The relatively large tongue, associated with:
      i. Muscle flaccidity in the anesthetized patient
      ii. Inadvertent displacement or compression of submental soft tissue and tongue by the anesthesiologist's fingers
      iii. Inadequate neck extension
      iv. Inadequate elevation of the mandible
      v. Premature removal of an artificial airway
   d. Regurgitated stomach contents—a common occurrence because of the frequency of feedings

Remember: Infants have large tongues and may be primarily nose-breathers. If the nasal airway is inadequate, an oral airway should be inserted without delay.

2. Ventilation may be compromised if the stomach becomes inflated, usually a result of
   a. Excessive inflation pressures
   b. Partial airway obstruction

   After protecting the airway with an endotracheal tube, pass a No. 10 or 12 suction catheter and aspirate stomach contents to reduce the possibility of aspiration.

3. Blood volumes are relatively small—significant hypovolemia may develop rapidly.

Routine Precautions

Preoperative

1. Be prepared to give atropine to all young children who are scheduled for laryngoscopy/tracheal intubation or to receive cholinergic drugs (i.e., halothane, succinylcholine), or have surgery that may elicit dangerous reflexes. Vagal reflexes are brisk and may lead to cardiac arrest. The longer you delay giving atropine, the longer it will take to have effect. (**N.B.** atropine does not correct hypoxemia.)
2. Always give 100% O_2 before intubating the trachea in children. (Desaturation occurs much more rapidly in children, particularly infants, than in adolescents.) Intubate the trachea as quickly and smoothly as possible.
3. Select the endotracheal tube size carefully, secure it firmly, and check its position; confirm $EtCO_2$ and listen to both sides of the chest. Position and support the tracheal tube so that it cannot kink. (These procedures are critical in children.)

Perioperative

1. Carefully maintain a patent airway and adequate ventilation.
2. Monitor the following constantly:
   a. Heart and lung functions by stethoscope, ECG and NIBP.
   b. SaO_2 and $EtCO_2$ (Do not disable alarms.)
   c. Body temperature
   d. Blood loss
3. Measure carefully all gases, vapors, and drugs; always read the drug label.

4. Measure fluid losses accurately and replace as indicated. (Even a small loss is significant in a small child). Ensure that you have a reliable, generous sized, IV route before you allow surgery to start.
5. Remember that rapid infusion of blood products may cause hyperkalemia or hypocalcemia (especially into a central vein in small infants).
6. Prevent unintentional pressure on the chest and abdominal wall from dressings, hands, surgical assistants leaning on drapes, and so on.
7. If problems arise, advise other members of the team (especially the surgeon) immediately.

Postoperative
Note: Cardiac arrest in the postanesthesia care unit (PACU) is as likely as in the operating room.

1. For all infants and all seriously ill children: do not extubate the trachea unless and until the child is reacting vigorously.
2. If possible, all children should be transported to the PACU in the lateral position, with the upper leg flexed at the hip and knee and the neck moderately extended (the tonsil or recovery position).
3. In the PACU:
    a. Immediately monitor SaO_2, NIBP and ECG.
    b. Provide a full report to the PACU nursing staff regarding underlying medical problems, surgical problems, medication doses and time of administration, and anticipated possible PACU problems.
    c. Ensure that the child remains safely positioned with a clear airway.
        i. Order humidified O_2 by mask until the child is responding well.
        ii. Ensure that vital signs are recorded and reported to you.
    d. Do not leave until you are assured vital signs are stable and have handed over care of your child to a nurse.
    e. Before discharge from the PACU, ensure that the danger of drug-induced respiratory depression has passed and that the child is fully conscious.
    f. Some neonates and infants need to be disturbed frequently to stimulate respiration.
    g. All former preterm infants of less than 60 weeks conceptual age and those with a history of chronic respiratory disease should be monitored on an apnea alarm for at least 12 hours apnea-free or 24 hours (Chapter 2, page 19).
    h. Children with obstructive sleep apnea (OSA) require extended observation and monitoring and may be sensitive to the respiratory depressant effects of opioids (see Chapter 10, page 283).

Treatment of Arrhythmias

Arrhythmias that cause hemodynamic compromise or those that might progress to cardiac arrest must be promptly treated. The advice of a pediatric cardiologist should be obtained whenever this is possible.

Supraventricular Tachycardia (SVT)

a. SVT may be difficult to differentiate from sinus tachycardia, but the history and the heart rate (SVT rates greater than 220 bpm in infants or greater than 180 bpm in children) usually clarify this.

b. Early consultation with a pediatric cardiologist is recommended for hemodynamically stable VT. Vagal maneuvers (Valsalva maneuver or ice applied to face) are recommended as initial therapy. Adenosine may be administered and if this is unsuccessful amiodarone may be indicated (page 560 for dosing). If circulatory instability is present, immediate synchronized electrical cardioversion (0.5 to 1 joule/kg) is recommended.

Ventricular Tachycardia (VT) and Fibrillation (VF)

a. For VT with hypotension but with a palpable pulse immediate synchronized cardioversion is recommended. Children with less hemodynamic compromise should be assessed for the cause of the VT and may be sedated before cardioversion.

b. For pulseless VT and VF, very prompt defibrillation is recommended. If this is unsuccessful or VT recurs, amiodarone 5 mg/kg may be considered.

Non-shockable Rhythm (asystole & PEA (pulseless electrical activity))

Asystole and PEA are the most common ECG findings in cardiac arrest in infants and children. PEA is a cluster of slow, wide QRS complexes in the absence of palpable pulses. CPR should be continued, defibrillation is not indicated. Underlying causes should be sought.

CARDIOPULMONARY RESUSCITATION

The guidelines for cardiopulmonary resuscitation and neonatal resuscitation are based on peer reviewed scientific publications that are critically analyzed to derive a consensus. This appendix incorporates the recommendations from their most recent International Liaison Committee on Resuscitation (ILCOR) deliberations (2005).

Basic Life Support

N.B. For basic life support in hospitals, use a bag and mask as soon as possible to prevent risk of infection to hospital personnel. Make sure that such equipment is immediately available and functioning in all patient-care areas. In rare instances, it may be necessary to resort to mouth-to-mouth resuscitation.

Do not leave the child. Call for help and equipment (including a defibrillator).

Begin with the ABCs:

A. Airway: check patency, apply jaw thrust.
B. Breathing (four ventilations) preferably with bag and mask.
C. Cardiac activity: check with stethoscope—alternatives brachial artery in an infant, femoral or carotid artery in a child.

When called to resuscitate a child, assess the situation immediately according to the following priorities:

A. Check Ventilation
   1. *If there are respiratory efforts:*
      a. Position the child in the lateral position (recovery position) to provide a clear airway and decrease the risk of aspiration should vomiting occur.
      b. Give O_2 by mask as soon as it becomes available.
   2. *If respiratory efforts are present, but evidence of airway obstruction is present* (breath sounds absent, intercostal retraction, flaring of lateral chest margins, cyanosis):
      a. Pull the tongue or mandible forward (by pressing behind the mandibular condyles) and remove any foreign matter from the pharynx, keeping the mouth slightly open.
      b. Extend the neck if necessary (Caution if neck injury—but remember that ventilation is the first priority.)
      c. Give O_2 by mask.
      d. Check for improved chest movement and breath sounds.
B. If There Is No Respiratory Effort or Ventilation Appears Inadequate
   1. Begin positive-pressure ventilation at once.
   2. Ventilate directly, mouth to mouth if necessary, until resuscitation equipment is placed in your hand. (The small infant face necessitates application of your mouth to the infant's mouth and nose). An infant's tidal volume is small (8 to 10 ml/kg); therefore only puffs are necessary.

As soon as possible, begin ventilation using a bag and mask with oxygen. Assure adequate expansion of the chest with each breath.

C. If cardiac activity is undetectable by auscultation, or by femoral, carotid, or brachial artery palpation (or if the heart rate is <60 bpm despite ventilation and oxygenation and there are signs of poor perfusion[pallor, cyanosis]).

1. Start external cardiac compression at once ("Push Hard, Push Fast"):
   a. The site of compression in an infant is one finger-breadth below the intermammary line; in a child, it is over the lower sternum, one finger-breadth above the xiphisternum. In an infant, two fingers may be used. In a child, the heel of the hand should be used.
   b. Depth of compression: one third to one half of the anteroposterior diameter of the chest; between compressions, release completely to allow the chest wall to fully recoil
   c. Rate of compression: infants, children, and adolescents, 100/min.
   d. Rate of ventilation (basic life support—unintubated airway):
      i. Single-person technique: 2 ventilations for 30 compressions
      ii. Two-person technique: 2 ventilations to 15 compressions
      iii. For intubated airways, a rate of 100 cardiac compressions per minute and 8 to 10 ventilations with 100% O_2 per minute should be initiated immediately. Prevent hyperventilation.
      iv. Do not interrupt the compressions for ventilation.
      v. Apply cardiac compressions to infants by encircling the chest with your hands (Figure II-1). This method results in a larger cardiac output than anterior sternal compression alone.

Defibrillation

Early defibrillation is recommended for children who have ventricular fibrillation or pulseless ventricular tachycardia. These are more likely when there has been a sudden unexpected arrest.

1. For infants and children weighing less than 20 kg, use pediatric defibrillator plates (diameter of 4.5 cm for infants and 8 cm for children).
2. Set the machine to deliver shocks appropriate to the child's size (to maximize the chance of success and minimize the danger of electrically induced myocardial damage); 2 joules (watt-seconds)/kg should be the initial setting. If this is unsuccessful, the dose should be doubled.
3. Give one shock and then immediately resume CPR.
4. Many AED's have the potential to detect pediatric "shockable" rhythms and can be adjusted to deliver appropriate energy to each shock. Ensure that AED's installed in a pediatric care environment conform to these requirements.

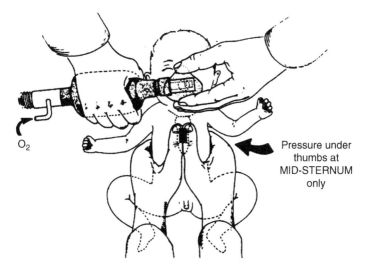

Figure II-1 Two-handed method of external cardiac compression. Note how both hands encircle the chest and how both thumbs are used for cardiac compression. (From Todres D, Rogers MC: Method of external cardiac massage in the newborn infant. J Pediatr 86:781, 1975, with permission.)

5. Children who are digitalized should be treated with the reduced power settings initially; then the power setting is gradually increased. Normal doses of countershock may cause irreversible cardiac arrest in the presence of bound digitalis in the heart muscle.

ADVANCED LIFE SUPPORT

The foregoing provides only basic interim resuscitation. Most children also require:

1. Ventilation with O_2 as soon as it is available. Ventilation and oxygenation are the first line of therapy for the acidosis that accompanies cardiac arrest.
2. Establish an airway by intubating the trachea, a cuffed tube may be used when appropriate to protect the airway. (The laryngeal mask airway may be useful in some instances). Exhaled CO_2 detection is recommended for early confirmation of successful intubation and to ensure adequate pulmonary circulation with chest compressions.
3. Definitive ECG diagnosis of cardiac activity and defibrillation if indicated (see previous discussion).

4. Establish an intravenous or intraosseous route for drug administration. Intratracheal drug administration is no longer recommended.
5. Supportive drugs, primarily epinephrine (see later discussion).
6. Further pharmacologic and medical treatment, including fluid replacement, as indicated.
7. Consideration of the possibility of lung injury by aspirated acidic gastric contents.
8. Early assessment of neurologic function—plan early and continue treatment to minimize and prevent further hypoxic-ischemic brain damage.

DRUG THERAPY

Although subsequent drug therapy is necessarily individualized, a standard initial protocol is advantageous.

1. Epinephrine: To be maximally effective, it must be given intravenously (preferably into a central vein) or, if this is not possible, by the intraosseous route.
   a. Initial and subsequent doses: 10 μg/kg (0.1 ml/kg of a 1:10,000 solution).
   b. High dose (100 μg/kg) epinephrine is no longer recommended (except possibly in the treatment of ß-blocker overdose).
2. Vasopressin has been successful in some cases of prolonged cardiac arrest but has not resulted in increased survival to a neurologically intact hospital discharge.
3. Dopamine infusion may be required for continued hypotension and poor tissue perfusion; 5 to 20 μg/kg/min may be titrated to achieve the desired effect.
4. Sodium bicarbonate administration is no longer recommended as a routine; but it might be considered in prolonged cardiac arrest for documented continuing severe metabolic acidosis despite adequate ventilation, oxygenation, and chest compressions. It may also be useful in the treatment of hyperkalemia, hypermagnesemia, or tricyclic antidepressant overdose.
N.B. Administration of excessive doses of sodium bicarbonate produces hyperosmolarity, hypernatremia, hypokalemia, decreased ionized calcium, impaired cardiac action, and possibly severe alkalosis after recovery.
5. Calcium is no longer recommended except as the definitive treatment for hyperkalemic-induced arrhythmias or arrest and citrate-induced hypocalcemia.

6. Glucose: Documented hypoglycemia should be treated by glucose infusions. Otherwise, avoid any glucose administration because hyperglycemia (glucose >200 mg/dl) may compromise neurologic outcome after a hypoxic event.

Route of Administration of Drugs

Inject epinephrine into a central line, if one is available; otherwise, use a peripheral intravenous or intraosseous line. The tracheal route is only used as a last resort.

Intracardiac injections should not be made. Damage to the heart and coronary arteries and/or a pneumothorax may result.

Fluid Replacement

1. Insert a large-bore intravenous cannula as soon as possible:
   a. To provide a route for drug therapy.
   b. For rapid replacement of fluid. (In cardiac arrest, hypoxic capillaries leak rapidly, diminishing the circulating blood volume.)
2. Replace losses initially with crystalloids and later with colloids (plasma or blood) as indicated.

   N.B.:

   a. Even a child previously in congestive heart failure needs infusions totaling at least 10% of the expected blood volume (EBV; equal to approximately 1% of body weight).
   b. With recovery, the extravasated fluid returns slowly to the vascular compartment, giving time for assessment of fluid volume and a decision as to whether diuretic therapy is necessary.
3. Avoid the use of dextrose-containing solutions. They may cause hyperglycemia, which may compromise cerebral survival. If hypoglycemia is suspected, it should be confirmed by blood glucose determination and treated accordingly.

Postresuscitation Care

Emphasis is placed on this as being critical to a favorable outcome.

1. Hyperventilation may be harmful and should be avoided maintain normocapnia.
2. Induced hypothermia (32 °C to 34 °C) for 12 to 24 hours should be considered for children who remain comatose after CPR.

3. Prevention of hyperthermia is recommended.
4. Hemodynamic support using vasoactive drugs (e.g., dopamine) should be considered to improve the circulatory status.
5. Target blood glucose levels to normal levels.
6. Restrict fluid replacement: avoid large infusions of crystalloid solutions once cardiovascular stability is ensured.
7. Treat seizure activity with phenobarbitone and/or phenytoin (Dilantin).
8. Obtain an early neurologic consultation.
9. Maintain cerebral perfusion pressure.

Suggested Reading

American Heart Association. 2005 American Heart Association (AHA) guidelines for cardiopulmonary resuscitation (CPR) and emergency cardiovascular care (ECC) of pediatric and neonatal patients: pediatric basic life support. Pediatrics 117(5):e989–e1004, 2006.

International Liaison Committee on Resuscitation. The International Liaison Committee on Resuscitation (ILCOR) consensus on science with treatment recommendations for pediatric and neonatal patients: pediatric basic and advanced life support. [Journal Article. Practice Guideline] Pediatrics 117(5):e955–e977, 2006.

Berg MD, Nadkarni VM, and Berg RA: Cardiopulmonary resuscitation in children. Curr Opin Crit Care 14(3):254–260, 2008.

Dingeman RS, Mitchell EA, Meyer EC, et al: Parent presence during complex invasive procedures and cardiopulmonary resuscitation: a systematic review of the literature. Pediatrics 120(4):842–854, 2007.

Sharman M and Meert KL: What is the right dose of epinephrine? Pediatr Crit Care Med 6(5):592–594, 2005.

NEONATAL RESUSCITATION

The anesthesiologist is frequently called upon to assist at or manage the care of the neonate immediately after birth.

Neonatal resuscitation must be based on a detailed knowledge of the normal physiologic changes that occur during transition to extrauterine life (see Chapter 2) plus a recognition of the pathologic processes in the mother or the fetus that may affect the infant at this time.

Most infants require little help. Those born at term, with clear amniotic fluid, who are crying or breathing and have good tone should be dried and kept warm. No further interventions are necessary.

Others, however, require rapid intervention if serious sequelae are to be prevented. Preexisting maternal or fetal disease and/or events during labor may affect the neonate's status after delivery. Frequently, infants at risk may be recognized before birth, and preparations can then be made for their immediate resuscitation on delivery. However, some infants who have demonstrated no antenatal signs of distress may need urgent intervention after birth.

Immediate Assessment of the Neonate

A rapid assessment must be made to determine the extent of stepwise treatment that is required. This determination is made on the basis of respirations, heart rate, and color. The steps in resuscitation are:

A. Clearing the airway, positioning, stimulating
B. Ventilation
C. Chest compressions
D. Medications or volume expansion

Procedures for Neonatal Resuscitation

These are the latest recommendations (ILCOR 2005) with some background information:

1. Assess Respirations
If the infant is breathing but cyanotic give oxygen; if cyanosis persists, then ventilate.
If the infant has apnea or HR less than 100, then ventilate.
2. Assess Heart Rate
If heart rate is less than 60 bpm, continue to ventilate and apply chest compressions.
Reassess heart rate; if heart rate remains less than 60 bpm, despite effective ventilation and compressions, then:
Administer epinephrine (10 to 30 μg/kg IV)
Augment blood volume (10 ml/kg isotonic crystalloid)

Some Notes

If bag-mask ventilation is unsuccessful in achieving good ventilation, intubate the trachea immediately. (In some instances, a laryngeal mask airway may be useful as an alternative)

Initial Resuscitation: Oxygen vs. Room Air

Whether to use supplementary oxygen or air to ventilate the lungs in the neonate is controversial. The use of oxygen has been associated with potentially adverse pulmonary and cerebrovascular effects, and may result in tissue damage from oxygen free radicals. Oxygen use during neonatal resuscitation has been linked to the development of childhood cancer. The results of animal studies are conflicting. However, human studies suggest that the results of resuscitation with room air are equal to or better than those when oxygen is used. Hence current recommendations are:

1. If respiratory efforts are absent or inadequate, priority should be given to lung inflation/ventilation.
2. If the heart rate remains low after ventilation is established, priority should be given to support cardiac output with chest compressions.
3. Supplementary oxygen should be considered for infants with continuing central cyanosis. Monitor SpO_2 to prevent hyperoxia.
4. Excessive oxygen may cause damage and should be avoided, especially in the preterm.
5. Avoid overventilation and hypocapnia.

Ventilation Strategies

Initial breaths of the neonate establish the functional residual capacity (FRC). The peak pressures and inflation time required to initiate ventilation and establish the FRC in the apneic neonate have not been determined. Pressures varying from 30 to 60 cm H_2O and ventilation rates of 30 to 60 per minute have been used successfully in reported series. Preterm lungs may be damaged by overinflation. Continuous positive airway pressure (CPAP) may help stabilize and improve lung function in sick neonates and may be useful in preterm infants, decreasing the need for intubation.

Current recommendations are:

1. Establishing effective ventilation is the primary objective.
2. If bradycardia is present, an increase in heart rate is the primary index of adequate ventilation.
3. Chest wall movement should be assessed if heart rate does not increase.
4. If airway pressure is being monitored, an initial inflation pressure of 20 cm H_2O may be effective but some full-term infants may require 40 cm H_2O.
5. For preterm infants, prevent excessive distention of the lungs as evidenced by chest wall movement. Initial inflation pressures of 20 to 25 cm H_2O are usually adequate.

Self-inflating bags, flow inflating bags, or T-piece systems can be used. The LMA is not recommended as a primary airway device but may be useful if intubation is unsuccessful or "not feasible." No recommendations are made regarding the use of CPAP in resuscitation.

Chest Compressions

Chest compressions are indicated for a heart rate less than 60 bpm despite adequate ventilation with supplementary oxygen for 30 seconds.

1. Compressions should be delivered at a rate of 90 per minute over the lower third of the sternum, preferably using the chest encircling/ thumbs compressing technique.
2. Ventilation to compression ratio should be 1:3, coordinated to prevent compression during an inspiratory phase of ventilation.
3. Check the heart rate every 30 seconds (stethoscope).
4. Compressions should continue until the spontaneous heart rate equals 60 bpm.

Medications

These are rarely indicated in neonatal resuscitation and there is a lack of data regarding the value of drugs in improving outcomes. High doses of epinephrine may reduce survival rates and increase neurologic damage. Naloxone, if given to an infant of opioid addicted mother, may cause seizures.

1. Epinephrine may be indicated if the heart rate remains less than 60 bpm despite adequate ventilation and cardiac compressions. The IV route is recommended (0.01 to 0.03 mg/kg); high doses are not recommended. The intratracheal route is not recommended.
2. Naloxone is not recommended for initial neonatal resuscitation. Depressed ventilation should be treated with bag and mask.
3. Sodium bicarbonate is not recommended.

Volume Expansion

Volume expansion is indicated for infants when blood loss is suspected, if the infant appears pale with a weak pulse, and has not responded fully to other measures.

4. Isotonic crystalloid solution, 10 ml/kg, is recommended and may need to be repeated.
5. Caution: In preterm infants, large volumes rapidly infused have been associated with intraventricular hemorrhage.

Meconium

Intrapartum suctioning has not been demonstrated to reduce the incidence of meconium aspiration syndrome and is no longer recommended.

Tracheal suctioning should be performed on meconium stained depressed infants before stimulation.

Meconium stained vigorous infants do not require suctioning.

Postresuscitation Care

1. Temperature control; hyperthermia is bad and increases the risk of mortality and morbidity. Selective head cooling may decrease the incidence of cerebral morbidity following encephalopathy.
2. Check blood glucose level and treat hypoglycemia.

The Preterm Infant

Some special considerations are necessary for the very small infant:

1. Special care must be taken to prevent heat losses; immediately dry and place the infant on a warm mattress under a heating lamp. Use humidified oxygen.
2. Infants weighing greater than 1000 g should be given O_2, suctioned, and stimulated.
3. Infants weighing less than 1000 g are very likely to require early intubation and ventilation. Be prepared to intervene rapidly unless the infant obviously is in satisfactory condition.
4. Any preterm infant displaying respiratory difficulty should be intubated to provide for optimal ventilation and oxygenation.

Suggested Reading

International Liaison Committee on Resuscitation: Part 13: Neonatal Resuscitation Guidelines, Circulation 112(Suppl 24):IV 118–IV 195, 2005.

O'Donnell CPF, Gibson AT, David PG: Pinching, electrocution, raven's beaks, and positive pressure ventilation: a brief history of neonatal resuscitation, Arch Dis Child 91:69–73, 2006.

Wyllie J: Resuscitation of the depressed newborn, Semin Fetal Neonatal Med 11:158–165, 2006.

Drug Doses

PREOPERATIVE PERIOD

N.B. Avoid giving drugs intramuscularly (IM) if possible. IM injections are painful and children do not like them. If IM drugs are necessary and more than one has to be given, combine them in the same syringe whenever possible.

Drugs for Premedication

Anticholinergics

Atropine: IV-0.02 mg/kg at induction (maximum dose, 0.6 mg); IM-0.02 mg/kg 30 to 60 minutes preoperatively (maximum, 0.6 mg). PO-same dose, 60 to 90 minutes preoperatively.
Glycopyrrolate: 0.01 mg/kg IV or IM.

Sedatives

Midazolam (Versed): 0.5 to 0.75 mg/kg PO, or 0.2 mg/kg intranasally, or 1.0 mg/kg PR, or 0.1 mg/kg IM, or 0.05 to 0.1 mg/kg IV (in a monitored area).
Clonidine: 4 µg/kg oral, or 1 to 2 µg/kg intranasal.

Dexmedetomidine: 2.5 µg/kg oral or 1 µg/kg intranasal. (N.B. No data on neurotoxicity for intranasal injection)

Lorazepam (Ativan): for adolescents, 1 to 2 mg PO.

Midazolam/ketamine mixture: 0.3 to 0.5 mg/kg midazolam plus 2 to 6 mg/kg; ketamine plus 0.02 mg/kg atropine PO (This combination may result in considerable sedation—use in a monitored setting).

Antacids: H_2-Histamine blocking agents

Cimetidine: 10 mg/kg PO, or 30 mg/kg PR, or 5 mg/kg IV.

Ranitidine: 2 to 5 mg/kg PO, or 1.5 mg/kg IV or IM.

Sodium citrate: 0.4 ml/kg PO.

Drugs to Speed Gastric Emptying

Metoclopramide: 0.15 mg/kg IV. (**Note:** Atropine blocks the effect of metoclopramide and should be withheld until induction of anesthesia.)

Topical local anesthetics

EMLA (eutectic mixture of local anesthetics): Prilocaine (2.5%) and *Lidocaine* (2.5%). Apply to skin 60-90 min. before procedure. Cover with occlusive dressing. Caution: metabolism of prilocaine may result in methemoglobinemia in neonates: limit application to 1 gm EMLA cream over 10 cm² skin.

Amethocaine Gel (Ametop): Tetracaine (4%). Apply to skin 45 minutes before procedure. Cover with occlusive dressing. Caution: not recommended for infants < 1 month.

Ela-Max (4% Lidocaine): Apply to skin 30 min. before procedure. Cover with occlusive dressing.

S-Caine Patch: Eutectic mixture of 70 mg *lidocaine* and 70 mg *tetracaine* in each patch. Apply 20 min. before procedure. Cover with occlusive dressing.

INTRAOPERATIVE PERIOD

Induction Agents

Thiopental sodium (Pentothal): neonates (younger than 1 month), up to 3 to 4 mg/kg; infants (1 month–1 year), up to 7 to 8 mg/kg; children, up to 5 to 6 mg/kg.

Etomidate: 0.25 to 0.3 mg/kg

Methohexital: up to 2 mg/kg IV or 15-25 mg/kg of a 1% or 20-30 mg/kg of a 10% solution PR

Propofol (Diprivan): infants 1.5 to 2 mg/kg, children 2.5 to 3.5 mg/kg.

Ketamine: 2 mg/kg IV or 4 to 8 mg/kg IM (plus atropine 0.02 mg/kg IM/IV)

Drugs for Intubation

Succinylcholine: infants, 2 mg/kg IV; older children, 1 mg/kg IV or 4 to 5 mg/kg IM.

Rocuronium: 0.3 to 1.2 mg/kg IV.

(**N.B.** Large doses of rocuronium in infants may result in prolonged blockade)

Vecuronium: 0.1 mg/kg IV.

(**NB:** Do not inject rocuronium or vecuronium immediately after thiopental; thiopental precipitates and may occlude IV.)

Cis-*atracurium:* 0.1 to 0.2 mg/kg.

Pancuronium: 0.1 mg/kg.

Topical lidocaine for laryngeal spray: maximum dose 4 mg/kg.

Maintenance

Fentanyl: Bolus doses 1 to 2 µg/kg IV prn
  IV infusion for major surgery; loading dose 5 µg/kg, infuse at 2 to 4 µg/kg/hr.

Hydromorphone: 0.01-0.02 mg/kg IV

Morphine: 10 to 100 µg/kg IV or intravenous infusion (for children older than 5 years of age); loading dose 100 µg/kg over 5 minutes, infusion at 40 to 60 µg/kg/hr.

Remifentanil: IV loading dose—0.5 to 2 µg/kg.
  IV Infusion—0.05 to 0. 3 µg/kg/min.

Acetaminophen: 30 to 40 mg/kg single dose PR followed by 20 mg/kg q6h (maximum daily dose 90 to 100 mg/kg)

Neuromuscular Blocking Drugs

1. Usual route of administration IV; only administer IM succinylcholine in emergency situation.
2. Give initial and repeat doses preferably as indicated by nerve stimulator, especially in infants (whose response to these drugs is extremely variable).
3. Remember that potent volatile agents (especially sevoflurane and isoflurane) reduce the dose requirement of nondepolarizing drugs.

4. Infusion rates are given as a guide only and should be modified as indicated by neuromuscular blockade monitoring.

Cis-atracurium: initial dose 0.1 mg/kg, repeat dose 0.03 mg/kg.
  Infusion: loading dose 0.1 mg/kg, infusion at 2 to 3 µg/kg/min.

Pancuronium: initial dose 0.06 to 0.1 mg/kg; repeat doses should not exceed one sixth of the initial dose.

Rocuronium: initial dose 0.3 to 1.2 mg/kg, incremental doses 0.15 mg/kg;
  Infusion: rate: 10 to 12 µg/kg/min.

Vecuronium: loading dose 0.1 mg/kg, incremental doses 0.02 mg/kg.
  Infusion rate 0.1 mg/kg/hr.

Antagonism of Neuromuscular Blockade

Atropine 0.02 mg/kg or *glycopyrrolate* 0.01 mg/kg mixed with *neostigmine* 0.05 mg/kg-administer slowly; use a nerve stimulator to monitor effect; **OR**

Atropine 0.02 mg/kg, followed by *edrophonium* 1 mg/kg.

POSTOPERATIVE PERIOD

Analgesics

Acetaminophen (Tylenol): 10 to 20 mg/kg q4-6h PO or 30 to 40 mg/kg dose PR followed by 20 mg/kg q6h (maximum daily dose 90 to 100 mg/kg)

Acetaminophen with codeine elixir: each 5 ml contains 120 mg acetaminophen + 12 mg codeine

Volume of elixir to administer should be equivalent to 1 mg/kg codeine PO q4h

Codeine (useful for minor surgery): 1 to 1.5 mg/kg IM. (Note: Codeine must not be given intravenously.)

Diclofenac: 1 mg/kg PO or PR.

Hydromorphone (Dilaudid): Bolus dose: 0.01-0.02 mg/kg IV q3 to 4h
  Continuous infusion rates: 3 to 5 µg/kg/hr
  Caudal analgesia: 10 µg/kg

Morphine, IM or IV: children, 0.05 to 0.1 mg/kg; infants, 0.05 mg/kg.
  Morphine infusion: children, 10 to 30 µg/kg/hr. To prepare a solution mix: [0.5 × the child's weight (kg)] mg morphine in 50 ml saline. The solution then contains 10 µg/kg/ml. Infuse at 1 to 3 ml/hr for postoperative analgesia (equivalent to 10 to 30 µg/kg/hr).

For infants, give 5 to 15 µg/kg/hr (i.e., 0.5 to 1.5 ml/hr).
Caudal or epidural morphine: 30 µg/kg single dose.
Spinal morphine (preservative free): 10 µg/kg single shot.
Oxycodone: 0.1 to 0.2 mg/kg PO q4h.

Opioid Antagonist

Naloxone (Narcan): 0.5 to 2 µg/kg IV or IM. This drug should be titrated
slowly until undesired opioid effects are reversed. Rapid administration of an excessive dose results in loss of analgesia, pain, and extreme
restlessness. The same dose of naloxone (µg IV) that resulted in desired
effect, should then be given IM to prevent recrudescence.

Prophylaxis Against PONV

First Line Medications

Dexamethasone: 0.0625 to 0.15 mg/kg (maximum 8 mg)
Ondansetron: 0.05 to 0.15 mg/kg
Granisetron: 40 µg/kg IV
Dolasetron: 0.35 mg/kg IV (max. 12.5 mg)
Metoclopramide: 0.15 mg/kg

Second Line Medications

Dimenhydrinate (Gravol, Dramamine): 1 mg/kg IV or 2 mg/kg PR

Ancillary Drugs

Antibiotics

The dose given is that for a single intraoperative intravenous administration. The smaller dose should be given to neonates under 1 week (limited
neonatal liver and renal function). The usual maximum daily dose for
children is given in parentheses. Antibiotics should be infused over several
minutes only (i.e., *never* give antibiotics as IV boluses!) to minimize the
possibility of adverse reactions. Some must be given over a greater period
(e.g., vancomycin). Regimens for antibiotic prophylaxis against subacute
bacterial endocarditis are listed on page 462.

Ampicillin*: 25 to 100 mg/kg (300 mg/kg)
Cefazolin: 20 to 40 mg/kg (100 mg/kg)
Cefoxitin: 20 to 40 mg/kg (160 mg/kg)

---

* Use caution in children with renal failure.

Cefuroxime: 20 to 50 mg/kg (240 mg/kg)
Clindamycin: 5 to 10 mg/kg (30 mg/kg)
Cloxacillin: 12 to 25 mg/kg (100 mg/kg)
Erythromycin: 2.5 to 5 mg/kg (20 mg/kg)
Gentamicin: 2.0 mg/kg (7.5 mg/kg)
Benzyl penicillin*: 30,000 to 50,000 IU/kg (250,000 IU/kg)
Vancomycin*: 10 mg/kg (60 mg/kg) (must be given over a period of at least 1 hour)

Adrenocorticosteroids

Dexamethasone (Decadron): 0.2 to 0.5 mg/kg IV (maximum, 10 mg)
Methylprednisolone (Solu-Medrol): 5 to 25 mg/kg IV slowly over 10 minutes
Hydrocortisone sodium succinate (Solu-Cortef): 1 to 5 mg/kg IV over 8 to 10 minutes

Cardiovascular Drugs (titrate infusions to effect) (see below for infusion setup)

Adenosine: 100 µg/kg as a rapid IV bolus. Repeat up to max. dose 0.3 mg/kg or 12 mg.
Amiodarone: loading dose 5 mg/kg (over 30 to 60 minutes)
Amrinone: loading dose 0.75 mg/kg; infusion 3 to 5 µg/kg/min in neonates, 5 to 10 µg/kg/min in children
Calcium chloride: 5 to 15 mg/kg
Calcium gluconate: 10 to 30 mg/kg
Dopamine: 5 to 20 µg/kg/min infusion
Dobutamine: 5 to 20 µg/kg/min infusion
Epinephrine: 0.1 to 1 µg/kg/min infusion
Esmolol: 100 to 500 µg/kg IV, 50 to 100 µg/kg/min infusion
Hydralazine: 0.1 to 0.2 mg/kg IM or IV
Isoproterenol (Isuprel): 0.025 to 0.1 µg/kg/min infusion
Lidocaine: 1 to 2 mg/kg
Milrinone: 50 to 100 µg/kg loading dose over 15 to 30 min, (reduce loading dose if hypotension occurs) followed by 0.5 to 1.0 µg/kg/min infusion
Norepinephrine (Levophed): 0.1 to 1 µg/kg/min
Nitroglycerin: 1 to 10 µg/kg/min infusion
Phenoxybenzamine: loading dose 0.25 mg/kg × 4 over 2 to 4 hours; maintenance, 0.25 mg/kg q6h

---

* Use caution in children with renal failure.

Phentolamine: 0.2 mg/kg IV
Phenylephrine: 0.1 to 1 µg/kg/min infusion
Procainamide: 5 to 15 mg/kg IV
Propranolol: 0.01 to 0.1 mg/kg IV over 10 minutes
Prostaglandin E_1: 0.05 to 0.1 µg/kg/min (starting dose). (Maintenance infusion rate, e.g., after PDA open, may be between 0.005 and 0.4 µg/kg/min)
Sodium nitroprusside: 0.5 to 10 µg/kg/min
Verapamil: 0.1 to 0.3 mg/kg IV. (Do not give to infants younger than 1 year of age.)

Diuretics

Ethacrynic acid: 0.5 to 1 mg/kg
Furosemide (Lasix): 1 mg/kg
Mannitol: 0.5 to 1.0 g/kg (give over several minutes to prevent transient hypotension)

Anticonvulsants

Diphenylhydantoin (Dilantin): loading dose 15 to 20 mg/kg IV slowly; maintenance, 2.5 to 5 mg/kg bid IV or PO
Phenobarbital: loading dose 10 mg/kg IV; maintenance, 1.5 to 2.5 mg/kg bid IV

Bronchodilators

Salbutamol (Albuterol): loading dose 5 to 6 µg/kg IV; infusion 0.1 to 1.0 µg/kg/min; inhaled aerosol 100 µg dose q6h (delivery of aerosol through pediatric tracheal tubes is only 3% to 10%; to deliver a more effective dose, activate the canister (during inspiration); (1) into a spacer, (2) through a catheter inserted part way down the tube, or (3) after inserting it into the barrel of a 60 ml syringe that is connected to the CO_2 port and reinserting the plunger into the barrel).
Aminophylline: loading dose 5 mg/kg over 30 minutes; infusion 1 mg/kg/hr (if no recent doses). Monitor blood levels (therapeutic range, 10 to 12 µg/ml).

Local Anesthetics

Recommended safe maximum doses:

Lidocaine plain: 5 mg/kg
Lidocaine with epinephrine: 7 mg/kg
N.B. The maximum recommended dose of epinephrine to be infiltrated during halothane anesthesia is 10 µg/kg.

Bupivacaine: 2.5 mg/kg
Ropivacaine: 2.5 mg/kg

DRUGS INFUSIONS FOR INFANTS AND CHILDREN

These formulas are designed to permit medications to be infused with limited fluid volumes. (N.B. Weight = the child's weight in kilograms)

Dopamine or dobutamine:
  (Weight × 6) mg of drug in 100 ml; then 1 ml/hr = 1 µg/kg/min
  In the case of neonates and infants <10 kg use:
  (Weight × 30) mg of drug in 100 ml; then 1 ml/hr = 5 µg/kg/min
Epinephrine:
  (Weight × 0.6) mg of drug in 100 ml; then 1 ml/hr = 0.1 µg/kg/min
Sodium nitroprusside or nitroglycerin:
  (Weight × 6) mg of drug in 100 ml; then 1 ml/hr = 1 µg/kg/min
Isoproterenol:
  (Weight × 0.15) mg of drug in 100 ml; then 1 ml/hr = 0.025 µg/kg/min
Prostaglandin:
  (Weight × 60) µg of drug in 20 ml; then 1 ml/hr = 0.05 µg/kg/min

DRUGS TO REDUCE BLEEDING

Desmopressin: May improve platelet function and reduce bleeding in some platelet diseases. Dose: 0.3 µg/kg by slow infusion over 20 minutes after weaning from cardiopulmonary bypass. Monitor cardiovascular parameters carefully during infusion.

ε-Aminocaproic acid (Amicar): Used to treat fibrinolytic states. May reduce postoperative bleeding, especially in cyanotic children. Should be administered before sternotomy. Loading dose: 100 to 200 mg/kg (maximum 5 g) diluted and infused slowly over 1 hour followed by continuous infusion during surgery at 10 to 15 mg/kg/hr.

Tranexamic acid: a synthetic drug that forms a reversible complex with both plasminogen and plasmin by combining at lysine binding sites—inhibits fibrinolysis and reduces bleeding. Loading dose 100 mg/kg to followed by infusion during surgery at 10 mg/kg/hr.

Index

Note: Page numbers followed by f and t indicate figures and tables, respectively.

Printed and bound by CPI Group (UK) Ltd, Croydon, CR0 4YY

03/10/2024

01040848-0001